Occupational Therapy and Mental Health

For Elsevier:

Commissioning Editor: Dinah Thom, Rita Demetriou - Swanick
Development Editor: Catherine Jackson
Project Manager: Elouise Ball
Designer: George Ajayi
Illustrations Buyer: Merlyn Harvey
Illustrator: Richard Morris

Occupational Therapy and Mental Health

Edited by

Jennifer Creek MSc DipCOT FETC

Freelance Occupational Therapist, North Yorkshire, UK

Lesley Lougher BScSoc DipCOT

Freelance Occupational Therapist working in the voluntary sector, Peterborough, UK

Foreword by

Hanneke Van Bruggen

Executive director of ENOTHE, Amsterdam

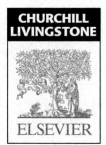

CHURCHILL LIVINGSTONE

ELSEVIER

EDINBURGH LONDON NEW YORK OXFORD PHILADELPHIA ST LOUIS SYDNEY TORONTO 2008

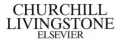

First published 2008
  Reprinted 2008

ISBN: 978 0 443 10027 7

British Library Cataloguing in Publication Data
A catalogue record for this book is available from the British Library.

Library of Congress Cataloging in Publication Data
A catalog record for this book is available from the Library of Congress.

Note
Knowledge and best practice in this field are constantly changing. As new research and experience broaden our knowledge, changes in practice, treatment and drug therapy may become necessary or appropriate. Readers are advised to check the most current information provided (i) on procedures featured or (ii) by the manufacturer of each product to be administered, to verify the recommended dose or formula, the method and duration of administration, and contraindications. It is the responsibility of the practitioner, relying on their own experience and knowledge of the patient, to make diagnoses, to determine dosages and the best treatment for each individual patient, and to take all appropriate safety precautions. To the fullest extent of the law, neither the Publisher nor the Editors assume any liability for any injury and/or damage to persons or property arising out of or related to any use of the material contained in this book.

The Publisher

Working together to grow
libraries in developing countries

www.elsevier.com | www.bookaid.org | www.sabre.org

ELSEVIER   BOOK AID International   Sabre Foundation

ELSEVIER your source for books, journals and multimedia in the health sciences
www.elsevierhealth.com

Printed in China

The publisher's policy is to use **paper manufactured from sustainable forests**

Contents

Contributors

Lynne Barr DipCOT MBA MSc
Professional Lead and Strategic Advisor for the
Integrated Occupational Therapy Service
(South Tees) and Teeside Community Equipment
Service, Middlesbrough, Teeside, UK

Clare Beighton BSc(Hons)
Occupational Therapist,
Tees, Esk and Wear Valleys NHS Trust, UK

Sheena E E Blair EdD MEd DipOT FHEA
Head of Division of Occupational Therapy,
Glasgow Caledonian University, Glasgow, UK

Mary Booth DipCOT BSc(Hons)
Associate Director of Allied Health Professionals,
Tees, Esk and Wear Valleys NHS Trust, UK; College
of Occupational Therapists Council Member for
Mental Health and Learning Disabilities

Alison Bullock BSc(Hons) BA(Hons) MSc
Occupational Therapy Clinical Lead,
St Lukes Hospital, Middlesbrough, UK

Jenny Butler PhD BSc(Hons) DipCOT TCert(HE)
Professor of Occupational Therapy,
Oxford Brookes University, Oxford, UK

John Chacksfield DipCOT PGCE
Head of Therapies and Social Inclusion, Senior
Management Lead for Forensic Addictions
Programme, Chadwick Lodge & Eaglestone View
Hospitals, Priory Secure Services,
Milton Keynes, UK

Fiona Cole MSc BSc DipCOT PGCL THE
Senior Lecturer, School of Rehabilitation and
Public Health, University of Cumbria, UK

Marilyn B Cole MS OTR/L FAOTA
Professor Emeritus, Quinnipiac University,
Hamden, Connecticut, USA

Jennifer Creek MSc DipCOT FETC
Freelance Occupational Therapist,
North Yorkshire, UK

Edward A S Duncan PhD BSc(Hons) Dip. CBT
Clinical Research Fellow, Nursing, Midwifery
and Allied Health Professions Research Unit,
University of Stirling, Stirling, UK

Alan Evans BA(Hons) DipCOT PostgradDip
(Art Therapy)
Head Occupational Therapist,
Leicester Partnership NHS Trust, UK

Jon Fieldhouse DipCOT BA(Hons) MSc
Department of Allied Health Professions
School of Health and Social Care
Senior Lecturer, Faculty of Health and Life
Sciences, University of the West of England,
Bristol, UK

Anne Fleming DipCOT BSc
Head Occupational Therapist,
Forth Valley Primary Care NHS Trust, UK

Donna Guest BSc(Hons)
Specialist Paediatric Occupational Therapist,
ADHD Team, Neurodevelopmental Service,
Peterborough District Hospital, Peterborough, UK

Robert Hawkes BSc(Hons)
Specialist Occupational Therapist,
The Stephenson and Cook Centres,
Mental Health Unit, North Tees University
Hospital, Stockton on Tees, UK

Simon Hughes DipCOT PGDip MA
Consultant Occupational Therapist,
Rehabilitation and Recovery Services,
Tees, Esk and Wear Valleys NHS Trust, UK

Clephane A Hume MTh BA FCOT
Retired. Formerly Lecturer in Occupational
Therapy, Queen Margaret University,
Edinburgh, UK

Deborah Hutton DipOT MA
Formerly Head Occupational Therapist, CAMHS,
Cambridgeshire and Peterborough Mental Health
NHS Trust, UK

Irene Ilott FCOT BA MEd PhD
Research Associate, Institute of Work Psychology,
University of Sheffield, UK

Valerie Johnstone BSc OT SROT
Senior Occupational Therapist,
Northumberland, Tyne and Wear NHS Trust, UK

Frank Kronenberg BSc BAEd
International Guest Lecturer, Occupational
Therapy without Borders, Zuyd University,
The Netherlands and University of the Western
Cape, South Africa; Head Development
and Marketing RAVE Experiences – Ishabi
Transformative Tourism (*www.ishabi.com*);
Co-founder, Shades of Black Productions

Jenny Lancaster DipCOT
Senior Occupational Therapist, Central and
North West London Mental Health NHS Trust,
London, UK

Kee Hean Lim MSc DipOT PGCE HEd
Lecturer in Occupational Therapy, Education
Officer COTSSMH, Kawa Model Associate,
School of Health Sciences and Social Care,
Brunel University, Middlesex, UK

Lesley Lougher BScSoc DipCOT
Freelance Occupational Therapist working in the
voluntary sector, Peterborough, UK

Marion Martin DipCOT BSc(Hons) MA (Ed) PhD
Senior Lecturer, School of Health Professions,
University of Brighton, Eastbourne, UK

Cathy Ormston DipCOT PGDip
Trust Professional Lead for Occupational Therapy,
Lancashire Care NHS Foundation
Trust, Lancaster, UK

Catherine F Paterson MBE PhD MEd FCOT
Retired. Formerly Director of Occupational
Therapy, Robert Gordon University,
Aberdeen, UK

Nick Pollard BA DipCOT MA MSc
Senior Lecturer in Occupational Therapy,
Sheffield Hallam University, UK

Jackie Pool DipCOT
Occupational Therapy Consultant in Dementia
Care, Southampton, UK

Mary Roberts MSc OT DipCOT SROT FETC
Assistant Team Manager, West Berkshire
Community Care and Housing Physical
Disability Team, UK

Sue Wheatley MA DipCOT PGCert
Senior Lecturer, School of Health Professions,
University of Brighton, Eastbourne, UK

Lynne Yarwood
Head Occupational Therapist for Working Age
Adult Services, Northumberland, Tyne and Wear
NHS Trust, UK

Acknowledgements

The editors would like to acknowledge the influence of Cathy Ormston during the planning stages of the book.

DEDICATION

This book is dedicated to the memory of Elsie May, who lived her short life to the full and brought great joy to the people who loved her.

Foreword

When I was asked to write the foreword for the fourth edition of *Occupational Therapy and Mental Health* I did not have to think long in order to react in a positive way to this request.

I immediately thought of the enormous challenges for mental health in the next decade and what contribution occupational therapists can make if we are alert to the important changes in policies.

Why is mental health important?
There is no health without mental health. Good mental health is important for citizens as well as for society. At individual citizen level, good mental health enables people to realise their intellectual and emotional potential to find and fulfil their roles in social, school and working life. At society level, good mental health contributes to social cohesion, a better social and economic welfare, solidarity and social justice. (EC 2005) on the other hand mental ill health imposes immense costs, losses and burdens on citizens, their families and wider environment and communities.

Global facts are:

- 450 million people experience mental or neurological disorders around the world. These disorders constitute 5-10 leading causes of disability worldwide
- Mental disorders can be diagnosed and treated cost-effectively

- In many parts of the world, mental health is still not acknowledged as important and remains a low health priority. Access to effective treatments is limited (WHO 2005).

For Europe the main facts are:

- More than 27% of adult Europeans are estimated to experience at least one form of mental ill health during any one year
- The most common forms of mental ill health in the EU are anxiety disorders and depression. By 2020, depression is expected to be the highest ranking cause of disease in the developed world
- Currently, in EU, some 58,000 citizens die from suicide every year, more than the deaths from road accidents, homicide, or HIV/AIDS (EC 2005).

In terms of policy priorities the European Ministers of Health have in 2006 endorsed the WHO Mental Health Action Plan for Europe.
The following priorities have been set out for the next decade:

i. Foster awareness of the importance of mental well-being;
ii. Collectively tackle stigma, discrimination and inequality, and empower and support people with mental health problems and their families to be actively engaged in this process;

iii. Design and implement comprehensive, integrated and efficient mental health systems that cover promotion, prevention, treatment and rehabilitation, care and recovery;

iv. Address the need for a competent workforce, effective in all those areas;

v. Recognise the experience and knowledge of service users and carers as an important basis for planning and developing services. (WHO 2005).

The fourth edition of *Occupational Therapy and Mental Health* is complying very well with the above mentioned policies, as I will show hereafter.

Since 1990 the book has been the authoritative publication in the field of mental health and occupational therapy.

A major change in the new edition is the use of consistent terminology fully based on the concept of occupation. As director of ENOTHE (European Network of Occupational Therapy in Higher Education), I was very pleased to discover that the project 'Terminology' has contributed to several of the terms used. For students all over Europe this terminology will be recognisable.

The philosophical assumptions, the concepts and knowledge base of occupational therapy clearly articulate awareness of the importance of mental well-being, because people are occupational beings and engaging in occupation is healthy. In the new chapter 2: Occupational perspectives on mental health and well-being, the Scottish Public Mental Health Alliance (2002 p4) is quoted as saying that positive mental health is a resource that strengthens the ability to cope with life situations: 'being mentally healthy implies having the ability to cope with changes and life transitions, to adapt to circumstances, set realistic aims, reach personal goals and achieve life satisfaction.'

The use of the words *citizen* and *society* in the mental health strategy of the European Union confirm the commitment to place mental health on the mainstream agenda and to incorporate the notion of equal rights for every citizen.

This strategy is reflected in the new chapter 30 on working with people on the margins, by Kronenberg and Pollard. They explain that the experiences of occupational apartheid (Kronenberg & Pollard 2005), occupational injustice (Townsend

and Wilcock 2004) and occupational deprivation (Whiteford 2000) are leading to the marginalised position of persons with mental ill health. New approaches in occupational therapy are proposed, where stigma is challenged and people are enabled to exercise their rights in order to enjoy full rights as a citizen.

Attention to the prevention of ill health and promotion of mental well-being is in this new edition underpinned with concepts and ideas of occupational science. It provides a basic understanding of how occupation can affect mental health and well-being.

In the chapter on roles and settings, an emphasis is placed on the role occupational therapists have to play in various multi-professional settings, with attention to social outcomes or participation in all life areas. At the same time, expansion in the roles of other established disciplines, such as nursing, in for instance developing healthy lifestyles is mentioned as a cause for more competition in the field.

This leads us to the next policy priority of the WHO, addressing a competent and effective workforce. The section on ensuring quality and the chapter on the developing student practitioner in this new edition, as well as the renewed subchapter on core skills, are answering this need.

Jennifer mentions those core skills related to the occupational therapy process, like collaboration with the client, assessment, enablement etc., listed by the College of Occupational Therapists (2004); they are complex and made up of sub-skills such as interpersonal and cognitive skills. She adds two kind of thinking skills essential to effective practice: clinical reasoning and reflection. Thinking skills are 'the mental actions used by the therapist in framing problems and working out the best solutions'.

In the chapter on clinical governance and clinical audit, the personal development portfolios, demonstrating change in skills, knowledge and attitudes, and continuing education are seen as essential conditions in ensuring that practitioners are competent for practice.

Considering research integral to effective practice and learning to be a research informed practitioner are other important aspects of a competent occupational therapist. Both themes are systematically approached in the chapter on research, evidence based practice and professional effectiveness. The author, Irene Ilott, encourages further studies and reading and suggests a rich variety of literature and Internet gateways about evidence-based practice and critical appraisal.

Very remarkable in this edition is the recognition of service users. Three different service users have reviewed different chapters.

The review of the chapter The knowledge base of occupational therapy, by a mental health service user, points out that client-centredness and focus on the individual's experience of illness in occupational therapy are important tools to reassure clients that they are human beings.

Other strong points are the recognition of the complexity of human beings and the change of roles, throughout life and within different environments, which each present different pressures.

The fact that this service user is mentioning that in occupational therapy the individual can begin to change their own life without feeling dependent on the profession sounds very rewarding.

The review on the research chapter is reflecting a criticism that is representing the voice of many service users nowadays. Sarah King very properly observed that involvement of service users in research should start with *them* setting the agenda, seeing the outcomes of research improving *their* road to recovery and *their* quality of life. *They* want to be doing and/or contributing to research themselves. (Creek,…)

A last chapter which adds an extra value to this new edition is the chapter on working in a transcultural context. Nowadays nearly every occupational therapist is working in a multicultural environment and therefore all occupational therapists need to develop cultural competences, which involves 'an awareness of, sensitivity to, and knowledge of the meaning of culture, including a willingness to learn about cultural issues, including one's own bias' (Dillard et al 1992).

The chapter explores the transcultural context of occupational therapy, promoting cultural awareness and exercises for self awareness and discussing culturally sensitive models and approaches, illustrated with case studies.

This new edition promotes a strong relationship between theory, practice and research in occupational therapy and it offers the reader a wealth of structured information, approaches and very useful references.

I wish to congratulate the editors with their remarkable job in gathering eminent writers in the occupational mental health area and in pulling together this wide array of subjects in a cohesive whole and responding to the WHO mental health action plan.

I hope that this book, launched in the European Year of Equal Opportunities for All, will contribute to the profile and competences of the occupational therapists in the European and global mental health area, promote quality mental health and social care through occupation, facilitate participation in society of people with mental health problems and prevent occupational exclusion.

Amsterdam,
September 2007

Hanneke van Bruggen
Executive director of ENOTHE

EC 2005 Green paper: Improving the mental health of the population: Towards a strategy on mental health for the European Union. Luxembourg: Office for Official Publication of the European Communities. Com (2005)484. (Brussels 14.10.2005)

Kronenberg F, Pollard N 2005 Overcoming occupational apartheid: a preliminary exploration of the political nature of occupational therapy. In Kronenberg F, Simo Algado S, Pollard N, (eds) Occupational therapy without borders: Learning from the spirit of survivors, Elsevier/Churchill Livingstone, Oxford, p1-13

Townsend E, Wilcock A 2004 Occupational justice and client-centred practice: A dialogue-in-progress. Canadian Journal of Occupational Therapy, 71:75-87

WHO 2005 Information sheet no 1

WHO European Ministerial Conference on Mental Health 2005 Mental Health Action Plan for Europe, Facing the challenges, building solutions- EUR/04/5047810/7

Whiteford G 200 Occupational Deprivation. Global challenge in the new millennium, British Journal of Occupational Therapy 63 (5) 200-204

Preface

Jennifer Creek and Lesley Lougher

Jennifer has been editing *Occupational Therapy and Mental Health* since the first edition, which was published in 1990. Updating the book at intervals has necessitated keeping up to date with changes both within the profession and in the external environment as it impacts on occupational therapy practice. For the fourth edition, she decided to share the workload with a co-editor and was fortunate to be able to tempt Lesley into the role.

Lesley and Jennifer first met when they began their secondary education in Leeds, at the age of 11. Lesley was the person who introduced Jennifer to the idea of becoming an occupational therapist. During the past 40 years, we have worked together on various projects, finding compatibility both in our passion for occupational therapy and in our perspective on the profession. For both of us, it is a real pleasure to have this opportunity to collaborate on a major rewrite of the book as we come to the end of our professional lives.

There are challenges for occupational therapists working in a world where resources are never sufficient to satisfy the demand for high-quality health and social care and, for some, where the contribution of occupational therapy is not appreciated. But we have been inspired by many of the developments taking place within the profession worldwide: in particular, the emergence of a community development/health promotion role for occupational therapy, the expansion of the profession into Eastern Europe and the international development of a consistent occupational therapy terminology.

Since the last edition of the book was published, in 2002, there have been important changes in how health and social care services are delivered, which have influenced how we approached the task of producing a fourth edition. Our aim has been to build on the strengths of previous editions while adapting to changing circumstances and needs. Some of the people who contributed to past editions have retired or moved to different fields of practice, so we have recruited new contributors who have brought fresh perspectives and up-to-date experience. One of the strengths of the book has always been that the practice chapters are written or co-written by people who are currently working in the field, and this has been continued. However, an innovation has been to invite people who use occupational therapy services to comment on some of the chapters. Three people have written personal commentaries on chapters 3, 4 and 10, offering a critique of occupational therapy theory from the service user perspective.

The book follows the same format as previous editions, although there has been some minor reorganisation. The first section describes the philosophy and theory base of the profession, in three chapters. Chapter 1, *A short history of occupational therapy in psychiatry*, has been updated by Catherine Paterson, herself a notable contributor to the development of occupational therapy education in Scotland. Chapter 2, *Occupational perspectives on mental health and well-being*, has been revised to strengthen the health promotion content, reflecting an expanding role for occupational therapists in this field. Chapter 3, *The knowledge base of occupational therapy*, has also been revised to incorporate the latest developments in professional theory and terminology. Many definitions of key occupational therapy terms have been taken from the work of the European Network of Occupational Therapy in Higher Education terminology project, an ambitious undertaking that is reaching consensus on the meanings of terms across all the major European language groups. This chapter also introduces the political dimension of occupational therapy, which is further developed in Chapter 30.

The second section of the book describes the occupational therapy process, in four chapters. The writing of this section was strongly influenced by a College of Occupational Therapists publication, *Occupational Therapy Defined as a Complex Intervention* (Creek 2003). This approach to occupational therapy intervention acknowledges the unpredictability and messiness that are often features of working in the field of mental health. Chapter 4, *Approaches to practice*, looks at what constitutes the content of practice, outlines the occupational therapy process and describes three frames of reference used by occupational therapists. Further frames of reference and models for practice are described in other chapters throughout the book. Chapter 5, *Assessment and outcome measurement*, takes the reader through the assessment stages of the occupational therapy process, giving the purposes of assessment, highlighting what is assessed and describing a range of assessment and outcome measurement tools and techniques. Chapter 6, *Planning and implementation*, has been extensively rewritten to capture the complexity of occupational therapy interventions in the real world. The reader is taken through the process of identifying needs and setting goals with the client, planning how to achieve those goals and implementing the plan. Some of the core skills of the occupational therapist are described: task analysis, activity analysis, activity adaptation and activity selection. A new section on the context of treatment implementation illustrates the multitude of external influences on the therapist's clinical reasoning during this process. Chapter 7, *Record keeping*, stresses the importance of keeping accurate and up-to-date records of all

interventions and gives the basics of how to do this effectively and efficiently. The chapter has been updated to take account of developments in electronic care records.

The third section of the book consists of three chapters that look at how the quality of occupational therapy services is ensured and monitored. Chapter 8, *Clinical governance and clinical audit*, takes the reader through the seven pillars of clinical governance: patient, service user, carer and public involvement; risk management; clinical audit; clinical effectiveness; staffing and staff management; education, training and continuing personal and professional development, and use of information to support clinical governance and health-care delivery. Chapter 9, *Management*, describes budget control, management roles and management structures, clarifying the differences between management and leadership, explaining what is meant by management and addressing its application and importance to the profession of occupational therapy. Chapter 10, *Research, evidence-based practice and professional effectiveness*, has been rewritten to highlight research principles and how they can be used to help fulfil the professional obligation to base practice on the best available evidence.

The fourth section of the book describes the context of occupational therapy practice. Chapter 11, *Ethics*, has been written by two occupational therapists for the first time: in previous editions, this chapter was written by a moral philosopher. This change perhaps reflects how occupational therapists are becoming more confident in their understanding of theory. The chapter is organised around three stories of the kind of dilemmas that occupational therapists are likely to encounter in their daily practice. Chapter 12, *Roles and settings*, addresses the changing context of the treatment of mental ill health. There is a stronger emphasis on treatment in the community, which reflects a greater concern about the social exclusion of people with mental illness. Changes in the workforce require occupational therapists both to take on more generic roles and to develop programmes to facilitate recovery through engagement in activities. Chapter 13, *The developing student practitioner*, challenges the myths and stereotypes some students may have accepted about mental illness. It highlights the differences between mental health and physical placements, introduces the student to the need for self-awareness and suggests how to develop therapeutic relationships within professional boundaries. Chapter 14, *Working in a transcultural context,* explores changing conceptual and contextual factors that dictate the need for a more culturally sensitive and inclusive approach to health and social care provision. The chapter suggests ways to develop cultural awareness and cultural competency.

The fifth section of the book describes some of the occupations that are the focus of occupational therapy intervention in the field of mental health. These are the same six areas that were covered in previous editions but the chapters have been extensively revised or rewritten. Chapter 15, *Mental health and physical activity,* explores the value of physical activity in the occupational lives of people with mental health problems, and the role of occupational therapy in enabling participation. The chapter also explores the evidence base for links between mental and physical well-being. Chapter 16, *Cognition and cognitive approaches in occupational therapy,* describes the use of a cognitive behavioural frame of reference and Allen's Functional Information-Processing Model in the assessment and treatment of people with cognitive impairments. Chapter 17, *Client-centred groups,* includes both a practical guide to facilitating groups and some of the theory base for group therapy. It offers a structure for occupational therapy groups and guidelines for designing group interventions. Chapter 18, *Creative activities,* describes the use of creative activities as therapy, outlines an occupational therapy theory of creativity and gives an example of a creative activity group. Chapter 19, *Play,* defines play and its function for people of all ages, examines theories of play and discusses the use of play as therapy with children and families. It also looks at the effects of the mental illness of a mother on her ability to play with her child. Chapter 20, *Life skills,* explains how people develop skills and how mental illness can cause skills deficits. It looks at skills training from the perspective of four occupational therapy models and describes some of the training methods that occupational therapists use.

The final section of the book describes the main client groups with whom occupational therapists work. Chapter 21, *Loss and grief,* looks at the types of loss and reactions to loss that might cause someone to seek professional help. Guidelines are given for working with people who are experiencing grief. Chapter 22, *Acute psychiatry,* examines the changing role of occupational therapy in this field, as there is a growing recognition of the importance of meaningful activities on wards and a debate between two approaches to mental ill health and well-being: recovery/hope and crisis/compulsion. Chapter 23, *Approaches to severe and enduring mental illness,* discusses more recent approaches to mental illness, such as the stress-vulnerability and recovery models, and the impact that these have on occupational therapy. It also examines the occupational therapist's role in work rehabilitation as greater opportunities are created for return to employment. Chapter 24, *Older people,* explores organic and functional mental disorders in old age and their impact on occupational performance and functional disability. The chapter takes the reader through the occupational therapy process with older people with mental disorders, highlighting some of the techniques used in this area of practice. Chapter 25, *Child and adolescent mental health services,* describes the different levels of intervention, from mental health promotion to inpatient admission, and includes a section on the use of a sensory integrative approach for children with attention deficit hyperactivity disorder (ADHD). Chapter 26, *Learning disabilities,* describes how the occupational therapy process is applied with this client group, then discusses specific areas of intervention, including profound and multiple impairment, older people with a learning disability, dual diagnosis, challenging behaviour and forensic services. Chapter 27, *Community mental health,* explores the issues of social inclusion, social capital and recovery for community-based occupational therapists, so that working *with* the community increases effectiveness *within* the community. It also looks at the role of the occupational therapist in the community mental health team. Chapter 28, *Forensic occupational therapy,* introduces specific issues relating to working in a secure environment – the increased level of risk assessment required and the occupational deprivation of the patients. It outlines methods of assessment and intervention suitable for patients in this setting. Chapter 29, *Substance misuse,* discusses the nature and extent of substance misuse and offers an occupational perspective on why people take drugs and the types of problems experienced. Specific occupational therapy intervention strategies for problem drug and alcohol users are described. Chapter 30, *Working with people on the margins,* expands on the political dimension of occupational therapy, describing how certain social groups are marginalised and proposing a political role for occupational therapy in addressing this issue. Examples of work undertaken with marginalised groups are offered to illustrate possible ways in which occupational therapists might enter this emerging field of practice.

The completion of this edition has been set against a backdrop of major life events for most of the authors. There have been births, marriages, divorces, new relationships, illnesses and deaths, both expected and untimely. People have found new jobs, moved house, retired and yet have managed to write and rewrite their chapters. On several occasions we doubted that a chapter could be completed but it was – so thanks are due to all those who overcame their personal circumstances to contribute to this edition.

REFERENCES

Creek J 2003 Occupational therapy defined as a complex intervention. College of Occupational Therapists, London

SECTION 1

Philosophy and Theory Base

SECTION CONTENTS

Chapter **1**

A short history of occupational therapy in psychiatry

Catherine F. Paterson

INTRODUCTION

History is interesting for its own sake but also facilitates understanding of contemporary roles and relationships. Just as our sense of personal identity is rooted in family history, so our professional identity and understanding of the contexts in which we work are enhanced by knowledge of their development. Although the concept of the therapeutic use of occupation dates back to antiquity, the term 'occupational therapy' was not coined until early in the 20th century and the first training course in the UK was not started until 1930. Occupational therapy has been developed in many different areas of practice but only the history of occupational therapy in the field of mental health is reviewed here. However, it can only be considered in the wider context of the social and medical history of psychiatry and the development of the profession as a whole.

This chapter briefly surveys some of the earliest references to occupation as treatment, explores the moral movement in psychiatry and other philosophical influences in the late 18th and early 19th centuries, discusses the contribution of psychiatrists Adolf Meyer, David Henderson and Elizabeth Casson to the founding of the profession of occupational therapy, and identifies some of the major developments in psychiatry and occupational therapy in the 20th century. Finally, there is a brief discussion of the professional organisations, training and state registration which are important to the professionalisation of occupational therapy.

PSYCHIATRY AND OCCUPATION BEFORE THE 19TH CENTURY

Throughout history, the social and medical care of the mentally ill has been dependent on public attitudes and medical opinion of the times. What constitutes 'normal' and 'abnormal' behaviour and what is considered 'mad' or 'bad' has varied throughout the ages. Beliefs about the causes of mental illness have had a significant influence on the way sufferers have been treated. Prevailing ideas of causation have included possession by evil spirits, overstimulation of the senses, brain disease, genetic inheritance, psychological trauma and faulty biochemistry. Finally, the national economy and society's willingness to pay have dictated limitations to the provision of services. Consequently the therapeutic use of occupation has fluctuated in relation to social, medical, political and economic factors.

From the very earliest surviving manuscripts and throughout the ages, in both Eastern and Western culture, we find reference to the belief that occupation in the form of exercise, work, recreation and amusements can both influence and be used to improve mental and physical health and well-being. The Greek physician Hippocrates, in the 4th century BC, taught that the brain was the seat of the mind and described how mental health depended on a balance of four bodily humours: blood, choler, phlegm and bile (Digby 1985). Galen, the most influential of the Roman physicians, followed the methods of Hippocrates, especially when mental aberrations occurred in the course of somatic disease. Seigel (1973) outlined Galen's psychotherapeutic concepts, stating: 'Since he treated mostly well-to-do patients, he advised good nursing care; demanded kindness with the emotionally ill; employed as physical methods hydrotherapy, showers, sweating, local application of heat and sunbathing … In milder cases he recommended travel, occupational therapy and, for the educated, an increasing participation in lectures, discussions, reading and in pastime creative activities'.

While the idea that madness was caused by evil spirits, witchcraft, sin or divine intervention dominated popular thinking throughout the Dark and Middle Ages, physicians in Europe continued to accept Hippocrates' and Galen's explanation of the humoral basis of madness well into the 18th century (Porter 1999).

In Britain at that time, the rich person with a mental illness would probably be attended at home by a physician or placed in a private madhouse. On the other hand, the mad poor were most likely to be treated no differently from other social deviants, being classed with the destitute, vagrants and criminals. Some were incarcerated in prisons or workhouses or in one of the few hospitals for pauper patients, such as Bethlem Hospital in London (Dickenson 1990). The conditions in which the mentally ill were kept, whether at home or in an institution, usually included the use of physical restraint, often by manacles and chains. There was usually no heat or lighting, little food, clothing, bedding or sanitation, no segregation of the violent from the quiet and withdrawn, and no meaningful occupation. There was even wrongful confinement, by their relatives, of people who were not in fact mentally ill. Traditional medical remedies were aimed at re-establishing humoral balance and included special diets, bleeding, purging, emetics and blistering, often on a seasonal basis (Jones 1972).

Eventually scandals, changes in public opinion and the example of a few asylums run on humanitarian principles led to a period of reform. Of particular significance were the Act of 1808 and the Select Committee of 1815–1816. The Act, for 'the better Care and Maintenance of Lunatics, being Paupers or Criminals, in England', laid down detailed specifications for the construction and maintenance of county asylums and the Select Committee investigated allegations of maltreatment in public institutions of the insane (Jones 1972). However, the transformation of the treatment of pauper lunatics made slow progress until the great expansion of the county asylum system in the 1840s (Walton 1981).

PSYCHIATRY AND OCCUPATION IN THE 19th CENTURY

THE MORAL MOVEMENT

At the beginning of the 19th century, the two asylums most celebrated for introducing reforms were the Bicêtre in Paris, under Dr Philippe Pinel

(1745–1826), and the York Retreat, founded by layman William Tuke (1732–1822). Pinel and Tuke became internationally acclaimed for their introduction of moral treatment for the mentally ill; that is, psychological rather than physical treatment (Paterson 1997).

Pinel was appointed to the medical staff of the Bicêtre in 1794, during the French Revolution, when the institution housed upwards of 200 male patients, who were regarded not only as incurable but also as extremely dangerous. Instead of blows and chains, he introduced light and fresh air, cleanliness, workshops and areas for walking but above all kindliness and understanding (Batchelor 1975). Pinel wrote in his 1801 treatise on insanity:

> It is no longer a problem to be solved, ... that in all public asylums as well as prisons and hospitals, the surest, and perhaps, the only method of securing health, good order, and good manners, is to carry into decided and habitual execution the natural law of bodily labour, so contributive and essential to human happiness ... I am convinced that no useful and durable establishments ... can be founded excepting on the basis of interesting and laborious employment. (Pinel 1962)

William Tuke and the Society of Friends founded the Retreat at York in 1796 on the Quaker principles of compassion and humanity. The central emphasis was on trying to help the patient gain enough self-discipline to master his illness. To this end, it was thought important to create a comfortable, domestic environment in which the patient could experience normal civilised daily living conditions, which would help the process of self-control. Anne Digby (1985) summarised the regime as follows:

> The need to balance the emotions and distract the patient from painful thoughts and associations led to the central feature of the Retreat's moral therapy: the creation of varied employment and amusements. ... the key to moral treatment lay in the quality of personal relationships between staff and patients. This is what makes the term moral treatment so elusive, and also made the treatment so difficult to translate successfully from the Retreat to other institutions in the mid-nineteenth century.

By 1839 it was reported that patients at the Retreat were cultivating a 2-acre field with potatoes and turnips under the supervision of an attendant employed for the purpose. There were also attempts to occupy the patients along the lines of their former posts; a surveyor's assistant made a survey of the estate, while a watch repairer and a carpenter were employed in their customary tasks. By 1844 two carpenter's shops had been set up to provide a greater variety of occupation for men. There were also opportunities for convalescent patients to go shopping or attend meetings in York, or to take tea with local Quakers. Some patients looked after kittens and birds, while others found pleasure in the grounds. Outdoor amusements were also available, from helping in the hayfield to archery or cricket. At Christmas, the carol singers visited the Retreat and, on Plough Monday, the Morris dancers. Indeed, Digby reported that the Lunacy Commissioners commented in 1847 that 'every means of amusement and occupation appear to be provided for the patients' (Digby 1985).

Although Pinel and Tuke are most frequently credited with the introduction of moral treatment, there were other asylum superintendents at the beginning of the 19th century who were particularly interested in the therapeutic use of occupation as part of a humane regime of care. These included William Hallaran (1765–1825), the first physician of the Cork Asylum, Sir William C Ellis (1780–1839), medical superintendent of the Hanwell Hospital, and William A F Brown (1805–1885), the first medical superintendent of the Crichton Institution at Dumfries.

Hallaran published a book in 1810 in which he laid stress 'On the Cure of Insanity', especially by suitable occupation for 'the convalescent maniac', combining 'corporeal action, with the regular employment of the mind'. He was the first physician to recognise the danger of institutional neurosis and gave the first account of the benefit derived from being allowed to paint (Box 1.1). He concluded that this case proved the need to introduce a systematic arrangement of daily labour which could help convalescent patients to become useful members of society once more (Hunter & MacAlpine 1963).

Box 1.1 From W Hallaran, *On the Cure of Insanity (1810)*

A young man ... came under my care in a state of acute mania, and continued so full three months without any intermission. The symptoms having at length given way, he was treated as a convalescent patient, and every means tried to encourage him to some light work, merely as a pastime, but all to no purpose. Though the maniacal appearances had totally subsided, he still betrayed an imbecility of mind that bordered closely on dementia, and it was found impossible to excite in him the smallest interest ... when by accident he was discovered in the act of amusing himself, with some rude colouring, on the walls of his apartment. ... he was questioned as to his knowledge of drawing, and he, having signified some acquaintance with that art, was immediately promised colours of a better description, if he would undertake to use them. This evidently gave immediate cheerfulness to his countenance, ... he immediately commenced a systematic combination of colours, and having completed his arrangements, he requested one of the attendants to sit for him. ... The portrait was an exact representation of the person who sat before him, and in a few days there were several other proofs of his skill in this line, which bore ample testimony to his ability. He soon became elated with the approbation he had met with, and continued to employ himself in this manner for nearly two months after, with progressive improvement as to his mental faculties, when he was dismissed cured. (Hallaran 1810, reprinted in Hunter & MacAlpine 1963)

Another of the early medical superintendents who championed the use of occupation was William Ellis. Ellis was appointed to the newly opened Wakefield Asylum in 1818, with his wife as matron. He later became medical superintendent at Hanwell (later St Bernard's Hospital, Southall), where he paved the way for his successor, John Conolly (1794–1866), renowned for the abolition of all physical restraint (Hunter & MacAlpine 1963). Samuel Tuke (1841), grandson of William Tuke, credited Ellis with:

the first extensive and successful experiment to introduce labour systematically into our public asylums. He carried it out ... with a skill, vigour, and kindliness towards the patients which were alike creditable to his understanding and his heart. He proved, that there was less danger from putting the spade and the hoe into the hands of a large proportion of insane persons, than from shutting them up together in idleness, though under the guards of straps, strait-waistcoats, or chains. (Tuke, cited by Hunter & MacAlpine 1963)

While the men at Hanwell were encouraged either to follow their own trade or to learn a new one, Lady Ellis organised the female patients under a 'work-woman' to make 'useful and fancy articles' which were sold at bazaars and outside the asylum:

She borrowed of the treasurer twenty-three pounds eighteen shillings: this she laid out in the purchase of a few articles in the first instance as patterns, and in buying the requisite materials. These are made up and worked by the patients, and sold by the workwomen to visitors at the bazaar, or are sent off to order. The scheme has answered beyond the most sanguine expectations ... It is hardly possible to conceive the benefit which the patients derived from this employment. (Ellis 1838, reprinted in Hunter & MacAlpine 1963)

The foremost of the moral physicians in Scotland was W A F Browne. His first position was as medical superintendent at the Montrose Asylum, where in 1837 he wrote an influential treatise entitled 'What asylums were, are and aught to be'. He wrote extensively on the prescription of occupation:

It is not enough to have the insane playing the part of busy automatons, or to wear out their muscular energies vicariously, in order to relieve the drooping heart of its load. There must be an active, and, if possible, intelligent and willing participation on the part of the labourer and such portion of interest, amusement, and mental exertion associated with the labour, that neither lassitude not fatigue may follow. The more elevated, the more useful the description of the occupation provided then, the better. (Browne 1837)

Browne was able to put many of his ideas into practice in the establishment of the well-endowed Crichton Institution in Dumfries, where the use of occupations is well recorded in all the annual reports. He appointed a superintendent of outdoor recreations and a superintendent of the workroom, where they made not only the 'usual articles of bed and body clothing' but also 'articles of embroidery and fancy work' (Easterbrook 1940).

GROWTH OF THE ASYLUMS IN THE 19TH CENTURY

The Victorian era in Britain was characterised by the building of large public asylums on the outskirts of every large town in response to the legislation of 1808 for the 'better care and maintenance of lunatics'. Many of these asylums became the mental hospitals which were later closed or contracted in response to the Care in the Community legislation of the 1990s. These institutions were, themselves, the product of social reforms, at a time when the urban industrialised working class in Britain lived in conditions of squalor and grinding poverty (Jones 1972).

However, the optimism that cures could be effected through treatment in an asylum could not be sustained. Patients became quieter and more manageable but most were still unable to return to their former situations. The success of the asylums led to the admission of more and more inmates, so that their very size – many containing 2000 or more patients – made them the antithesis of the domestic surroundings necessary for treatment on moral principles. Many asylums found it impossible to attract the number and calibre of attendants required to manage disturbed patients without resorting to measures of restraint. Thus, during the latter half of the 19th century, the individualised prescription of occupation gave way to the widespread use of the physically fit patients for work in the kitchens, laundry, farm and gardens of the asylums, as much for economic as for therapeutic reasons (Jones 1972).

Wilcock (2001) has explored in detail the origins of all aspects of the profession, including mental health, up to the end of the 19th century, in the first volume of *Occupation for Health*.

DEVELOPMENTS IN THE 20TH CENTURY

INSTITUTIONALISATION AND DEINSTITUTIONALISATION

At the beginning of the 20th century the most important influences on psychiatry were the theories of Sigmund Freud (1856–1939) and his associates Alfred Adler (1870–1937) and Carl Jung (1875–1961), who developed psychoanalysis and psychotherapy. Although these new disciplines had a significant influence on the way people thought about mental processes and on consulting room practice, they had little effect on regimes within British asylums. Denis Martin (1968) described asylums as benignly authoritarian, in that the satisfactory running of the hospital depended on the submission of the patients to authority with the minimum of resistance. Methods of dealing with those who were unable to submit included locked doors, various forms of mechanical restraint, segregation of the sexes, heavy sedation, electroconvulsive therapy, prolonged sleep and prefrontal leucotomy, which were administered as treatment but which could be perceived or even used as punishment. However, the same authority was benevolent since the hospital provided security and met the patients' physical needs, so that the final result was 'institutionalisation' (Martin 1968).

During the early part of the 20th century, conditions remained largely unchanged in the hospitals. However, the move beyond the asylum can be traced back to the changes in practice during the First World War, when the problem of shell-shock required a new response to mental distress (Stone 1985). The Mental Treatment Act of 1930 provided a further impetus for the development of outpatient clinics and aftercare services as well as admission of patients on a voluntary basis (Jones 1972).

The 1950s saw the introduction of the first effective antipsychotic and antidepressant drugs and subsequently the beginning of a sustained debate about the legitimacy of custodial care. The criticisms were led by psychiatrists Ronald Laing, David Cooper and Thomas Szasz – collectively dubbed 'antipsychiatrists' – and by Erving

Goffman, whose seminal work *Asylums*, published in 1961, drew attention to the dangers of the 'total institution' (Pilgrim & Rogers 1993). The ideological and financial pressures on the psychiatric hospitals, together with the continuing development of effective medication, expedited the deinstitutionalisation movement which began slowly in the 1960s and finally gained momentum with the Care in the Community legislation in the 1990s. The widespread reliance on drugs to control symptoms also re-established the somatic basis of mental illness as the dominant view, alongside precipitating psychological and social factors (Shorter 1997).

THE BEGINNING OF THE PROFESSION OF OCCUPATIONAL THERAPY IN THE USA

At the end of the 19th century, in the USA as in Britain, the asylums were suffering from overcrowding and economic pressures. However, there was a resurgence of interest in reform and in structuring the patient's day in a more productive manner, stimulated by various antecedents. These antecedents – ideologies, movements and schemes – included: pragmatism (Breines 1987, Cutchin 2004), the mental hygiene movement (Loomis 1992), the arts and crafts movement (Levine 1987), work cures in tuberculosis (Creighton 1993) and scientific management (Creighton 1992), as well as the legacy of the use of occupation as an integral aspect of moral treatment (Paterson 1997).

A major influence on psychiatry on both sides of the Atlantic was Dr Adolf Meyer (1866–1950), who emigrated from Switzerland to America in 1892. According to Rowe & Mink (1993), Meyer viewed mental illness as the outcome of a person's maladaptive interaction with the environment. His emphasis on objective observation of patient behaviour and on habit was compatible with the psychology of learning that was being developed by American psychologists, especially William James (1842–1910) and John Dewey (1859–1952), the founders of pragmatism, and his views anticipated the biopsychosocial model adopted by many psychiatrists in the late 20th century (Rowe & Mink 1993).

As early as 1892, Meyer observed that 'the proper use of time in some helpful and gratifying activity appeared to me a fundamental issue in the treatment of any neuropsychiatric patient'. In 1895, Meyer's wife, a social worker, introduced a systematic type of activity into the wards of the state institution in Worcester, Massachusetts, so that: 'A pleasure in achievement, a real pleasure in the use and activity of one's hands and muscles and a happy appreciation of time began to be used as incentives in the management of our patients'. Meyer considered that:

> The whole of human organization has its shape in a kind of rhythm. ... night and day, of sleep and waking hours, of hunger and its gratification ... work and play and rest and sleep, which our organism must be able to balance even under difficulty. The only way to attain balance in all this is *actual doing*, *actual practice*, a program of wholesome living as the *basis* of wholesome feeling and thinking and fancy and interests. (Meyer 1922, reprinted 1977)

Meyer is generally regarded as one of the founders of occupational therapy in the USA, along with other professionals who were developing the use of occupation quite independently. These were Susan E Tracy, a nurse, Eleanor Clarke Slagle, a social worker, William Rush Dunton Jnr, another psychiatrist, and, finally, Thomas B Kidner and George Barton, who both originally trained as architects. Barton became an advocate after his own illness, when he experienced the beneficial effects of directed occupation. He founded an institution in Clifton Springs, where people with chronic ill health could be retrained or adjusted to gainful living by means of occupation. It is Barton who is credited with introducing the term 'occupational therapy' at a meeting in 1914 and it was at Clifton Springs in 1917 that the National Society for the Promotion of Occupational Therapy was formed, with Barton as its first president. In 1923, the name was changed to the American Occupational Therapy Association (Licht 1967).

THE BEGINNING OF THE PROFESSION OF OCCUPATIONAL THERAPY IN SCOTLAND

Professor Sir David K Henderson (1884–1965) (Fig. 1.1), a prominent Scottish psychiatrist during the first half of the 20th century, was much

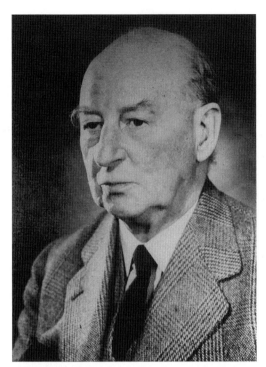

Figure 1.1 Professor Sir David K Henderson.

influenced by Meyer, with whom he had worked in New York and Baltimore. On returning to Scotland, Henderson's first position was at the Gartnavel Royal Hospital in Glasgow (Figs 1.2, 1.3), where he employed, in 1922, Dorothea Robertson, the first instructress in occupational therapy in Britain (Henderson 1925). Miss Robertson, although a graduate of Cambridge University, did not have the benefit of any training in occupational therapy but, within months, she had made sufficient impact for the Commissioners of the General Board of Control for Scotland to report that:

> For many years the advantages of farm and garden work for men and domestic work for women have been recognised from curative and ameliorative aspects and many patients have been so employed. There are, however, many patients not physically fitted for these strenuous labours or whose mental disorder such, for instance, as epilepsy, requires that they be under constant supervision. In all such cases the occupational therapy is being tried with excellent results. Patients were seen under a competent instructress making baskets, toys, rugs, etc.

> So successful has the treatment been that it is proposed to erect a special building within the grounds of the establishment where manifold light occupations can be carried out. (General Board of Control for Scotland 1923)

Henderson considered that mental disorder, whatever its underlying reason, resulted in patients being unable to adapt. This made patients, for the time being, social failures so that, no matter how they attempted to compensate, their innermost reaction was one of hopelessness. In a lecture to the Scottish Division of the Medico-Psychological Association in 1924, Henderson emphasised that:

> there is nothing which will sooner and more satisfactorily increase a person's self-esteem than his ability to accomplish something ... It is therefore our duty to attempt to establish well co-ordinated, purposeful ways of doing things, instead of idleness, apathy, or inadequate reaction. We must plan and organise our patient's day, so that adequate time is provided for work and rest and play, so that interests are stimulated and to borrow a word from Meyer – exteriorized. Even although the patient has been a failure in the world at large, we must attempt to make him a success in the hospital environment. (Henderson 1925)

Henderson was an influential figure in the development of occupational therapy in Scotland, particularly in his encouragement of the founding of the Scottish Association of Occupational Therapy in 1932 and in the reconstitution of the Association after the war in 1946, when he became its president (Groundes Peace 1957).

The first qualified occupational therapist to work in Britain was Margaret Barr Fulton (1900–1989) (Fig. 1.4), who became interested in occupational therapy during a holiday in the USA and who trained in Philadelphia. At first, Miss Fulton found it difficult to find a position; however, she was eventually given an introduction to Henderson in Glasgow. Unable to employ her himself, Henderson referred her to a former colleague, Dr R Dods Brown, medical superintendent of the Royal Aberdeen Mental Hospital, who secured her services immediately (Paterson 1996).

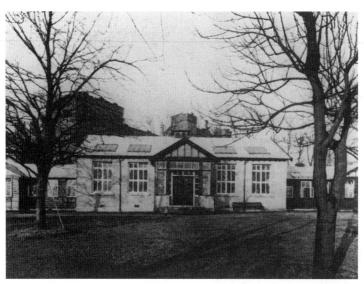

Figure 1.2   The Occupational Therapy Pavilion, Gartnavel Royal Hospital, Glasgow, 1923, with permission from **NHS** Greater Glasgow & Clyde Archives.

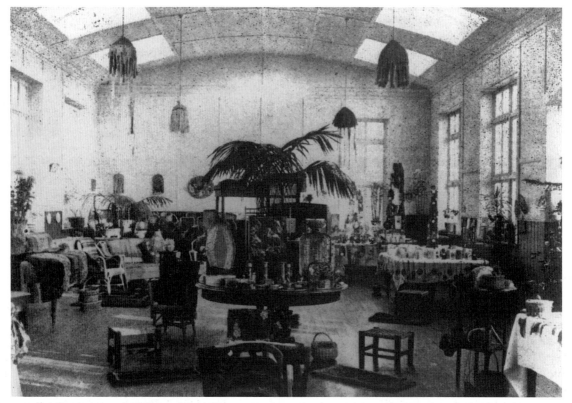

Figure 1.3   The interior of the Occupational Therapy Pavilion, Gartnavel Royal Hospital, Glasgow, with permission from **NHS** Greater Glasgow & Clyde Archives.

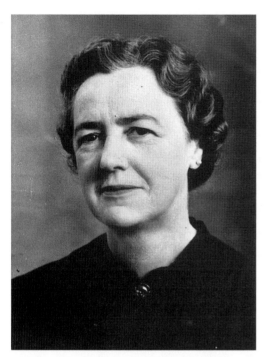

Figure 1.4   Miss Margaret Barr Fulton MBE.

In 1929, Dods Brown published an article entitled 'Some observations on the treatment of mental diseases' in which he gave a description of occupational therapy, which was based in an army hut erected in the grounds of his hospital. His paper was illustrated with case material, including the reports in Box 1.2.

Following the appointment of Miss Robertson and Miss Fulton, it appears that many Scottish mental hospitals followed suit in appointing instructresses in arts and crafts, most of whom held art college diplomas. By 1932, there were 15 such ladies who, under the direction of Miss Fulton and with the encouragement of Dr Henderson, formed themselves into the Scottish Association of Occupational Therapy (SAOT) (Paterson 2002).

Although Miss Fulton continued to work at the Royal Aberdeen Mental Hospital until her retirement in 1963, her influence was considerable both throughout Scotland and worldwide in her capacity as one of the founders in 1952 of the World Federation of Occupational Therapists and as its first president (Paterson 1996).

THE BEGINNING OF THE PROFESSION OF OCCUPATIONAL THERAPY IN ENGLAND

Among the delegates at the conference where Henderson described the occupational therapy department at the Gartnavel Royal Hospital in 1924 was Dr Elizabeth Casson (1881–1954) (Fig. 1.5), who was also destined to play an important role in the development of occupational therapy in Britain. Casson qualified as one of the first women doctors at Bristol in 1919 and chose to specialise in psychological medicine. In 1926, while on holiday in America, she visited an occupational therapy department at Bloomingdale Hospital, New York, and the Boston School of Occupational Therapy, where the idea of an English school on similar lines was implanted in her mind (Casson 1955).

At that time Casson was employed at the Holloway Sanatorium, where there was a tradition of many forms of occupation including games, entertainments, competitions and the annual sports. One of the instructresses, Alice Constance Tebbit (1906–1976), later Mrs Glyn Owens, obtained a scholarship at the Philadelphia School of Occupational Therapy and qualified in 1929 (Casson 1955).

By this time, Casson had fulfilled her ambition of founding a residential clinic for women psychiatric patients at Dorset House in Bristol, to which was attached the first school of occupational therapy in the UK, which opened on 1 January 1930 with Miss Tebbit as its first principal. The school later moved to Dorset House in Oxford, where it is now part of the Oxford Brookes University. At the Bristol clinic, Dr Casson:

> decided to establish a treatment centre where each patient's daily life would be so planned that it fitted the individual's need like a well tailored garment. She planned that each member of the household, whether patient or staff, should feel an integral part of the whole and each would contribute, according to capacity, to the welfare of the whole. There would be no sharp social or professional distinctions between members of staff and every patient would be made to eradicate any unnecessary dividing line between the patients and the staff. In this community everyone would be essential and therefore would feel valued and valuable. (Owens 1955)

12 PHILOSOPHY AND THEORY BASE

> ## Box 1.2 From Dods Brown, *Some observations on the treatment of mental diseases*
>
> A man, aged 69, had been in hospital for several months, during which time he did not improve. He spoke to no-one and would not employ himself in any way. He seemed to be deteriorating rapidly and to be passing into dementia. He was sent to 'The Hut' every day but for more than a week he showed not the slightest interest in anything he saw nor what was said to him. Later he was induced to do a little sandpapering, which he did in an entirely mechanical way. After a time he was given a fret saw to use and this seemed to arouse some interest in him. As the days passed it was apparent that his interest was growing more and more, not only in the work but also in his personal appearance, because one day he objected to the sawdust getting on his clothes. As time went on he was given more difficult work to do and in this he became thoroughly interested and indeed enthusiastic, and when his discharge was being discussed, he was reluctant to leave the institution. He made a thoroughly good recovery.
>
> A woman who had been in a depressed and somewhat agitated condition and who had maintained almost complete silence for about two years and who, on account of delusions of unworthiness, had refused her food and had been tube-fed for several months, was put to the occupational therapy department. From that time she began to converse and to take an interest in things outside herself. She improved steadily and rapidly and was discharged recovered. (Dods Brown 1929)

These last sentiments anticipated the concept of the therapeutic community developed after the Second World War by Maxwell Jones and Denis Martin. Early in the 1930s, there was also a 6-month course at the Maudsley Hospital for state-registered nurses for training in occupation work (Board of Control 1933) and schools of occupational therapy were opened in London and in Edinburgh in 1937 (Jay et al 1992).

Dr Casson was a source of inspiration and encouragement to occupational therapists throughout her life, which is commemorated by the Casson Memorial Lecture delivered at the annual conference of the College of Occupational Therapists.

ASSOCIATIONS OF OCCUPATIONAL THERAPY

While the Scottish Association of Occupational Therapy (SAOT) had been formed in 1932, the Association of Occupational Therapists (AOT), covering the rest of the UK, had its inaugural meeting in 1935, when Mrs Owens was elected chairman. In the few years leading up to the Second World War, the Association organised the first national examinations in occupational therapy, which initially allowed students to qualify in either physical or psychiatric practice, and launched a journal (Anon 1955, Hume & Lock

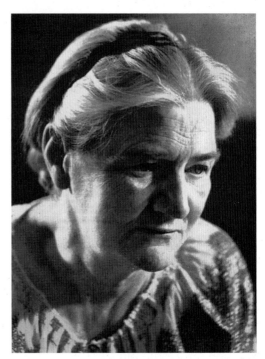

Figure 1.5 Dr Elizabeth Casson OBE.

1982). From 1939 to 1945 the Association was immersed in the war effort, including the organisation of shortened courses for occupational therapy auxiliaries for the military hospitals and the development of a realistic form of treatment in the physical field. Evelyn Mary Macdonald

(1905–1993), a recent graduate at the time and later principal of Dorset House, recalled that:

> While Occupational Therapy was receiving this impetus in the physical field, the work in mental hospitals was sadly curtailed. Departments were taken over for emergency beds, materials were difficult to obtain and priority of supplies went to hospitals dealing with physically disabled civilian and service cases. The Occupational Therapists doing psychological work struggled on bravely … It is interesting to note the trends in occupations at this time. In the physical field the choice was controlled largely by the materials made available through the special government priority system. These were mainly those for 'handicrafts' – in some cases almost too light and diversional in the eyes of keen therapists. A second controlling factor was that the occupations were deliberately limited by the government to 'crafts' and excursions in the realms of 'trade' were not permitted. In the psychological field, however, the Occupational Therapists, without the materials required for much of the usual craft work, turned the patients' interests to other and what might be termed more mundane but realistic occupations. This was in fact a progressive step and these are proving useful and acceptable in the treatment in both fields to-day. (Macdonald 1957)

After the war, in 1948, the whole management of health-care services was revolutionised by the formation of the National Health Service, when all psychiatric services, except some small homes, became a national rather than a local authority responsibility, with services being free at the point of delivery. Most occupational therapists became employees of the NHS (Paterson 1998).

A commission was soon set up to consider the staffing and training requirements of the new service, and representatives of the AOT and SAOT became involved in protracted negotiations with the Ministry of Health and the British Medical Association (BMA) on how occupational therapy should be regulated. The BMA wanted to continue to control the 'auxiliary professions', including occupational therapy, while the professions themselves wanted autonomy. The outcome was a compromise. The Professions Supplementary to Medicine Act (1960) provided for a board for each of the eight professions, regulated by a council (CPSM) responsible to the Privy Council. The boards and council had strong medical representation, albeit not sufficient to outvote the professions (Mendez 1978).

The Act was significant in that it recognised the need for properly qualified and registered occupational therapists to work in the NHS, and the Occupational Therapists Board recognised the diplomas of the two associations as qualifications for entry to the Register. The CPSM was replaced by the Health Professions Council in April 2002.

In 1952, Mrs Owens, then Principal of the Liverpool School, hosted a meeting to form the World Federation of Occupational Therapists (WFOT). The constitution drawn up required that the AOT and SAOT should be jointly represented on the WFOT Council, which led to the Joint Council of the Associations of Occupational Therapy in the UK. Co-operation between the two associations inevitably led to amalgamation and to the formation of the British Association of Occupational Therapists in 1974 (Hume & Lock 1982).

One of the outcomes of this amalgamation was revision of occupational therapy training, particularly the phasing out of the national diploma examinations, a system which had become unwieldy with increasing numbers of students. The new system of validation of courses paved the way for the development of degree courses, the first being approved in Belfast and Edinburgh in 1986. By 1994 the profession had achieved all-graduate entry and by 2007 there were 31 educational establishments in the UK providing a variety of routes to qualification.

A detailed account of the development of the profession during the 20th century can be found in the second volume of *Occupation for Health* (Wilcock 2002).

SUMMARY

Historically, the use of occupation as an integral aspect of treatment has fluctuated in relation to prevailing ideas about the causes of mental illness and other social and political factors. Of particular importance was the moral treatment developed in small asylums in the early 19th century, where individualised programmes of work and leisure and good interpersonal relationships between staff and patients were paramount.

From the inspiration of three psychiatrists and a handful of remarkable pioneering occupational therapists, the profession in Britain has developed in the relatively short period of about 80 years so that by 2007 there were over 29,000 registered occupational therapists. Having been involved in the treatment of the most intractable patients in psychiatric hospitals before the introduction of effective drugs in the 1950s, and the gradual deinstitutionalisation of patients since then, the profession has an even greater challenge in the 21st century. Occupational therapists are now required to provide services to a wide range of clients, from the young to the very old, in diverse settings and fulfilling varying roles within treatment teams. In the ever-changing organisation and structure of the health and social services, they need to be proactive in the provision of effective services for people with mental health problems wherever they may be. Occupational therapists should continue to be mindful of the humanistic ideals on which the profession was founded: the belief in the therapeutic value of meaningful occupation and the importance of satisfying interpersonal relationships and balance in the daily routines of work, self-care and leisure.

References

Anon 1955 Dual qualification. Occupational Therapy 18(3):131

Batchelor IRC 1975 Henderson and Gillespie's textbook of psychiatry. Oxford University Press, London

Board of Control 1933 Memorandum on occupation therapy for mental patients. HMSO, London

Breines E 1987 Pragmatism as a foundation for occupational therapy curricula. American Journal of Occupational Therapy 41(8):522-525

Browne WAF 1837 What asylums were, are and aught to be. Reprinted in: Scull A 1991 The asylum as Utopia: W A F Browne and the mid-nineteenth century consolidation of psychiatry. Tavistock/Routledge, London

Casson E 1955 How the Dorset House School of Occupational Therapy came into being. Occupational Therapy 18(3):92-94

Creighton C 1992 The origin and evolution of activity analysis. American Journal of Occupational Therapy 46(1):45-48

Creighton C 1993 Graded activity: legacy of the sanatorium. American Journal of Occupational Therapy 47(8):745-748

Cutchin MP 2004 Using Deweyan philosophy to rename and reframe adaptation-to-environment. American Journal of Occupational Therapy 58(3):303-312

Dickenson E 1990 From madness to mental health: a brief history of psychiatric treatments in the UK from 1800 to the present. British Journal of Occupational Therapy 53(10):419-424

Digby A 1985 Moral treatment at the Retreat, 1796-1846. In: Bynum W, Porter R, Shepherd M (eds) The anatomy of madness: essays on the history of psychiatry, Tavistock, London

Dods Brown R 1929 Some observations on the treatment of mental diseases. Edinburgh Medical Journal 36(11):657-686

Easterbrook CC 1940 The chronicle of Crichton Royal. Courier Press, Dumfries

General Board of Control for Scotland 1923 Tenth Annual Report. HMSO, Edinburgh

Groundes Peace Z 1957 An outline of the development of occupational therapy in Scotland. Scottish Journal of Occupational Therapy 30:16-43

Henderson DK 1925 Occupational therapy. Journal of Mental Science 71(292):59-73

Hume CA, Lock SJ 1982 The golden jubilee, 1932-1982: an historical survey. British Journal of Occupational Therapy 45(5):151-153

Hunter R, MacAlpine I 1963 Three hundred years of psychiatry, 1535-1860. Oxford University Press, London

Jay P, Mendez A, Monteath HG 1992 The diamond jubilee of the professional association, 1932-1992: an historical review. British Journal of Occupational Therapy 55(7): 252-256

Jones K 1972 A history of the mental health services. Routledge and Kegan Paul, London

Levine RE 1987 The influence of the Arts-and-Crafts Movement on the professional status of occupational therapy. American Journal of Occupational Therapy 41(4):248-254

Licht S 1967 The founding and founders of the American Occupational Therapy Association. American Journal of Occupational Therapy 21(5):269-277

Loomis B 1992 The Henry B. Favill school of occupational therapy and Eleanor Clarke Slagle. American Journal of Occupational Therapy 46(1):34-37

Macdonald EM 1957 History of the Association Chapter IV, 1942-1945. Occupational Therapy June: 30-33

Martin DV 1968 Adventure in psychiatry. Bruno Cassirer, Oxford

Mendez MA 1978 Dr Elizabeth Casson Memorial Lecture. Processes of change: some speculations for the future. British Journal of Occupational Therapy 41(7):225-228

Meyer A 1922 The philosophy of occupation therapy. Archives of Occupational Therapy 1: 1-10. Reprinted in: American Journal of Occupational Therapy 1977 31(10):639-642

Owens C 1955 Recollections, 1925-1933. Occupational Therapy 18(3):95-97

Paterson CF 1996 Margaret Barr Fulton MBE (1900-1989) pioneer occupational therapist. In: Adam A, Smith D, Watson F (eds) To the greit support and advancement of helth. Aberdeen History of Medicine Publications, Aberdeen

Paterson CF 1997 Rationales for the use of occupation in 19th century asylums. British Journal of Occupational Therapy 60(4):179-183

Paterson CF 1998 Occupational therapy and the National Health Service, 1948-1998. British Journal of Occupational Therapy 61(7):311-315

Paterson CF 2002 Celebrating small beginnings. British Journal of Occupational Therapy 65(10):439

Pilgrim D, Rogers A 1993 A sociology of mental health and illness. Open University Press, Buckingham

Pinel P 1962 A treatise on insanity (trans. D D Davis) Hafner, New York (published 1806)

Porter R 1999 The greatest benefit to mankind: a medical history of humanity from antiquity to the present. Fontana Press, London

Rowe CJ, Mink WD 1993 An outline of psychiatry. Brown and Benchmark, Madison

Seigel RE 1973 Galen on psychology, psychopathology and function and diseases of the nervous system. S Karger, Basel

Shorter E 1997 A history of psychiatry: from the era of the asylum to the age of Prozac. John Wiley, New York

Stone M 1985 Shellshock and the psychologists. In: Bynum WT, Porter R, Shepherd M, (eds) The anatomy of madness, vol. 2 Routledge, London

Walton J 1981 The treatment of pauper lunatics in Victorian England: the case of the Lancaster Asylum, 1816-1870. In: Scull A (ed) Madhouses, mad-doctors and madmen: the social history of psychiatry in the Victorian era, Athlone Press, London

Wilcock AA 2001 Occupation for health – a journey from self health to prescription, vol. 1. British Association of Occupational Therapists, London

Wilcock AA 2002 Occupation for health – a journey from prescription to self health, vol. 2. British Association of Occupational Therapists, London

Chapter **2**

Occupational perspectives on mental health and well-being

Sheena E. E. Blair, Clephane A. Hume, Jennifer Creek

INTRODUCTION

The beginning of the 21st century is characterised by an increased interest in the prevention of mental ill health and the promotion of well-being. All professions involved in health and social care have explored ways of broadening their remit, perhaps encouraged by the shift of working contexts in the United Kingdom, which are now largely community based. The World Health Organization (WHO) (2001) has more formally linked ideas of activity and participation within the *International Classification of Functioning, Disability and Health*. In Scotland, a link between policy and services is apparent, for example in the *National Programme Action Plan 2003–2006 to improve mental health and wellbeing in Scotland* (2001). In turn, this is part of a broader Scottish Executive policy initiative that includes attention to health improvement, social justice, education and lifelong learning.

Until recently, the responsibility for health promotion lay within the field of public health. Now, more attention is being given to health promotion within health-care policies; for example, *The Health of the Nation* (DoH 1992), *Saving Lives* (DoH 1999) and the *National Programme for Improving Mental Health and Well-Being* (Scottish Executive 2003). These policies give priorities for action, such as dementia awareness; suicide reduction; eliminating stigma and discrimination in minority ethnic groups, and the mental health of children and young people. Policies designed to integrate spirituality into health care, together with other publications such as *Caring for the Spirit* (South Yorkshire Workforce Development Confederation 2003), have led to changes in education for staff that broaden the focus of health promotion and health education.

These policy initiatives have implications for occupational therapists throughout the UK and Creek (2004) predicted that the profession will continue to have a much higher profile within health promotion. Those occupational therapists who have accepted the challenge of exploring the relationship between occupation and health, and of working towards occupation-centred practice, are finding this an exciting time. The discipline of occupational science has boosted knowledge generation in this area and the ideas of people as occupational beings, whose complex actions and interactions significantly impact on health, have stimulated the enthusiasm of students, educators, practitioners and researchers (Wilcock 1998). Occupational science has also encouraged a broader vision of the contribution of occupation to social justice, with the notion of occupational justice (Wilcock & Townsend 2000).

This chapter begins with an exploration of the terminology used to refer to mental health, mental disorder and the promotion of positive mental health. There is then a discussion of the personal characteristics, events and experiences that have been found to promote or inhibit positive mental health: protective factors and risk factors. The third section describes strategies and interventions used to promote positive mental health in individuals and communities. It concludes with some thoughts on the role of occupational therapy in promoting mental health and well-being.

UNDERSTANDING THE TERMINOLOGY

There are many terms used in the field of health promotion and disease prevention, each one given a variety of different meanings. These key terms can be found in published papers and glossaries, and are frequently heard in occupational therapy seminars and conferences. It is particularly interesting to note that language usage by occupational therapists has changed over the past decade from a preponderance of medical terminology to a more client-centred and occupation-focused style. The concepts defined here are health, mental health, well-being, health promotion, disease prevention, health education, mental health promotion, wellness, lifestyle and quality of life.

HEALTH

Defining health is a complex matter and the concept defies neat description. The occupational scientist, Wilcock (1998), offered an occupational perspective on health in which she explored the relationship between occupation and health and the importance of this relationship for public health. Wilcock acknowledged the enduring nature of the WHO (1946) definition of health: 'Health is a state of complete physical, mental and social well-being, and not merely the absence of disease or infirmity'.

However, there have been many criticisms of this definition; for example, Webb (1994) noted that it implies a static rather than a dynamic phenomenon. In contrast, the moral philosopher David Seedhouse (1986, p61) offered a definition that acknowledges the dynamic nature of health and recognises individual differences:

> A person's optimum state of health is equivalent to the state of the set of conditions which fulfil or enable a person to work to fulfil his or her realistic chosen and biological potentials. Some of these conditions are of the highest importance for all people. Others are variable dependent upon individual abilities and circumstances.

The WHO has been moving towards an understanding of the dynamic relationship between what people do and their health. The *Ottawa Charter for Health Promotion* (WHO 1986, p1) stated that health is 'a resource for everyday life, not the objective of living … it is a positive concept emphasizing social and personal resources, as well as physical capacities'. The *International Classification of Functioning, Disability and Health* (WHO 2001) has a focus on activity and participation that locates occupation as a major domain within health.

MENTAL HEALTH

The concept of mental health can be problematic, not least because it may be understood very differently in different cultural contexts (Fernando 1993). Indeed, it has been said that 'every definition of mental health has inherent cultural assumptions' (Chwedorowicz 1992, cited by Tudor 1996, p22), which means that no one definition will be appropriate for all purposes.

Mental health can be defined as the absence of objectively diagnosable disease – a deficit model – or as a state of physical, social and mental well-being – a positive model (mentality 2004). Current definitions of mental health usually incorporate both personal characteristics and the influence of environmental and social conditions. In other words, mental health is an interaction between the individual and her or his circumstances.

The Health Education Authority (1997) defined mental health as: 'the emotional and spiritual resilience which enables us to survive pain, disappointment and sadness. It is a fundamental belief in our own and others' dignity and worth'. The Scottish Public Mental Health Alliance (2002, p4) suggested that positive mental health is a resource that strengthens the ability to cope with life situations. It went on to say that the 'core individual attributes of positive mental health include the ability to:

- develop self-esteem/sense of personal worth
- learn to communicate
- express emotions and beliefs
- form and maintain healthy relationships
- and develop empathy for others'.

Being mentally healthy implies having the ability to cope with changes and life transitions, adapt to circumstances, set realistic aims, reach personal goals and achieve life satisfaction. In contrast, mental health problems disrupt people's capacity to think and feel in a way that is normal for them, interfere with the ability to make decisions and shatter people's sense of well-being.

WELL-BEING

The state of well-being, like health, is a multifaceted phenomenon. The *Oxford English Dictionary* (Brown 1993) definition links it with both health and welfare: 'healthy, contented or prosperous condition; moral or physical welfare'. An Australian occupational therapist, Therese Schmid (2005, p7), emphasised that the state of well-being is a subjective experience consisting of: 'feelings of pleasure, or various feelings of happiness, health and comfort, which can differ from person to person'. Wilcock (2006, p36) agreed that 'Health, happiness and prosperity have more than an intuitive fit with well-being'.

The American occupational therapist Betty Hasselkus (2002, p60) wrote that 'Research on the human state of well-being is permeated by the belief that a person's ability to engage in life's daily activities is a key ingredient'. She referred to the work of two psychologists, Ryff & Singer (1998, cited by Hasselkuss 2002, p61), who suggested that well-being can be defined by two core features: '1) leading a life of purpose, and 2) quality connections to others'. This description is reminiscent of Winnicott's idea of reciprocity as a necessary precursor to well-being.

The psychotherapist Donald Winnicott is reputed to have pronounced that 'health was more difficult to deal with than disease' (Phillips1989, p612). Certainly, changes have to be made in attitude, ideology and delivery of practice to accommodate the values of client education and enablement, which are central to the promotion of health. For over 40 years, Winnicott's work charted influences on personal growth and development, and one of his key themes was the metaphor of a containing space or holding environment as a necessary precursor to health and well-being. For him, health was concerned with nurturing relationships and reciprocity. Occupation tends to engage people in mutual endeavour where such reciprocal relationships can develop and, therefore, offers real possibilities for the promotion of healthy individuals and of healthy communities where people can live and learn together.

HEALTH PROMOTION

Since the mid-1980s, a confusing array of terms has been used in this area, including health promotion, health education, disease prevention and health protection. For example, Downie and colleagues (1993, p59) defined health promotion as 'effort to enhance positive health and prevent ill-health, through the overlapping spheres of health education, prevention and health protection'. They emphasised that the health promotion approach involves a sense of individual control.

Seedhouse (1997, p61) also defined health promotion in terms of effort, and helpfully attempted to unpick some of the terms used within his definition:

> Health promotion comprises efforts to enhance ways of acting and believing based on conservative political values and to prevent disease and illness, through a co-ordinated plan to influence individual behaviour in specific ways (health education), providing and strongly promoting the uptake of medical surveillance (disease prevention), and by legislating to guarantee or firmly enforce some behaviours in order to reduce some morbidities (health protection).

The WHO (1986, p1) definition is useful for occupational therapists because it views health promotion as a process of enablement: 'Health promotion is the process of enabling people to increase control over, and to improve, their health'.

DISEASE PREVENTION

The prevention of mental disorders, or the prevention of relapse, is often seen as one of the aims of mental health promotion strategies (WHO 2002). The WHO (2002) pointed out that the idea of primary disease prevention as a way of preventing disease from developing does not work well in the field of mental health, where it can be difficult to determine the exact time of onset or even to agree on a definite diagnosis. Rather, the *primary prevention* of mental disorders involves interventions at three levels.

- *Universal prevention* targeting a whole population group; for example, advertising on television the safe limits of alcohol consumption.
- *Selective prevention* targeting subgroups at high risk; for example, providing free nursery places for the children of single parents.
- *Indicated prevention* targeting individuals at high risk; for example, offering counselling to the children of mothers with depression.

Secondary prevention refers to all treatment-related strategies designed to reduce the prevalence of mental disorder, and *tertiary prevention* refers to interventions that reduce disability, mitigate the severity of disease, prevent relapse or contribute to rehabilitation and recovery.

HEALTH EDUCATION

All health-care professionals have a responsibility in terms of health education, which has been described by Downie and colleagues (1993, p28) as 'communication activity aimed at enhancing positive health and preventing or diminishing ill-health in individuals and groups, through influencing beliefs, attitudes and behaviour of those with power and of the community at large'. Health education can also be targeted at different levels (Draper et al 1980).

1. Health education about the body and its maintenance, for example at school.
2. Health education involving information about access to and appropriate use of health services, such as radio advertisements about sexual health advice lines.
3. Health education within a wider context that includes education about national, regional and local politics that have ramifications for health.

MENTAL HEALTH PROMOTION

Interest in the promotion of mental health has a history of more than 100 years, dating back to the formation of the Finnish Association for Mental Health in 1897. The World Federation of Mental Health was founded in 1948 to promote better understanding of mental illness and to serve as a means of drawing attention to mental health. More recently, an initiative between the European Commission and the WHO (WHO 1999) acknowledged that issues surrounding mental health problems contribute to five of the 10 leading causes of disability worldwide and that, while ongoing improvements in physical health can be detected, this is not the case for mental health.

Mental health promotion is about 'improving quality of life and potential for health rather than the amelioration of symptoms and deficits' (WHO 2002, p8). It consists of actions taken to enhance the mental well-being of individuals, families, organisations and communities (mentality 2004).

There are several complementary models of mental health promotion which acknowledge both individual and broader socio-economic determinants of mental health. A common feature of these models is recognition of the need to broaden mental health promotion programmes and interventions beyond those targeting the individual. For example, community interventions that focus on building social capital or policy-level interventions which widen participation in education have also been identified as mental health promotion.

A public mental health approach, that supports the enhancement of well-being or the promotion of positive mental health, reflects a public health ethos which looks beyond individuals to the physical, social and environmental context for health (DoH 2001). The logical endpoint of this approach is the design and delivery of interventions and programmes to promote the mental health of organisations and communities with a view to fostering a mentally healthy society.

WELLNESS

In 1986, an American occupational therapist, Jerry Johnson, wrote a book about wellness, which she described as 'a context for living' (Johnson 1986, p13). By this, she meant that wellness is a process of caring for oneself, including care for the body, the emotions, personal identity and the spiritual self.

The WHO definition of wellness includes both individual characteristics and social integration:

> Wellness is the optimal state of health of individuals and groups. There are two focal concerns: the realization of the fullest potential of an individual physically, psychologically, socially, spiritually and economically, and the fulfilment of one's role expectations in the family, community, place of worship, workplace and other settings. (Smith et al 2006, p344)

Wellness requires that a harmony is sought between mind, body and spirit and also between the individual and society. Occupational therapists would also suggest that a balance of occupations contributes to a state of wellness.

LIFESTYLE

Lifestyle has been defined as 'the particular way of life of a person or group' but the term is often used to refer to 'health-related behaviour such as smoking, drinking, diet and exercise' (Ewles & Simnett 2003, p337). Occupational therapists think more broadly about lifestyle as being the configuration of an individual's activities that links with both personal needs and the expectations of society. For example, Mayers (2003) designed a lifestyle questionnaire that covers self-care, living situation, looking after others, being with others, work or education, beliefs and values, choices, finances and desired activities.

QUALITY OF LIFE

It is difficult to agree on what constitutes quality of life, since it can mean different things to different people. Mayers (1995) searched the literature and found that, while the concept of quality of life was widely used, there were few attempts to define it. Common features of existing definitions included subjective satisfaction, choice, sense of well-being, fulfilment of hopes and spiritual satisfaction. Mayers (2000) suggested that quality of life is concerned with both the satisfaction of needs and the ability to meet personal priorities.

Since quality of life is a subjective experience, it should be measured using self-completed questionnaires or rating scales (Mayers 1995).

FACTORS CONTRIBUTING TO MENTAL HEALTH AND ILL HEALTH

Many factors have been found to influence the mental health of individuals and communities, including both individual coping mechanisms and social support. These factors can be divided into three categories: biological, psychological and sociological/environmental. Some examples of each are given in Box 2.1.

Box 2.1 Factors that may affect mental health

BIOLOGICAL	PSYCHOLOGICAL	SOCIOLOGICAL/ENVIRONMENTAL
Biochemical	Stressful life events	Deprivation and poverty, including
Cerebrovascular accident	Learned behaviour	homelessness
Trauma, e.g. head injury	Relationships	Social status
Genetic	- expressed emotion	Unemployment
Toxins, e.g. alcohol	- double bind	Gender/sexual orientation
Deafness	Loss	Racism
Physical ill health	Loneliness	Vandalism
Pollution	Abuse	Migration
Nuclear contamination	Experience of being a	Climate
	refugee	Noise
		Natural disasters
		Terrorism

The rapid pace of change in modern society, along with increased geographical and social mobility, is putting stress on people while weakening supportive social structures, such as the extended family. When the normal balance of life is disturbed by external or internal factors, the relationship between stress and the ability to cope with the demands of everyday life can be depicted in the form of a curve, in which performance increases while the individual is in a state of ever-heightening arousal. This arousal prevents attention to the warning signs of fatigue, culminating in physical or psychological ill health. A model of how interacting demands can contribute to illness is shown in Figure 2.1.

Across the lifespan, everyone experiences a range of transitions such as leaving home, starting work, marrying or retiring. These transitions will be challenging but are regarded as normal stages within development (see Box 2.2). People in general have considerable capacity to withstand the stresses of transitions and other traumatic events. Many years ago, Holmes & Rahe (1975) identified life events which were significant and rated these according to the stress which they provoke. Events relating to loss, such as bereavements, unemployment and ill health, are examples of significant crisis situations. However, more positive events such as the formation of partnerships are not without stress!

Unexpected life events and normal transitions, such as those shown in Box 2.2, have important implications for health and well-being. How individuals manage such events depends upon a complex mix of personal, social and economic factors. The robustness of personality plus sound support systems usually enable people to negotiate transitions, but anxiety and depression can result from major life cycle changes such as marriage, parenthood, unemployment, retirement or loss.

Occupational therapists are interested in the ways in which occupations change over the course of the lifespan and correspond to life events. A sense of continuity is an important element in understanding an individual's strengths and coping capacity when faced with transitions in life. Kaplan & Sadock (1991), in a general text on psychiatry, included a section on 'phase of life problem'. It is recognised that stresses in the life cycle, due to life changes and transitions, can be key aspects of a presenting problem.

The context in which life events occur is obviously of importance – the widower with young children who is made redundant will not experience the same reactions as the older man with a grown-up family. Perceived support is one of the key factors in ability to cope when life events threaten a person's sense of well-being. One person's stress is another person's motivation to continue and many people operate at high stress levels, producing excellent work.

Stress is a process in which perceived demands (internal or external) severely tax or exceed available coping resources. This leads to a vicious cycle in which mood (depression) influences feelings

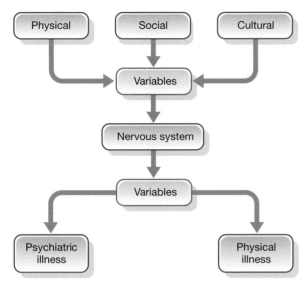

Figure 2.1   Factors Contributing to illness.

('I am useless') and tends to alter behaviour (not participating in activities) which, in turn, increases the level of depression. External events are more likely to conquer someone's adaptive ability if:

- they are unexpected
- the events are numerous
- the resulting stress is chronic and unremitting
- one loss triggers many other necessary adjustments.

Those people who are able to engage successfully with the conditions that life presents to them, including adverse circumstances and stressful

---

Box 2.2 Transitions and life events

POSSIBLE CRITICAL TRANSITION POINTS	UNANTICIPATED LIFE EVENTS
Birth	Accidents
Adolescence	Life-threatening
Marriage/partnership	disorders
Pregnancy	Natural disasters
Separation/divorce	Wars
Unemployment/retirement	Physical/mental
Dying	illness
	Loss of status/
	prestigious role
	Bereavement

---

events, are called *emotionally resilient*. Emotional resilience is the name given to the range of protective mechanisms and processes that enable people to withstand the potentially damaging effects of stress and to maintain high self-esteem and self-efficacy in the face of adversity (Rutter 1987).

PROTECTIVE FACTORS

Factors that have been found to protect against the damaging effects of stress and adversity fall into four main groups: individual factors, family factors, life experiences and community factors.

- **Individual factors (including personal characteristics).** The individual with an easy temperament is more likely to have harmonious interactions with others, and this has been shown to contribute to resilience. An easy temperament is characterised by equable mood, mild-to-moderate intensity of emotional reactions, malleability, predictable behaviour, openness to new situations and a sense of humour (Rutter 1987). Other personal characteristics that protect against the damaging effects of stress include above-average intelligence or an aptitude for a particular skill, good problem-solving skills, an internal locus of control, effective social skills, optimism, moral beliefs and high self-esteem. People who are more active, physically and/or mentally, are also more likely to be emotionally resilient. Other factors include personal awareness of strengths and limitations, a belief that one's own efforts can make a difference and an ability to empathise with others (Newman 2002). Additional individual factors in childhood include attachment to the family, adequate nutrition and school achievement (DoH 2001).
- **Family factors.** Families that promote positive mental health are secure, stable and harmonious. They also tend to be small, with more than 2 years' age difference between siblings. Other protective factors within the family include strong family norms and morality and at least one supportive, caring parent or a supportive relationship with another adult during childhood (DoH 2001). Where there is parental disharmony, a close relationship with one or other parent is a

protective factor. A supportive extended family and a valued role for the child within the family, such as doing household chores, are further protective factors (Newman 2002).

- **Life experiences.** Three types of experience have been shown to increase the chances that a person will grow up with feelings of high self-esteem and self-efficacy. The first is secure early attachments to parents or parental figures. The second is successful task accomplishment. This can include academic success, taking positions of responsibility, social success, employment and success in non-academic pursuits such as sports or music. There is evidence that feelings of self-esteem and self-efficacy, while initially formed in early childhood, can be modified by later life experiences (Rutter 1987). The third type of experience is opportunities at critical turning points in life, when doors to new, positive experiences are opened.
- **Community factors.** Positive mental health is promoted by a sense of connectedness with the community and attachment to community networks. This may be through participation in a particular community group, such as a faith group. Healthy communities have a strong cultural identity and pride, and there are strong norms against violence (DoH 2001).

RISK FACTORS

Factors that inhibit positive mental health are called risk factors. These can be divided into the same four categories as protective factors: individual factors, family factors, life experiences and community factors (DoH 2001).

- **Individual risk factors.** These include prenatal brain damage or birth injury, prematurity, low birth weight, poor health in infancy, physical or intellectual disability, low intelligence, a difficult temperament, impulsivity, poor social skills and low self-esteem.
- **Family and social risk factors.** These include having a teenage mother and/or a single parent, absence of father in childhood, large family size, antisocial role models, family disharmony and violence, poor supervision

and monitoring of the child, long-term parental unemployment, parental mental disorder and/or criminality, a harsh or inconsistent disciplinary style, social isolation and lack of warmth and affection.
- **Life events and situations.** The factors that create risk include physical, sexual and emotional abuse, divorce and family break-up, death of a family member, poverty or economic insecurity, school transitions and war or natural disaster.
- **Community risk factors.** These include socioeconomic disadvantage, social or cultural discrimination, social isolation, neighbourhood crime and violence, poor housing and lack of community facilities such as transport, shops and recreation centres.

Mental health promotion strategies may be targeted at any or all of these areas. It has been shown that prevention and early intervention are far more effective for mental health than treating illness once it has become established.

PROMOTING POSITIVE MENTAL HEALTH

Over the last 50 years, traditional Western health care has been challenged many times in terms of its ideology, management and interventions. Dissatisfaction with the medicalisation of health has promoted new philosophies which, since the mid-1980s, have placed health care in the context of the community. Consequently, the challenge for all health-care professionals has become a quest for more proactive approaches to promote and maintain sound physical and mental health for people within their communities. Inherent in the new philosophies of care are ideas of individual responsibility, self-determination, empowerment and a more equitable partnership between client and health professional.

In 1986, the first International Conference on Health Promotion was held in Ottawa, primarily to acknowledge changing worldwide expectations for a new emphasis in the public health movement. The Ottawa Charter was the outcome of this and it endorsed the need to work towards healthy communities and a reorientation of health services, including changes in health research and in professional education. In the same year, the Division of Health Psychology of the British Psychological Society was established, again with a focus on health rather than on illness and a drive towards a psychology of prevention rather than treatment (Niven 1989).

Health education also shifted in emphasis away from the traditional imparting of sensible information, which had been criticised for its assumption that people are rational human beings who are free to choose health-related lifestyles. Health education has become part of a broader approach to promoting health which incorporates efforts to change political, social and economic conditions for individual groups and communities. This implies co-operation between agencies in both the statutory and voluntary sectors.

Mental health promotion functions at different but interconnected levels (DoH 2001, Health Education Authority 1997).

- **Level of the individual**: increasing emotional resilience through interventions designed to promote self-esteem, life skills and coping skills, for example communicating, negotiating, relationship skills and parenting skills. This is the level with which occupational therapists are most familiar.
- **Level of the community**: increasing social support, social inclusion and participation, improving neighbourhood environments, anti-bullying strategies at school, workplace health, community safety, childcare and self-help networks. Occupational therapists are increasingly moving into this area of work.
- **Structural/policy level**: developing initiatives to reduce discrimination and inequalities and to promote access to education, meaningful employment, affordable housing, health, social and other services which support those who are vulnerable. Occupational therapists are not yet working at this level, except in isolated projects.

Strategies for promoting mental health operate through one or more of four processes (Newman 2002).

- **Altering perceptions of or exposure to risk**. For example, poor social skills are a risk factor so social skills training programmes can promote positive mental health.
- **Reducing the chain reaction that takes place when risk factors compound each other and multiply**. For example, many young people who drop out of school come from unstable families, have literacy and numeracy problems, are involved with the police, take drugs, engage in risky sexual behaviour and so on. A 10-week programme for these young people was designed to teach them basic social and personal skills in order to reduce or remove some of these risk factors.
- **Improving self-esteem and self-efficacy**. For example, a drop-in creative activity group was provided in a community centre on a large housing estate. Participants gained in self-confidence and self-esteem through making items that they valued and that were admired by friends and family.
- **Creating opportunities for change**. For example, a supported employment scheme can assist someone with limited work experience to retain a job while learning the necessary skills.

Some mental health promotion strategies have been found to be more effective than others. A review of the literature identified eight features that are characteristic of the most effective programmes (Sure Start 2004).

- **Comprehensiveness:** no single type of intervention has been found to prevent multiple high-risk behaviour, so successful programmes involve a combination of intervention methods and aim to influence a combination of several risk or protective factors.
- **System orientation:** successful interventions aim to change institutions as well as individuals, and involve the social network of the individual or group.
- **Relatively high intensity and long duration**: short-term programmes tend to have time-limited benefits, especially with high-risk groups. Long programmes (years rather than months) have an impact on more risk factors and have more lasting effects. The most

successful programmes intervene at a range of different times rather than once only.

- **Structured curriculum**: successful interventions are targeted at risk and protective factors rather than at problem behaviours.
- **Early commencement**: this is essential. Intervention during pregnancy brings additional benefits.
- **Specific to particular risk factors**: prevention needs to be disorder, context and objective specific. Generic prevention programmes have less impact.
- **Specific training**: there is no evidence about what qualifications are needed for effective mental health promotion. All people who work with young children and their carers should have skills in this area.
- **Attention to maintaining attendance**: the people who most need intervention are likely to be those who need most support if they are to stay in a programme.

OCCUPATIONAL THERAPY AND HEALTH PROMOTION

Christiansen & Baum (1997, p600) defined occupational therapy as 'a health discipline concerned with enabling function and well-being' and Brown (1987) considered that occupational therapy was an 'unrecognised forerunner in the wellness movement'. While few occupational therapists in the UK work comprehensively with the well population. they have been involved in working with carers, offering support, advice and education, for many years.

The values underpinning the promotion of sound mental health have always been implicit within occupational therapy and they have become more explicit since the renaissance of occupation as a core construct within research, theory and practice. Some of the assumptions made by occupational therapists about the relationship between occupation and health are as follows.

- People are occupational beings.
- Engagement in occupation is healthy.
- People need a healthy balance of occupation.
- There are links with purpose and meaning.

- Occupation is a tool for healthy participation in life.
- Occupation can act as a barometer for gauging health.

An understanding of the value of activity is central to the profession's philosophy and its focus on occupational performance. The health-promoting value of purposeful participation in activity is inherent in the concept of self-actualisation: through *doing*, people are confronted with the evidence of their ability to function competently and take control of their lives as far as they are able. Personal dignity and beliefs are enhanced and a sense of self-worth is developed. For example, Argyle (1987) suggested that Scottish country dancing epitomises the totality of an enhancing activity in which there is social contact, skill, exercise and involvement in culture. Gardening can be understood in the same light; although different in pace, it provides the participant with closeness to the seasons and the rhythm of life. It enhances the quality of life by the provision of colour, smell, experiences and the produce which results from careful tending.

Giving people opportunities to take part in demanding and challenging activities makes them less sensitive to risk and more able to cope with physical and emotional demands (Newman 2002). A person needs to experience demands that are within his capabilities, or that stretch him slightly, in order to develop a sense that he can manage. If the demands are too great, leading to repeated failure, or too light, so that skills are not developed, then the individual will not be able to trust in his ability to cope (Antonovsky 1993).

OCCUPATIONAL THERAPY AND WELL-BEING

The occupational therapy process, as outlined by Reed & Sanderson (1992), focuses on leisure, personal care and occupation in relation to the physical, psychological, social, economic and spiritual aspects of a person's life. External factors, both sociological and environmental, are taken into account and there is an emphasis on enhancing the competence of the individual rather than highlighting areas of disability or malfunction. The philosophy underpinning this approach, which is essentially holistic and focused towards empowerment, is compatible with health promotion and the concepts of personal responsibility and control.

The wellness and holistic health movement in America, which emerged from the human potential and counter-culture movements in the 1960s and 1970s (Johnson 1986), fitted well with philosophies in occupational therapy that acknowledge the dynamic interaction of mind, body, spirit and social context. The focus on spiritual well-being encompasses the values of the individual and recognises the need for self-esteem and affirmation. Without some sense of spirituality, there is a lack of meaning in life, which can often be identified in loneliness, depression and feelings of powerlessness (Neuhaus 1997).

A client-centred focus will in itself help to combat problems. Many people lack experience of warm and supportive relationships and the therapist can facilitate the expansion of social networks to enhance feelings of well-being.

Some of the factors which promote a sense of well-being are reflected in the following six Cs.

- **Contribution**. An old Indian proverb states that the smile you send out returns to you. A sense of being able to give to others is an essentially healthful phenomenon.
- **Comfort with change in life**. Self-regard and acceptance of one's lot lead to being at ease in one's surroundings. Parallel with this is the ability to change and adapt so that the individual does not sink into stagnation.
- **Contact/companionship**. Involvement and social networks are essential for human survival and the degree of support which a person perceives he is receiving from others is a crucial factor in the ability to cope. Empathy with others is an aspect of this.
- **Choice**. Also significant is the degree to which the person feels in control, having a sense of empowerment and choice.
- **Competency**. The ability to cope builds a positive self-concept which reinforces a sense of competency. Carrying out activities proficiently promotes self-esteem.
- **Commitment**. This brings a sense of purpose and belonging and of direction in life.

THE CONTRIBUTION OF OCCUPATIONAL SCIENCE

The discipline of occupational science is concerned with the form, function and meaning of occupation. While its relationship with the practice of occupational therapy is a robust one, it draws its knowledge base from diverse interdisciplinary sources. This provides a rich contribution to our understanding of how occupation affects mental health and subsequent well-being. Yerxa (1993) was an early proponent of this new science, believing that it offered a new way to comprehend the occupational nature of human beings and how this could enhance human potential and personal growth.

A number of theorists (for example, Clark 1993, Townsend 1997, Watson & Swartz 2004) have extended these ideas and offered a type of qualitative research methodology in the form of narrative analysis which has revealed how engagement in meaningful activities can be a transformative experience. Further, occupational patterns and routines provide a sense of coherence and balance (Ekelman et al 2003). Mental well-being can be enhanced by the significant social, spiritual, psychological and biological features which a balanced occupational life offers (Wilcock 2006). Occupational balance is the result of healthy resolution of occupational deprivation, alienation and injustice, through the achievement of occupational justice (Townsend 2003, Whiteford 2000, Wilcock 1998).

SUMMARY

Prevention of ill health and the promotion of mental well-being are now regularly featured within the media. In one popular evening newspaper in the East of Scotland, on one night alone, there were features concerning volunteering to promote good mental health, an article advertising a module to assist police officers to recognise the signs of dementia in the course of their work and a feature on ways of combating depression in young men.

This chapter has explored some of the concepts and ideas that underpin the promotion of mental health and well-being. It has identified the factors that have the potential to promote or inhibit positive mental health and looked at some of the strategies and interventions used in mental health promotion programmes. It finished by considering the role of occupational therapy in the promotion of health and well-being, and the contribution that occupational science is making to the field.

The early years of the new millennium have been exciting ones for the profession of occupational therapy in relation to ideas of health, wellness and well-being. Occupational perspectives of health are now more confidently articulated, whether in relation to micro, meso or macro aspects of society. The underlying philosophy of occupational therapy is consistent with models of health which focus on the empowerment of individuals by acquiring life skills to achieve a greater sense of control. It is concerned with the constellation of activities which give meaning to life by determining roles, relationships and routines. These give shape and purpose to our lives and provide the vital ingredients that contribute to a sense of well-being.

References

Antonovsky A 1993 The sense of coherence as a determinant of health. In: Beattie A, Gott M, Jones L et al (eds) Health and wellbeing: a reader. Macmillan, Basingstoke

Argyle M 1987 The psychology of happiness. Methuen, London

Brown KL 1987 Wellness: past visions, future roles. In: Cromwell F (ed) Sociocultural implications in treatment planning in occupational therapy. Howarth Press, London

Brown L (ed) 1993 The New Shorter Oxford English Dictionary. Clarendon Press, Oxford

Christiansen C, Baum C 1997 Enabling function and well-being, 2nd edn. Slack, New Jersey

Clark F 1993 Occupation embedded in a real life: interweaving occupational science and occupational therapy. American Journal of Occupational Therapy 47(17): 1067-1078

Creek J 2004 Health promotion in the United Kingdom. WFOT Bulletin 49: 9-12

Department of Health 1992 The health of the nation. HMSO, London

Department of Health 1999 Saving lives: our healthier nation. HMSO, London

Department of Health 2001 Making it happen: a guide to delivering mental health promotion. Department of Health, London

Downie RS, Fyfe C, Tannahill A 1993 Health promotion models and values. Oxford University Press, Oxford

Draper P, Griffiths J, Dennis J et al 1980 Three types of health education. BMJ 281: 493-495

Ekelman B, Bazyk S, Dal Bello-Haas V 2003 Occupation, participation and health. Occupational Therapy Journal of Rehabilitation 23(4): 130-142

Ewles L, Simnett I 2003 Promoting health: a practical guide, 5th edn. Baillière Tindall, London

Fernando S 1993 Mental health for all. In: Beattie A, Gott M, Jones L, Sidell M (eds) Health and wellbeing: a reader. Macmillan, Basingstoke

Hasselkuss B 2002 The meaning of everyday occupation. Slack, New Jersey

Health Education Authority 1997 Mental health promotion: a quality framework. Health Education Authority, London

Holmes TH, Rahe RH 1975 The social readjustment rating scale. Journal of Psychosomatic Research 11: 213-218

Johnson JA 1986 Wellness: a context for living. Slack, New Jersey

Kaplan H, Sadock BJ 1991 Synopsis of psychiatry. Williams and Wilkins, Baltimore

Mayers C 1995 Defining and assessing quality of life. British Journal of Occupational Therapy 58(4): 146-150

Mayers C 2000 Quality of life: priorities for people with enduring mental health problems. British Journal of Occupational Therapy 63(12): 591-597

Mayers C 2003 The development and evaluation of the Mayers' Lifestyle Questionnaire (2). British Journal of Occupational Therapy 66(9): 388-395

mentality 2004 Know-how that works. NeLH in collaboration with mentality: www.nelh.co.uk

Neuhaus B 1997 Including hope in occupational therapy practice: a pilot study. American Journal of Occupational Therapy 51(3): 228-234

Newman T 2002 Promoting resilience: a review of effective strategies for child care services. Centre for Evidence-based Social Services, University of Exeter

Niven N 1989 Health psychology. Churchill Livingstone, Edinburgh

Philips A 1989 Winnicott: An introduction. British Journal of Psychiatry 155: 612-618

Reed KL, Sanderson SN 1992 Concepts of occupational therapy, 2nd edn. Williams and Wilkins, Baltimore

Rutter M 1987 Psychosocial resilience and protective mechanisms. American Journal of Orthopsychiatry 57(3): 316-331

Schmid T 2005 Promoting health through creativity: an introduction. In: Schmid T (ed) Promoting health through creativity for professionals in health, arts and education, Whurr, London

Scottish Executive 2003 National Programme for Improving Mental Health and Well-being. Stationery Office, Edinburgh

Scottish Public Mental Health Alliance 2002 With health in mind: improving mental health and wellbeing in Scotland. Scottish Council Foundation, Edinburgh

Seedhouse D 1986 Health: the foundations for achievement. Wiley, Chichester

Seedhouse D 1997 Health promotion: philosophy, prejudice and practice. Wiley, Chichester

Smith BJ, Tang KC, Nutbeam D 2006 WHO health promotion glossary: new terms. Health Promotion International 21(4): 340-345

South Yorkshire Workforce Development Confederation 2003 Caring for the spirit: a strategy for the chaplaincy and spiritual healthcare workforce. South Yorkshire Workforce Development Confederation, Sheffield. Available online at: www.southyorkshire.nhs.uk/chaplaincy/documents/Workforce_Strategy.pdf

Sure Start 2004 What works in promoting children's mental health: the evidence and the implications for Sure Start local programmes. DfES Publications, Nottingham

Townsend E 1997 Occupation: potential for personal and social transformation. Journal of Occupational Science Australia 4(1): 18-26

Townsend E 2003 Reflections on power and justice in enabling occupation. Canadian Journal of Occupational Therapy 70(2): 74-87

Tudor K 1996 Mental health promotion: paradigms and practice. Routledge, London

Watson R, Swartz L (eds) 2004 Transformation through occupation. Whurr, London

Webb P (ed) 1994 Health promotion and patient education, Chapman and Hall, London

Whiteford G 2000 Occupational deprivations: global challenge in the new millennium. British Journal of Occupational Therapy 63(5): 200-204

Wilcock AA 1998 An occupational perspective on health. Slack, New Jersey

Wilcock AA 2006 An occupational perspective of health. 2nd edn. Slack, New Jersey

Wilcock AA, Townsend G 2000 Occupational therapy interactive dialogue: occupational justice. Journal of Occupational Science 7(2): 84-86

World Health Organization 1946 Constitution. World Health Organization, Geneva

World Health Organization 1986 Ottawa Charter for Health Promotion. World Health Organization, Geneva

World Health Organization 1999 Fact sheet No. 220. World Health Organization, Geneva

World Health Organization 2001 International classification of functioning, disability and health. World Health Organization, Geneva

World Health Organization 2002 Prevention and promotion in mental health. World Health Organization, Geneva

Yerxa E 1993 Occupational science: a new source of power for participants in occupational therapy. Journal of Occupational Science 1(1): 3-10

Chapter 3

The knowledge base of occupational therapy

Jennifer Creek

INTRODUCTION

In the first chapter we looked at the development of occupational therapy into a modern-day profession. Using this information as a background, we can now look more closely at the current philosophical and theoretical base of occupational therapy. We will do this by analysing the following:

- the development of professional philosophy in the modern age
- the philosophical assumptions that underpin practice today
- the key concepts that are used in occupational therapy
- theories of occupation
- the relationship of the theoretical base to the practice of occupational therapy.

THE PHILOSOPHICAL DEVELOPMENT OF THE MODERN PROFESSION

As described in Chapter 1, the profession of occupational therapy as we know it today dates from about 1917. Since that time the profession has undergone, and is still undergoing, changes in its outlook and philosophy. Professional philosophy is the system of shared beliefs and values held by members of a profession; for those whose profession is occupational therapy, this includes beliefs about the nature of human beings, society, health and ill health, the nature and purpose of occupational therapy and the relationships between these various elements.

THE EARLY YEARS

When the profession of occupational therapy began, it operated with a pragmatic and humanistic view of human beings and their relationship with occupation. Some of the main proponents of this philosophy of pragmatism, such as John Dewey and George Herbert Mead, worked in Chicago, where the first occupational therapy course was started in 1908. Pragmatism 'recognizes the inextricable influences on each other of the mental and physical aspects of human beings, their artifacts, their environments,

and the societies and times in which they live' (Breines 1995, p16). This philosophy permeated early writings on occupational therapy; for example, Adolph Meyer (1917, cited by Young & Quinn 1992, p118) argued that mental disorders can be understood only 'in the context of the total personality, and in the light of the many interacting factors that conspire to bring them about'.

Humanism views people as 'growing, developing, creating being(s), with the ability to take full self-responsibility' (Cracknell 1984, p73). This includes taking responsibility for maintaining their own health and for making choices that determine what they become.

These beliefs in the mind–body–environment–time interrelationship and in the capacity of human beings to achieve health through what they do led occupational therapists to use broad and balanced programmes of activity to treat mental health problems.

In 1922, Meyer wrote about the value of occupation in the management of psychiatric patients. Although he did not attempt to define occupational therapy, Meyer was aware that 'the proper use of time in some helpful and gratifying activity appeared to be a fundamental issue in the treatment of the neuropsychiatric patient'. He also outlined his philosophy as a recognition of:

> the need of adaptation and the value of work as a sovereign help in the problems of adaptation
> ...our conception of man is that of an organism that maintains and balances itself in the world of reality and actuality by being in active life and active use ...

> ... Our role [as occupational therapists] consists in giving opportunities rather than prescriptions
> ... Man learns to organise time and he does it in terms of doing things. (Meyer 1922, reprinted 1977)

Key concepts from the foundation of the profession which still inform practice today include taking a temporal perspective of the client and being concerned with the balance of activities in an individual's life over time, not just with single activities. Occupational therapists are concerned not only with the person as he is now, at the moment of intervention, but also with how he functions at different times and in different environments. We are interested in the person's past, how he functioned previously, and in his future, what he expects to do after the intervention is finished and for the rest of his life.

The whole-person approach is still considered to be a crucial aspect of occupational therapy intervention. Mattingly & Fleming (1994) described this as a concern with 'the patient's relationship with the disease ... with disability as a meaningful experience, especially inasmuch as it has affected the patient's capacity to move through the world, and to take up the occupations that have shaped his or her life and given it significance'.

THE INFLUENCE OF REDUCTIONISM

Throughout the 1950s and 1960s, occupational therapy gradually changed its philosophy under the influence of the reductionist model of science which was then being adopted by all the life sciences in an attempt to become scientifically respectable. Reductionism is based on the belief that the structure and function of the whole can best be understood from a detailed study of the parts by observation and experiment (Smith 1983). Reilly (1962) said that each person's need to be occupied should not be inferred from global generalisations but was being rigorously investigated under laboratory conditions. This comment sat uncomfortably within a model which emphasised a view of human beings as complex organisms developing and functioning within their own environments, and demonstrates some of the confusion of identity that occupational therapists were experiencing at that time.

Shannon (1977, p231) claimed that occupational therapists at this period not only lost sight of the beliefs of the founders of the profession but also adopted the medical model with 'its focus on pathology ... and on the minute and measurable'. Medicine is concerned with acute illness or with the acute phase of illness, whereas occupational therapy is traditionally and most usefully concerned with the needs of people with chronic health problems. Therapy began to focus on pathology and on the therapeutic techniques used rather than on the person, and became concerned with reducing symptoms and working with people who could be 'cured' rather than those with complex, long-term needs.

With the increasing use of technology and accompanying need for specialisation, the focus moved from health to illness and the responsibility for wellness moved from the individual to the medical profession. Occupational therapy, in accepting this change, lost its humanistic perspective and began to prescribe activities for patients rather than giving them opportunities to influence their own health through occupation.

By adopting the reductionist model, occupational therapists were able to develop a great depth of expertise in various fields of practice – for example, many therapists became highly skilled in the use of projective media in analytic group psychotherapy – but the profession as a whole suffered from role diffusion and loss of identity (Kielhofner & Burke 1977).

REASSESSING OUR BELIEFS

The 1970s and 1980s saw a conscious effort on the part of occupational therapists to reassess the original philosophy of the profession, which had become obscured during the 1950s and 1960s. West (1984) suggested that society was moving from a mechanistic view of man and health to a systems view which is congruent with the pragmatic and humanistic perspective of occupational therapy: 'Health care of the future will consist of restoring and maintaining the dynamic balance of individuals, families and social groups, and it will mean people taking care of their own health individually, as a society, and with the help of therapists'.

The profession attempted to reassert the validity of occupational therapy traditions and values without losing the very real advances in theory and practice made during the reductionist era. The areas of belief which were examined and agreed to be still relevant to occupational therapy practice in mental health can be summarised as follows:

- a concern with the person as a physical, thinking, emotional, spiritual and social being, who has a past, present and future, and who functions within physical and social environments

- a belief in intrinsic motivation – an innate predisposition to explore and act on the environment and to use one's capacities
- a recognition of each person's need for a balance of occupations in his life in order to: facilitate development, give meaning to life, satisfy inherent needs, realise personal and biological potentials, adapt to changing circumstances and maintain health
- an acceptance of the social nature of people and of the importance of social interaction in shaping what we become
- a recognition of the influence of what we do on what we become – the primacy of function over structure
- a view of health as a subjective experience of well-being, resulting from being able to achieve and maintain a sense of meaning and balance in life
- a belief in the responsibility and capability of people to find healthy ways of adapting to changing circumstances by what they do
- an acceptance of the role of occupational therapists in serving the occupational needs of people in order to help them restore meaning and balance to their lives
- a belief in occupation as the central organising concept of the profession and in the use of activity as the main treatment medium.

WORKING WITH COMPLEXITY

In the latter years of the 20th century, there was an emerging recognition that organic systems cannot be fully understood through traditional scientific analysis, but require new ways of understanding and new methods of enquiry. This is because organic systems are complex, in that they can only be understood by looking at the relationships between components, not by studying those components separately. The study of complexity crosses many diverse disciplines, such as chemistry, biology, neurology, population dynamics, meteorology, economics (Lewin 1999) and health promotion (McQueen 2000). Complexity theory has much to offer occupational therapy because people are complex, illness and disability are complex and occupational therapy itself is a complex process (Butler 2004, Creek et al 2005, Royeen 2003).

What is *complexity*? In a complex system, the interactions between components are such that the system as a whole cannot be fully understood simply by analysing those components (Cilliers 1998). Patterns of interaction change over time so that the system evolves in a non-linear way. This means that small changes in any aspect of the system can lead to dramatically large consequences overall, or to no effect at all on the whole system. For example, weather systems are non-linear and notoriously unpredictable.

It is tempting to think that *complex* is the opposite of *simple* but the distinction is not necessarily a clear one. The South African philosopher Cilliers (1998) suggested that 'Many systems appear simple, but reveal remarkable complexity when examined closely … Others appear complex, but can be described simply' (p2). Occupational therapy can look simple to the outsider but it is difficult to define or explain.

In 2003, the College of Occupational Therapists published a document defining occupational therapy as a complex intervention (Creek 2003). This publication marked a critical shift from using general systems theory as an organising framework for knowledge to 'acknowledging the complex, multifaceted and contextual nature of occupational therapy' (College of Occupational Therapists 2006a, p17). This will be described in more detail later in this chapter.

The continuing search for a clearer understanding of occupational therapy is not an academic exercise but a response to major changes both in society and within the profession. The remainder of this chapter is a brief review of three aspects of occupational therapy:

- the philosophical assumptions underpinning current practice
- the theoretical base of the profession
- the ways in which theory is linked to practice.

PHILOSOPHICAL ASSUMPTIONS

A professional philosophy is a system of shared beliefs and values held by members of a profession. Philosophical assumptions are the basic beliefs which make up this system and which show how members of a particular profession view people and the profession's goals and function (Mosey 1986). In occupational therapy, we accept as true certain beliefs about the nature of people, for example that 'All people experience the need to engage in occupational behaviour because of their species common combination of anatomical features and physiological mechanisms. Such engagement in occupation is an integral part of complex health maintenance systems' (Wilcock 1995, p69). Without this belief we would not be convinced of the value of occupation as therapy. This sharing of fundamental beliefs contributes to our sense of identity as a profession.

The three areas of belief central to occupational therapy are concerned with:

- the nature of human beings
- the nature of health and illness
- the nature and purpose of occupational therapy.

VIEW OF HUMAN BEINGS

Occupational therapy is essentially person centred. The individual is seen 'not as an object or thing to be manipulated, controlled or made to conform but as a unique individual whose very humanness entitles him to choices in determining his own destiny' (Yerxa 1967, p7). This belief in the right of the individual to be himself is made up of three separate beliefs:

- a concern with the whole person within his environment
- a belief in intrinsic motivation to be active
- an understanding of the social nature of people.

Concern with the whole person

Occupational therapists see each person as a unique individual whose body, mind and spirit function together and cannot be seen or understood as separate entities. People change, according to this view, if they are separated from the environmental influences that have shaped who they are. These influences include the physical environment, cultural environment, societal factors and social support (Christiansen 1997).

The whole-person approach assumes that people can only be understood by seeing the relationships between body, mind, spirit and environment over time. Occupational therapists are concerned with the person as he is now, at this moment, and with how he functions at different times and in different environments. We are concerned with the balance of occupations in the individual's life over time, not just with single activities. Meyer wrote, in 1922, that 'the culminating feature of evolution is man's capacity of imagination and the use of time with foresight based on a corresponding appreciation of the past and the present'. Occupational therapists are interested in the person's past, how he functioned previously, and with his future, what he expects to do with the rest of his life.

People as initiators of action

Western medical science is founded on the principle that human life should be preserved if possible. Occupational therapy takes the principle that human function should be preserved or restored where possible. It is the basic premise of our profession that being able to function in a range of occupations is a desirable condition (Reilly 1962).

Indeed, it can be argued that human life and human function are the same thing. People have an intrinsic motivation to act on the environment in order to discover their own potential and to develop their capacities. We do not wait for the environment to impinge on us and then respond; we are able to visualise the ends we wish to achieve and act to realise them. West (1984) summarised the writings on philosophy of several occupational therapists as follows:

> Activity is the essence of living and is significantly interrelated with high morale ... to some degree life itself is seen as purposeful occupation – that is to say, as activity, as task, as challenge ... it is the purposefulness of behaviour and activity that gives human life order ... the basic philosophy of occupational therapy speaks to Man as an active being and to the use of purposeful activity as Man's interaction with and manipulation of his environment.

People as social animals

People do not act in isolation. We are essentially social animals who develop and live in the context of a group. Human interaction stimulates biological, psychological, emotional and social development, and people deprived of human company do not thrive. There is a long period of physical and emotional dependency in childhood, and it is both normal and healthy to retain some emotional dependence on others once physical maturity is reached.

Social groupings take different forms in different cultures but, within all cultures, a small and stable social group is considered most desirable. We do not cope well with living in groups that are too large for us to know everyone else and we have had to devise coping strategies, for example for living in cities.

VIEW OF HEALTH

Occupational therapists do not view health as merely the absence of disease, or disease as the absence of health. Health, as defined by occupational therapists, is:

> A dynamic, functional state which enables the individual to perform her/his daily occupations to a satisfying and effective level and to respond positively to change by adapting activities to meet changing needs. (Creek 2003, p54)

The individual is seen as healthy when he has learned the skills necessary for successful participation in the range of roles he is expected to play throughout his life. These roles change throughout the life cycle and there may be times when existing skills lag behind new needs. Dysfunction occurs when the individual is unable to maintain himself within his environment because he does not have the skills necessary for coping with the current situation. Dysfunction is very individual. For a violinist, the loss of a finger could be a major disability; for a singer, the same injury may be only a minor inconvenience.

The World Health Organization (WHO 2001, p19) described a dynamic relationship between health and activity:

> an individual's functioning in a specific domain is an interaction or complex relationship between the health condition and the contextual factors (i.e. environmental and personal factors). There is a dynamic interaction among these entities: interventions in one entity have the potential to modify one or more of the other entities.

Not only do occupational therapists believe that health can be defined by what we are able to do, we also believe that what we do makes us healthy or unhealthy. Occupational therapists believe that occupation is the highest level of human function, that it develops and integrates the individual's potentials of body, mind and will through the process of doing. What people do creates functional demands that drive neuroplastic changes and organisation, and therefore occupations shape what we become: physically, mentally, socially and spiritually.

Why dysfunction occurs

Dysfunction is 'a temporary or chronic inability to meet performance demands adaptively and competently and to engage in the repertoire of roles, relationships and occupations expected or required in daily life' (Creek 2003, p52). Causes of dysfunction fall into four main groups:

- failure to develop and mature normally due to physical abnormality or environmental deprivation, for example chromosomal abnormality or emotional abuse
- environmental or personal changes that the individual cannot cope with, such as war or bereavement
- new physiological or psychological needs which cannot be met using existing skills, such as parenthood
- pathology or trauma causing loss of skills, for example schizophrenia or head injury.

When the individual encounters a new situation, he uses his existing skills to try to master it. If these fail, he will try to learn effective new skills. Eventually, if the situation still remains outside his control, he will experience disequilibrium or crisis.

The pace at which change occurs is important for maintaining equilibrium; too fast a pace means that new skills are not learned quickly enough, adaptation is disturbed and a state of dysfunction may occur (Mosey 1968). The degree and pace of change that a person can manage without losing equilibrium are dependent on both internal factors (e.g. the ability to learn new skills quickly) and external factors (e.g. the amount of support available in the social environment).

VIEW OF THE PROFESSION

The uniqueness of the occupational therapy approach to psychosocial dysfunction lies in the philosophical view that human beings have the ability to influence their own health through what they do. 'Occupational therapy practice in the field of mental health is based on an understanding of the relationships between occupation, health and wellbeing and a belief in the potential of people with mental health problems to learn and grow' (College of Occupational Therapists 2006b, p9).

Occupational therapy is concerned with the consequences of disease or injury as they affect a person's ability to function, rather than with the primary pathology. For example, the occupational therapist will try to slow down the process of dementia by involving the client in a balanced programme of activities to maintain physical and cognitive functioning, rather than by tackling the disease itself.

The main aim of intervention is to develop each person's potentials to his highest possible level, to enhance his quality of life and sense of well-being, to increase his satisfaction in daily living and to improve access to opportunities for participation in life situations. The core of occupational therapy practice is activity analysis, adaptation, synthesis and application. The outcome of intervention should be that the client is able to enact a satisfying range of occupations 'that will support recovery, health, well-being, satisfaction and sense of achievement' (Creek 2003, p32).

Domain of concern

Occupational therapists work with people of all ages who have problems with carrying out the activities and occupations that they expect or need to do, or with carers or care staff who oversee the daily activities and occupations of clients. Intervention may be at an early stage of the client's difficulties, in order to mitigate or prevent any ongoing adverse effects, or may be appropriate at any stage of a long-term health condition.

Occupational therapy is often concerned with multiple and complex needs and problems but can also be of benefit to people who have minor coping difficulties or for those who wish to maintain and promote their well-being (Creek 2003).

Client–centred practice

Occupational therapists recognise that their interventions are most effective when the client is involved and engaged in the process of setting and realising goals. It is a requirement of the *Code of Ethics and Professional Conduct* (College of Occupational Therapists 2005, p6) that the therapist should 'at all times recognise, respect and uphold the autonomy of clients, and advocate client choice and partnership working in the therapeutic process'.

Client-centred occupational therapy intervention is a collaborative process in which the therapist, client and other interested parties negotiate and share choice and control. This can be at two levels:

- **the level of the intervention**: throughout the occupational therapy process, the focus is on the client's needs, wishes and goals rather than on the requirements of the health or social care system. This includes determining the need for occupational therapy, assessment and data gathering, setting goals, working in partnership to attain goals and evaluating the outcomes of intervention (Sumsion 1999)
- **the level of service planning, delivery and evaluation**: service users are represented and take an active role in those committees and working groups responsible for the design, delivery and evaluation of services.

When the client is too ill or disabled to participate fully in the intervention process, the therapist may have to take responsibility for making decisions on his behalf. In this case, the therapist remains aware of the risk of imposing her own goals and values on the client, and actively tries to avoid this. One of the goals of intervention will be 'to work towards increasing client understanding, autonomy and choice' (Creek 2003, p30).

VIEW OF THEORY

The theoretical foundation of the occupational therapy profession is made up of selected theories from various disciplines and fields of inquiry (Mosey 1981). A theory is not reality but is a conceptual system or framework that is used to organise knowledge and to understand or shape reality. A theory is constructed for a particular purpose and a good theory will fulfil the purpose for which it was designed.

A theory for practice is made up of four aspects. These are illustrated here with the example of functional assessment using a person/environment/occupational performance model (Hagedorn 2000):

- **a description of a set of phenomena**: functional assessment enables the occupational therapist to describe the client in terms of his abilities and limitations
- **an explanation of how and under what circumstances the phenomena occur**: the functional assessment should include consideration of the conditions under which the client is being assessed and the environment in which he would normally function
- **a demonstration of how these conditions relate to each other**: the therapist needs to identify how the client's impairments, his personal characteristics and environmental factors work together to determine his level of function
- **a prediction about what actions will change the situation**: the therapist has to know what intervention will make it possible for the client to achieve his optimum level of function.

Nixon & Creek (2006, p77) suggested that theory is not something that practitioners learn and then apply in practice:

In occupational therapy, theorising is an integral aspect of practice. We do not contribute to theory by first understanding what theory is and then developing a theory of our own. We *do* theory by

developing collaborative models of thoughtful practice that challenge assumptions and suggest new lines of inquiry; we *do* theory by learning how to align thoughtfulness and practice within specific contexts that require constant negotiation across complex professional, cultural and social boundaries.

This view of theory shows the therapist continually thinking about what she is doing, reasoning about the most appropriate course of action, reflecting on the effects of her interventions, negotiating with the client and others to reach agreement on the way forward. Formal theories, learned from lectures and books, are only one part of theorising in complex, client-centred interventions.

The most basic level of theory is naming theory or concept formation (Dickoff et al 1968). This is the level at which the mind creates concepts and categories of concepts. *Concepts* are 'mental representations of objects or ideas' (Creek 2003, p32). For example, *activity* is a concept that can be differentiated from other concepts that are not activity. Naming concepts makes it possible 'to point out, denote, or attend to conceptually a factor within the mind's consciousness' (Dickoff et al 1968, p420). In a sense, until something is given a name it does not exist.

CONCEPTS: THE BUILDING BLOCKS OF THEORY

In order to build theories to support the practice of occupational therapy, it is necessary to identify key concepts and agree on their precise meaning. Clearly defined concepts allow us to think and communicate about occupational therapy, to describe what we see and what we are doing, and to explain why certain situations or actions lead to change in one direction or another.

Key concepts for occupational therapists are shown in Box 3.1. Many of these terms have been defined by the European Network of Occupational Therapy in Higher Education (ENOTHE) and translated into all the major European languages, facilitating communication between occupational therapists across many countries.

Box 3.1 Key occupational therapy concepts

Occupation	Temporal adaptation	Engagement
Activity	Routine	Participation
Task	Habit	Motivation
Role	Environment	Volition
Occupational performance	Context	Independence
Function	Setting	Autonomy
Ability		Capacity
Skill		

OCCUPATION

The words *activity* and *occupation* are often used synonymously by occupational therapists but it is important to clarify the difference. Reilly (1962) suggested that the very existence of occupational therapy depends on our knowledge of the difference between the two terms and our capacity to act on that knowledge.

Hagedorn (2000) described a hierarchical taxonomy, in which social role is the highest level, followed by occupation, routine, activity, task, task stage, performance unit and actions, with skills components at the lowest level. Each term represents a different type of performance, and each level of the hierarchy incorporates the lower levels so that, for example, activities are combined into routines which contribute to occupations.

A different approach to understanding the relationships between occupation, activity and task was suggested by ENOTHE, using complexity theory as the organising framework. In this conceptualisation, a piece of performance can be an occupation, an activity or a task, depending on the perspective of the person doing the action. For example, cooking might be an occupation for a chef, an activity for a housewife and a task for a detained patient undergoing rehabilitation.

The ENOTHE (2006) definitions of occupation, activity and task are shown in Box 3.2.

Occupations are frequently classified into three different categories:

Box 3.2 ENOTHE definitions

Occupation: 'a group of activities that has personal and sociocultural meaning, is named within a culture and supports participation in society. Occupations can be categorised as self-care, productivity and/or leisure'. An occupation is enacted through the activities that are its doing aspects. For example, the main work occupation of a nurse is nursing. Some of the activities that she might perform as part of this occupation include observing patients, communicating with colleagues, overseeing meals and writing notes.

Activity: 'a structured series of actions or tasks that contribute to occupations'. An activity is not a random series of actions but is a doing process that is structured towards a goal. For example, the activity of doing the household shopping consists of a series of tasks – making a shopping list, getting ready to go out, reaching the shops, purchasing the items on the list, returning home and unpacking the shopping. If these tasks are not performed in a logical sequence or if a key task is missed out, the activity will not be completed successfully.

Task: 'a series of structured steps (actions and/or thoughts) intended to accomplish the performance of an activity'. For example, the first task in doing the household shopping might be to check what supplies are running low.

- self-care
- play/leisure
- productivity/work.

These are artificial differentiations, since an occupation can move from one category to another or belong in more than one category at the same time. For example, cooking a meal may be self-care if it is to satisfy an individual's hunger, it may be work if it is to feed a family, it may be leisure if it is to give a dinner party to friends, or it may serve more than one purpose.

Self-care

Self-care activities enable the individual to survive and to promote and maintain health. They include:

- basic physical functions such as eating, sleeping, excreting, keeping clean and keeping warm

- survival functions such as cooking, dressing, shopping, maintaining one's living environment, and keeping fit. Many of these functions have become specialised and have been delegated to members of society who have special skills, such as builders and bakers, but some remain with the individual.

Play/leisure

Man is a very adaptable species. This adaptability has been achieved by developing flexible behaviour rather than specialised behaviour (Kielhofner 1980). Play is the medium through which the child is able to learn and rehearse a wide range of skills that will enable him to respond appropriately and adaptively in different situations. Even in adult life, new skills are learned more thoroughly and integrated more successfully into the pattern of daily life if the individual approaches learning in a playful and explorative manner.

In adult life, play is usually called *leisure* and is often used to satisfy individual needs that are not met by either self-care or work occupations. For example, amateur dramatics can improve the physical well-being of a person who has an otherwise sedentary lifestyle, provide intellectual stimulation for a full-time mother of small children, create social contacts for an unemployed person or enhance the status and self-esteem of someone who has a low-level position at work.

Productivity/work

Work is any productive activity, whether paid or unpaid, that contributes to the maintenance or advancement of society as well as to the individual's own survival or development. Work may help to maintain society (e.g. housework) or contribute to its advance (e.g. theoretical physics).

The work in which a person spends most of his time usually becomes an important part of his personal identity and a major social role, giving him his position in society and a sense of his own value as a contributing member. Different jobs are given different social values so that people in certain jobs are considered to be more important than others, irrespective of how necessary their work is to the continuation of society. For example, the work of a doctor is more highly valued in Western society than that of a housewife.

Work serves many functions for the individual.

- It gives the person a major role in society and a social position.
- It usually provides the person with a means of livelihood.
- It gives a structure to time around which other activities can be planned.
- It can give a sense of purpose and value to life.
- It can be an important part of an individual's personal identity and a source of self-esteem.
- It can be a forum for meeting people and building different types of relationships.
- It can be an important interest and a source of satisfaction.

Anyone who is unable to work misses all these benefits and is, in addition, usually seen as making a negative contribution to society.

ROLE

Each person fulfils a number of roles during his lifetime. At any one time the individual may adopt a variety of roles, and these roles will change at different stages of life. For example, a child may have the roles of: daughter, sibling, school pupil, friend, Brownie, niece, dog owner. A decade later, some of these roles will have been dropped and new ones taken up, so that she is now: daughter, sibling, student, friend, flatmate, lover, waitress, and so on.

An occupation and a social role may share the same name, although a role is more likely to be described by a noun and an occupation by a verb. For example, *mother* is a role while *mothering* is an occupation. The concept of occupation is mainly concerned with the actions that a person takes to achieve his purposes while the concept of role is mainly concerned with social expectations and the mechanisms by which society shapes the actions of individuals.

Roles are social constructs that carry behavioural expectations and contribute to a person's self-image and sense of identity. They are 'the socially defined attributes and expectations associated with social positions' (Bond & Bond 1994, cited by Blair 1998 p42). Roles are allocated by society and adopted by the individual; that is, a role is both a social position and a set of tasks performed by the individual. Each person will interpret a role in a unique way. For example, the role of mother carries expectations about the care and nurturing of children. Women in the UK normally play a major part in bringing up their own children because that is the expectation in Western society. Different women will interpret the role in different ways, perhaps delegating some aspects to a relative or a paid childminder. If society feels that a woman is not fulfilling her role adequately, then it may be taken away from her and her children given into the care of others. Or a woman may choose not to accept the role of mother and may give her children into some form of care.

Social role is linked to social status, which refers to the position of the individual within the social structure. The status we achieve through our major social roles influences both the way that other people in our social group treat us and our expectations of how we will be treated. If we have a high social status, we are more likely to expect to be treated with respect and consideration.

Roles carry both rights within society and obligations to that society. For example, a university student has the obligation to attend a certain number of teaching sessions, to behave in an acceptable way during those sessions, to make an effort to learn the topics presented and to complete a prescribed number of assignments within a given timescale. In return, the student is given money, a position in society and the possibility of paid employment at the end of the programme of study.

OCCUPATIONAL PERFORMANCE

The word *occupation* is used to refer to both the performance of an activity and the pre-existing format that guides or structures that performance (Nelson 1988). For example, there is an established format of rules, procedures, equipment and environment for playing football. This is the *occupational form*, which is socially constructed and exists independently of performance. Football has a physical environment which includes materials, location, human context and temporal context.

It also has a sociocultural reality that depends on a social or cultural consensus and allows the occupational form to be interpreted differently in different social contexts, such as the major differences between a game of football for schoolchildren and an FA Cup championship match.

Christiansen & Townsend (2004a, p278) defined *occupational performance* as 'the task-oriented, completion or doing aspect of occupations, often, but not exclusively, involving observable movement'.

Playing football, the *doing*, is occupational performance. The way in which we perform within a given occupational form also depends on our level of competence and the meanings that we give to the occupation. For example, a professional goalkeeper may deliberately allow the ball into the net if he is trying to encourage a young child to learn the game, or he may do his best to keep it out to help his team win an international match.

Christiansen (1997) described intrinsic factors that enable or support occupational performance, calling them *performance enablers*. These include the sensory and motor systems, physical health and fitness, cognitive skills, self-concept, self-esteem and emotional state. Environmental factors also influence how an occupation is performed. These include the physical properties of environments, culture and the social context.

FUNCTION

The word *function* has two related meanings for occupational therapists and this can lead to misunderstandings. Function is 'the underlying physical and psychological components that support occupational performance' (ENOTHE 2006). It is being used in this sense in the phrase 'upper limb function'. Function also means 'the ability to perform competently the roles and occupations required in the course of daily life' (Creek 2003, p53). It is being used in this sense in the phrase 'function in personal activities of daily living'.

Effective function depends on abilities and skills. An *ability* is 'an innate characteristic that supports occupational performance' (ENOTHE 2006). For example, a child might have the ability to sing in tune.

A *skill* is 'a specific ability or integrated set of abilities (e.g. motor, sensory, cognitive or perceptual) which evolve with practice' (Creek 2003, p59). For example, the child with a talent for music can develop that ability through practice.

Occupational therapists commonly assess function in order to determine whether or not someone will be capable of living independently, to estimate the level of support they will need or to plan for intervention.

TEMPORAL ADAPTATION

Each person engages in many occupations in the course of his life. These fit together in what Bateson (1997, p7) called 'the framework of a life'. Self-care, play and work exist in a balance that is not static but changes at different stages of the life cycle and varies from individual to individual. People are not pre-programmed to follow a daily routine of activities; they continually make choices about what to do with their time and how to structure their daily routine. 'The net effect is engagement in a daily blend of occupations, each of which may be experienced as work, rest, play, leisure or self-care and which shape, in part, one's perception of the quality of life' (Yerxa et al 1989).

The term *temporal adaptation* is used to refer to the normal use of time in a purposeful daily routine of activities. A *routine* is 'an established and predictable sequence of tasks' (ENOTHE 2006). The healthy individual has his daily life activities organised into a satisfying and flexible pattern that meets his needs and is socially acceptable. Some routines are repeated in the same way until they become habitual and do not require conscious thought. A *habit* is 'a performance pattern in daily life, acquired by frequent repetition, that does not require attention and allows efficient function' (ENOTHE 2006).

The balance of occupations in a person's life is determined by personal interests and abilities, social expectations, age, environment and personal circumstances. For example, a professional woman with no children may find that she enjoys a variety of social and sporting activities that keep her fit, relieve the stress of working and enable her to meet people. A single mother with four children and a low-paid job, on the other hand, may not have the resources of time, energy or money to engage in a range of leisure activities.

Some patterns of activity can be seen to be unbalanced. For example, the 40-year-old man who works up to 12 hours a day, rarely sees his children, has no social life outside work and has no other important interests could not be said to have a healthy balance of occupations. If he loses his job, he may develop serious health problems. For occupational therapists, the balanced use of time in daily living activities not only influences health but is an indicator of health.

Occupational therapists are not so much concerned with a person's ability to carry out specific tasks at particular points in time as with the way in which he uses and organises time in daily life. In order to achieve a balance, the individual must have an awareness of time and of himself within time. Using time adaptively requires remembering past experiences and acting on them, being aware of likely future consequences of actions, planning ahead, acting on those plans and monitoring the effects of actions.

ENVIRONMENT

Occupational performance takes place within a variety of environments, contexts and settings that influence how the person performs. An *environment* is 'the human and non-human surroundings of the individual, including objects, people, events, cultural influences, social norms and expectations' (Creek 2003, p52). A person's environment will include physical, social, cultural, economic and political influences.

Hagedorn (2000) described three levels of environment, as shown in Box 3.3.

Occupational therapists also talk about settings and contexts, sometimes using these words interchangeably with each other and with environment. A *context* is 'a set of circumstances or conditions' (Creek 2003, p51). For example, we say that the meaning of an action changes depending on the context. The WHO (2001) stated that context is made up of two components: environmental factors and personal factors. Environmental factors are external influences on functioning and disability that facilitate or hinder activity and participation. Personal factors are the attributes of the person that impact on functioning and disability.

Box 3.3 Hagedorn's environmental levels

Resource area: this is all the places, objects and people that are familiar to the individual and with which he interacts regularly. It includes the *immediate environment* (the area within reach), the *near environment* (the area within a few steps of the individual) and the *used environment* (all the other areas that the individual uses regularly).

Exploratory area: this is all the other areas to which the individual has access. As the individual explores new areas, some of them will become part of the resource area. For example, a person attending a course at the local college could meet a fellow student with whom he gets on so well that they remain friends after the course finishes.

Closed area: this is the parts of the world that the individual does not know about or cannot access. These closed areas can be 'real or imagined, physical or metaphysical' (Hagedorn 2000, p43).

A *setting* is the immediate surroundings of the person, including both place and time, that equates to Hagedorn's immediate environment. For example, we talk about the influence of the treatment setting on how the client performs.

ENGAGEMENT

We have already noted that it is important for the client to be engaged in the process of therapy if the intervention is to be fully effective. *Engagement* is 'a sense of involvement, choice, positive meaning and commitment while performing an occupation or activity' (ENOTHE 2006).

Engagement in activity suggests attention and commitment to what is being done, not simply being present in body. When someone is engaged in an activity, his attention is focused on a goal and/or on the experience, not on the skills and effort required. He is absorbed in the activity and pays minimal attention to extraneous thoughts and feelings or to his physical state (Creek 2007).

It is possible to participate in an activity without being fully engaged, but engagement is not possible without participation. *Participation* is defined by the WHO (2001, p10) as 'involvement in a life situation'. Occupational therapists add that this involvement takes place 'through activity within a social context' (ENOTHE 2006).

Two personal factors determine the extent to which a person becomes engaged in an activity: motivation and volition. *Motivation* is 'a drive that directs a person's actions towards meeting needs' (ENOTHE 2006). *Volition* is 'exercise of the will, the mental action of consciously willing or resolving something; or making of a choice or decision regarding a course of action; the conscious awareness, during an activity, of its being performed voluntarily' (Creek 2003, p61). These two concepts are discussed in more detail in Chapter 6.

INDEPENDENCE

Independence has sometimes been described as the goal of occupational therapy interventions but, in recent years, the concept of interdependence has been gaining ground (Baum & Christiansen 1997). *Independence* is 'the position of not being dependent on authority; not relying on others for one's opinions or behaviours; being able to do things for oneself; having choice, control and participation in society' (Creek 2003, p54). Baum & Christiansen (1997) pointed out that no person who lives in a community is truly independent because we all collaborate and co-operate with each other. They also suggested that:

> The concept of interdependence is embodied within the idea of occupational therapy as a helping profession. That is, by working with our clients and their families, we can achieve goals that we could not achieve working independently. (p35)

The occupational therapist may work towards increasing the client's independence or interdependence – the goal will be determined by what the client wishes. When the client is not able to make such decisions for himself, it may be that his autonomy is compromised. *Autonomy* is 'the capacity to think, decide, and act on the basis of such thought and decision freely and independently and without … let or hindrance' (Gillon

1985/1986, p60). The ability to make and enact choices rests on three types of autonomy:

- **autonomy of thought**: being able to think for oneself, to have preferences and to make decisions
- **autonomy of will**: having the freedom to decide to do things on the basis of one's deliberations
- **autonomy of action**: the capacity to act on the basis of reasoning.

It is possible to make autonomous decisions without compromising healthy interdependence. For example, an individual with severe physical disabilities may take the decision to be dependent on others for his self-care so that he can put his energy into pursuing an interesting career.

Another term that is used when referring to people's ability to take decisions for themselves is *mental capacity*. This is a legal term that denotes competence. Hagedorn (2000, p308) defined *competence* as 'Skilled and adequately successful completion of a piece of performance, task or activity'. However, she pointed out that it can also mean being adequately qualified to perform a task.

The 2005 Mental Capacity Act makes provision for people who are thought to lack the capacity to make their own decisions in the areas of finance, social care, medical treatment, research and so on. Each decision is treated separately, so that someone can be deemed to have mental capacity in some areas of life but not in others.

Having explored the meanings of the key concepts used in occupational therapy, we will now look at theories of occupation. Since occupational therapy is primarily a practical profession, rather than an academic discipline, it is likely that we will continue to develop our theoretical base by drawing on the work of other disciplines. Occupational therapists need to be skilled in selecting, adapting and applying new knowledge, from whatever source, as it becomes available, while continuing to develop the understanding of occupation that is our core concern.

THEORIES OF OCCUPATION

The profession of occupational therapy was founded on the belief that people can influence their own health by being proficient in occupations which allow them to explore and interact with their environment in an adaptive way. In order to understand this interaction and its effects, it is necessary to develop a theory of occupation, including both the individual and the political dimensions of occupation.

First, we will acknowledge the contribution to the occupational therapy knowledge base of the academic discipline of occupational science.

Occupational science

Although occupational therapy was founded on a set of beliefs about the occupational nature of people, it is only relatively recently that the profession has begun to formulate its own theories about occupation. Occupational science is an academic discipline that studies people as occupational beings (Yerxa 2000). It brings together knowledge from different disciplines with the intention of providing a knowledge base in occupation for the practice of occupational therapy.

The discipline was established in the last decade of the 20th century to study the nature of occupation, to develop theories to explain why people choose certain activities over others and to explore the complexity of factors that influence why, where and how people decide to live their lives in relation to work, rest and play (Clark et al 1991). Elizabeth Yerxa, the founder of the first doctoral programme in occupational science at the University of Southern California, claimed that occupational science would 'address some of the major dilemmas of occupational therapy practice' (Yerxa 1993, p3).

In less than 20 years, occupational science has contributed to the knowledge base of occupational therapy at all levels, from elucidating key concepts, such as occupational alienation (Townsend & Wilcock 2004a), through building theories to explain why people choose particular occupations, such as theories of meaning (Primeau 1996), to developing appropriate research methodologies (Carlson & Clark 1991) and carrying out research into the effects of occupation on health (Iwarsson et al 1997).

Many of the theories described in this section have been developed under the banner of occupational science. They are organised under two headings: the individual and the political dimensions of occupation.

THE INDIVIDUAL DIMENSION OF OCCUPATION

As described above, occupations are enacted by individuals within physical and social environments that influence how they are performed. This section looks at four aspects of individual occupational performance:

- occupational behaviour and occupational choice
- the meaning of occupation
- the functions of occupation
- the relationship between occupation and health.

Occupational behaviour and occupational choice

The term *occupational behaviour* was coined to refer to active engagement in occupation. Occupational behaviour has been defined as 'the entire developmental continuum of play and work' (Reilly 1969) that evolves throughout the life cycle. Children learn the rules for acceptable behaviour in society through play, and their play experiences lead on to choice of occupations in adult life. The major occupation of many adults is work, and the process of choosing a job or career is called *occupational choice*.

Ginzberg and colleagues (1951) studied how people choose their main work occupation, finding that such an important decision is not made in one step but is the culmination of many smaller decisions made over many years. This long process of decision making allows the individual to accumulate knowledge of what he likes doing, what he does well and what activities he values. Ginzberg and his associates described occupational choice as a series of choices and the elimination of choices, as changes occur in the individual and the environment, which lead eventually to a narrowing of choice and to decisions being made. They identified four elements that influence the occupational choices made by individuals:

- awareness of one's own capacities
- interests
- personal goals and values
- time perspective of occupations.

In addition, the opportunity for making a particular choice must be present. The range of choices is determined by social factors, such as public disapproval, and by the physical environment, such as the location of sport and leisure facilities. In order to choose to do something, the individual also has to be aware of what his choices are. This awareness includes knowing what activities are available and knowing how to access them. It also implies having the capacity to see opportunities for action and having enough information on which to base choices.

The meaning of occupation

It is the nature of human beings to be active, therefore activity has always been a part of human life. However, the activities which have purpose and meaning for people and which take up a large part of their time have changed over the ages, from the physical activities of hunter/gatherer societies to the more passive, sedentary lifestyle of modern Western people. Breines (1995) called this evolution of human activity *occupational genesis*: 'Occupational genesis describes the evolving adaptive process in which humans engage in purposeful activities that are meaningful to their lives as their world and their experiences change'.

Purpose is 'the reason for which something is done or made, or for which it exists' (Creek 2003, p58). Activity may be for a particular purpose, irrespective of who is carrying it out. For example, cleaning the kitchen maintains food hygiene and safety, whoever does it. Purpose can also be found in the intentions of the person carrying out the activity. For example, a woman decides to walk upstairs in order to keep fit and there would be no point in someone else doing the activity for her (Creek 1998).

The *meaning* of an activity is the significance or importance that it has for an individual or a social group (Creek 2003). Some meanings are shared within a culture or subculture while others are personal. Meaning can be conceptualised as a continuum, with self-definitions of meaning at one end and social definitions of meaning at the other end (Reker & Wong 1988, in Hasselkuss 2002). The balance of personal and social meaning in any activity will be influenced by various factors, including the individual's prior experience and personality but also social and cultural expectations.

An American occupational therapist, Betty Hasselkuss (2002), linked finding meaning in life with health and well-being, describing meaning as 'an essential for life' (p1). People search for meaning or try to create meaning and become uncomfortable when a situation or event seems unintelligble to them. Hasselkuss stressed the importance of activity in the construction of meaning: 'it is through *peformance* that we enter a life of understanding, because when we perform we interpret, and interpretation is the source of comprehension' (2002, p5). Children naturally try to engage actively with new experiences, stimulated by curiosity to explore and so to understand their world. 'Human beings [are] dynamical systems that are self-organised, engaged in self-directed actions and creating their unique experiences' (Lazzarini 2004, p343).

Engagement in activities that are appropriate to age and culture can ground the individual in his own community and lead to a sense of connectedness with others. Conversely, an inability to perform the activities that are considered normal in society, or that the individual would consider appropriate for himself, can lead to feelings of exclusion and worthlessness. The occupational therapist needs to understand which activities will enhance a sense of belonging and worth in the client.

The functions of occupation

People have a basic need to engage in activity that has meaning and value for them. Reilly (1962) claimed that 'man has a vital need for occupation and that his central nervous system demands the rich and varied stimuli that solving life problems provides him'. Occupations, and the activities by which they are enacted, can serve various functions in daily life.

- Occupations provide for the essential needs of the organism (Wilcock 1998a, b).
- People develop and maintain function through being active (Baum 1995).

- Physical, cognitive and emotional development are influenced by the physical and mental activity of the growing child (Passmore 2003, Rogoff 2003, Watson & Fourie 2004).
- People relate to the human and material worlds through what they do (Breines 1989).
- Occupations form an important part of each person's social identity and social status, and they influence social development (Watson & Fourie 2004).
- Occupations contribute to an individual's personal sense of identity (Hasselkuss 2002).
- People create meaning in their lives through what they do (Creek 1998).
- Activity is a tool for exploring and learning, and for developing competence (Passmore 2003).
- Occupations promote social inclusion (Passmore 2003).
- The health and well-being of the individual are influenced by what he does (Christiansen & Townsend 2004b, Hasselkuss 2002).

The potential of occupations and activities to bring about healthy changes in a person will be explored in more detail in the next section.

The relationship between occupation and health

Occupational therapists claim that there is a link between occupation and health but there has been, until recently, no strong theory to explain this link. In the 1990s, an Australian occupational therapist, Wilcock, published a series of papers and a book outlining a theory of the relationship between occupation and health (Wilcock 1995, 1998a, b).

Wilcock (1998a, p5) argued that humans are occupational beings with a central nervous system that has the capacity to 'analyse, organise, understand, produce, judge, plan, activate, formulate and execute complex occupation'. Occupations are, therefore, innate human behaviours that encompass all the things that people do, serving both a social and a biological function. Humans have evolved as occupational beings and it is through occupation that we adapt to, or insulate ourselves from, our physical, cultural and social environments.

Wilcock (1998a) further suggested that the two evolutionary functions of occupation are survival and health. It is through occupations that we meet our basic survival needs of safety, food, water, warmth and shelter. Health, which can be seen as the natural state for a person to be in, is also achieved through occupation, first by having all the basic survival needs met and then by 'having physical, mental and social capacities maintained, exercised and in balance' (p6).

Health can be a positive experience of well-being and not just the absence of disease or infirmity. Wilcock (1998b, p103) described mental well-being as a condition in which people can 'be creative and adventurous as they experience all human emotions, explore and adapt appropriately, and without undue disruption meet their life needs'.

Three occupational factors that can cause a breakdown of health are occupational imbalance, deprivation and alienation (Wilcock 1998b). *Occupational imbalance* is a lack of balance between work, rest and play, causing a loss of harmony between internal bodily systems and between the person and the environment. *Occupational deprivation* arises when external circumstances prevent the individual from using his capacities to the full, leading to imbalance and failure to develop or maintain normal functioning. *Occupational alienation* occurs when a person engages in activity which is not in accordance with the occupational nature of the species or the individual. The results are frustration, boredom, unhappiness and stress.

Occupational therapy can intervene at the level of the individual, usually in health or social care settings, or at the level of society, as in health promotion or community development, in order to counteract the negative effects of occupational imbalance, deprivation and alienation. Wilcock's theory of the occupational nature of health suggests that the most appropriate arena for the work of the occupational therapist is not in secondary or tertiary health-care systems but in prevention and public health.

THE POLITICAL DIMENSION OF OCCUPATION

As described in the last section, it is not always possible for people to engage in a range of occupations that lead to personal satisfaction,

social inclusion, health and well-being. Wilcock (1998b) introduced the concepts of occupational imbalance, occupational deprivation and occupational alienation to represent three of the ways in which participation in occupations can become dysfunctional.

Occupational imbalance, deprivation and alienation

People have an occupational nature. This means that people seek to be occupied and that occupation fulfils many functions for the individual, including promoting survival and health. However, occupation also has a social dimension. Societies determine how people should perform their occupations, which occupations are socially useful or acceptable and what occupations are available to particular groups of people.

Ideally, a wide range of occupations would be available to each person throughout the lifespan, so that an individual occupational profile can be developed through the choices made. However, individual and social factors can sometimes combine to block access to an adequate number of occupations, so that the person may experience occupational imbalance, occupational deprivation or occupational alienation.

A healthy balance of occupations includes a variety of physical, mental and social occupations, so that the individual is able to develop and exercise his capacities in all these areas. The balance may also be 'between chosen and obligatory occupations; between strenuous and restful occupations; or between doing and being' (Wilcock 2006, p343). Each person seeks a balance that is comfortable for him and that promotes health and well-being. This balance may be disrupted if a person does not have access to enough occupations, leading to empty times in the day when there is nothing worthwhile to do. Or the imbalance may be due to 'an undue focus on one occupation or category of occupation to the exclusion of others' (Creek 2003, p56); for example, someone working long hours in a sedentary job may find it hard to find time for physical exercise.

Townsend & Wilcock (2004b) pointed out that occupational imbalance is also seen in societies, where some people are overoccupied and others are underoccupied. This is often in the area of work, where some sectors of the population are overemployed while other sectors are either under-employed or unemployed. Townsend & Wilcock described this as unjust because 'in part, the hierar-chical classification of occupations drives a labour market in which those with particular skills and knowledge are paid well and have lots of work, while others are unable to find paid work at all'.

Wilcock (2006, p164) listed some of the social factors that can lead to people being deprived of access to a broad range of occupations: 'technol-ogy, the division of labour, lack of employment opportunities, poverty or affluence, cultural val-ues, local regulations, and limitations imposed by social services and education systems, as well as the social consequences of illness and disability'. Examples of occupational deprivation due to social factors include the closure of coal mines in the UK in the 1980s, leading to a massive loss of employment in some areas, and compulsory detention in hospital under the Mental Health Act with little for people to do on the wards.

Whiteford (2004) suggested that when occupa-tional deprivation is a temporary phenomenon, such as during a period of mourning, and when it is due to personal rather than social factors, such as a broken leg, it should be called disruption rather than deprivation. *Occupational disruption* is 'a transient or temporary condition of being restricted from participation in necessary or mean-ingful occupations, such as that caused by illness, temporary relocation, or temporary unemploy-ment' (Christiansen & Townsend 2004a, p278).

When people experience daily life as lack-ing meaning or purpose, either because they cannot find anything important to do or they have to spend all their time and energy on tasks that they do not value, the outcome is *occupa-tional alienation* (Townsend & Wilcock 2004a). Occupational alienation refers to 'a sense of isola-tion, powerlessness, frustration, loss of control, or estrangement from society or self that results from engagement in occupations that do not satisfy inner needs' (Christiansen & Townsend 2004a, p278). Some occupations are experienced as spir-itually and mentally enriching, in addition to hav-ing more practical functions. These occupations provide opportunities for choice and individual

expression, and often have an element of creativ-ity. Other occupations are confining, regimented and lack meaning, leading to boredom and aliena-tion. Having to spend a lot of time performing occupations that do not enhance, or even dimin-ish, a person's sense of self can damage personal identity (Townsend & Wilcock 2004a).

Occupational justice

The concepts of occupational imbalance, depriva-tion and alienation draw attention to inequalities between people who have access to a satisfying, personally enriching range of occupations and those who do not. Townsend & Wilcock (2004a) described this as an issue of *occupational justice*. Occupational justice refers to 'justice related to opportunities and resources required for occu-pational participation sufficient to satisfy per-sonal needs and full citizenship' (Christiansen & Townsend 2004a, p278).

The idea of occupational justice is based on two beliefs: that people have the potential to grow towards the highest level of personal development through what they do, and that they have rights in relation to occupation. These can be summarised as (Townsend & Wilcock 2004b) the right to:

- experience occupation as meaningful and en-riching
- participate in occupations for health and social inclusion
- exert autonomy through choice of occupations
- benefit from diverse participation in occupa-tions.

The concept of *occupational injustice* draws attention to the many ways in which participation in occupations can be 'barred, confined, restricted, segregated, prohibited, undeveloped, disrupted, alienated, marginalized, exploited, excluded or otherwise restricted' (Townsend & Wilcock 2004b, p77).

Occupational apartheid

In 2005, three occupational therapists working with marginalised populations in different areas of the world extended the concept of occupa-tional injustice by confronting more explicitly the issue of power relationships (Kronenberg et al 2005). They coined the term *occupational apartheid*, which they defined as the 'more or less chronic established environmental (systemic) conditions that deny marginalized people rightful access to participation in occupations that they value as meaningful and useful to them' (Kronenberg & Pollard 2005, p65).

Kronenberg & Pollard (2005) stated that: 'occupational apartheid refers to the segregation of groups of people through the restriction or denial of access to dignified and meaningful participation in occupations of daily life on the basis of race, colour, disability, national origin, age, gender, sexual preference, religion, political beliefs, status in society, or other characteristics' (p67). The implication is that the people who have control over the distribution of work, money and status determine which groups will be allowed access to these benefits.

Occupational therapists have traditionally worked with those groups who are marginalised in society: people with severe physical, intellectual or emotional disabilities, those with enduring mental illness, older people and people detained in institutions for whatever reason. The role of the occupational therapist has been to help people to learn effective survival skills, adjust to their life circumstances and move towards social inclusion and integration. Taking a more overtly political stance would redefine occupational therapists as agents of social change, raising public awareness of occupational injustice and working towards the creation of a more occupationally just world (Duncan & Alsop 2006).

OCCUPATIONAL THERAPY THEORY INTO PRACTICE

Occupational therapists use theories from a variety of disciplines, as shown above. The breadth of the theoretical base and the complexity of some of the theories we use could seem overwhelming. However, not all occupational therapists need to know all the theories that make up the total body of knowledge of the profession. We use different theories depending on the area in which we work, the kind of problems we encounter in that setting and our own knowledge, skills and preferences.

In this section, we look first at the vocabulary used when talking about theories for practice: frame of reference, approach, model and paradigm. We then look at how the different concepts relate to each other in a theoretical framework (Fig. 3.1).

TERMS USED WHEN TALKING ABOUT THEORY

Theories that work well together and that can be applied within a particular field of practice can be organised as frames of reference that, in turn, are translated into practice through various approaches and models. These terms are explained here.

Frame of reference

A frame of reference is an individual's 'personal notion of reality, their cultural, social, and psychological biases, their values and beliefs, and how these factors influence the practice of occupational therapy' (Krefting 1985). So, in its widest sense, a frame of reference is the way a person sees the world.

Creek (2003, p53) offered a narrower definition for occupational therapists: 'a collection of ideas or theories that provide a coherent conceptual foundation for practice'. A frame of reference, therefore, is made up of selected theories that are compatible with each other and that can be applied within a particular field of practice. Bruce & Borg (1993) wrote that a frame of reference refers to the principles behind practice with particular client groups.

Within occupational therapy there are many frames of reference, some of which can be used in more than one field and some of which are for very specific purposes. The choice of a frame of reference is influenced by the presenting problems of the client, the ethos of the unit where the intervention takes place and the knowledge of the therapist (Hurff 1985).

Approach

The terms 'frame of reference' and 'approach' are often used synonymously. A simple definition of an approach is 'the methods by which theories are put into practice and treatment is administered' (Creek 2003).

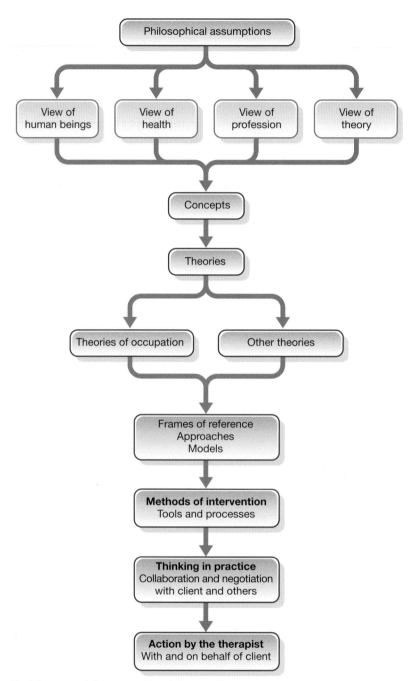

Figure 3.1   Theoretical Framework for occupational therapy theory.

Model

A *model* is a simplified description or representation of something. However, different writers use the term in different ways. Krefting (1985) suggested that there are generic models, which encompass all aspects of the profession, and models which have a narrower focus and are only relevant within a particular field of practice. A *model for practice* is 'A simplified representation of the structure and content of a phenomenon or system that describes or explains certain data or relationships and integrates elements of theory and practice' (Creek 2003). During the 1980s and 1990s, a large body of literature was developed on models for practice in occupational therapy.

Paradigm

Mosey (1986) used the term *model* in the way that most other occupational therapy writers use the term *paradigm*, to refer to:

> the particular way in which a profession perceives itself, its relationship to other professions, and its association with the society to which it is responsible ... the reservoir of the collected knowledge and beliefs of a profession. It is characterised by a description of the profession's philosophical assumptions, ethical code, body of knowledge, domain of concern, the nature of and principles for sequencing the various aspects of practice, and the profession's legitimate tools.

Creek & Feaver (1993) suggested that a paradigm is 'the profession's world view that encompasses philosophies, theories, frames of reference and models for practice'.

FRAMEWORK FOR OCCUPATIONAL THERAPY THEORY

Philosophies, theories, frames of reference and models for practice can be organised into a flexible framework that depicts the relationships between each of these components of occupational therapy and shows how they influence practice (see Fig. 3.1).

Philosophical assumptions about the nature of the world and, more specifically, about the nature of people, occupation and health determine how occupational therapists view their professional domain of concern, goals and legitimate methods of intervention. This world view can be described using terms that are selected and defined by occupational therapists: health, occupation, role, occupational performance, function, temporal adaptation, environment, engagement and independence. These terms represent key concepts that are the building blocks of occupational therapy theory. Occupational therapists draw theories of occupation such as occupational behaviour, occupational choice, an occupational perspective of health and occupational injustice, many of which were developed within the discipline of occupational science.

Occupational therapists learn formal theories, including the theories of occupation described above, and theories selected from other disciplines. These theories act as guides to practice by offering explanations of what the therapist observes and making it possible to predict the outcomes of interventions. For example, the theory of occupational choice tells us that increasing someone's insight into their own capacities will improve their ability to make realistic choices about what to do.

Theories are organised into frames of reference, approaches and models that can be used in different areas of practice. For example, the cognitive behavioural frame of reference is widely used in the field of adult mental health, the rehabilitative approach is used in the field of severe and enduring mental illness and the process of change model is applied in the field of health promotion. Frames of reference and approaches describe the principles of practice, enabling the therapist to be consistent in her way of working. Models for practice give more guidance to the inexperienced therapist as they suggest a more structured procedure and tools for intervention. Some of the frames of reference and models used in occupational therapy are described in Chapter 4.

The therapist's methods of intervention, that is, the tools and processes of therapy, are determined by the frame of reference, approach or model being used. For example, projective techniques are tools for assessment and treatment used within a psychodynamic frame of reference. Some of the assessment tools used by occupational therapists are described in Chapter 5 and treatment methods are described in Chapter 6.

Philosophical assumptions, concepts, theories, frames of reference, approaches and models give coherence and consistency to the practice of occupational therapy. They can guide the inexperienced therapist through the process of intervention with a client and offer alternative perspectives to the expert therapist whose practice is guided by her experience. However, in a dynamic, complex practice, no theory can offer an infallible guide to action. It is essential for the therapist to develop a range of thinking skills if she is to take into account the many factors that impinge on the client's function when reaching a decision about the best course of action (Creek 2003). Some of the thinking skills used by occupational therapists are described in Chapter 4.

SUMMARY

In this chapter, a concise overview was given of the knowledge base of occupational therapy. Specialist textbooks on the different subjects will provide more details.

There was first a discussion of the changes that have taken place in the beliefs and values espoused by members of the profession during the past 90 years. The philosophical assumptions underpinning present-day practice were briefly reviewed under the headings of view of human beings, view of health and dysfunction, view of the nature and purpose of the occupational therapy profession and view of theory.

The knowledge base of occupational therapy is drawn from a wide range of disciplines. The various theories of occupation that have been and are still being developed, many under the banner of occupational science, were described in this chapter. It was emphasised that, although occupational therapists are now developing their own theories of the relationships between people, health and occupation, occupational therapy will continue to benefit from drawing on new theories from other disciplines, as it has always done.

In conclusion, a framework was offered for understanding how the various components of occupational therapy fit together to allow theory to be translated into practice.

References

Bateson MC 1997 Enfolded activity and the concept of occupation. In: Zemke R, Clark F (eds) Occupational science: the evolving discipline. FA Davis, Philadelphia

Baum CM 1995 The contribution of occupation to function in persons with Alzheimer's disease. Journal of Occupational Science: Australia 2(2):59-67

Baum C, Christiansen C 1997 The occupational therapy context: philosophy – principles – practice. In: Christiansen C, Baum C (eds) Occupational therapy: enabling function and well-being, 2nd edn. Slack, New Jersey

Blair SEE 1998 Role. In: Jones D, Blair SEE, Hartery T, Jones RK (eds) Sociology and occupational therapy: an integrated approach. Churchill Livingstone, Edinburgh, pp41-53

Breines EB 1989 Making a difference: a premise of occupation and health. American Journal of Occupational Therapy 43(1):51-52

Breines EB 1995 Occupational therapy activities from clay to computers: theory and practice. FA Davis, Philadelphia

Bruce MA, Borg B 1993 Psychosocial occupational therapy: frames of reference for intervention, 2nd edn. Slack, Thorofare, New Jersey

Butler J 2004 The Casson Memorial Lecture 2004: the fascination of the difficult. British Journal of Occupational Therapy 67(7):286-292

Carlson ME, Clark FA 1991 The search for useful methodologies in occupational science. American Journal of Occupational Therapy 45(3):235-241

Christiansen C 1997 Person–environment occupational performance. In: Christiansen C, Baum C (eds) Enabling function and well-being. Slack, New Jersey

Christiansen CH, Townsend EA 2004a Glossary. In: Christiansen CH, Townsend EA (eds) Introduction to occupation: the art and science of living. Prentice Hall, Upper Saddle River, New Jersey

Christiansen CH, Townsend EA 2004b An introduction to occupation. In: Christiansen CH, Townsend EA (eds) Introduction to occupation: the art and science of living. Prentice Hall, Upper Saddle River, New Jersey

Cilliers P 1998 Complexity and postmodernism: understanding complex systems. Routledge, London

Clark FA, Parham D, Carlson ME et al 1991 Occupational science: academic innovation in the service of occupational therapy's future. American Journal of Occupational Therapy 45(4):300-310

College of Occupational Therapists 2005 Code of ethics and professional conduct: College of Occupational Therapists, London

College of Occupational Therapists 2006a Recovering ordinary lives: the strategy for occupational therapy in mental health services 2007-2017, literature review. College of Occupational Therapists, London

College of Occupational Therapists 2006b Recovering ordinary lives: the strategy for occupational therapy in mental health services 2007-2017, a vision for the next ten years. College of Occupational Therapists, London

Cracknell E 1984 Humanistic psychology. In: Willson M (ed) Occupational therapy in short-term psychiatry. Churchill Livingstone, Edinburgh, pp73-88

Creek J 1998 (ed) Occupational therapy: new perspectives. Whurr, London

Creek J 2003 Occupational therapy defined as a complex intervention. College of Occupational Therapists, London

Creek J 2007 Engaging the reluctant client. In: Creek J (ed) Contemporary issues in occupational therapy: reasoning and reflection. Wiley, Chichester

Creek J, Feaver S 1993 Models for practice in occupational therapy, part 1: defining terms. British Journal of Occupational Therapy 56(1):4-6

Creek J, Ilott I, Cook S, Munday C 2005 Valuing occupational therapy as a complex intervention. British Journal of Occupational Therapy 68(6):281-284

Dickoff J, Jamess P, Wiedenbach E 1968 Theory in a practice discipline: Part 1. Practice oriented theory. Nursing Research 17(5):415-435

Duncan M, Alsop A 2006 Practice and service learning in context. In: Lorenzo T, Duncan M, Buchanen H, Alsop A (eds) Practice and service learning in occupational therapy: enhancing potential in context. Wiley, Chichester, pp7-19

ENOTHE 2006 www.enothe.hva.nl

Gillon R (1985/1986) Philosophical medical ethics. Wiley, Chichester

Ginzberg E, Ginsberg SW, Axelrad S et al 1951 Occupational choice: an approach to a general theory. Columbia University Press, New York

Hagedorn R 2000 Tools for practice in occupational therapy: a structured approach to core skills and processes. Churchill Livingstone, Edinburgh

Hasselkuss BR 2002 The meaning of everyday occupation. Slack, Thorofare, New Jersey

Hurff JM 1985 Visualisation: a decision-making tool for assessment and treatment planning. Occupational Therapy in Health Care 1(2):5-12

Iwarsson S, Isacsson Å, Persson D et al 1997 Occupation and survival: a 25-year follow-up study of an aging population. American Journal of Occupational Therapy 52(1):65-70

Kielhofner G 1980 A model of human occupation, part 2: ontogenesis from the perspective of temporal adaptation. American Journal of Occupational Therapy 34(10): 657-663

Kielhofner G, Burke JP 1977 Occupational therapy after 60 years: an account of changing identity and knowledge. American Journal of Occupational Therapy 31(10): 675-689

Krefting LH 1985 The use of conceptual models in clinical practice. Canadian Journal of Occupational Therapy 52(4):173-178

Kronenberg F, Pollard N 2005 Overcoming occupational apartheid: a preliminary exploration of the political nature of occupational therapy. Kronenberg F, Algado SS, Pollard N (eds) Occupational therapy without borders: learning from the spirit of survivors Elsevier Churchill Livingstone, Edinburgh, pp58-86

Kronenberg F, Algado SS, Pollard N (eds) 2005 Occupational therapy without borders: learning from the spirit of survivors. Elsevier Churchill Livingstone, Edinburgh

Lazzarini I 2004 Neuro-occupation: the non-linear dynamics of intention, meaning and perception. British Journal of Occupational Therapy 67(8):342-352

Lewin R (1999) Complexity: life at the edge of chaos, 2nd edn. Phoenix, London

Mattingly C, Fleming F 1994 Clinical reasoning: forms of inquiry in a therapeutic practice. FA Davis, Philadelphia

McQueen DV 2000 Perspectives on health promotion: theory, evidence, practice and the emergence of complexity. Health Promotion International 15(2):95-97

Meyer A 1922 The philosophy of occupation therapy. Archives of Occupational Therapy 1: 1-10. Reprinted in: American Journal of Occupational Therapy 1977 31(10):639-642

Mosey AC 1968 Recapitulation of ontogenesis: a theory for the practice of occupational therapy. American Journal of Occupational Therapy 22(5):426-438

Mosey AC 1981 Occupational therapy: configuration of a profession. Raven Press, New York

Mosey AC 1986 Psychological components of occupational therapy. Raven Press, New York

Nelson DL 1988 Occupation: form and performance. American Journal of Occupational Therapy 42(10): 633-641

Nixon J, Creek J 2006 Towards a theory of practice. British Journal of Occupational Therapy 69(2):77-80

Passmore A 2003 The occupation of leisure: three typologies and their influence on mental health in adolescence. OTJR: Occupation, Participation and Health 23(2):76-83

Primeau LA 1996 Running as an occupation: multiple meanings and purposes. In: Zemke R, Clark F (eds) Occupational science: the evolving discipline. FA Davis, Philadelphia

Reilly M 1962 Occupational therapy can be one of the great ideas of 20th century medicine. American Journal of Occupational Therapy 16(1):1-9

Reilly M 1969 The educational process. American Journal of Occupational Therapy 23(4):299-307

Rogoff B 2003 The cultural nature of human development. Oxford University Press, Oxford

Royeen CB 2003 Chaotic occupational therapy: collective wisdom for a complex profession. American Journal of Occupational Therapy 57(6):609-624

Shannon PD 1977 The derailment of occupational therapy. American Journal of Occupational Therapy 31(4):229-234

Smith AG 1983 Holistic philosophy and general systems theory: an overview for occupational therapy. Journal of the New Zealand Association of Occupational Therapists 34(1):13-18

Sumsion T 1999 The client-centred approach. In: Sumsion T (ed) Client-centred practice in occupational therapy: a guide to implementation. Churchill Livingstone, Edinburgh

Townsend E, Wilcock A 2004a Occupational justice. In: Christiansen CH, Townsend EA (eds) Introduction to occupation: the art and science of living. Prentice Hall, Upper Saddle River, New Jersey

Townsend E, Wilcock A 2004b Occupational justice and client-centred practice: a dialogue in progress. Canadian Journal of Occupational Therapy 71(2):75-87

Watson R, Fourie M 2004 Occupation and occupational therapy. In: Watson R, Swartz L (eds) Transformation through occupation. Whurr, London, pp19-32

West WL 1984 A reaffirmed philosophy and practice of occupational therapy for the 1980s. American Journal of Occupational Therapy 38(1):15-23

Whiteford G 2004 When people cannot participate: occupational deprivation. In: Christiansen CH, Townsend EA (eds) Introduction to occupation: the art and science of living. Prentice Hall, Upper Saddle River, New Jersey, pp221-242

Wilcock AA 1995 The occupational brain: a theory of human nature. Journal of Occupational Science: Australia 2(1):68-73

Wilcock AA 1998a A theory of occupation and health. In: Creek J (ed) Occupational therapy: new perspectives. Whurr, London

Wilcock AA 1998b An occupational perspective of health. Slack, Thorofare, New Jersey

Wilcock AA 2006 An occupational perspective of health, 2nd edn. Slack, Thorofare, New Jersey

World Health Organization 2001 International classification of functioning, disability and health. World Health Organization, Geneva

Yerxa EJ 1967 Authentic occupational therapy. American Journal of Occupational Therapy 21(1):1-9

Yerxa EJ 1993 Occupational science: a new source of power for participants in occupational therapy. Occupational Science: Australia 1(1):3-10

Yerxa EJ 2000 Confessions of an occupational therapist who became a detective. British Journal of Occupational Therapy 63(5):192-199

Yerxa EJ, Clark F, Frank G et al 1989 An introduction to occupational science, a foundation for occupational therapy in the 21st century. Occupational Therapy Health Care 6(4):1-17

Young ME, Quinn E 1992 Theories and principles of occupational therapy. Churchill Livingstone, Edinburgh

Service user commentary

Reading this chapter from a service user perspective, I found it interesting to see what an occupational therapist's perspective is of a person with mental health difficulties. It was reassuring to read that service users are still treated like individuals, with individual needs which are met through a structured approach involving both the professional and the client. This is very different to the medical model, which still seems to be the main focus when treating people with mental health problems; through the use of psychiatry and medication.

Through being client centred, occupational therapy allows the individual to stay in control of their illness at a time when they feel very vulnerable; often it is the case that they only see themselves through the illness rather than as an individual of any worth. Occupational therapy has a solid ground base which focuses on the individual's experience of their illness and not on their diagnosis. This is a very useful tool when dealing with individuals who only see the label(s) they have been given; it reassures them that they are still human beings and that the feelings they are experiencing are acceptable and valid, and so too are the resulting symptoms.

An individual could experience many thoughts or feelings that impact on their life as a result of mental health difficulties. Because of this, it is useful that occupational therapy does not just focus on one area of life but recognises the complexity of human beings and spans all areas of life, including self-care, social, work, leisure, culture, spirituality, etc. It is possible that through solving a problem in one area, other issues may seem diluted. For example, roles are recognised within occupational therapy and it is accepted that these change throughout life, and even within different environments, each presenting with different pressures. So a mother can also be a teacher and a friend and would maybe need different support in the different areas to help her fulfil her roles. And by solving a work-related problem, the pressures at home may seem to ease.

Through educating clients about their condition during intervention, and through the resulting actions, the individual can begin to change their own life and does not feel dependent on the profession, as can occur so often in the medical model, for example with medication. This gives control back to the person and raises self-esteem. The knowledge gained by the individual also becomes invaluable after discharge, perhaps being used to synthesise coping strategies in new situations, and also to avoid relapse through recognition of triggers and early signs of illness.

I think another strong point of occupational therapy, which has become apparent from reading the chapter, is that people often want to achieve their maximum potential and that occupational therapy will support this where other professions perhaps don't. For example, the occupational therapist would do as much as possible to keep an older person in their own home instead of taking the easier option of a residential care home.

Through all these points I think the occupational therapist ensures that the client feels valued with or without their condition and I think this is perhaps the most valuable aspect of occupational therapy which stands out for me.

Melanie Hart, mental health service user

SECTION 2

The Occupational Therapy Process

SECTION CONTENTS

Chapter **4**

Approaches to practice

Jennifer Creek

INTRODUCTION

Chapter 3 described some of the theories that occupational therapists use and a framework was offered for understanding how theory relates to practice. In this chapter, we will look in more detail at how theory informs practice. The chapter is in five parts: the content of practice; the core skills of the occupational therapist; the nature of occupational therapy practice; the process of intervention, and frames of reference used in the field of mental health.

CONTENT OF PRACTICE

A definition of the structure and scope of occupational therapy practice should derive from the philosophy and theoretical base of the profession, not from the constraints and demands of the service setting, although the way the intervention is carried out will be influenced by such external factors. Practice can be defined as the actions taken by the therapist to serve the needs of the client (Argyris & Schön 1974). Only if these actions are based on a coherent philosophical and theoretical framework can the therapist make skilled predictions about outcomes.

We will look at the content of practice under four headings:

- domain of concern
- goals and desired outcomes
- population served
- legitimate tools.

DOMAIN OF CONCERN

The concern of occupational therapy is with the things that people do in their daily lives, the meaning that people give to what they do and the impact that doing has on their health and well-being. This broad focus on occupation, 'the ordinary and extraordinary things that people do every day' (Watson 2004a, p3), means that occupational therapists can not only contribute to the restoration of health and function but can also meet people's needs within a broader social context.

The purpose of occupational therapy has been described as 'helping people cope with the challenges of everyday living imposed by congenital anomalies, physical and emotional illnesses, accidents, the ageing process, or environmental restriction' (Baum & Christiansen 1997, p28). This involves more than simply working to remediate impairments or improve function. Occupational therapy is as much concerned with building people's occupational identities as it is with restoring physical and mental function; it pays as much attention to building healthy communities that can include all their members as it does to helping people to change in order to fit better into society.

The American anthropologist Cheryl Mattingly (1994, p37) described how occupational therapists work with both the physical body and the person:

> One of the most interesting features of occupational therapy practice is that it tends to deal with functional problems that fall nicely within biomedicine (treating physical injuries with specific treatment techniques), as well as problems going far beyond the physical body, encompassing social, cultural and psychological issues that concern the meaning of illness or injury to a person's life.

GOALS AND DESIRED OUTCOMES

A *goal* is 'a concise statement of a desired outcome or specific result to be attained at a particular stage in an intervention' (Creek 2003, p54). The major goal of occupational therapy is 'for the client to achieve a satisfying performance and balance of occupations, in the areas of self care, productivity and leisure and that will support recovery, health, well-being and social participation' (op cit, p32). The goals of occupational therapy include process goals, such as developing a therapeutic relationship with the client, and outcome goals, such as enabling the client to return home after a period in hospital.

An outcome goal is sometimes called a *predetermined outcome*: 'an agreed, clearly defined, expected or desired result of intervention' (Creek 2003, p56). The *actual outcome* of therapy is 'the result of therapeutic processes, which may be different from the initial objectives' (op cit, p56). Outcome goals can be expressed at different levels:

- **skills**: for example, the client will pay attention for up to 10 minutes to a demonstration of a craft activity within a small group setting
- **tasks**: for example, the client will follow a demonstration and verbal instructions to produce a craft item to his own satisfaction within a 2-hour group session
- **activities**: for example, the client will participate in a 2-hour creative activity group
- **occupations**: for example, the client will find a creative leisure activity that he wants to pursue at home
- **social participation**: for example, the client will visit a craft exhibition at a local gallery in the company of a small group.

Learning skills or completing tasks can be intermediate or short-term goals on the way to achieving the main outcomes that are expressed in terms of occupations and social participation.

In client-centred practice, clients' goals and desired outcomes are the focus of intervention. The therapist listens respectfully to what the client says and negotiates with him to reach agreement on the goals they will work towards.

POPULATION SERVED

The premise that people can influence their own health by their actions can be applied to a wide range of problems once the appropriate specialist knowledge and skills to support it have been acquired. Anyone who has problems of doing, whatever the person's age, gender or diagnosis, is a potential client of occupational therapy. In practice, occupational therapists work in two main areas: institutional services and settings, and public health and community development.

Institutional services and settings

The client traditionally encountered occupational therapy in a medical setting, which predetermined, to some extent, the range of problems seen, the degree of dysfunction the client was experiencing and the amount of time the therapist could spend on treatment. As the profession

has expanded into new areas, clients are also being encountered in other settings, such as social services departments, educational settings, health centres, day centres, prisons, community centres, the workplace and people's own homes.

Occupational therapists may be employed in health or social services, in education, in the prison service or in the voluntary sector. Increasingly, they work across service boundaries, in partnership with other agencies or other professionals to provide integrated services for clients (College of Occupational Therapists 2006).

Public health and community development

Public health is concerned with health promotion and the prevention of disease. Mental health promotion is an emerging area of practice for occupational therapists (see Chapter 2). It is concerned with 'improving quality of life and potential for health rather than the amelioration of symptoms and deficits' (World Health Organization 2002, p8). In 2004, the UK Treasury published a report on the determinants of health in England and the projected cost of improving the health of the whole population (Wanless 2004). The report concluded that 'health services must evolve from dealing with acute problems through more effective control of chronic conditions to promoting the maintenance of good health' (p10).

Community development is a population approach that involves the therapist working in partnership with the community to bring about internal and external change (Watson 2004b). It focuses on raising people's awareness of the possibilities for change so that they are able to take control and be 'active contributors in their own world and for their own benefit' (p57). Occupational therapists in some countries around the world are already working in this field and there is the potential for occupational therapists in the UK to move into community development (College of Occupational Therapists 2006).

LEGITIMATE TOOLS

The occupational therapist uses various techniques and media during the treatment process. Mosey (1986) described the permissible means of carrying out occupational therapy as the profession's 'legitimate tools'. These tools are: the self, activities and the environment.

Therapeutic use of self

The relationship between the therapist and client is an important part of the therapeutic process, from first meeting with a new client, through coping together with the successes and setbacks of the intervention process, to ending the programme on a positive note. Ideally, the relationship is a partnership or collaboration between therapist and client in which the goals and methods of intervention are negotiated throughout the therapeutic process. If a client is unable to take a full part in the process because of illness or disability, the therapist has a responsibility to facilitate that person's involvement as far as possible and to protect his interests to the best of her ability. Further information about the therapeutic use of self can be found in Chapter 13.

The term *enablement* is sometimes used to describe the therapist's role in 'helping the individual to achieve what is important to her/him, to respond to her/his circumstances, to assert her/his individuality and establish her/his goals' (Creek 2003, p52).

Mosey (1986) identified 11 elements that contribute to the therapist's ability to relate effectively to clients:

- a perception of individuality – recognition of each person as a unique whole
- respect for the dignity and rights of each individual
- empathy – ability to enter into the experience of another person without losing objectivity
- compassion or sympathy
- humility – recognition of the limits of one's own knowledge and skill
- unconditional positive regard – concern for the client without moral judgements on his thoughts and actions
- honesty – telling the truth to clients is an aspect of respect for persons
- a relaxed manner
- flexibility – ability to modify behaviour to meet the demands of a situation

- self-awareness – ability to reflect on one's own reactions to the world and on the effect one is having on the world in any given situation
- humour – a lightness of approach, used appropriately, can facilitate the therapeutic process.

Peloquin (1998) described the occupational therapist as *being with* the client by *doing with* the client and identified empathy as the most important element of the therapeutic relationship. Empathy involves turning to the client in a genuine attempt to make a positive relationship, recognising what the therapist and client have in common, recognising the client's uniqueness, entering into the experience of the client, connecting with the client's feelings and being able to recover from that connection so that the therapist is not damaged by the therapeutic encounter.

The therapist can use interpersonal skills to deal with a whole range of needs, such as engaging the initial interest of someone with a volitional disorder, supporting a bereaved client through the grieving process, helping someone to express difficult feelings appropriately, valuing a client with chronic low self-esteem and helping carers to work out how best to balance their own and the client's needs. The therapist herself can be the most valuable resource in an intervention.

Activities as therapy

Activity is a flexible and adaptable treatment medium that can be used with all clients in many different contexts to achieve diverse outcomes. The use of activity as a therapeutic tool requires that the therapist has a range of skills, including the following.

- **Activity analysis**. This is 'a process of dissecting an activity into its component parts and task sequence in order to identify its inherent properties and the skills required for its performance, thus allowing the therapist to evaluate its therapeutic potential' (Creek 2003, p49).
- **Activity selection and activity synthesis.** The therapist selects activities that have the greatest potential to meet the client's needs, develop his skills and engage his interest. Alternatively, activity components may be combined into new

activities (activity synthesis) that will better achieve these goals. For example, a craft activity could be done in a group so that interpersonal demands are added to the other skills required for the performance of the activity.

- **Activity adaptation.** An activity may be adjusted or modified to suit the client's needs, skills, values and interests. For example, a traditional craft such as macramé could be done with modern materials to produce a modern piece of jewellery that the client finds attractive.
- **Activity grading** and **sequencing**. Grading is adapting an activity so that it becomes progressively more demanding as the client's skills improve or less demanding as the client's function deteriorates. For example, walking can be done for longer or over more difficult terrain to build the client's stamina. Activity sequencing means 'finding or designing a sequence of different but related activities that will incrementally increase the demands made on the individual as her/his performance improves or decrease them as her/his performance deteriorates. It is used as an adjunct or alternative to activity grading' (Creek 2003, p38).

These skills are described in more detail in Chapter 6.

Environment

People function within human and non-human environments that Jenkins (1998, p29) called their 'lifeworld context'. Aspects of the client's normal environments must be taken into account when planning treatment so that the outcome of intervention is a comfortable match between the abilities of the person and environmental demands. The goal of intervention may be to help the client to adapt to his environments or to adapt those environments to suit the client's needs and abilities. Many interventions involve both the client making changes and adaptations being made to the physical or social environment.

The occupational therapist analyses the environment in terms of:

- content – the physical and human elements in the environment

- demands – the effect the environment has on performance
- potential for adaptation (Hagedorn 1995).

The therapeutic encounter also takes place within environments that can be manipulated to achieve the desired outcomes, whether within a specialised treatment setting or the client's own living place or workplace.

CORE SKILLS

The *core skills* of the occupational therapist are 'the expert knowledge and abilities that are shared by all occupational therapists' (College of Occupational Therapists 2006, p5). They can be categorised as *generic*, that is, those skills shared by other health-care professionals, and *profession specific*, that is, those skills that are peculiar to occupational therapists.

Examples of generic skills include communication and team working. Some generic skills are extended by occupational therapists so that they become profession specific. For example, many health and social care professionals are skilled in group facilitation but occupational therapists have particular skills in planning and facilitating activity groups.

The College of Occupational Therapists (2004) listed the core skills of the occupational therapist as follows.

- **Collaboration with the client:** involves building a relationship with the client in which decisions are shared and actions negotiated. The aim of a collaborative relationship is to promote the client's autonomy and engage him in the therapeutic process.
- **Assessment:** a collaborative process through which the therapist and client are able to identify and explore the client's functional potential, limitations, needs and environmental conditions.
- **Enablement:** the process of helping the client to identify what is important to him, set his own goals and work towards them, thus taking more control of his life.
- **Problem solving:** a process involving a set of cognitive strategies that are used to identify

occupational performance problems, resolve difficulties and decide on an appropriate course of action.

- **Using activity as a therapeutic tool:** as described above, the therapist uses a range of skills to transform everyday activities into treatment media. These skills include activity analysis, synthesis, adaptation, grading, sequencing and facilitation.
- **Group work:** involves planning, organising, leading and evaluating activity groups.
- **Environmental adaptation:** involves assessing, analysing and modifying physical and social environments to increase function and social participation.

All these core skills are complex and made up of component subskills, such as interpersonal skills and cognitive skills. Thinking skills and thought processes have been identified as essential to effective occupational therapy practice, especially in client-centred occupational therapy (Creek et al 2005).

THINKING SKILLS

Occupational therapists use different types of thinking as they work with clients, depending on the purpose of their thinking or in response to particular features of what they are thinking about (Fleming 1994). Thinking skills are 'the mental actions used by the therapist in framing problems and working out the best solutions' (Creek 2007). Sinclair (2007) classified them into five categories.

- **Evidence discovery** means gathering data in order to name and frame problems. It involves sensing what problems might be relevant for the client, recognising relevant clinical cues and formulating the problems to be addressed.
- **Theory application** is the use of formal and personal theory to direct practice. Sinclair (2007) pointed out that practice cannot always be guided by theory but requires other forms of thinking as well.
- **Decision making** involves evaluating the situation, planning what to do, setting priorities for action and predicting the outcomes of possible actions.

- **Judgement** is the ability to draw conclusions from the available evidence. Judgement involves recognising the potential consequences of decisions and actions and taking responsibility for them.
- **Ethics** includes awareness of the moral dimension of issues, sensitivity to one's own impact on other people and the will to implement the best solutions (see Chapter 11).

The main terms used to describe the types of thinking used by occupational therapists are reasoning and reflection. These are discussed here.

Clinical reasoning

At each stage of the process of intervention, the occupational therapist has to make decisions about what to do, taking into account a multiplicity of factors. This thinking process is called *clinical reasoning*, which is: 'the mental strategies and high level cognitive patterns and processes that underlie the process of naming, framing and solving problems and that enable the therapist to reach decisions about the best course of action' (Creek 2003, p51).

The American clinical reasoning study (Mattingly & Fleming 1994) identified three different types of clinical reasoning, each used for working through different types of problem. Fleming (1991) described these thinking strategies as follows.

- **Procedural reasoning.** This is the type of thinking used when considering the patient's disability and how to remediate it. It involves identifying problems, setting goals and planning treatment.
- **Interactive reasoning.** This type of thinking occurs when the therapist is working face to face with the client, building a relationship and trying to understand his experience.
- **Conditional reasoning.** This is used when the therapist is thinking broadly about the client in his temporal and lifeworld contexts and about the consequences of possible interventions. The therapist builds an image of the client's past, present and future in order to make predictions about what will work best.

Two other terms used to describe aspects of clinical reasoning are narrative reasoning and ethical reasoning. *Narrative reasoning* structures therapy as an unfolding story within which therapy is seen as a chapter of the client's longer life story (Fleming & Mattingly 1994). *Ethical reasoning* is a process of thinking about the moral dimension of a situation in order to reach the best decision. What is clinically the best course of action may not necessarily be morally the best course of action. For example, in Janet's story in Chapter 11, the therapist has to decide between taking what she thinks is the most ethical course of action and doing what she thinks will bring about the best clinical outcome.

Reflection

Reflection is subjective awareness and appreciation of activity and its impact on the individual and the environment. For the therapist, reflection is a way of making sense of those situations, commonly encountered in practice, that are characterised by complexity, uncertainty and uniqueness. It involves standing back from practice and taking time to evaluate it, judge the quality of what is being done and seek to make improvements. Reflection-in-action is a process of questioning and adapting habitual ways of working so that therapy becomes more responsive and person centred (Schön 1983). Reflection after the event involves recalling the experience and re-evaluating it.

THE OCCUPATIONAL THERAPY PROCESS

Occupational therapy is a process, in the sense that intervention and change take place over time. Occupational therapy is also a process in the sense that the therapist's actions follow a recognisable sequence. There is an accepted first step to occupational therapy intervention, followed by a logical second step and so on. There is general agreement on the steps that make up the process, although not all the steps are carried out in every case and the process is not necessarily a linear one. The more experienced therapist modifies the process to suit the client and the context of the intervention.

The 11 steps of the occupational therapy process are shown in Figure 4.1. Nine of them are implemented in partnership with the client but, in many cases, the first two stages are carried out by the therapist alone, often before she meets the client (Creek 2003). The occupational therapy process is outlined here but more details of the different stages can be found in Chapters 5, 6 and 7.

REFERRAL

Occupational therapists come into contact with their clients through various routes. In some settings, the therapist sees only those people who are referred to the service or identifies potential clients during team meetings. The ward-based or day centre-based therapist usually sees everyone who is admitted to the service and makes her own decisions about whom to work with. Some therapists work in drop-in centres or other settings where there is no formal system of referral.

Depending on the setting, the therapist may or may not receive good information about the client. Whether or not there is a formal referral, the therapist will want to know certain things about the client before making a decision about intervention and, preferably, before meeting him.

INFORMATION GATHERING

Certain information is necessary for the therapist to determine whether the referral is appropriate or whether someone will benefit from occupational therapy intervention. If she decides that the referral is not appropriate, she informs the referring agent of her decision and the reasons for it.

The sort of information that could be useful includes the person's medical history and presenting problem, social history and present social situation, work history and current work status, reason for referral to occupational therapy, other services that are involved and any risk factors. This information may be gleaned from case notes, other staff, the referring agent, family and carers and the person himself.

If the referral seems appropriate or the therapist judges that someone might benefit from occupational therapy intervention, she will carry out an initial assessment.

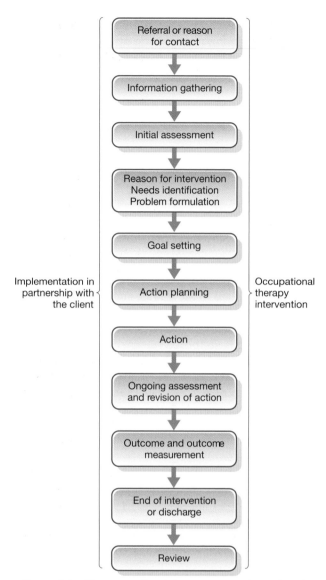

Figure 4.1 The occupational therapy process (reproduced with permission from Creek 2003).

ASSESSMENT

Assessment is the basis for all intervention and must be both thorough and valid in order to ensure that treatment is appropriate. Assessment is in two stages:

1. initial assessment
2. detailed assessment.

Assessment begins from the moment a referral is received or the therapist starts to identify those clients who could benefit from occupational therapy. The initial assessment is a screening process to determine the main areas of need of the client and whether or not occupational therapy can be of any value in this case. Factors influencing whether or not a referral is accepted include:

- the needs of the client
- the client's goals, expectations and views about occupational therapy
- the resources available, including manpower and expertise
- the client's personal support systems and social networks
- the reason for referral
- the treatment contract.

Once a client is accepted, a more detailed assessment is carried out to determine the client's needs, strengths, interests and goals. Effective assessment will lead directly to setting measurable goals or defining expected outcomes of intervention and choosing appropriate treatment methods. It also establishes the baseline from which change can be measured.

There may be no clear division between assessment and treatment in occupational therapy, where clients are often assessed by being observed participating in activities which also have therapeutic value. However, at some stage the therapist and client will formulate problems, establish goals and agree on a plan of action.

PROBLEM FORMULATION

People are complex and it is usually possible to formulate problems or needs in different ways. For example, if a woman has severe depression, the main focus of intervention could be to reduce the risk of suicide, to improve her mood or to increase her level of activity.

The occupational therapist formulates the desired outcomes of intervention as goals, problems or needs. The way in which problems are formulated influences the actions taken to achieve desired outcomes.

GOAL SETTING

In client-centred practice, the therapist and client negotiate and agree the goals of intervention. The goals are the desired outcomes of the intervention. An actual outcome is the extent to which goals have been met following the intervention.

A review date should be set at the time when the goals of treatment are set. This is the date when measurement occurs. The more precisely a goal is defined, the easier it will be to measure when it has been reached.

Goals can be expressed on different levels (Creek 2003):

- **developing skills**: for example, the client will be able to use a computer for writing documents
- **carrying out tasks**: for example, the client will find out the times when he can use a computer at his local library
- **engaging in activities**: for example, the client will write a short story
- **performing occupations**: for example, the client will read his own stories to his children as part of their bedtime routine
- **participating in life situations**: for example, the client will join the editorial board of his local community magazine.

The client may want to achieve several outcomes, in which case it will be necessary to decide which ones to work on first. When a client is too ill to express a view about what the priority should be, the therapist has to make a decision about initial goals. If possible, this should be discussed with colleagues, family and carers.

ACTION PLANNING

Once the client's problems have been identified, goals set and priorities agreed, the therapist and client plan what approach to use and what actions to take to achieve the desired outcomes. The preliminary action plan should be formulated by the therapist and client together, if the client is capable of making a contribution to the process at this stage. Other significant people, such as carers, may also be involved.

The action plan will include goals of treatment or desired outcomes, methods to be used, an individual programme and a list of the people who need to be informed about the programme. Occupational therapy interventions are usually designed to meet several goals or achieve several outcomes.

In client-centred practice, each programme of intervention is highly individualised. Factors taken into account in drawing up the treatment plan include:

- the client's needs, values and preferences
- the client's circumstances and environments, including social circumstances
- the therapist's style of working and preferences
- the quality of the relationship between the therapist and client
- the treatment setting, including resources available and what is expected of the therapist
- the evidence base for intervention
- local and national policies and standards.

ACTION

Most occupational therapy interventions involve partnership working with other professionals, community workers or volunteers and carers. As far as possible, the therapist and client negotiate what action to take and how the results can be interpreted so that the client shares control over the process (Creek 2003).

Occupational therapy intervention usually involves the client in activity. The client and therapist may engage in activity together or they may discuss activities that the client will carry out elsewhere. For example, the client may attend a cookery group run by the therapist or decide to join a cookery class at his local college.

There is an element of risk in all occupational therapy interventions and respecting the client's choices can seem particularly alarming, especially for the inexperienced therapist. Assessing and managing risk is an essential aspect of intervention.

When the occupational therapist delegates interventions to others, such as students or support workers, she remains responsible for the client, which will include ensuring that they are competent to carry out the procedures and providing sufficient direction or supervision (Creek 2003).

ONGOING ASSESSMENT AND REVISION OF ACTION

The client's progress is continually monitored, both during treatment sessions and over time, in order to measure progress towards the agreed goals and to ensure that the intervention is being effective. The therapist and client discuss and agree modifications to the programme in response to assessment findings. Minor changes can be agreed without having to organise a full review or alter the action plan.

Throughout the process of intervention, a close liaison is maintained with other disciplines involved so that any changes or problems can be shared. If the treatment setting allows for a long period of intervention, regular reviews are held to evaluate the need for more radical programme changes. Clear and regular records of treatment sessions are kept to assist in the review process (see Chapter 7).

OUTCOME MEASUREMENT

Change is measured by comparing the results of assessment following intervention with the baseline assessment. There are four possible results of intervention:

- the expected outcome is achieved
- the outcome falls short of what was expected
- the outcome is better than expected
- the client's performance is worse than before the intervention.

If the expected outcome has been achieved, the therapist and client may set new goals or, if they feel that enough has been done, the discharge procedure may be started. If goals have been partially met, then the treatment programme may be upgraded. If goals have not been met or the client's performance has deteriorated, then goal setting and action planning may have to be revisited.

DISCHARGE

Planning for the end of an occupational therapy intervention should take place from the moment a referral is received or the therapist first meets the client. If a person has been in hospital or other place of residential care, discharge is planned so that his resettlement takes place as smoothly as possible.

Ideally, the therapist and client recognise when goals have been reached or outcomes achieved and agree on the best time for the intervention to end. However, it is not always possible to reach agreement between the client, the multidisciplinary team and the carer, so compromises have to be made. This may involve some form of follow-up so that the client does not experience the termination as too abrupt.

REVIEW

Reviewing and evaluating interventions and services is a way of safeguarding standards and ensuring that services are fit for purpose. Evaluation is essential to demonstrate the effectiveness of intervention for the client, the therapist, the referring agent and other interested parties. Evaluation should be a part of the whole occupational therapy process, for example, through self-appraisal, professional supervision, peer review and client feedback. Formal evaluations of particular aspects of the service, such as groups, or of the service as a whole may be carried out at intervals in the form of an audit. Clinical audit is discussed in more detail in Chapter 8.

Evaluation of services should be carried out by occupational therapists themselves against their own standards of performance. Such evaluation may lead to changes in skill mix in a department, to a request for improved resources, to a restructuring of the way the service is delivered or to a complete change of focus, such as relocating staff from specialist community teams to primary care.

FRAMES OF REFERENCE

In Chapter 3, a frame of reference was defined as: 'a collection of ideas or theories that provide a coherent conceptual foundation for practice' (Creek 2003, p53). As the knowledge base of occupational therapy has expanded, theories have been organised into an increasing number of frames of reference, approaches and models. In 1946, a textbook on the theory of occupational

Table 4.1 Frames of reference used in mental health occupational therapy

Frame of reference	Example of a model for practice	Reference
Psychodynamic	Occupational therapy as a communication process	Fidler & Fidler 1963
Human developmental	Recapitulation of ontogenesis	Mosey 1968
Cognitive behavioural	Cognitive therapy	Beck 1976
Occupational behaviour	Model of Human Occupation (MOHO)	Kielhofner & Burke 1980
Health promotion	Transtheoretical model	Prochaska & DiClemente 1983
Cognitive	Functional information-processing model (cognitive disability)	Allen 1985
Rehabilitative	Recovery model	Deegan 1988
Occupational performance	Canadian Model of Occupational Performance (CMOP)	Canadian Association of Occupational Therapists 1993

NB: Original references have been given to highlight the sequence of development of the models for practice. All these models are still used by occupational therapists, some more widely than others, therefore there have been more recent developments and publications on all of them.

therapy (Haworth & MacDonald 1946) described one approach to therapy (rehabilitation) and offered one chapter on occupational therapy in the treatment of mental disorders, which focused on engaging patients in activities to improve or maintain health. In 2002, the third edition of this book referred to seven frames of reference: rehabilitative, psychodynamic, behavioural, occupational behaviour, human developmental, cognitive behavioural and cognitive disability (Creek 2002). New developments in theory and practice may result in further frames of reference being developed in the future, for example, a community development frame of reference.

A frame of reference delineates the field and the theoretical base for practice while a model gives more precise directions for putting theory into practice. Some models for practice are associated with more than one frame of reference. For example, Cole's Seven Steps, which are a model for group leadership, draw on elements of the client-centred, the cognitive behavioural and the developmental frames of reference (Cole 2005). Other models draw their theory from a single frame of reference, for example, adaptation through occupation (Reed & Sanderson 1992) developed within the occupational behaviour frame of reference. Table 4.1 shows seven frames of reference and examples of models that are associated with them.

Three frames of reference are described below: psychodynamic, human developmental and occupational performance. Each one is described in terms of: basic assumptions about the nature of people that underpin the approach, the knowledge base, how function and dysfunction are conceptualised, how change occurs, the client group, goals of intervention and techniques for assessment and intervention.

PSYCHODYNAMIC FRAME OF REFERENCE

In the 1950s, Azima & Wittkower (1957, p1), two psychiatrists at McGill University in Canada, carried out a survey of psychiatric occupational therapy in 15 departments in Canada and the USA. They concluded that 'too much emphasis has been put upon the diversional and occupational aspects of activities to the neglect of psychodynamic problems of the individual receiving occupational therapy'. Two years later, Azima & Azima (1959) published their outline of a dynamic theory of occupational therapy. This paper suggested a theoretical base for occupational therapy, drawing on psychodynamic theory and, in particular, object relations theory. This work was taken up and expanded by Fidler & Fidler (1963) in their book *Occupational Therapy: A Communication Process in Psychiatry*. These publications represented the first systematic attempts by occupational therapists to develop their own knowledge base for practice in the field of mental health.

Basic assumptions about people

Psychodynamic theory and the psychodynamic approach developed from the work of Sigmund Freud and his followers. Freudian thinking views people as having both a conscious and an unconscious mind. Behaviour is largely influenced by material in the unconscious mind, therefore people are usually not aware of why they act in particular ways and their actions are not always under conscious control. Actions are taken to gratify needs but not necessarily the needs of which the individual is consciously aware.

Fidler & Fidler (1963) described basic assumptions about the relationship of people with activity. People have an innate drive to be active that is directed towards achieving gratification of basic needs and making satisfactory relationships. Action is used to express and communicate feelings and thoughts. It arises from mental images, and feedback about the results of action allows these images to be modified to match external reality.

The infant strives for competence in actions that will both meet his needs and increase his sense of personal identity and integrity. A sense of self-worth comes from intrinsic satisfaction in doing well in the particular areas of life that he values. The more situations and actions the child is able to experience, the greater will be his knowledge of his own potential and limitations, leading to greater adaptability. Knowledge of what patterns of action are most useful and acceptable in the individual's culture is gained through interaction with the social environment.

Knowledge base

A number of different psychodynamic theories evolved, as many of Freud's followers developed their own approaches to psychotherapy. The occupational therapist working within a psychodynamic frame of reference will have knowledge and understanding of:

- psychiatry
- psychoanalytic theory

- psychopathology
- group dynamics
- the symbolic potential of activities and materials
- object relations theory.

The psychodynamic approach is concerned with both intrapersonal aspects of the person, that is, how the individual relates to himself, and interpersonal aspects, how he relates to other people (Atkinson & Wells 2000). For the occupational therapist, a third dimension is how the individual relates to activity, using activity to create himself, express himself and interact with the world.

One of the most important psychodynamic theories for occupational therapists, and one that was taken up by Fidler & Fidler (1963), is object relations theory: 'The term "object relations" refers to the investment of emotions and psychic energy in objects for the purpose of satisfying needs ... Objects are any human being (including the self), abstract concept, or non-human thing which has the potential for satisfying needs or interfering with need satisfaction' (Mosey 1986, p55).

Objects have both actual meanings and symbolic meanings. For example, a woman wraps a woollen shawl over her coat in winter when she is using public transport because it keeps her warm. This is the real and practical meaning of the shawl. But it also creates a symbolic barrier between her and the distracting environment of public transport. This is part of the shawl's symbolic meaning and value for her.

Symbols play a part in 'connecting the inner life and the consciousness of the individual with the collective belief systems of his or her culture' (Fine 1999, p13) and hence can be used by the therapist as a route to understanding the meaning that activity has for individuals and how they use it to relate to their human and non-human environments.

Function and dysfunction

There are several ways of conceptualising dysfunction, depending on which psychodynamic theory is being used. For example, in Freudian theory, the ego has to balance the conflicting demands of reality, the id and the superego. Conflicts that are not dealt with as the individual grows and develops may be retained in the unconscious mind and surface as anxiety. The ego defends against anxiety by using ego defence mechanisms. This takes up psychic energy so that it is no longer available for other uses. Dysfunction occurs when the individual is unable to contain the anxiety because the conflicts are too great, or ego defence mechanisms are not working effectively and material from the unconscious interferes with function.

In object relations theory, as applied to occupational therapy by the Fidlers (1963), dysfunction is characterised by immature object relationships which may be the result of a failure to develop healthy object concepts or may be due to psychopathology and regression. For example, a person experiencing psychological disorganisation in severe psychosis may have difficulty recognising himself as separate from others. A functioning individual is one who has an integrated self-identity and a realistic concept of others, who continues to grow and develop throughout his life, who is able to satisfy his basic needs and who contributes to the welfare of others. A well-organised personality has a positive and realistic sense of self and good object concepts.

How change occurs

Since dysfunction is believed to arise from unresolved conflicts located in the unconscious mind, change can be initiated by bringing these conflicts into the conscious mind so that they can be verbalised and shared. Once the difficult or painful material has been accessed, the therapist can help the client to find alternative ways of coming to terms with the feelings it arouses or dealing with it in a more adaptive way. Alternatively, the therapist may decide not to engage in exploration of the unconscious mind but deal with anxiety by supporting the client's existing coping mechanisms and finding new ways of gratifying needs.

Mosey (1986) pointed out that resolution of conflicts does not necessarily lead to the client spontaneously learning the skills needed for successful functioning. The psychoanalytical frame of reference may have to be used in conjunction with, or followed by, a more pragmatic approach to facilitate the acquisition of these skills.

Client group

The psychodynamic approach is appropriate for use with people of all ages and for treating a wide range of psychosocial disorders. It has been most widely used with adults and adolescents with acute disorders but is also appropriate for children and people with chronic illness. Traditional forms of psychotherapy require good verbal skills but occupational therapists can use non-verbal media, such as paint or music, to facilitate expression and communication.

Goals

There are two main approaches associated with this frame of reference. An explorative approach assumes that the content of the unconscious can best be dealt with by bringing it into the conscious mind so that it can be shared and examined. The individual can then find ways of resolving conflicts and accepting difficult or painful feelings so that more adaptive ways of meeting needs can be achieved. A supportive approach aims to keep unresolved conflicts and painful feelings hidden in the unconscious mind and to strengthen the client's ego defence mechanisms so that material does not 'leak' into the conscious mind and cause problems.

Whichever approach is used, the goals of intervention may be to:

- assist in finding ways to gratify frustrated basic needs
- reverse psychopathology
- provide conditions for normal psychosexual and psychosocial development
- facilitate the development of a more realistic view of the self in relation to action and to others
- help to build a more healthy and integrated ego.

Assessment and intervention

Within a psychodynamic frame of reference there may be no clear distinction between assessment and treatment. The activities that help to bring unconscious material into the conscious mind allow for a clearer understanding of underlying conflicts while at the same time beginning the process of resolving those conflicts. The client's progress is apparent in the way he responds to the activities provided as treatment.

Examples of assessment tools used within this frame of reference include the meaning of objects interview (Fidler 1999a) and observation of relationships in groups (Finlay 2002).

In both the supportive and explorative approaches, the therapeutic elements of occupational therapy are:

- actions of the client
- objects used in, or resulting from, action
- human and non-human environments
- interpersonal relationships.

During intervention, close liaison with other team members is essential, especially if an explorative approach is being used. Treatment planning takes account of the amount of support and structure available to the client and therapist outside treatment sessions. Activities are selected for their symbolic potential as well as the potential to provide an appropriate level and type of social interaction and to match the client's needs. Activity analysis is in terms of the psychodynamics of activity, the symbolic potential of materials and actions, interpersonal aspects and sociocultural significance (Fidler 1999b). The choice of activities may be made by the therapist or by the client, depending upon the client's needs. However, the client must be an active participant in the therapeutic process if it is to be of value to him.

Treatment may be individual or in groups but the group should always be small enough to allow the individual to relate closely to everyone in it (8–10 members is usually considered to be the optimum size). A supportive psychotherapy group would aim to:

- offer encouragement
- provide opportunities for mutual support
- provide a forum for exchanging information about resources
- provide a place to air problems
- help to relieve anxiety
- give opportunities to consider new ways of dealing with problems.

Explorative psychotherapy was traditionally a talking therapy, either one to one or in small groups. Occupational therapy has contributed activity to the process, with the use of creative arts as ego-explorative activities (Blair & Daniel 2006). This involves:

- the presentation of stimuli to which the client can respond with feelings or thoughts (e.g. a piece of music or a poem), or
- the creation of a piece of work through which the client can express feelings or thoughts (e.g. a painting or a piece of free clay modelling).

At the beginning of the 21st century, few occupational therapists are working solely within a psychodynamic frame of reference. However, a knowledge of psychodynamic theories and processes can deepen the therapist's understanding of how people relate to activity and to the world through activity and so enhance any therapeutic approach.

HUMAN DEVELOPMENTAL FRAME OF REFERENCE

A developmental approach to human function and dysfunction fits well with the temporal perspective taken by occupational therapists. The two names most closely associated with the human developmental frame of reference in occupational therapy are Anne Cronin Mosey and Lela A Llorens. Mosey's 1968 paper 'Recapitulation of ontogenesis: a theory for the practice of occupational therapy' outlined a developmental model which can be used in the field of mental health. She subsequently expanded and developed the model, drawing out general principles of a human developmental frame of reference. Llorens (1970) wrote a paper entitled 'Facilitating growth and development: the promise of occupational therapy' for the Eleanor Clarke Slagle lecture in 1969. In it she outlined a framework for intervention, based on developmental theory, that had grown out of her work in the fields of psychiatry, paediatrics and community health. This was followed by a series of publications expanding and clarifying the model and looking at aspects of its application.

This outline of the human developmental frame of reference draws on the work of both Mosey and Llorens, as well as on the work of some other occupational therapy theorists.

Basic assumptions about people

People are seen as dynamic, developing organisms whose life cycles go through predictable stages of growth and decline that necessitate adaptation by the individual. Developmental achievements are not necessarily permanent; regression to an earlier level can occur and maladaptive or incomplete development can be remediated.

Development takes place in a sequence that is common to everyone, although the pace may vary widely. Each stage of development can only proceed normally if the preceding stages have been completed successfully. Incomplete development in one area of skill, or in one life stage, will influence subsequent development. Age ranges can be suggested for particular skills to be mastered but these are not absolute and are mainly useful for checking whether development in all skill areas is proceeding at the same pace. Early patterns of development influence the personality structure of the adult but growth and development continue into adulthood and middle age, especially in the areas of changing responsibilities and relationships.

Fidler & Fidler (1978, p305) proposed that purposeful action 'is viewed as enabling the development and integration of the sensory, motor, cognitive and psychological systems'. However, people's activities and hence their development are influenced by environmental opportunities and barriers. Development will not proceed normally if the child is deprived of a normal range of purposeful activities.

Llorens (1970) based her model of human growth and development on 10 premises, as follows.

1. A person develops in parallel the areas of neurophysiological, physical, psychosocial and psychodynamic growth, social language, daily living and sociocultural skills.
2. All these areas continue to develop throughout the person's life.
3. Mastery of skills to an age-appropriate level in all areas of development is necessary to the achievement of satisfactory coping behaviour and adaptive relationships.
4. Such mastery is usually achieved naturally in the course of development.
5. Intrinsic factors and external stimulation received within the family environment interact to promote early growth and development.
6. The later influences of the extended family, community and social groups assist in the growth process.
7. Physical or psychological trauma can interrupt the growth and development process.
8. Such interruption will cause a gap in the developmental cycle resulting in a disparity between expected coping behaviour and the skills necessary to achieve it.
9. Occupational therapy can provide growth and developmental links to assist in closing the gap between expectation and ability through the skilled application of activities and relationships.
10. Occupational therapy can provide growth experiences to prevent the development of maladaptive behaviour and skills related to insufficient nurturance.

Knowledge base

The developmental frame of reference is based on theories of human development in and across all skill areas:

- Physical
- Cognitive
- Psychological
- Emotional
- Psychosocial.

Different aspects of developmental theory are used with different client groups. For example, the occupational therapist working with children with learning difficulties may draw on knowledge of language, cognition, emotional, psychosexual, social and sociocultural development. If the child has multiple impairments, the therapist may also draw on knowledge of physical, sensorimotor and perceptual development. The occupational therapist working with adults in an acute psychiatric setting may use theories of personality, emotional, moral, psychosexual, psychosocial, social and sociocultural development.

Function and dysfunction

Function and dysfunction are a continuum. A functioning individual is one who achieves satisfactory coping behaviour and adaptive relationships by developing appropriate skills, abilities and relationships at each stage of the lifespan. These adaptive behaviours allow the individual to adjust to both internal needs and external demands. Growth and development can be disrupted or delayed by congenital or acquired disease or injury, or by absence of the conditions for normal growth and development.

Dysfunction occurs when the developmental level of the individual, in any area, is unequal to the age-related demands made on him. Some of these expectations will be for skills common to all people, such as walking by a certain age, while others will be culturally determined, such as social skills.

Trauma at any age can interrupt the developmental process and inhibit the development of adaptive skills or cause regression to an earlier developmental level. A major disruption in any one area will affect all other areas and the longer the disruption continues, the more gaps there will be in the developmental process. However, Mosey (1986) pointed out that people may complete a delayed developmental stage at a later time, when the conditions are right, or may compensate for developmental delay by learning certain higher level skills without the underpinning of more basic ones.

How change occurs

Skills are learned in the normal developmental sequence so that higher level skills are integrated with lower level skills in the same area and with other skills areas developing in parallel. If higher level skills are not integrated with more basic ones then they may be lost when the individual is under stress, and regression to an earlier level of development may occur.

An individual is able to move from one stage of development to the next when the requirements of the earlier stage have been met and the conditions for further development are in place. As the individual's physical and psychological needs change and as new environmental demands are made, the person experiences disequilibrium. This motivates him to learn the skills needed to re-establish a state of equilibrium. New skills are acquired through practice of relevant activities in a facilitating environment until competence is achieved. Once a basic skill has been learned, the individual refines and elaborates it through use.

Client group

Occupational therapists are concerned with promoting development at all ages, therefore this frame of reference is applicable throughout the lifespan. It can be used with people suffering from any kind of chronic or acute mental disorder, as well as those with delay in physical or cognitive development.

Goals

The occupational therapist uses activities and relationships, applied with knowledge and skill, to facilitate growth and development. The overall goal of intervention is to increase skills in all areas, with emphasis being placed on the main area of deficit, so that the gap between expected coping behaviour for the individual's chronological age and actual adaptive ability is closed or narrowed. Short-term goals are to learn the skills needed for the next stage of development.

Occupational therapy is also concerned with maintaining health and preventing maladaptation through early detection of problems and early intervention. This will allow the individual to continue the growth process with a minimum of disruption or maladaptation.

Assessment and intervention

The individual's developmental level in the different skill areas is assessed to find where normal development has been disrupted or has ceased. Appropriate assessment methods include interviews, general observation, observation in tasks designed to elicit specific skills, review of records, projective techniques and testing.

Intervention takes the client's present level of development and ability as the starting point and builds on existing skills. Llorens (1970) stated that it is necessary to meet an individual's needs at his present developmental level if further development is to take place. Bruce & Borg (1993, p130) pointed out that 'confrontation with change creates tension, disequilibrium and stress' but that 'this process is not, of itself, pathological and in fact is often a necessary part of the change process ... a history of successful adaptation promotes future success in meeting challenges'.

If development in the different skill areas has proceeded unevenly, so that one or more areas lag behind the others, then intervention is started in the area where development is most delayed. When that area has caught up, attention is transferred to the next most delayed area so that development across the skills areas proceeds relatively evenly. Intervention is continued until the client has attained an age-appropriate level of adaptive skill in all areas or has attained sufficient skill to be able to function adequately in his expected environment, or has reached what seems to be his highest possible level of achievement.

Treatment techniques include activities and relationships. Activities are analysed and selected for their potential to facilitate the development of particular skills and are combined with a suitable type and level of interpersonal interaction to achieve the maximum benefit.

OCCUPATIONAL PERFORMANCE FRAME OF REFERENCE

The development of a frame of reference focusing on occupation was initiated by Mary Reilly who, from 1959, was chief of the Rehabilitation Department of the Neuropsychiatric Institute at the University of California at Los Angeles (UCLA) (Van Deusen 1988). Early in her career, Reilly became interested in the relevance of the central nervous system to human performance. Through her work on developing patient skills and competence, she began to construct a frame of reference that would combine knowledge of the neurosciences with theories of intrinsic motivation and social psychology and with the ideas of Meyer, one of the founders of the occupational therapy profession. This was the occupational behaviour frame of reference, which had a major influence on occupational therapy theory and practice in the latter half of the 20th century

and was a forerunner of the occupational performance frame of reference.

Following on from Reilly, several occupational therapy theorists began to develop conceptual frameworks to support occupation-focused practice (for example, Christiansen & Baum 1997, Kielhofner & Burke 1980, Reed & Sanderson 1980). One of the most influential of these has been the Canadian Model of Occupational Performance, which was developed by a working group convened by the Canadian Association of Occupational Therapists in conjunction with Health Canada (Canadian Association of Occupational Therapists 1993). Most occupational therapists today would acknowledge the influence of the occupational performance frame of reference on their practice, even if it is not the only approach they use.

Basic assumptions about people

People are occupational beings who have evolved to be adaptable and flexible in what they do, engaging in a wide range of occupations that enable them to survive in almost any environment on earth (Wilcock 2006). Achieving competent occupational performance is a lifelong process of adaptation to internal and external demands that occur naturally within the context of person–environment–occupation interactions (Schkade & Schultz 1998).

There are four components of occupational performance through which the person interacts with the environment: spiritual, physical, cognitive and affective (Sumsion & Blank 2006). People live and occupy themselves in communities, so that their environments are both human and non-human. Through what they do, people are able to adapt to these environments but environments also shape what they do, and what they become, in a two-way process.

Wilcock (2006) put forward the idea that the primary role of the human brain is healthy survival, describing it as both 'an occupational brain and a healing brain' (p70). Survival is the primary drive of all animals and survival depends on health. People's occupational brains allow them to engage in a wide variety of occupations that support health and thus enable survival.

Knowledge base

The discipline of occupational science has contributed much to the occupational performance theory base, from clarifying basic concepts to carrying out research into the relationship between occupation and health. Some of the knowledge base is also drawn from longer established disciplines, such as biology, sociology, social psychology, neurology and anthropology.

This frame of reference integrates an understanding of the structure and functions of the body with awareness of the person. We talk about the health of the body but we use the term *well-being* to refer to the state of the person.

People are thinking, feeling, spiritual and social beings who express themselves, transform themselves and relate to the world through occupation. The occupations that a person performs at any stage of his life are shaped by his own abilities and preferences but also by his environments and opportunities. Occupations develop throughout the lifespan and shape the person as much as the person shapes his occupations.

Occupational performance environments include physical objects, spaces, people, events, cultural influences, social norms and attitudes (Creek 2003). The cultural environment includes values, beliefs, customs and behaviours (Christiansen & Baum 1997). The human environment also includes politics, economy and the law.

Wilcock (2006) spoke of being, doing and becoming.

- **Being** refers to who the person is, his essential nature, which shapes and is shaped by his occupations.
- **Doing** refers to occupational performance, to the engagement of the person in all the occupations that make up the framework of his everyday life.
- **Becoming** refers to growth and development which takes place through occupational performance.

Specific areas of knowledge that fall within the occupational performance frame of reference include theories of:

- occupation and health
- adaptation
- types of occupation
- the components of occupational performance
- motivation
- meaning and values
- volition and engagement
- occupational development and occupational choice
- occupational balance and temporal adaptation
- performance environments
- role and identity
- culture.

Function and dysfunction

People have the capacity to influence the state of their own health through what they do and a balance of rest, play and work in daily life is necessary to maintain physical and mental health. People are in a state of function when they have the range of skills and level of competence necessary to perform a balanced variety of occupations that satisfy their needs and support their health and well-being.

Dysfunction occurs when people are unable to carry out the occupations they need to do, want to do or are expected to do due to disease, injury or environmental conditions (Law et al 1994).

How change occurs

Human beings have a very large and complex brain that gives them highly developed capacities for abstraction, insight, learning, curiosity and exploratory behaviour (Wilcock 2006). These capacities make people very adaptable and, although much adaptation to specific environments takes place in childhood, people retain the ability to change in response to changing circumstances throughout their lives.

Change occurs through people learning or relearning skills to support the performance of their desired range of occupations, or putting in place support to enable them to perform those occupations, or finding alternative occupations to meet their needs and maintain health and life satisfaction.

Client group

The occupational performance frame of reference has a very wide applicability because it is concerned with what people do in their daily lives, at any age, in any circumstances and in any environment. It can be used in traditional health and social care settings, in other institutions, such as prisons, and in health promotion or community development projects.

Goals

The task of the occupational therapist is to enable occupational performance in the presence of impairment, disability or any other barrier. Reilly (1969, p300) stated: 'It is the task of medicine to prevent and reduce illness; while the task of occupational therapy is to prevent and reduce the incapacities resulting from illness'. The main process goal of occupational therapy is for the client to become the agent of therapeutic change (Schkade & Schultz 1998) so it is important to elicit the client's perception of his needs and desired level of performance. The goal of intervention is that the client will be able to carry out the occupations he wants to do, needs to do or is expected to do in order to support health and well-being.

Assessment and intervention

The occupational therapist begins by identifying the occupations that the client expects to do in daily life and the areas where he is having problems. Examples of assessment techniques include the interview, the Canadian Occupational Performance Measure (Law et al 1994), environmental analysis (Hagedorn 2000) and observation of the client's occupational performance.

When the problem areas have been identified, the therapist and client together identify barriers to and enablers of occupational performance. Intervention is targeted at removing or overcoming barriers or putting in place more effective enablers. This may involve developing skills to a level of competence that supports occupational performance, solving occupational performance problems or adapting environments to facilitate performance.

Within the occupational performance frame of reference, interventions are usually individualised because each person has a unique range of occupations and environments. Effective intervention depends on matching the client's performance to the demands of his physical and social environments and his occupations.

Intervention techniques can be categorised as:

- using activity as a therapeutic medium: for example, developing self-confidence and self-esteem through creative activities
- education and training strategies: for example, teaching social skills
- modification of the physical environment: for example, buying a microwave oven to make cooking easier
- modification of the human environment: for example, joining a course at the local college in order to meet people.

SUMMARY

This chapter looked at the components of occupational therapy practice, other than the knowledge base which was discussed in Chapter 3. It began by outlining the content of practice, including the domain of concern, professional goals, population served and legitimate tools of the profession. The next section identified the core skills of the occupational therapist, including thinking skills.

The third section described briefly the occupational therapy process, which is discussed in more detail in Chapters 5, 6 and 7. The chapter finished by examining the way in which occupational therapy knowledge is organised into frames of reference. Three examples were given: psychodynamic, human developmental and occupational performance.

The next chapter looks at aspects of occupational therapy assessment and outcome measurement.

References

Allen CK 1985 Occupational therapy for psychiatric diseases: measurement and management of cognitive disabilities. Little, Brown, Boston

Argyris C, Schön DA 1974 Theory in practice: increasing professional effectiveness. Jossey-Bass, San Francisco

Atkinson K, Wells C 2000 Creative therapies: a psychodynamic approach within occupational therapy. Stanley Thornes, Cheltenham

Azima H, Azima FJ 1959 Outline of a dynamic theory of occupational therapy. American Journal of Occupational Therapy 13(5):215-221

Azima H, Wittkower ED 1957 A partial field survey of psychiatric occupational therapy. American Journal of Occupational Therapy 11(1):1-7

Baum C, Christiansen C 1997 The occupational therapy context: philosophy – principles – practice. In: Christiansen C, Baum C (eds) Occupational therapy: enabling function and well-being, 2nd edn. Slack, Thorofare, New Jersey

Beck AT 1976 Cognitive therapy and the emotional disorders. International Universities Press, New York

Blair SEE, Daniel MA 2006 An introduction to the psychodynamic frame of reference. Duncan EAS (ed) Foundations for practice in occupational therapy, 4th edn. Elsevier Churchill Livingstone, Edinburgh, pp233-253

Bruce MA, Borg B 1993 Psychosocial occupational therapy: frames of reference for intervention, 2nd edn. Slack, New Jersey

Canadian Association of Occupational Therapists 1993 Occupational therapy guidelines for client-centred mental health practice. Canadian Association of Occupational Therapists, Canada

Christiansen C, Baum C 1997 Person–environment occupational performance: a conceptual model for practice. In: Christiansen C, Baum C (eds) Occupational therapy: enabling function and well-being. Slack, Thorofare, New Jersey, pp47-70

Cole MB 2005 Group dynamics in occupational therapy. Slack, Thorofare, New Jersey

College of Occupational Therapists 2004 COT/BAOT briefing no. 23: definitions and core skills for occupational therapy. College of Occupational Therapists, London

College of Occupational Therapists 2006 Recovering ordinary lives: the strategy for occupational therapy in mental health services 2007-2017, literature review. College of Occupational Therapists, London

Creek J 2002 Approaches to practice. Creek J (ed) Occupational therapy and mental health, 3rd edn. Churchill Livingstone, Edinburgh, pp73-92

Creek J 2003 Occupational therapy defined as a complex intervention. College of Occupational Therapists, London

Creek J 2007 The thinking therapist. In: Creek J, Lawson-Porter A (eds) Contemporary issues in occupational therapy: reasoning and reflection. Wiley, Chichester

Creek J, Ilott I, Cook S et al 2005 Valuing occupational therapy as a complex intervention. British Journal of Occupational Therapy 68(6):281-284

Deegan PE 1988 Recovery: the lived experience of rehabilitation. Psychosocial Rehabilitation Journal 11(4):11-19

Fidler GS 1999a The language of objects. In: Gidler GS, Velde BP (eds) Activities: reality and symbol. Slack, Thorofare, New Jersey

Fidler GS 1999b Deciphering the message: the activity analysis. Fidler GS, Velde BP (eds) Activities: reality and symbol. Slack, Thorofare, New Jersey, pp47-58

Fidler GS, Fidler JW 1963 Occupational therapy: a communication process in psychiatry. MacMillan, New York

Fidler GS, Fidler JW 1978 Doing and becoming: purposeful action and self-actualisation. American Journal of Occupational Therapy 32(5):305-310

Fine SB 1999 Symbolization: making meaning for self and society. Fidler GS, Velde BP (eds) Activities: reality and symbol. Slack, Thorofare, New Jersey, pp11-25

Finlay L 2002 Groupwork. In: Creek J (ed) Occupational therapy and mental health, 3rd edn. Churchill Livingstone, Edinburgh, pp245-264

Fleming MH 1991 The therapist with the three-track mind. American Journal of Occupational Therapy 45(11): 1007-1014

Fleming MH 1994 The therapist with the three-track mind. Mattingly C, Fleming MH, (eds) Clinical reasoning: forms of inquiry in a therapeutic practice, FA Davis, Philadelphia, pp119-136

Fleming MH, Mattingly C 1994 Giving language to practice. In: Mattingly C, Fleming MH (eds) Clinical reasoning: forms of inquiry in a therapeutic practice. FA Davis, Philadelphia, pp3-21

Hagedorn R 1995 Occupational therapy: perspectives and processes. Churchill Livingstone, Edinburgh

Hagedorn R 2000 Tools for practice in occupational therapy: a structured approach to core skills and processes. Churchill Livingstone, Edinburgh

Haworth NA, MacDonald EM 1946 Theory of occupational therapy, 3rd edn. Baillière Tindall and Cox, London

Jenkins M 1998 Shifting ground or sifting sand? In: Creek J (ed) Occupational therapy: new perspectives. Whurr, London

Kielhofner G, Burke JP 1980 A model of human occupation, part 1. Conceptual framework and content. American Journal of Occupational Therapy 34(9):572-581

Law M, Baptiste S, Carswell A et al 1994 Canadian occupational performance measure. Canadian Association of Occupational Therapists, Ottawa

Llorens LA 1970 Facilitating growth and development: the promise of occupational therapy. American Journal of Occupational Therapy 24(2):93-101

Mattingly C 1994 Occupational therapy as a two-body practice: The body as machine. In: Mattingly C, Fleming MH (eds) Clinical reasoning: forms of inquiry in a therapeutic practice. FA Davis, Philadelphia

Mattingly C, Fleming MH (eds) 1994 Clinical reasoning: forms of inquiry in a therapeutic practice. FA Davis, Philadelphia

Mosey AC 1968 Recapitulation of ontogenesis: a theory for the practice of occupational therapy. American Journal of Occupational Therapy 22(5):426-438

Mosey AC 1986 Psychosocial components of occupational therapy. Raven Press, New York

Peloquin SM 1998 The therapeutic relationship. In: Neistadt ME, Crepeau EB (eds) Willard and Spackman's occupational therapy, 9th edn. Lippincott, Philadelphia

Prochaska JO, DiClemente CC 1983 Stages and processes of self-change in smoking: towards an integrative model of change. Journal of Consulting and Clinical Psychology 51:390-395

Reed KL, Sanderson SN 1980 Concepts of occupational therapy. Williams and Wilkins, Baltimore

Reilly M 1969 The educational process. American Journal of Occupational Therapy 23(4):299-307

Schkade JK, Schultz S 1998 Occupational adaptation: an integrative frame of reference. In: Neistadt ME, Crepeau EB (eds) Willard and Spackman's occupational therapy, 9th edn. Lippincott, Philadelphia, pp529-535

Schön DA 1983 The reflective practitioner: how professionals think in action. Basic Books, New York

Sinclair K 2007 Exploring the facets of clinical reasoning. In: Creek J, Lawson-Porter A (eds) Contemporary issues in occupational therapy: reasoning and reflection. Wiley, Chichester

Sumsion T, Blank A 2006 The Canadian model of occupational performance. Duncan EAS (ed) Foundations for practice in occupational therapy, 4th edn. Elsevier Churchill Livingstone, Edinburgh, pp109-124

Van Deusen J 1988 Mary Reilly. In: Miller BRJ, Sieg KW, Ludwig FM et al (eds) Six perspectives on theory for the practice of occupational therapy. Rockville, Aspen, Colorado

Wanless D 2004 Securing good health for the whole population: final report. HM Treasury, London

Watson R 2004a New horizons in occupational therapy. In: Watson R, Swartz L (eds) Transformation through occupation. Whurr, London, pp3-18

Watson R 2004b A population approach to transformation. In: Watson R, Swartz L (eds) Transformation through occupation. Whurr, London, pp51-65

Wilcock AA 2006 An occupational perspective of health. 2nd edn. Slack, Thorofare, New Jersey

World Health Organization 2002 Prevention and promotion in mental health. World Health Organization, Geneva

Service user commentary

In this chapter of Jennifer Creek's new book I discovered the work of a highly competent academic intent on carefully and diligently passing on the received wisdom of her chosen profession to the new entrant. She does this in an engaging way that even included me, someone who has availed herself of the skills of occupational therapy over many years.

Jennifer has the best interests of the new recruit at heart in an age of sometimes careless and even crass experimentation. She treads a careful and measured path, carefully explaining, defining and referencing every concept. She says it once, then she says it again with an unswerving logic and clarity of thought which is admirable. As a teacher and writer myself, I recognise the long hours of research that have gone into this document.

I am comforted to have in my hands part of a book which welcomes the budding occupational therapist into a profession that is clearly underpinned by a well-thought through philosophy and set of scientific theories. This must inform practice and hence contribute to credibility in a highly competitive world. The chapter contains a wealth of knowledge and I was particularly interested in the section on core skills, examples of which include the skills of communication and team working. These she describes as both generic, i.e. shared by other health professionals, and profession specific in that they are peculiar to occupational therapists charged with planning and facilitating activity groups. As is to be found throughout, this section on complex core skills is backed up by the work of others and leads on to a very relevant and clear discussion on the importance to the occupational therapist of thinking skills, clinical reasoning and reflection.

As someone charged with helping to monitor the services of a primary care trust, I was particularly drawn to the section on clinical governance. Jennifer herself describes this as 'a framework ... through which organisations are accountable for continuously improving the quality of their services and safeguarding high standards of care' (Creek 2003, p 50). A range of quality initiatives is listed and reference is made to the responsibilities of health and social care organisations re policies and procedures that ensure that services are delivered in the most clinically effective, cost effective and efficient ways possible.

I was also particularly drawn to the three 'frames of reference', each described succinctly in terms of basic assumptions about the nature of people that underpin the approach, the knowledge base, how function and dysfunction are conceptualised, how change occurs, the client group, goals of intervention and techniques for assessment and intervention. I enjoyed being able to read a concise introduction followed by a more detailed, but not overly long, explanation clearly referenced to the experts in the field.

I hope I have done justice to Ms Creek's work. I regard Jennifer Creek as an expert in her field and I can only wonder at the thoroughness with which she has tackled her task - to produce a state-of-the-art book for new entrants into a profession whose high standards she obviously cares about.

Marian Moore BA CertEd

February 2007

Chapter 5

Assessment and outcome measurement

Jennifer Creek, Alison Bullock

INTRODUCTION

Assessment and outcome measurement are integral parts of the occupational therapy process. An initial assessment is used to evaluate the client's strengths, identify problem areas, determine whether or not occupational therapy intervention is appropriate, set the desired outcomes of intervention and establish a baseline prior to beginning programme planning. Ongoing assessments show any changes that have taken place during treatment, enable further investigation of specific areas and demonstrate when outcome goals have been reached. Later assessments provide a picture of residual problems, which can be measured against the client's life demands in order to make recommendations about discharge and to plan follow-up.

Assessment is measurement of the quality or degree of the various factors in a situation or condition. For occupational therapists, it is 'the process of collecting accurate and relevant information about the client in order to set baselines and to monitor and measure the outcomes of therapy or intervention' (Creek 2003, p50). In clinical practice, assessment is used to measure the assets and deficits of the client that relate to his referral for therapy.

Outcomes are the intended or expected results of intervention. The desired outcome is the result that the client and therapist want to achieve, or their goal. For example, the desired outcome for someone with agoraphobia might be to be able to do her weekly supermarket shopping independently. The actual outcome is the measurable result of the intervention. Outcome measurement is the evaluation of the extent to which an outcome goal has been reached (Creek 2003). Ways of recording outcomes are discussed in a later section.

The process of assessment and outcome measurement is invoked when a client is referred to the occupational therapist because some change is judged to be necessary in the person's situation. Assessment is not something that is done *to* the client. It involves the client's active co-operation, both in providing information and in helping to interpret it. Outcomes are identified in collaboration with the client. They may be long-term outcomes or short-term specific, measurable and realistically achievable steps towards meeting an agreed longer term goal. They should be in a form that is readily understood by the client, therapist and others involved.

This chapter will discuss the part that assessment and outcome measurement play in the occupational therapy process. It will consider what is assessed, methods of assessment, how to set realistic outcomes, different approaches to measuring outcomes and how to determine the validity of results.

THE ASSESSMENT AND OUTCOME MEASUREMENT PROCESS

The assessment process, as shown in Figure 5.1, relates to the occupational therapy process as a whole. Assessment and outcome measurement take place in three stages.

- **Initial assessment** takes place at the start of the intervention. It provides an opportunity for the client to find out what he might expect from occupational therapy and begin to get to know the therapist. It enables the therapist to gather information about the client on which to base decisions about intervention.
- **Ongoing assessment** occurs throughout the intervention process, enabling the therapist and client to monitor progress and, if necessary, to gain further specific information, modify interventions or review planned outcomes.
- **Final assessment** takes place at the end of the intervention. It is used for measuring whether or not outcome goals have been reached and planning for appropriate follow-up. The way in which an occupational therapy intervention ends is as important as how it begins if the client is to gain maximum benefit from the experience.

During the process of assessment, the therapist's focus of attention shifts between different aspects of the client's performance: skills, tasks, activities and occupations (Creek 2003). An initial assessment usually begins with the therapist asking the client about the occupations he performs in daily life. Once the main problem area has been identified, the assessment will focus in on the activities that the client is having difficulty with. It may

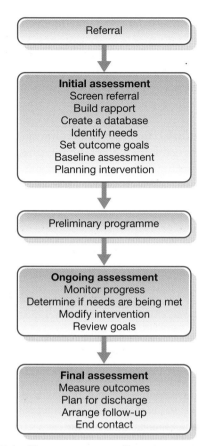

Figure 5.1   The assessment and outcome measurement process.

then be necessary to carry out a more detailed assessment of the activity that is problematic, perhaps focusing on particular tasks that the client is unable to perform and identifying the skills that are lacking or insufficient. Once an intervention has been implemented, the therapist again assesses the client's skills, the effect on tasks and activities and, finally, whether this means that the individual is now better able to perform his usual range of occupations.

Assessment and outcome measurement techniques are designed to work within particular theoretical perspectives or frames of reference. When assessing clients, we do not take account of every factor in their situation; rather, we select certain factors as being important, depending on our philosophical and theoretical perspective. For example, an occupational therapist working in a vocational rehabilitation service will focus on

those aspects of the client's performance that could impact on his ability to find and retain work.

INITIAL ASSESSMENT

Initial assessment can be described as the art of defining the problem to be tackled or identifying the goal to be achieved. When a referral is received, the first step in the occupational therapy process is to collect and organise information about the client from a variety of sources in order to identify problems, set outcome goals and plan treatment effectively (see Box 5.1). Methods of information gathering will be discussed in more detail in the section on methods of assessment.

The steps of the initial assessment process described here may not be carried out in the same sequence with every client, depending on the client's needs and wishes, the context of the intervention and other constraints.

The initial assessment has several functions.

1. It gives the therapist and client an opportunity to judge whether or not the client will benefit from occupational therapy intervention (screening).
2. It provides an opportunity to begin to build rapport and engage the client's interest and co-operation.
3. It creates a database of information about the client.
4. It gives a picture of the client's overall functional ability and problem areas so that the need for intervention can be established.
5. It enables the therapist and client to identify what they want to achieve from the intervention (problem formulation and goal setting).
6. It establishes the client's present level of functioning from which change can be measured (baseline assessment).
7. It identifies the client's strengths, which can be used to promote engagement and goal achievement.

Screening referrals

The outcome of an initial assessment may be a decision *not* to provide an occupational therapy intervention. The main reasons why this decision might be taken are as follows.

- The client's problem does not come within the domain of concern of the occupational therapist. For example, if the reason why someone is unable to do her own shopping is a foot problem, the therapist will refer her to a podiatrist.
- The client could not benefit from occupational therapy intervention at this particular time. For example, a person with alcoholism needs to acknowledge that he has a drink problem before he can benefit from intervention.

- The resources of the department cannot meet the client's needs at this particular time. For example, someone with poor interpersonal skills would benefit from attending a social skills training group but there is none being run due to staff shortages.

Occupational therapy intervention only contributes directly to the treatment process when the programme is based on an assessment procedure that clearly indicates the need for such intervention.

Box 5.1 Initial assessment with Helen

Helen is a 20-year-old woman with a diagnosis of emotionally unstable personality disorder who was referred to occupational therapy by her psychiatrist. The reason given for referral was 'chaotic lifestyle and lack of structure to week'. A CPA baseline assessment had already been completed and had led to Helen's appointment with the psychiatrist. A Mayers' Lifestyle Questionnaire (see p103) and introductory letter were sent to Helen, along with an appointment for 2 weeks ahead. Helen did not attend her appointment or return her questionnaire so, following a team discussion, an appointment was sent to coincide with her next psychiatry appointment.

Helen did attend this appointment; however, she reported having lost the forms sent out previously. The occupational therapist began by asking Helen to fill in the form whilst she was present, explaining the purpose of the form fully and offering assistance where necessary. The completed questionnaire helped the occupational therapist to gain information about general aspects of Helen's occupational performance and also the level of choice and control she felt she had over this. It also enabled Helen to identify and prioritise immediately those areas she was most concerned about.

Helen identified a large number of priority areas but, following discussion with the therapist, it became apparent that her housing status was of immediate and significant impact. She was being verbally and physically abused by drug dealers and was immersed in a drug culture that extended to her physical environment, friends, acquaintances, financial situation, own drug taking and a feeling of inability to change her life.

Due to the immediate risks and the impact of this situation on Helen's ability to begin making positive change in other areas of her life, the initial goals of intervention were negotiated around section 2 (living situation) of the Lifestyle Questionnaire. The overall aim was agreed: to help Helen feel that she could change her answers from 'No' to 'Yes' for the following questions.

- Do you like where you live?
- Do you have the level of privacy you would like?
- Do you feel safe in your home?

Specific, smaller goals were set with Helen. Both her level of responsibility in reaching these goals and the therapist's role in helping her to reach them were clearly identified. Goals were split into two groups: 'For Helen to ....' and 'For the occupational therapist to ....'.

Goals were carefully set in order to maintain Helen's engagement whilst also promoting her independent action (thus, also beginning to work from the start on Helen's role in making her own choices and emphasising the control that she had over her own situation – an area in which Helen had given poor responses).

Building rapport

Establishing a rapport with the client during the initial meeting is important to the client–therapist relationship. It can take a great deal of courage for someone to admit that he needs help and the experience of attending a hospital or clinic, or having a visit from a health-care professional, can be very traumatic, particularly if this is the first contact with secondary services. Older clients, in particular, may be distressed by having to share their difficulties with a younger person and may resent being asked to carry out activities if they cannot see their point. The client may be acutely ill and have difficulty concentrating on what is being said. The therapist needs to appreciate these feelings and not feel personally threatened if a client is unco-operative at first.

The essential ingredients in building rapport with a client are as follows.

- **Respect** for the person, whatever the problems are. The client is a person first and a client only temporarily.
- **Empathy**. It is not possible to like everyone with whom we come into contact, but the therapist should be able to empathise with most of the problems encountered. Most importantly, the therapist does not make value judgements about the client. If there is a real personality clash, which cannot be overcome with help from the supervisor, then it may be advisable to pass the client to another therapist.
- **Honesty** on the subject of what occupational therapy is about and what it can offer. It may be tempting to promise great results or to try to sound mysterious and potent but, in the long run, full co-operation can only be engaged if the client understands the therapeutic process and feels in control.
- **Sharing power** with the client by genuinely working in partnership to identify needs, agree goals, select methods of intervention and evaluate outcomes.

Creating a database

Basic information, such as the client's name, age, sex and marital status, can usually be found in the case notes. A comprehensive initial assessment has often been completed on the client's first contact with a service by a member of the multidisciplinary team, for example, Single Assessment Process (SAP), Care Programme Approach (CPA) initial assessment or Health of the Nation Outcome Scales (HONOS). In some community settings, it may be appropriate to ask the client for this information or it may be preferable to wait until it is volunteered or until some rapport has been developed. Additional information will emerge during the intervention process, the initial assessment being only a starting point from which the general direction of treatment is determined.

The information is used to:

- determine the need for occupational therapy intervention
- identify the client's needs and assets
- build a database of information about the client
- identify which areas need further investigation
- suggest methods of intervention.

Recording the results of investigations is the starting point for interpretation and, as such, is part of treatment planning. Methods of recording data are discussed in Chapter 7. The process of organising information, which should be carried out as far as possible with the active co-operation of the client, is used to:

- produce a list of problems and strengths
- agree on goals of intervention
- suggest strategies and methods of intervention.

Identifying needs

Through the assessment process, the therapist and client build up a picture of the client's functional ability, identifying strengths and interests as well as problem areas. Function has been defined as 'the capacity to use occupational performance components to carry out a task, activity or occupation' (ENOTHE 2006). Function means different things to different people at different times and must be measured in relation to the client's age, cultural background and expected environment (Mosey 1986).

Functional analysis, or functional assessment, is the part of the assessment process which looks at how the individual manages the normal range of daily life activities. The occupational therapist begins by asking about the occupations that the client wants to do, those that are necessary in his life and those that are expected of him. For example, a woman wants to get physically fit, she has to look after her baby and she is expected to cook dinner for her husband who is at work all day.

Functional analysis is a wide-spectrum assessment that allows the therapist and client to identify the client's strengths, problems, sociocultural environment and personal view of life before beginning more focused assessments of particular aspects of function. Mattingly & Fleming (1994) described functional analysis as an important part of the occupational therapist's whole-person approach:

> The functional assessment, which is the occupational therapy equivalent of the doctor's diagnosis, generally requires that the therapist go beyond gathering information and assessing the patient's physiological condition. It requires that the therapist pay some attention to the patient's unique life history and to how the patient sees and understands her or his condition. (pp74–75)

Functional analysis is a process that takes place in three stages:

1. data collection
2. data analysis
3. identification of areas of dysfunction.

Methods of functional analysis will be described in the next section.

Once a picture has been formed of the client's usual occupations, the therapist and client work together to identify which of those occupations are problematic or unsatisfactory and require intervention. If several areas need to be addressed, the therapist and client will decide which ones to work on first. Having agreed on the areas of function that the client wants to or needs to improve and the priorities for intervention, they set goals for meeting the identified needs, using the client's strengths and abilities where possible.

Setting outcome goals

The purpose of an occupational therapy intervention can be expressed as goals to be attained, problems to be resolved, needs to be met or aims to be achieved (Spreadbury & Cook 1995). Whichever mode of formulation is used, it is important that the desired outcome of the intervention is clearly formulated and recorded.

The therapist and client together determine the purpose of intervention and produce a set of outcome goals although, if the client's problems are severe, the occupational therapist may be concerned with the direction of change rather than with setting clear and measurable outcomes (Creek 2003). As far as possible, the client and carer are actively involved in negotiating and agreeing goals.

The purpose of setting outcome goals is twofold:

- the therapist, the client and others with an interest in the client's progress are clear about the purpose of the occupational therapy intervention, and
- everyone knows whether and when the goals have been reached.

Outcome goals can be expressed on different levels: adapting to fixed deficits, developing skills, carrying out tasks, engaging in activities, performing occupations or participating in life situations (Creek 2003). For example, the client's goal might be to listen to the news on the radio instead of buying a newspaper (adaptation), learn to read (skill), walk to the shop to buy a newspaper every day (activity) or keep abreast of current affairs by reading the newspaper every day (occupation/participation).

If the overall goal of intervention is likely to take some time to achieve, it can be broken down into a sequence of short-term goals that represent the steps to be taken towards reaching the long-term goal. For example, the client's long-term goal may be to find full-time, paid employment. If he has not worked for a long time, a first goal on the way to achieving this might be to establish a regular pattern of sleeping at night and waking at the same time every morning.

Outcome measurement involves comparing the client's level of function after intervention with what he was able to do before. Therefore, before beginning intervention, it is necessary to establish the client's current level of function.

Baseline assessment

During the initial assessment process, the therapist and client identify problem areas and agree on the priorities for intervention. Once the goals of the intervention have been agreed, a more focused assessment is carried out to establish a baseline from which change can be measured. The baseline should include information about:

- the client's activities and how they are performed, including skills, abilities, level of function and social behaviour
- the client's feelings and attitudes
- the client's level of knowledge and understanding
- the amount and type of assistance the client needs to perform activities, including equipment, physical assistance and physical and verbal prompting
- the length of time taken to complete activities
- features of the environment in which the client performs daily activities, including home, work and community (Spreadbury 1998).

Planning intervention

A programme is then planned and implemented. It may be necessary to start with a temporary programme while further data are collected, but this programme should be designed to help elicit the information required.

ONGOING ASSESSMENT

Ongoing assessment is a part of the treatment process and is used to monitor the client's progress, determine if needs are being met, identify if the intervention needs to be modified and review whether the original goals are still appropriate (see Box 5.2). This is sometimes called formative assessment (Opacich 1991). Formative assessment is used to build a dynamic picture of the client's progress and to shape the course of intervention and further assessment in a continuous process.

Monitoring progress

During the treatment programme, the therapist has many opportunities to observe the client's performance but the therapist and client may decide to carry out regular, more formal assessments. All clients should be reviewed regularly but the time between these assessments will depend on the type of service and expected length of the intervention. In an acute setting, the client's progress may be reviewed weekly while in a community support service the interval may be as long as 6 months.

The time interval for formal monitoring is usually agreed when outcome goals are set. For example, the client's goal might be to get in contact with his brother whom he has not seen for 5 years. He decides that it is realistic to do this within a month and arranges to see the therapist at the end of this time to review whether or not the desired outcome has been attained.

Determining if needs are being met

Ongoing assessment enables the therapist to judge whether or not the client is moving towards the desired outcomes. It also provides opportunities to check that the intervention is being delivered as planned and is still appropriate to the client's needs. When someone other than the therapist is carrying out the programme, such as a support worker, the therapist remains responsible for monitoring progress (Creek 2003).

Modifying the intervention

Minor adjustments can be made to the programme at any time on the basis of observation and discussion with the client. For example, the therapist observes that a client's concentration span has increased so that he now has no difficulty in staying for a half-hour painting session. The therapist points this out to the client and suggests the length of the session be increased to three-quarters of an hour. The client agrees to try, the relevant people are informed of the change and the new length of session is implemented.

More radical programme changes are usually discussed by all the people directly involved in the client's programme, if not by the whole team.

Box 5.2 Ongoing assessment with Helen

Whilst working on her initial goals in relation to housing, Helen also agreed to further functional assessment of her specific skills/abilities. Once she had moved to more appropriate accommodation, it was agreed that work should begin in relation to section 1 of the questionnaire (looking after yourself). Helen was able to see that there was one section of the questionnaire (living situation) where she now could not make any negative responses, although she continued to focus on the negative aspects of the questionnaire.

Although the questionnaire does not have a scoring system, Helen and the occupational therapist developed a scoring system that worked for Helen and that enabled her to monitor her progress easily. They also spent time discussing what score would be an acceptable optimum for Helen, given that 'life is rarely perfect'. They identified this as the point at which Helen would no longer require support from secondary mental health services. The occupational therapist also said she would monitor episodes of self-harm and overdose and the time between such episodes in order to also use this type of information to help Helen evaluate her progress.

Intervention continued in this way, with new goals being identified as earlier goals were reached. Specific goals were also set at regular intervals, providing just the right degree of challenge for Helen to eventually meet the more general aims of each question area.

Methods of intervention included the following.

- Education (firmly rooted in activity Helen perceived as valuable), for example, sleep, hygiene and activity scheduling.
- Discussion of Helen's behaviour and its consequences (altering behaviour to gain more positive outcomes).
- Working around specific activities and how they made Helen feel, in order to establish coping strategies based on purposeful activity.
- Practical skills training/education.
- Promotion of engagement in activity in the wider community, instead of within mental health services, where possible.

Throughout the intervention, the occupational therapist promoted the benefits of stability in engagement and routine and the effects that this would have on feelings of control and competence. She was careful to encourage Helen to take as much responsibility as possible, although Helen's motivation and engagement were initially very variable so that each goal had to be carefully considered and re-evaluated in order to promote progress most appropriately.

A case review may be routine or can be called by the therapist:

- because she feels the client is ready for it
- when there has been a significant change in circumstances, such as a change in the care setting
- in order to change the programme direction
- to enhance client involvement
- to increase client-centred team working, including across agencies
- as a mechanism to offer choice
- to emphasise progress or to give positive feedback from all those involved.

Reviewing goals

If the client is not making progress towards the agreed outcomes, it may be that those outcomes are unrealistic or no longer relevant at this time. Short-term goals are continually being met and updated and it may be necessary to change long-term goals in the light of new information acquired during therapy or if the client's progress does not match expectations.

The process of treatment, assessment, evaluation and modification of the programme and/or goals can take place as many times as is necessary for the client to reach his optimum level of functioning.

Box 5.3 Final assessment with Helen

Helen eventually began to comment that she could quote the Lifestyle Questionnaire to the therapist word for word. She began to measure her own progress and set her own goals, feeding back to the occupational therapist during visits what she had done and what she would be doing next, including how she would do this. The role of the occupational therapist became much more passive as Helen moved towards discharge, and mainly consisted of monitoring and positive reinforcement. The issue of completion of the intervention was raised on a regular basis during review of the Lifestyle Questionnaire, in relation to the goals originally agreed and with increased emphasis towards the end of therapy.

The occupational therapy process with Helen took $2\frac{1}{2}$ years, but she is now married and completing an access course at college with a view to doing a degree.

FINAL ASSESSMENT AND OUTCOME MEASUREMENT

At some stage, it will become apparent that either the desired outcomes have been attained or there are reasons why no further progress can be made at this time (see Box 5.3). The decision to terminate treatment is ideally taken by therapist and client together but it may be a one-sided decision in some cases. For example, the therapist may feel that the client could benefit from further practice in the relatively protected environment of the department but the client feels ready to take on his social responsibilities again and decides to leave.

Measuring outcomes

Change in the client's performance is measured by comparing the results of ongoing and final assessments with the baseline assessment results. The therapist records whether or not the desired outcomes have been achieved and any unexpected outcomes.

The process of measuring the outcomes of an intervention can provide an opportunity for both the therapist and client to reflect on the journey that they have undertaken together and can be a beneficial part of the intervention.

Planning for discharge

If the client has been in hospital or other temporary residential care during the occupational therapy intervention, discharge planning precedes his return to the community – to his own home, to a new place of residence or to some form of further care (Creek 2003). Planned discharge is the ideal but many factors may intervene to cause an intervention to be terminated before the client has attained maximum benefit. The occupational therapist does not necessarily make the final decision on how long a client remains in therapy, whether in the health or social services or in private practice. Planned discharge may include a period of monitoring which reduces in frequency to ensure that gains are maintained over time prior to final discharge. It can also help clients who have anxieties around discharge to make a successful transition.

If the discharge is planned, there will be time to write a discharge report. This can serve several purposes.

- It provides a record of outcomes achieved or progress towards those outcomes.
- It allows the client to see what changes he has made so that he can leave feeling positive about himself.
- It gives the occupational therapist an opportunity to evaluate the effectiveness of the treatment programme.
- A record of the intervention and outcomes goes into the case notes in the form of the discharge summary.
- Any gap between the client's existing level of skills and the skills he needs to carry out his expected roles and occupations is highlighted

so that recommendations can be made for further treatment, or advice given on where to find help.
- It can aid continuity of care or transfer to other services.

Arranging follow-up

On discharge, the client may feel confident of being able to cope without further support. In these circumstances, the therapist and client may agree that no follow-up is needed or may plan a single contact to ensure that all is going well. Other clients may need some form of ongoing support, either from the occupational therapist or through transfer to another service.

Ending contact

Eventual recovery and discharge should be discussed from the point of initial contact, if only generally. Throughout the intervention, reference should also be made to discharge, with discussion becoming more explicit as the client approaches this point in the intervention. As far as possible, the therapist ensures that the client's departure from the service is experienced as positive so that he feels optimistic about the future and confident that he could use the occupational therapy service again if needed.

WHAT IS ASSESSED?

The occupational therapist does not assess every aspect of a person's functioning but makes a general assessment of the client's range of occupations so that areas of need can be identified before a more focused, in-depth assessment is carried out. In some cases, the client will have a clear idea of what kind of help is needed and does not want a broad assessment; indeed, it may be perceived as irrelevant or even intrusive.

It is not possible or necessary to learn everything there is to know about a client; therefore data are collected and organised in the context of the purpose of the referral, the nature of the service offered and the frame of reference being used by the therapist.

The occupational therapy assessment covers the client and the client's environment, both physical and social.

THE CLIENT

Aspects of the client that are assessed include:

- occupations
- balance of activities in daily life
- abilities, strengths and interests
- problems or areas of dysfunction
- aspirations and expectations
- change and direction of change.

Occupations

Occupations exist in a balance that changes throughout the life cycle. A healthy balance is one that allows most of the individual's needs to be satisfied in ways that promote social inclusion and integration. This balance can be disrupted by illness or disability but, equally, an inability to participate in a range of chosen occupations can have a negative impact on health (Creek 2003).

The therapist wants to know:

- if the client's daily life needs are being met
- if the client is able to carry out the occupations he wants to do, needs to do or is expected to do
- any reduction or increase in the expected number of occupations
- any imbalance between self-care, work and leisure occupations
- the client's occupational history.

Balance of activities in daily life

Occupations are enacted through activities; for example, the occupation of mothering is expressed through such activities as bathing the child, feeding the child, playing with the child, reading to the child and answering the child's questions. The therapist will seek to discover what activities the client normally performs and whether or not these activities support a healthy range of occupations.

Daily activities are organised into routines that support the individual's sense of self and, if performed regularly, become habitual; for example, brushing one's teeth involves a sequence of actions that becomes habitual so that one does not have to think carefully about every stage of the operation. Routines and habits enable the individual to perform everyday tasks without having to remember consciously how to go about them. They are developed to suit the individual's needs at any one period of life; new habits are learned and old ones discarded as circumstances change.

The therapist assesses how clients organise their time; that is, whether they have useful habits or have to expend a lot of time and energy in deciding what to do and working out ways of performing. Habits may also have become too rigid to allow for necessary changes so that the client's behaviour no longer meets the needs of his situation. It is useful to take an occupational history to assess whether the individual's habits have been disrupted or whether he has never developed good habits. If possible, the therapist will identify the point at which habits broke down.

The therapist also looks at how the client uses time over the course of days and weeks – whether there are empty times or times when there is too much to do. It is also helpful to find out if time use has changed recently, perhaps with the loss of a major occupation or with the introduction of new demands. The most important measure of a successful balance of activities may be the client's own perception or, conversely, he may lack insight into what appears to others to be a problem.

Abilities, strengths and interests

Abilities, strengths and interests influence the range of occupations a person adopts and the way in which these occupations are performed.

Ability is the measure of the level of competence with which a skill is performed. In order to function effectively in a desired range of occupations, a person must have a variety of skills and be able to perform them competently. When assessing clients, it should be taken into account that competence is not an absolute concept; norms for competence vary with age and are to some extent socially defined (Mocellin 1988).

Strengths are the personal factors that enable the client to function effectively. They include skills, other personal attributes and social networks. The therapist assesses the client's strengths so that interventions can be designed to support and build on them.

Interest is the expectation of pleasure in an activity which is aroused by a combination of experience and some degree of novelty – experience tells us that we have enjoyed something similar in the past and novelty arouses in us the urge to try a new experience. It is important to know what the client's interests are so that interventions can be designed that are appropriate and that support his sense of self.

Areas of dysfunction

Function and dysfunction are not opposites but exist on a continuum; there is no clear line with function on one side and dysfunction on the other. Spencer (1988, p437) pointed out that:

> Temporary or permanent disability takes on a unique meaning for each individual. Age, developmental stage, previous ability, achievements, life-style, family status, self-concept, interests and general responsibilities affect attitudes such as understanding, acceptance, motivation and emotional response ... An accurate analysis of the biopsychosocial context by the therapist is essential to determine the functional implications of the patient's condition.

The ways in which function and dysfunction are conceptualised are determined by the frame of reference the occupational therapist is using. For example, using the adaptive skills model (Reed & Sanderson 1992), dysfunction is seen in terms of lack of mastery of the adaptive skills appropriate to the individual's age and stage of development. Within a cognitive behavioural frame of reference, dysfunction is seen in terms of faulty information processing, irrational thinking and distorted perceptions.

For simplicity, function is divided into skill areas that can be separated for the purpose of assessment but act together in the performance of activities. One classification of skill areas is that suggested by Reed & Sanderson (1992):

- sensorimotor skills (for example, hearing, hand–eye co-ordination)
- cognitive skills (for example, memory, concentration)
- psychosocial skills (for example, listening, taking turns).

Satisfaction with function is very individual and the therapist may have to accept that a client is happy with his own level of functioning in a particular occupation, even though the therapist believes that he has the potential to perform to a higher standard.

During assessment it is important to take a temporal perspective, considering the client's past level of functioning and expected future occupations as well as present capabilities, in order to find out whether he has lost skills or never developed competence in certain areas.

Aspirations and expectations

People have a basic urge to be active, to test their own potential and to have an impact on their surroundings, but the extent to which they act on that urge and the actions that they choose are influenced by life experiences. Fidler & Fidler (1978) stated that each person learns his own capacities by 'doing'. Successful doing leads to a sense of satisfaction and a sense of competence. Persistent failure, due to lack of skill or lack of opportunity to do, leads to a sense of incompetence and lack of control.

It is important that occupational therapy interventions match the client's aspirations and expectations, but someone's capacity to make realistic plans for the future can be affected by fear of failure or by illness. The assessment process is designed to elicit both what the client would like to achieve and how realistic those aspirations are.

Change and direction of change

Occupational therapists take an essentially optimistic view of human beings, believing that everyone has the potential to change and to influence the direction of that change by what they do. Seedhouse (1986, p73) argued that health is closely related to human potential:

> Except in extreme instances of illness or external control, people possess an indefinite number of potentials depending upon what they do and what happens to them ... This is true even of terminal patients in hospital, even until the time they finally lapse into unconsciousness ... people can change themselves and their environments for the better.

The extent of change will be limited by personal factors, such as personal goals, degree of disability and investment in maintaining existing coping methods. Change will also be influenced by external factors such as the goals of the family or carers, social support networks and social expectations. All these factors must be assessed and taken into account when setting or modifying goals.

THE ENVIRONMENT

People are never independent of their environment but learn how to adapt to it, or adapt it to themselves, to satisfy their needs. Through acting on the environment and receiving feedback about the effect of their actions, people learn how best to achieve their own aims. Skilled performance of actions is only developed through exploring the environment and acting on it. Failure to adapt to the environment leads to dysfunction.

A healthy environment allows individuals to act in ways that enable them to meet their needs. Sometimes people find themselves in an environment that they cannot adjust to in a healthy way or that does not give them opportunities to make changes. A person may become ill because of environmental factors and then discover that the illness allows him to meet his needs, either by removing him from a difficult environment or by changing the attitudes and behaviour of people around him. The costs of being ill are outweighed by the benefits, which then act to maintain the illness behaviour.

The environment includes both physical factors, such as poor housing or inadequate public transport, and social factors, such as poverty or working in an unsatisfying job.

Physical environment

The physical environment includes place of residence, workplace and community.

- **Place of residence**: type and quality of housing; temporary or permanent accommodation; access to the home; any problems, such as damp; facilities such as space, heating and garden; privacy; furnishings and organisation of household goods; comfort; where the home is situated; whether it is convenient for transport, shops, libraries and open spaces; distance from the workplace, and the character of the neighbourhood.
- **Workplace**: location in relation to home; transport; access; space, including characteristics of the working space and the total area of the workplace; facilities, such as canteen and health care; noise levels; heating and air conditioning; any hazards, and tools or equipment.
- **Community**: type of neighbourhood; community resources such as shops and leisure facilities; public transport infrastructure; access to health care, including GP, dentist and optician, and open spaces.

Social environment

The social environment consists of the people who make up the individual's social world, at home, at work and in other areas of life. This includes: neighbours; family; friends; work colleagues; casual contacts, such as shopkeepers and people met on public transport; social groups, such as co-religionists and club members, and Internet contacts. All these people influence and shape how a person feels about himself through the roles that are assigned to him and the expectations that go with those roles.

Roles are patterns of activity associated with social position. They are defined by society and assigned to individuals on the basis of such attributes as age, sex, relationships, possessions, education, job, income and appearance. For example, at work, a person takes on his work role; when going shopping, he takes a consumer role. Each role carries expectations of performance, which the individual who accepts the role attempts to carry out. A role contributes to the individual's sense of social and personal identity and influences the way in which occupations are performed.

A properly integrated role, supported by the skills and habits necessary for its performance, satisfies both society's expectations and the individual's needs. However, when a person is assigned a role that he is unable or unwilling to accept, then dissonance occurs between society's expectations and the person's performance. This can lead to social exclusion and stigma.

METHODS OF ASSESSMENT

Occupational therapists use a wide range of assessment tools, from interviews to assessment batteries. Some depend on the experience and skill of the tester, such as observation of performance in activities, while others are standardised and can, in theory, be applied objectively by anyone who has been trained in their use.

In thinking about which assessment tools to use, there are several points to consider.

1. What aspects of the client does the therapist wish to assess?
2. Have these aspects been defined in such a way that they can be measured accurately? (Reliability)
3. How can the desired function or performance be elicited for assessment?
4. Does the proposed assessment procedure measure what it is intended to measure? (Validity)
5. Does the assessment capture changes that have occurred as a result of intervention? (Outcome measurement)
6. Is there a clearly defined way of administering the assessment? (Standardisation of administration)
7. How are the results to be recorded and scored?
8. Can the results be compared with the normal results for a comparable population? (Standardisation)

Occupational therapists use two main methods of assessment: standardised and non-standardised. Both of these approaches can be used to measure the outcomes of interventions. Non-standardised outcome measures are individualised; that is, they are designed to be sensitive to the changes that the client wants to achieve.

OUTCOME MEASUREMENT

Outcome measurement is 'evaluation of the nature and degree of change brought about by intervention, or the extent to which a goal has been reached or an outcome has been achieved' (Creek 2003, p56). Change is measured by comparing assessment results before and after intervention; the difference between the two results is the amount of change that has taken place. An outcome measure is an assessment tool that is capable of detecting change over time.

Standardised outcome measures

Standardised outcome measures have been tested for reliability and validity with large groupings of particular populations. Scores for the population are published so that the results achieved from any assessment can be compared with the normal range for that population. For example, the Barthel Index is a standardised assessment of functional independence in personal care and mobility (McDowell & Newell 1996). Standardised outcome measures used by occupational therapists include the Allen Cognitive Level Screen (Allen 1985) and the Assessment of Motor and Process Skills (Fisher 1995).

It is important that standardised assessments are used with the population for whom they are designed and that they are administered following the exact standardised procedures. Some tools require that the therapist is trained and certified before they can be used, in order to ensure that they are used correctly. If a standardised assessment tool is modified, used with people other than those it was designed for or administered in a way that deviates from the standardised procedure, the results will be invalid.

Individualised outcome measures

Individualised outcome measures compare the client's performance after intervention with how he performed before intervention, rather than judging performance against a norm. These measures are sensitive to small changes and to those which may be important to the client (Spreadbury & Cook 1995). For example, the Canadian Occupational Performance Measure (COPM: Law et al 1994) is designed to detect changes in the client's own perception of his occupational performance over time and can be used with a wide range of people (Box 5.4).

Individualised outcome measures used by occupational therapists include the Binary Individualised Outcome Measure (Spreadbury & Cook 1995), Goal Attainment Scaling (Ottenbacher & Cusick 1993) and the COPM (Law et al 1994).

Some individualised outcome measurement tools, such as the COPM, are scaled; that is, they produce a score on a numerical scale. However, the scale does not represent a normal distribution and cannot be used to compare one client's performance with another.

Using an individualised outcome measure

The process of using an individualised outcome measure has four stages: goal setting, baseline assessment, intervention and reassessment. This process can be carried out as many times as is needed for the client to reach all his important goals.

Goal setting

The client and therapist identify problem areas, agree on the goals of intervention and decide which goals should be given priority. In order to be able to measure when goals have been reached, it is necessary to define the desired outcomes clearly, in a form that is:

- **specific**: the more specific the goal, the easier it will be to measure when it has been reached. The goals should include the activity to be performed by the client, the conditions in which it will be performed, the standard or level of performance to be reached and the time that performance will take (Spreadbury & Cook 1995). For example, the man who is trying to establish a healthy sleep pattern might set his first goal as: to be in bed, ready to sleep, by 11pm on Sunday to Thursday evenings
- **achievable and realistic**

Box 5.4 Canadian Occupational Performance Measure

The Canadian Occupational Performance Measure (COPM) was designed for use by occupational therapists in a variety of fields of practice. It is an individualised outcome measure which is appropriate for use within the individual programmes of care provided by occupational therapists (Spreadbury 1998).

The COPM (Law et al 1994) focuses on occupational performance and takes the form of a semi-structured interview. The client is assisted to identify occupational performance problems in the areas of self-care, productivity and leisure. He is then asked to rate each problematic activity for how important it is in his life on a 10-point scale from 1 (not important at all) to 10 (extremely important). The client is then invited to choose up to five activities that seem the most important for intervention. Each of these is rated on two further dimensions: performance and satisfaction. The client is asked to mark on a 10-point scale how well he thinks he performs the activity now, from 1 (not able to do it at all) to 10 (able to do it extremely well). He is also asked to rate how satisfied he is with the way he does the activity now from 1 (not satisfied at all) to 10 (extremely satisfied).

After an appropriate period of intervention, the client is asked to rate the activities again for performance and satisfaction. Changes in the scores demonstrate changes in performance and satisfaction.

The COPM has standardised instructions and methods for administration and scoring but it is not norm referenced (Pollock et al 1999). It is only intended to measure changes in individual performance and satisfaction.

- time limited
- measurable or observable.

Subjective goals, such as feeling more confident in social situations, can be operationalised by identifying performance indicators. That is, the therapist asks the client, 'What will you be able to do when you feel more confident?' The performance (what the client will be able to do) becomes the measurable outcome, rather than the subjective goal of feeling more confident, which is difficult to measure.

Baseline assessment

The client's current level of performance is assessed, using the chosen outcome measurement tool.

Intervention

The negotiated intervention is carried out for an agreed length of time before the client is reassessed.

Reassessment

The measurement tool used for the baseline assessment is applied again and the results are compared with the results before intervention to see what change has taken place.

RELIABILITY AND VALIDITY

Vague and inaccurate assessment leads to vague and imprecise goal setting and treatment. This is unacceptable for both ethical and practical reasons. The occupational therapist has a duty to use treatment that will benefit and not harm the client (see Ch. 11); therefore intervention must be based on accurate knowledge of the client's needs and abilities. The two most important concepts in ensuring accuracy of assessment procedures are reliability and validity.

Reliability

The first concern in legitimising an assessment procedure is whether or not it reliably elicits accurate information. There are two main ways of determining reliability.

1. **Test–retest.** The rater assesses the client and records the results. After a suitable interval to minimise the effect of practice, the test is given again and the results are compared. Obviously, results are more likely to be similar if the aspects being measured have been clearly defined and the testing procedure is standard.

2. **Interrater evaluation**. The assessment procedure is carried out on the same client by two or more raters and their results compared. This method is appropriate for evaluating procedures that involve observation. If possible, the raters observe the client doing the same activity, perhaps by using a videotape. The results are more likely to be similar if the testing procedure is standard and the raters have been trained in its use.

Validity

Establishing the validity of an assessment procedure is more difficult than establishing reliability, so it is only carried out on procedures that are known to be accurate and therefore worth validating.

Validation involves checking that the procedure measures what it is intended to measure; if we want to know whether a client is able to cook a meal on a gas cooker, there is no point in assessing the client's performance on the department's electric cooker.

There are three main types of validity:

1. **content or face validity**: analysing the assessment procedure to see if it measures what it purports to measure
2. **criterion-related or concurrent validity**: comparing the assessment results with an external criterion such as data collected from other sources
3. **construct validity**: looking at the accuracy of the assessment procedure in measuring the theories or hypotheses behind the intervention.

All assessment tools should be reliable and valid. When they have been tested for reliability and validity with a particular population, using a sufficiently large sample, they are said to have been standardised for that population.

STANDARDISED ASSESSMENTS

If an assessment procedure is found to be both accurate and reliable, then it may be appropriate and useful to standardise it for use in a particular way with the client group it was developed for. Establishing a clear and uniform procedure for applying the test is called standardisation of administration, and establishing the performance of a similar group of people for comparison is called standardisation of results, or norming.

Standardisation of administration

Standardised administration means that the procedure can be repeated in exactly the same way by different people, at different times and on different subjects. This involves defining the functions to be assessed very clearly and giving precise instructions about administering and scoring the test. Objective tests are easier to standardise than tests that require an observer to make a judgement. Observer bias must be minimised by training the rater (Garfield 1982).

Standardisation of results

This is a lengthy procedure that involves administering a reliable and valid assessment procedure to a large number of people who are matched for such factors as sex, age, cultural background and, possibly, disability. The results are presented as a numerical scale, representing the normal range of performance for that group, that can be used as a comparison with the scores of an individual.

Standardised assessments in occupational therapy

Occupational therapists use standardised assessments designed by other disciplines, such as Health of the Nation Outcome Scales for Mentally Disordered Offenders (Royal College of Psychiatrists 1999), and those designed by occupational therapists, such as the Structured Observational Test of Function (Laver & Powell 1995).

NON-STANDARDISED ASSESSMENTS

The first four assessment techniques described here (review of records, interview, observation and home visits) are used by other professionals as well as by occupational therapists. Techniques more specific to occupational therapy are those that focus on function and involve activity or occupation: functional analysis, checklists, performance scales, questionnaires and projective techniques.

Review of records

The therapist sometimes does not have easy access to case notes and other records, for example if she works in the community. In this case, a well-designed referral form or discussion with the referring agent can elicit the desired information before the client is seen. In some settings, such as outreach work, it is not possible for the therapist to find much information about the client in advance of meeting him.

It is sometimes suggested that therapists should not read clients' records before seeing them as this may influence their perceptions. However, it is very frustrating for clients to have to give the same information to many people and, if therapists are aware of the danger of bias, they can consciously try to avoid it.

Looking through medical and nursing records can be time-consuming, especially if the client has a long medical history, but familiarity with the way case notes are organised makes the search easier. Hemphill (1982) suggested that the therapist looks at:

- social history
- admission summary
- nurses' notes
- the psychologist's report
- the physician's reports
- any other pertinent reports.

Hemphill (1982) recommended a checklist to use when reading case notes to ensure that no relevant information is missed.

Information gained from the client's records can be used to plan an initial interview.

The interview

In most treatment settings occupational therapists are in constant, informal communication with their clients. However, a formal interview can often be a useful additional method of communication and assessment.

Interviews can be structured or unstructured. No interview is truly unstructured if it is to be of use but there is a difference between knowing what you want to elicit and having a list of set questions to ask. The structured interview tends to be more popular with less experienced therapists (Kielhofner 1988).

Unstructured interviews

Before the interview, the therapist collects together information about the client and decides what she wants to find out. Time need not be wasted during an interview in going over what the therapist already knows. If appropriate, the client is informed in advance about the time, place and purpose of the interview. The therapist may expect the client to turn up on time, may collect him or may go to where he is to carry out the interview, depending on the client's needs.

Where possible, the interview is carried out in an informal atmosphere without distractions or interruptions. If the therapist has some control over the environment, she will pay attention to details such as height and positioning of chairs, in order to gain maximum rapport. Comfortable but straight-backed chairs, placed at an angle of 90° to each other, are probably ideal since both parties can then see each other without effort. Interruptions can usually be avoided if staff or others are informed that the interview is taking place, where it is and how long it will take.

At the beginning of the interview the therapist calls the client by name and makes sure that the client knows the therapist's name and the purpose of the interview. The therapist may take a more or less directive role in the interview, depending on the client's mental state and the purpose of the interview, but a warm and accepting manner is usually most successful. The therapist is an active listener, paying respectful attention to what the client says and attempting to reach a good understanding of his intended meaning.

The length of the interview may be set in advance, especially if there are many constraints on time, or it may be determined by the course of events. A confused person may not be able to tolerate a long interview whereas a client in acute distress may benefit from the therapist's undivided attention until he feels calmer.

Upon termination of the interview, a brief summary by the therapist of its main points can help the client to continue thinking about it afterwards. The therapist then checks that the client knows where he is going and walks with him if it is appropriate. Notes are usually written up immediately after the interview.

Structured interviews

The structured interview format may be designed for use in a particular treatment setting if the therapist finds it useful to collect the same information about each client. Alternatively, it may be designed as part of a particular model; for example, an occupational history is often taken to collect information about a client's performance in past and present occupational roles for use within the Model of Human Occupation (Forsyth & Kielhofner 2006).

The structured interview consists of a series of questions designed to elicit the desired information. Such a series of questions could also be administered as a questionnaire if the therapist is confident that the client understands it fully, but an interview is more personal and allows rapport to be developed (Florey & Michelman 1982). It is often acceptable to take brief notes during a structured interview.

An interview may also be semi-structured; that is, the therapist has a number of questions to ask but allows for digressions if they seem useful. Florey & Michelman (1982) suggested that, while the questionnaire or structured interview are effective for gathering a history of discrete events such as childhood illnesses, the semi-structured interview is useful for taking a history of more abstract events.

Many of the histories and checklists used by occupational therapists could be administered as interviews, self-assessment instruments or computer programmes, depending on the needs and abilities of the client.

Content of the interview

During the interview the therapist can observe the client's:

- verbal and non-verbal communication skills
- sensory deficits (if any)
- quality of self-care
- mannerisms (if any)

- posture
- facial expression.

By asking questions, the therapist can find out the client's:

- level of cognitive functioning
- attitude to his current situation
- feelings about being involved in occupational therapy
- mood
- expectations of therapy.

Questions can be directed towards exploring a particular aspect of the client (e.g. relationships with other people).

The interview is also an opportunity for giving the client information and feedback. At the initial interview, rules and expectations within the occupational therapy department can be explained, including how violations of the rules are dealt with. A discussion of the general function of the department and its potential value helps the client to make more informed decisions about becoming involved in treatment. Clients frequently complain that they do not see how occupational therapy can help them and a clear explanation can enhance the value of therapy.

During later interviews the client can be given feedback on his performance and on any changes that have been observed. The client may also give feedback on how he feels about the programme. Modifications to the programme are discussed so that the client continues to be actively involved in his own treatment.

Observation

Observation involves noting and recording the type, frequency and duration of activities by the client and interpreting what is observed according to the model being used. The client may be observed performing activities individually or as a member of a group.

Mosey (1973) described three steps in using observation as a method of assessment.

1. **Observation**. Noting what the client does without ascribing meaning to it.
2. **Interpretation**. Using observed data to reach conclusions about the reasons for the client's actions.

3. **Validation**. Seeking to confirm the accuracy of interpretations by sharing them with the client or others who know the client well.

There are three main types of observation:

- general observation of the client during activities
- observation of specified performances
- observation of the performance of set tasks.

General observation

The range of activities within the domain of occupational therapy gives opportunities for observing clients under different circumstances so that a picture of their capabilities and deficits can be built up. However, clients' performance in their normal environment is often very different from when they are in the occupational therapy department or on a ward, so staff also benefit from spending time out of the institutional setting to observe clients.

Using a checklist to record what is observed can help to ensure accuracy and reduce subjectivity. Checklists make it possible to look at complicated areas of skills without becoming confused, although a description may also be needed to give additional information.

Much can be learned from the physical appearance of the client (physique, posture, facial expression, mannerisms, gait, grooming and dress). Some illnesses, such as severe depression, produce a characteristic stooped posture and flat expression. However, the use of certain drugs may mask symptoms of the underlying disorder with an array of side-effects; for example, obesity or rigidity may be due to phenothiazine medication.

Form and content of speech provide clues to the client's inner life, including mood, insight, cognitive functioning and thought disorder. A good rapport with the client is helpful in that clients will be more willing to share their thoughts in the context of a warm and trusting relationship.

The client's performance patterns can be observed in different situations and at different times of day to assess energy level, diurnal variations in energy, interaction with others, willingness to co-operate, initiative and skills. The client may respond in totally different ways to family, friends, junior staff, students and senior staff, so that everyone in contact with the client will have something to contribute to a total assessment.

Observation of specified performances

General observation tends to be descriptive and inevitably misses much of what happens. The occupational therapist is usually a participant observer, which can interfere with the observation of a client's performance. A more precise method of observation is to specify what is to be observed and ignore all other activity. This method is commonly used by psychologists but can be useful for occupational therapists, particularly within a behavioural model. The process consists of:

- deciding what to observe
- selecting an observation technique
- making the observation
- recording the observation
- analysing the recorded performance.

The therapist may wish to observe the number of times a particular activity is carried out (frequency) or the length of time the activity lasts (duration). The observation technique chosen will depend on what is to be observed but the three main methods are (Felce & McBrien 1987, Hogg & Raynes 1987):

- **event counting**: the therapist specifies the action she wishes to observe then counts the total number of times it occurs, either during the whole session or during a specified period of time
- **time sampling**: if the action to be observed occurs frequently, it may be more appropriate to take samples than to record it continuously. This can be done by noting the number of times the action occurs during brief, regularly spaced intervals of time, say, for 1 minute in every 10 (interval recording), or by making an observation at fixed intervals and noting if the action is occurring at that moment (time sampling)
- **duration recording**: this is used for actions that occur for longer periods or for variable periods of time. The easiest method is to use a

cumulative stopwatch to record the total amount of time spent on the action in a given period.

Event counting and time sampling are used to count the frequency of activities that are brief, discrete and easily identified, such as head-banging. Duration recording is used for activities that last for longer periods.

Set tasks

When further information is required about a particular area of functioning, such as cooking a meal or planning an outing, the client can be asked to participate in a task designed to measure that function. The task may demand practical skills, such as hand–eye co-ordination, or cognitive skills, such as problem solving. It may be a social task that requires interaction with others or it may be designed to highlight the client's attitudes by making unusual demands.

A careful and detailed analysis of the task ensures that it requires the skills that the therapist hopes to observe. Knowledge of what constitutes normal performance is also necessary so that the client's performance can be measured against it.

It is rarely possible to reproduce external conditions accurately within a hospital or clinic setting and it may be more appropriate to visit the client's home or workplace to assess its particular demands or to try out skills.

Home visits

Home visits may be made at any stage of treatment for the purpose of assessment or treatment, or both. Within a multidisciplinary team it is necessary to co-ordinate with other staff to limit the number of people who do home visits and to share information obtained.

Purpose

If the treatment setting is a hospital or day centre, the home visit can be an expensive use of staff time so it is important to establish the purpose clearly beforehand. The occupational therapist builds up a picture of the client's assets and needs from an assessment in the treatment setting, which she can use to determine what to assess in the home environment.

The home visit can be used to:

- gain a picture of the client's life demands and role expectations
- observe the client's level of functioning in his normal environment
- carry out specific assessments, such as using the kitchen
- observe the physical environment, including the home and its surroundings
- meet the client's family and neighbours on their own territory.

The emotional environment is more difficult to assess in a single visit since the family dynamics will be changed by the presence of a stranger. However, the therapist may learn something about stresses and supports within the home by observing the number of family members and the amount of personal space each one has. More difficult to assess, but very useful to know, is how emotionally close to each other the family members are, what roles they take within the family, what methods of communication they use and their attitudes to the person who is receiving treatment. Neighbours' attitudes are also relevant, especially if the client lives alone.

Carrying out a home visit

A date and time for the visit are set to suit the therapist, the client and the client's family, taking transport into account. It will be easier to determine the length of the visit if the aims are very clear and specific. The therapist should carry some form of identification for the benefit of the family.

Safety is an important consideration when carrying out home visits to clients and/or their families. It is important to let other staff know where you are going and when you expect to return so that they can check on you if you are late. A mobile phone may be carried so that any change of plan can be reported. If there are any anxieties about safety on a particular home visit, the therapist should take a colleague.

The purpose of the visit is clearly explained to the family, especially if the therapist has not met them before. Many families like to offer a cup of tea to a visitor and this can provide an opportunity for getting to know them in a relaxed way.

Further structuring of the visit depends on what the therapist wishes to assess.

After a home visit, the therapist can discuss with the client his level of functioning against his life demands. This can be the basis for deciding if any adjustments can be made to the environment or whether the client needs to make personal changes in order to cope.

Functional analysis

As described above, functional analysis is the part of the assessment process which looks at how people spend their time and at their capabilities and any problem areas. Over 200 different techniques have been devised for collecting data about how an individual functions in daily life (Unsworth 1993), but most of these focus only on activities of daily living (e.g. the Barthel Index and the Rivermead ADL Assessment) and most have been devised for use with elderly people.

The simplest way to collect data about function is probably to ask clients to say what they do in a typical day. The COPM (Law et al 1994) recommends the therapist to 'Encourage clients to think about a typical day and describe the occupations they typically do'. A form can be used, dividing the day into half-hour sections (Fig. 5.2), which the client fills in to give a record of a typical day. This can then be analysed in various ways to find out where areas of dysfunction are occurring. The COPM suggests that the client first identifies the activities he needs, wants or is expected to do and then identifies which ones he can do to his own satisfaction. This gives an indication of the performance areas the client is having problems with.

One of the purposes of the analysis is to find what meaning clients place on different aspects of life, what activities are important to them, what purpose they see the different activities serving, what motivates them and what their main goals are for therapy.

Other questions that might be asked about the typical day include:

- Which activities does the client find pleasurable, unpleasant or neutral? This will highlight the balance of pleasurable activities in the individual's life.

- Are there any problems in the overall balance of activities – empty times in the day or times when there is too much to cope with?
- What life roles do the day's activities represent? Is the range of roles appropriate to the client's age/developmental level?

The therapist will also be interested in the social, physical and cultural environment in which the client will be functioning and whether it will support the client in his chosen roles and occupations.

Functional analysis identifies areas of dysfunction as a starting point for deciding the focus of intervention. The client's own priorities should then be taken as a guide in selecting the area to work on first. Once the functional analysis has been completed, the therapist begins a more detailed assessment.

Checklists, performance scales and questionnaires

Occupational therapists have always used checklists for assessing skills such as activities of daily living (ADL) and work skills but over the last three decades there has been an increase in the number of assessment procedures developed for use within particular frames of reference. There has also been more interest in standardising assessments, although normative data have still to be collected for many tests that are in regular use.

Some checklists and performance scales measure directly observable performance, for example the ability to dress independently. Others assess functions which are more complex and may be more difficult to observe, for example the ability to participate in a mature group (Mosey 1986). In order to assess these functions, they can be tied to performances which indicate their presence or their absence (performance indicators). For example, Mosey (1986) suggested that the ability to participate in a mature group is indicated by 'comfort in heterogeneous groups and the ability to take a variety of membership roles'. Lack of the skill is shown by 'preference for same sex or other types of homogeneous groups and excessive preoccupation with task accomplishment or satisfaction of social-emotional need'.

NAME :		DATE :

Night hours	
05.00 am	
05.30 am	
06.00 am	
06.30 am	
07.00 am	
07.30 am	
08.00 am	
08.30 am	
09.00 am	
09.30 am	
10.00 am	
10.30 am	
11.00 am	
11.30 am	
12 noon	
12.30 pm	
01.00 pm	
01.30 pm	
02.00 pm	
02.30 pm	
03.00 pm	
03.30 pm	
04.00 pm	
04.30 pm	
05.00 pm	
05.30 pm	
06.00 pm	
06.30 pm	
07.00 pm	
07.30 pm	
08.00 pm	
08.30 pm	
09.00 pm	
09.30 pm	
10.00 pm	
10.30 pm	
11.00 pm	
11.30 pm	
12 midnight	
00.30 am	

Figure 5.2 Activities in a typical day.

There are other skills, such as level of cognitive ability, which are not directly observable (Allen & Allen 1987). Again, these skills can be assessed by linking them to observable performance. Allen & Allen (1987) suggested that the individual's level of cognitive disability is indicated by the activities he is unable to perform. A battery of craft activities was devised to measure precisely the level of disability.

Checklists can be used to make sure no skill area has been missed during the assessment. The types of checklist commonly used by occupational therapists include:

- broad assessments, such as the Occupational Therapy Development Analysis, Evaluation and Intervention Schedule (DAEIS)
- assessments of specific skill areas, such as ADL checklists and task inventories
- multidisciplinary assessments, such as the Personal Assessment Chart (PAC).

Performance scales may be norm referenced or criterion referenced. Norm-referenced scales are those in which a typical range of performance has been identified by administering the test to a broad sample. The client's performance is compared with this typical, or normative, performance. Criterion-referenced scales are those in which the client's performance is judged against the desired outcome of intervention. A criterion sets the standard of performance which the client hopes to achieve by the end of treatment.

Some of the many areas of performance that can be assessed by the use of checklists or performance scales include adaptive skills, sensory integration, past and present life roles, balance of occupations, motivation, interests, locus of control and time structuring. Three of these will be described here: the Mayers Lifestyle Questionnaire, the Interest Checklist and the Occupational Questionnaire. Readers are recommended to follow up references at the end of the chapter for details of further methods.

Mayer's Lifestyle Questionnaire

The Mayers' Lifestyle Questionnaire was developed by Mayers (2004) to enable people with enduring mental health problems to state their priority needs in terms of quality of life at the beginning of an occupational therapy intervention. It consists of nine sections:

- looking after yourself
- living situation
- looking after others
- being with others
- being in or out of work/attending college
- beliefs and values
- finances
- choices
- activities.

Some items require yes or no answers. Others are rated as 'independently', 'with difficulty' or 'with extreme difficulty'. The client completes the questionnaire either independently or with the aid of the therapist.

The questionnaire was formulated following completion and analysis of interviews with clients experiencing enduring mental illness and both a pilot study and main study have been completed to evaluate its use. The questionnaire can also be used as an outcome measure by comparing responses and positioning of ticks with copies of the questionnaire completed at an earlier stage of intervention.

The Interest Checklist

The Interest Checklist was developed by Matsutsuyu (1969) to assess clients' interests in order to facilitate the selection of therapeutic activities that would evoke and sustain interest throughout the treatment programme. It includes 80 items that the client can mark under the headings of 'casual interest', 'strong interest' or 'no interest'. These include activities such as cooking, gardening, solitaire, religion and swimming. There is space to add any other interests not included in the list and space for a written report on the client's interests from schooldays to the present.

Matsutsuyu suggested six propositions to describe the properties of the interest phenomenon.

- Interests are influenced by early experiences in the family.
- Interests are affective in nature and evoke positive or negative emotional responses.

- Making choices on the basis of interest leads to commitment to the roles chosen.
- Interest leads the individual to engage in activities that teach him how to act effectively to achieve his goals.
- Interest in a task can sustain action after the novelty of the task has worn off.
- Interests reflect the image a person has of himself.

These six propositions became the theoretical basis for designing an interest checklist.

The data from this checklist can be classified by intensity of interest felt, ability to express personal preference, ability to discriminate type and intensity of interests and categories of interest. All the items on the list can be classified as manual skills, physical sports, social recreation, activities of daily living or cultural/educational.

From this information it should be possible to select activities that will maintain the client's commitment to treatment for the attainment of either short-term or long-term goals.

The Occupational Questionnaire

This questionnaire was developed for use within the Model of Human Occupation (Kielhofner 1988). It consists of a daily timetable in half-hour blocks for the client to fill in to show his typical way of spending time on a working day or a non-working day. Each activity can then be rated by the client as being, in the client's perception:

- work
- a daily living task
- recreation
- rest.

The client is also asked to rate each activity on a five-point scale for:

- how well he thinks he performs it – personal causation
- how important he thinks it is – values
- how much he likes it – interest.

The questionnaire is designed to provide data about the client's habits, balance of activities, feeling of competence, interests and values, and to show up problems in any of these areas. Used in collaboration with the client, it can assist in setting therapeutic goals. The results can be displayed in various ways to give a visual picture that the client will understand, for example a pie chart or a profile, since it is necessary for the client to be involved in interpreting the results.

The questionnaire can also be filled in for a time when the client feels he was functioning effectively, so that a comparison can be made with present functioning.

Other versions of the questionnaire are now being developed to measure different aspects of the client; for example, one version highlights the amount of pain and fatigue the client is experiencing.

Projective techniques

Projective techniques were developed as a method of assessing emotions, motivations and values, none of which could be measured with existing tools. Early techniques included the Rorschach Inkblot Test, Morgan and Murray's Thematic Apperception Test and Cattell's Sentence Completion Test. All these tests present subjects with ambiguous stimuli to which they are asked to give meaning. Projective tests use standard stimuli that allow subjects to make their own interpretations. The theory behind them is that the subject does not know what is expected (i.e. what would constitute a good performance) and therefore performs spontaneously.

The material projected by the subject may be one of three types.

1. Projection was described by Freud as an ego-defence mechanism through which painful or unacceptable feelings are ascribed to someone else. This is an unconscious process.
2. Projection can also be a way of giving meaning to situations that are otherwise confusing by seeing them in terms of one's own motives and beliefs.
3. Projection may be an unconscious method of wish fulfilment; for example, a woman who does not find it easy to attract men may think that all men have designs on her (Munn 1966).

All three aspects of projection are involved in projective techniques.

The use of projective techniques by occupational therapists

Occupational therapists use projective techniques in two ways.

1. Creation of an object by the client, such as a painting, or presentation of a stimulus by the therapist, such as a poem, followed by a period of discussion in which the client is encouraged to express his feelings about the object freely. This is usually done in a group.
2. Presentation of a series of standard activities to the client with an assessment of how he copes with them.

Using projective techniques in groups

The distinguishing feature of occupational therapy as opposed to other therapies is the presence of objects that can be manipulated by the client. These objects may already be available or may be created by the client (Azima & Azima 1959). Thus, projective techniques are an appropriate method of assessment for occupational therapists because they involve doing as well as, or instead of, talking.

Most of the projective techniques used by occupational therapists involve a phase of creating, which can be structured or unstructured, and a phase of talking about the created object or free-associating about it. The technique is used as assessment and as a form of treatment simultaneously, in that therapists help clients to accept projected material as their own and gain insight into how their own perceptions are formed.

Projective tests developed by occupational therapists

Two projective tests developed by occupational therapists for individual use are the Azima Battery and the Goodman Battery.

The Azima Battery is a typical projective technique developed by an occupational therapist (Azima 1982). This utilises three tasks: a free pencil drawing, drawings of a person of each sex and a free clay model. These are presented to the client in a standard order and method. The client is given a set period of time to complete each task. During the 'doing' phase of the test, the therapist records the time taken, the client's behaviour, any verbalisations and the techniques used. When the work is finished the client is asked to describe his productions.

An evaluation scale is used to interpret the results of the battery. This includes organisation of mood, organisation of drives and organisation of object relations, all of which are inferred from aspects of the client's observed behaviour and content of speech. Findings are analysed and presented as a summary to be used in differential diagnosis, treatment planning and prognosis (Azima 1982).

The Goodman Battery was developed from the Azima Battery and differs from it in that the tasks given are progressively less structured, thus making it possible to assess cognition and ego functioning under decreasingly structured conditions. It was designed for use with young adults and adults suffering from psychiatric disorders.

The four tasks in the battery are: copying a mosaic tile, spontaneous drawing, figure drawing and free clay modelling. The tester assesses the client's ability to conceptualise, to organise and to plan procedures that will enable him to complete the tasks. The theory underlying this technique is that the individual's ability to carry out practical tasks will be affected by the presence of conflicts and defences that consume energy and by weak ego boundaries. When ego boundaries are weak, performance may be expected to deteriorate as the external structure becomes looser.

A guide has been developed to help in the recording and interpretation of findings, and rating scales are used for the different aspects of performance. These include ability to organise, independence and self-esteem (Evaskus 1982).

SUMMARY

This chapter has discussed the assessment and outcome measurement stages of the occupational therapy process. Assessment is an integral part of intervention, not a series of separate stages, and this should be borne in mind when reading the next chapter, planning and implementation.

References

Allen CK 1985 Occupational therapy for psychiatric diseases: measurement and management of cognitive disabilities. Little Brown, Boston

Allen CK, Allen RE 1987 Cognitive disabilities: measuring the consequences of mental disorders. Clinical Psychiatry 48(5):185-190

Azima FJC 1982 The Azima Battery: an overview. In: Hemphill BJ (ed) The evaluative process in psychiatric occupational therapy. Slack, New Jersey

Azima H, Azima F 1959 Outline of a dynamic theory of occupational therapy. American Journal of Occupational Therapy 13:1-7

Creek J 2003 Occupational therapy defined as a complex intervention. College of Occupational Therapists, London

ENOTHE 2006 European Network of Occupational Therapists in Higher Education Terminology Project. www.enothe.hva.nl

Evaskus MG 1982 The Goodman Battery. In: Hemphill BJ (ed) The evaluative process in psychiatric occupational therapy. Slack, New Jersey

Felce B, McBrien J 1987 Workshop: challenging behaviour in mental handicap. Stockport

Fidler GS, Fidler J W 1978 Doing and becoming: purposeful action and self-actualization. American Journal of Occupational Therapy 32(5):305-310

Fisher AG 1995 The Assessment of Motor and Process Skills (Manual and software package). Three Star Press, US

Florey LL, Michelman SM 1982 Occupational role history: a screening tool for psychiatric occupational therapy. American Journal of Occupational Therapy 36(5):301-308

Forsyth K, Kielhofner G 2006 The Model of Human Occupation: integrating theory into practice and practice into theory. In: Duncan EAS (ed) Foundations for practice in occupational therapy, 4th edn. Elsevier Churchill Livingstone, Edinburgh

Garfield M 1982 The principles of developing assessment tools. In: Hemphill BJ (ed) The evaluative process in psychiatric occupational therapy. Slack, New Jersey

Hemphill BJ (ed) 1982 The evaluative process in psychiatric occupational therapy. Slack, New Jersey

Hogg J, Raynes N V 1987 Assessment in mental handicap: a guide to assessment, practices, tests and checklists. Croom Helm, London

Kielhofner G 1988 Workshop: the model of human occupation. York

Laver AJ, Powell G 1995 The Structured Observational Test of Function. NFER-Nelson, Windsor

Law M, Baptiste S, Carswell A et al 1994 Canadian Occupational Performance Measure. 2nd edn. CAOT Publications ACE, Toronto

Matsutsuyu JS 1969 The interest checklist. American Journal of Occupational Therapy 23(4):323-328

Mattingley C, Fleming MH 1994 Clinical reasoning. Slack, Philadelphia

Mayers C 2004 The Mayers' Lifestyle Questionnaire (2). School of Professional Health Studies, York St. John College, York

McDowell I, Newell C 1996 Measuring health: a guide to rating scales and questionnaires, 2nd edn. Oxford University Press, New York

Mocellin G 1988 A perspective on the principles and practice of occupational therapy. British Journal of Occupational Therapy 51(1):4-7

Mosey AC 1973 Meeting health needs. American Journal of Occupational Therapy 27(1):14-17

Mosey AC 1986 Psychosocial components of occupational therapy. Raven Press, New York

Munn NL 1966 Psychology: the fundamentals of human adjustment, 5th edn. Houghton Mifflin, Boston

Opacich KJ 1991 Assessment and informed decision-making. In: Christiansen C, Baum C (eds) Occupational therapy: overcoming human performance deficits. Slack, Philadelphia

Ottenbacher KJ, Cusick A 1993 Discriminative versus evaluative assessment: some observations on goal attainment scaling. Alternative strategies for functional assessment. American Journal of Occupational Therapy 47(4):349-354

Pollock N, McColl MA, Carswell A 1999 The Canadian Occupational Performance Measure. In: Sumsion T (ed) Client-centred practice in occupational therapy: a guide to implementation. Churchill Livingstone, Edinburgh

Reed KL, Sanderson SN 1992 Concepts of occupational therapy, 3rd edn. Williams and Wilkins, Baltimore

Royal College of Psychiatrists 1999 Health of the Nation Outcome Scales for Mentally Disordered Offenders. Royal College of Psychiatrists, London

Seedhouse D 1986 Health: the foundations for achievement. Wiley, Chichester

Spencer EA 1988 Functional restoration: preliminary concepts and planning. In: Hopkins HL, Smith HD (eds) Willard and Spackman's occupational therapy, 7th edn. J B Lippincott, Philadelphia

Spreadbury P 1998 You will measure outcomes. In: Creek J (ed) Occupational therapy: new perspectives. Whurr, London

Spreadbury P, Cook S 1995 Measuring the outcomes of individualised care: The Binary Individualised Outcome Measure. Trent Regional Health Authority, Nottingham

Unsworth CA 1993 The concept of function. British Journal of Occupational Therapy 56(8):287–292

Chapter 6

Planning and implementation

Jennifer Creek, Alison Bullock

INTRODUCTION

In Chapter 5 we looked at the assessment stages of the occupational therapy process. This chapter looks in detail at planning and implementing interventions, starting from the point where the initial assessment has been carried out and the therapist and client are ready to begin identifying needs and setting goals for intervention, as shown in Figure 6.1.

The chapter describes the process of analysing the client's expected occupations and environments and identifying any functional problems that are interfering with occupational performance. This information enables the therapist and client to agree on the need for intervention and formulate the problems to be addressed. The next stage of the process is goal setting and this section covers setting long-term, short-term and intermediate goals.

Once the goals of intervention have been negotiated and agreed, the therapist and client plan the actions to be taken to reach them. This section describes methods of task analysis, activity

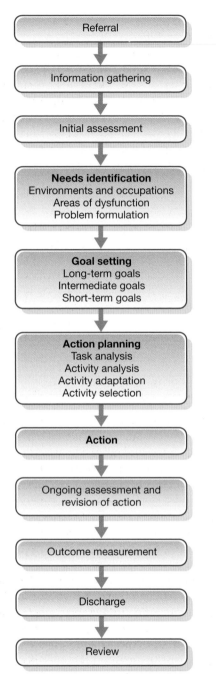

Figure 6.1 The treatment planning and implementation process.

achieving therapeutic goals, the therapist considers the client's motivation, volition and autonomy. An extended activity analysis format is given that can be used when considering aspects of activity that have the potential to engage the participant, together with a sample extended activity analysis.

The next section of the chapter looks at what is involved in putting the plan into action. The elements of intervention are the client, the therapist, the activity and the environment.

The chapter ends with a discussion of some of the practicalities and policies that make up the context in which occupational therapy interventions take place, including the multidisciplinary team, case management, case review, clinical governance, evidence-based practice and continuing professional development.

NEEDS IDENTIFICATION

Analysis of data obtained from the initial assessment produces two key areas of information that enable the therapist and client to identify areas of need and formulate the problems to be addressed:

1. the client's expected environments and occupations
2. areas of dysfunction that might interfere with the fulfilment of these occupations.

ENVIRONMENTS AND OCCUPATIONS

The client cannot be considered in isolation from his physical and social environments, since the skills he will require are determined by the demands of those environments, the occupations the client performs within them and the support available. The client may expect to return to his previous environments and previous level of functioning if the problem requiring intervention is an acute one. He may have recently been diagnosed with a serious illness, in which case there will be a lot of unknowns in his future. He may have a chronic disability that necessitates changes to the occupations that make up his life.

analysis and activity adaptation. A generic activity analysis format is given, with a sample activity analysis. In order to ensure that the activities selected are appropriate to the client, as well as

The therapist needs to be clear about what the client expects to do in the future and what skills he will need in order to cope. Dysfunction can only be defined relative to the client's expected occupations and environments; there is no universal standard of achievement for all clients.

AREAS OF DYSFUNCTION

A person usually requires occupational therapy intervention because he is unable to meet the demands of his physical or social environments, because the demands have changed, the client has changed or he has never been able to cope adequately. The therapist's task is to identify areas of dysfunction where there is a gap between the skills the client needs and the skills that he has. There may be a general deficit across several skill areas, for example problems with literacy, numeracy and social skills, or there may be a specific deficit, such as poor anger management.

Each person requires a range of skills in order to be able to perform his occupations. Lack of skills, or insufficient competence in skills, can lead to the individual being unable to perform the occupations that support his participation in society. For example, if someone has difficulty managing his time, so that he gets up at a different time every day, he may find it hard to hold down a job. Skills for living are discussed in more detail in Chapter 19.

In addition to looking at the range of skills the client has, the therapist assesses whether or not he has achieved a sufficient level of competence to carry out his expected occupations and whether skills have been organised into routines that allow for efficient use of time and energy. This assessment highlights the skill areas that must be developed if the client is to fulfil his expected occupations and leads on to setting goals for achieving those skills.

PROBLEM FORMULATION

When the therapist and client have identified the client's main problem areas and agreed which ones to work on first, the therapist formulates these problems in such a way that the goals of intervention are clear. *Problem formulation is* 'the process of identifying and recording the

difficulties an individual is having which may require action' (Creek 2003, p57).

Complex problems can be analysed in different ways, using a variety of theoretical perspectives, each of which will produce a different formulation. For example, the problem of the client who gets up at a different time every day could be seen as a skill deficit (poor time management), a task performance problem (it takes too much effort to leave the television and go to bed at night), an activity limitation (too many of his preferred activities take place during the night) or an occupational performance problem (he has never had a job or developed good work habits). The problem of sleeping during the day could be formulated in all these ways, each of which would potentially lead to a different approach to treatment.

Once the therapist and client have agreed on how the client's problems are to be recorded and on priorities for action, they can set specific goals for the intervention.

GOAL SETTING

Goals are the targets that the client hopes to reach through involvement in occupational therapy. They define both the outcomes to be achieved and the level of performance that will be acceptable. Goals must be within the client's capabilities and he must adopt them as his own. The involvement of clients is crucial in setting occupational therapy goals because people are experts in their own lives and know what they need to achieve in order to live those lives successfully.

When goals have been set, the client should know exactly what is expected of him and how he is to reach them. The client and the therapist can see what progress has been made by measuring the outcomes of therapy against the original goals. Goals must be couched in clear and specific terms so that the therapist, the client and any other interested parties understand the purpose of the intervention and know when it should be terminated. For example, 'getting fit' is too vague to be an outcome goal but 'walking the dog for at least 2 miles twice a day' is specific and measurable.

Attaching a performance indicator to the goal allows both the client and the therapist to see when it has been reached. For example, a woman with severe anxiety and social phobia has the overall aim of feeling less anxious in company. Her immediate goal is to be able to walk into a room with people in it and not feel anxious. The performance marker she identifies, that will enable her to tell when the goal has been attained to a standard that is satisfactory for her, is to be able to walk into the group room and initiate a conversation with someone within the first 10 minutes.

More information on setting outcome goals can be found in Chapter 5.

Client goals are usually set on two or three levels.

- **Long-term goals** are the overall goals of the intervention, the reasons why the client is being offered help and the expected outcome of intervention. Long-term goals are usually expressed in terms of occupational performance or participation in life situations.
- **Intermediate goals** may be clusters of skills to be developed, attitudes to be changed or barriers to be overcome on the way to achieving the main goals of therapy. In a crisis intervention or other acute episode of treatment, it may not be necessary to use intermediate goals; the fluid nature of the problem and the short intervention time allow problems to be tackled rapidly.
- **Short-term goals** are the small steps on the way to achieving major goals. The short-term goal is usually to learn a subskill or skill component of the adaptive skill that is needed for successful occupational performance (Mosey 1986). Short-term goals are organised into a sequence, with the most basic goal to be tackled first.

LONG-TERM GOALS

As discussed in the previous chapter, the occupational therapist and client produce from the initial assessment a general picture of the client's life situation, balance of occupations, areas of skills deficit and future needs. These data should suggest overall aims, or long-term goals, of intervention.

Whenever possible, the client's own perception of his needs is the guiding principle in setting aims, since he is the person who must achieve them. However, certain problems impair the ability to make rational decisions about the future. These may be temporary, as in severe depression, or permanent, as in dementia. In such cases the therapist may take a stronger lead in establishing goals, while recognising that these are subject to review as the client changes during the intervention and becomes able to express his opinions. If the therapist takes a strongly supportive role in the early stages it may be difficult to pass personal responsibility back to the client at a later stage, so one of the stated goals of intervention should be for the client to take responsibility for his own progress as and when he is able.

In many cases the client will expect to return to his previous occupations, so interventions are designed to restore lost skills, teach additional skills or improve the performance of existing skills in order to prevent recurrence of problems. In other cases the problem that caused the client to seek help is unlikely to be completely overcome, so that a change in occupations and the skills needed to support them can be anticipated.

The overall goals of the treatment team will also influence the goals set for occupational therapy intervention. The occupational therapy programme is a part of a wider treatment programme and will play a greater or lesser part in achieving its aims.

Box 6.1 Long–term goals

Julie, a young woman with a diagnosis of schizophrenia, lived alone in a flat and had not worked for several years. Her psychotic symptoms were controlled by medication but she had episodes of acute psychosis which sometimes resulted in a period of hospitalisation. She found that the episodic nature of her illness caused disruption in many areas of her life, including self-care, productivity and social activities. During an acute episode, whether or not she was hospitalised, she was not able to perform her usual range of activities. Afterwards, she found it hard to pick them up again and, over time, felt an increasing sense of failure.

Julie began to attend a weekly women's craft group run by two occupational therapists at a social services day centre. Her personal goals were to find ways of picking up her activities again after an episode of illness and to finish what she started.

INTERMEDIATE GOALS

Long-term goals may not take a long time to reach, particularly in an acute setting. However, in some cases they can take months or years to attain and may be modified to a greater or lesser extent during the process of intervention. In the latter case, it may be difficult for the client to imagine himself ever attaining his ultimate goals and it can be useful to set intermediate goals, which can be seen as easier to reach. These are smaller goals that lead towards attainment of long-term goals.

Certain disorders, such as dementia, interfere with the ability of clients to take a temporal perspective and therefore with their ability to plan for the long-term future. These clients will have difficulty in setting realistic long-term goals but may become involved in the planning process by setting smaller goals. The acute phase of illness may also interfere with a person's perception of his own potential and make his involvement in long-term goal setting impossible, although intermediate goals can still be discussed. For example, the therapist might feel that it is appropriate for a severely depressed client to aim to return home once the acute phase of the illness is over. During the acute phase, the client feels utterly hopeless about the possibility of ever leaving hospital but is able to accept intermediate goals of attending a supportive psychotherapy group twice a week and a creative activity group once a week.

Three main factors determine what the intermediate goals should be:

1. the client's wishes
2. any barriers to performance that need to be overcome, for example, an overprotective family who are reluctant to allow the disabled member to become more independent
3. the advantages of learning skills in a developmental sequence so that higher level skills are built on lower level skills.

SHORT–TERM GOALS

When long-term and/or intermediate goals have been agreed they can be broken down into a sequence of smaller steps. Each short-term goal needs to be realistically within the client's reach and a decision must be made about where to start. Short-term goals can be set or changed at any point in the process of intervention to meet changing needs. Each goal should be measurable, so that client and therapist know when it has been reached.

Once short-term goals have been agreed, a programme of activities that will lead to their achievement is planned. Knowledge of activity analysis and synthesis enables the therapist to identify or modify activities to incorporate all the skills, personal factors and environmental factors that will best bring about change.

Box 6.2 Intermediate goals

After attending four sessions of the women's group in order to find out what it could offer, Julie had a goal-setting interview with one of the occupational therapists. She agreed to attend the group for a further 8 weeks and set two goals to achieve in that time. The first was to return to the group if she had to have time off for health reasons. The second was to finish every item that she started making. Julie and the therapist recorded these goals and set a date to review progress in 8 weeks time.

Box 6.3 Short–term goals

Over the 8-week period that Julie was attending the group, she began to experience paranoid delusions. She discussed how she felt with the occupational therapist and they agreed that Julie could use the smoking room for time out if she became panicky during a group session. However, she had to return to the group room before the session ended. If Julie was unable to meet this condition, it was agreed that she would take some time off from attending the group until her florid symptoms settled down.

ACTION PLANNING

Occupational therapy interventions are individualised and programme planning is done with and for each client. It is a collaborative process that involves the therapist, the client, the carer and other professionals in devising a unique solution to the problems of this individual under a particular set of circumstances (Creek 2003).

Activity is the main tool that occupational therapists use to bring about changes in function. In order to select the most suitable activity to bring about the desired change, we need to know exactly what demands an activity will make on the client, what skills are required for the performance of the activity and how activities can be adapted to change those demands and skills. In addition to analysing activities for their performance demands, the therapist also considers their potential to engage the client's interest and contribute to a positive sense of self. This section looks in more detail at both these aspects of activity analysis.

Some activities are simple and can be analysed for all their components. For example, making a cup of tea is usually a simple activity. Other activities take place in a more complicated sequence of tasks that make different demands. For example, doing the household shopping involves finding out what is needed and making a shopping list, getting to the shops, buying what is on the list, bringing the shopping home and putting it away. Each stage of the activity has different performance requirements. If the activity is a complicated one, with each stage making different performance demands, the therapist will carry out a task analysis to identify the sequence of steps before carrying out a detailed activity analysis.

TASK ANALYSIS

Any activity is made up of steps or tasks that are performed in sequence. Discovering the task sequence of an activity is called *task analysis*. For example, in making a clay pinch pot the tasks are:

- cut an appropriately sized piece of clay
- wedge the clay
- shape clay into a ball
- push thumb into clay
- pinch the clay to the required thickness all over
- smooth the inner and outer surfaces
- add any embellishments or decoration
- leave to dry out before firing.

Any one of these steps could be analysed into a further series of tasks: for example, there is a sequence of steps involved in wedging a ball of clay. Task analysis is carried out for a purpose and the extent to which an activity is analysed into smaller and smaller tasks will depend on the purpose of the analysis. If a person has very specific difficulties it may be necessary to carry out a detailed task analysis to isolate the precise problem. On the other hand, if the therapist is analysing a fairly simple activity in order to teach it to a client, it may only be necessary to identify the main steps of the activity.

Task analysis may be carried out in order to:

1. select an appropriate teaching method for an activity, for example, backward chaining (teaching the last stage of the task first, so that the therapist carries out most of the activity and the client completes it)
2. select an appropriate activity to meet a therapeutic aim
3. adapt an activity to meet client needs by changing or eliminating a step
4. identify the precise part of an activity a client is having difficulty performing.

The therapist needs to be cautious about concentrating on a single step in the sequence of actions that make up an activity. Clients should be given opportunities to practise whole activities rather than single tasks because 'performance does not occur normally in a step by step approach but rather as an integrated continuous flow of behavioural performance. Failure to provide practice in the whole sequence may result in halting, awkward performance' (Reed & Sanderson 1992, p174).

ACTIVITY ANALYSIS

Activity analysis is 'a process of dissecting an activity into its component parts and task sequence in order to identify its inherent properties and the skills required for its performance, thus allowing the therapist to evaluate its therapeutic potential' (Creek 2003, p49). An activity can be analysed for all its component parts that come within the domain of the occupational therapist. Mosey (1986) called this the generic approach and pointed out that there is no universally accepted framework for doing this. An alternative approach is to study only those components that are relevant to the model or frame of reference being used; for example, activity analysis within a psychodynamic model focuses on the psychological functions and psychosocial interactions involved in performing an activity (Katz 1985).

The format presented here is a generic one that was developed from several different frameworks (Fidler & Fidler 1963, Hopkins & Tiffany 1988, Llorens 1976, Mosey 1986).

The performance of activities requires many skills that can be divided for the purpose of analysis into:

- physical
- cognitive
- psychological
- interpersonal.

In order to understand the effect that an activity might have on the client, the therapist needs to break it down into these skill areas and look at each one in detail.

Activity analysis also includes any potential for adapting the activity in order to allow for change in the client. Grading allows the client to move on to the next goal once a skill has been mastered. Grading may involve a gradual change in the nature of the activity by changing one or two components, or a complete change of activity.

Analysing an activity enables the therapist to:

- understand the demands the activity will make on the client; that is, the range of skills required for its performance
- assess what needs the activity might satisfy
- determine the extent to which the activity might inhibit undesirable behaviour
- determine whether or not the activity is within the client's capacity
- discover the skills that the activity can develop in the client; these may be specific skills, such as threading a needle, or more general, transferable skills, such as reading
- provide a basis for adapting and grading activities to achieve particular outcomes.

Table 6.1 shows a generic activity analysis format and Table 6.2 shows how it was used to analyse a particular activity, hill walking.

ACTIVITY ADAPTATION

The therapist and client together identify those activities that have the greatest potential to achieve the desired outcomes. For example, if the client's main goal is to improve his general fitness, they may decide that walking is the most appropriate activity to begin with.

Alternatively, activity components may be combined into new activities that will better achieve the desired goals. This is called *activity synthesis*. For example, the client's secondary goal may be to find a part-time job, so the therapist suggests that he walk to the library every day to look for jobs in the newspapers.

An activity may be adjusted or modified to suit the client's needs: this is called *activity adaptation*. For example, if the client is not fit enough to walk to the library and back, he could take the bus for part of the way.

An activity can be adapted in stages so that it becomes progressively more demanding as the client's skills improve or less demanding as the client's function deteriorates. This is called *activity grading*. For example, the client can walk more of the distance to the library each week as his strength and stamina improve.

Activity sequencing can be used as an alternative or adjunct to activity grading. *Activity sequencing* means 'finding or designing a sequence of different but related activities that will incrementally increase the demands made on the individual as her/his performance improves or decrease them as her/his performance deteriorates' (Creek 2003, p38). For example, as the client feels more confident about his fitness, he could join a walking group or take up swimming, cycling or dancing.

The elements in an activity that have potential for change to enable adaptation and grading are:

- the materials and equipment used (media)
- the environment, including other people involved
- the method of carrying out the activity.

Table 6.1 Activity analysis format

Name of activity	Appropriateness for different ages and sexes
Timing/length of time/number of sessions	Social and cultural appropriateness
Special features of the environment (space and setting)	Preparation (tools, equipment, materials, environment, partici-
Brief description of activity	pants, therapist)
	Precautions

Performance requirements

Physical	*Psychological*
Sensation	Expression of feelings
Sensory integration	Control of feelings
Perception	Frustration tolerance
Spatial awareness	Coping with pressure
Motor planning	Sublimation
Gross motor movement	Playing/exploring
Mobility	Tolerating risk
Balance	Trust
Fine motor movement	Independence
Repetition	Passive or active
Rhythm	Spiritual dimension
Co-ordination	Creativity
Strength	Exploration of feelings and motives
Endurance	Responsibility
Flexibility	Involvement
Range of movement	Sharing
Posture	Self-image
Types of movement	Body image
Speed	Identification
	Sexual identity
	End product
	Contrived or real experience

Cognitive	*Interpersonal*
Attention	Individual or group/size of group
Concentration	Mixed or segregated sexes
Discrimination	Communication
Generalisation	Co-operation
Use of symbols	Competition
Perceiving cause and effect	Negotiation
Abstract thinking	Sharing
Reality testing	Compromise
Choice	Leadership
Language	Structure
Following demonstration/instructions	Rules
Reading	Interaction
Writing	Isolation
Numbers	Variety of relationships
Spatial orientation	Involvement
Awareness of time	Role opportunities
Memory	
Range of knowledge	
Goal setting	

Table 6.1   Cont'd

Planning
Organisation
Number of processes
Imagination
Creativity
Logic
Problem solving

Potential for grading

Materials and equipment
Environment – human and non-human
Method
Related activities (for sequencing)

Table 6.2   Sample activity analysis: hill walking

Name of activity: Hill walking

   Timing/length of time/number of sessions: It is usually safer and more interesting to walk during the day, although some routes are traditionally followed at night. Time has to be allowed for getting to the start and returning after the walk. A hill walk could last from half an hour to a full day. It can be done as often as time and fitness allow.

   Special features of the environment: This is an outdoor activity that requires a lot of space. Open hills, such as moorland, are ideal for hill walking.

   Brief description of activity: The individual or group plan a linear or circular route to suit them and walk from the start to the finish, taking breaks as they wish.

   Appropriateness for different ages and sexes: Not suitable for very young children unless they can be carried all or part of the way. Can be enjoyed by both sexes.

   Social and cultural appropriateness: In most parts of the UK, this activity is more popular with older people and may not be attractive to young people. There are many organisations that plan and organise walks for groups of people, such as the Ramblers Association.

   Preparation: It is necessary to have good equipment for walking in open country, including walking boots, warm, light-weight and waterproof clothing and, if desired, sticks or poles. Maps and compasses are important for safety. Food, drink and extra clothing should be carried. The walker or group leader should be familiar with the route and should let someone know the route and expected time of return.

   Precautions: Check the weather forecast before setting out. Ensure that participants are medically fit for the exercise. Check that everyone has suitable boots and clothing. Count the number in the group at regular intervals during the walk to make sure no-one is lost.

Performance requirements

Physical

Good mobility for negotiating rough terrain.
Balance when walking on uneven paths or downhill.
Visual-spatial perception for finding the best place to step. Stamina when walking up hills.
Rhythmic walking on smoother surfaces.

Cognitive

Choosing and planning an appropriate route.
Selecting appropriate clothing and equipment.
Awareness of walking speed, personal stamina and distance that can be achieved within time available.
Attention to the terrain to avoid accidents.
Following a planned route, a map or a leader.
Ability to read signs and symbols marking pathways.
Use of compass to find direction, if necessary.

Table 6.2   Cont'd

Psychological

Ability to tolerate open spaces, risk of getting lost and physical effort.
There may be physical discomfort due to weather and/or terrain.
Opportunities to explore countryside and own physical abilities.
Can be an independent activity, could lead a group or could be a group member.
Need to trust group leader and own abilities.
Necessity of reaching the end of the walk even when tired or bored.
No concrete end product.

Interpersonal

Could be an individual or a group activity, usually 10–20 people.
Mixed sexes.
Group walking requires communication to agree on the route and make arrangements to meet.
Co-operation and compromise are needed for setting a pace that suits everyone and making sure no-one falls behind.
Not usually competitive.
Loose structure but everyone is expected to follow the leader and let him know if they intend to drop out.
Rules of the countryside include keeping to paths, not dropping litter and closing gates.
Interaction between group members is mostly optional but some conversation is expected.

Potential for grading

Materials and equipment

Walking poles or sticks.
Type and weight of bag carried.

Environment

Steepness and number of gradients.
Type of paths and number of stiles.
Weather.
Alone or in a group.
With or without a dog.

Method

Amount of guidance.
Speed of walking.
Distance.
Number of breaks.

Related activities

Urban walking.
Field walking.
Jogging.
Cycling.
Dancing.

These three dimensions can be manipulated to achieve the desired therapeutic result. For example, the activity of walking can be made easier by using a stick (equipment), using a companion's arm for support (environment) or walking slowly (method). Walking can be made more demanding by carrying a heavy rucksack (equipment), walking up hills (environment) or walking and talking at the same time (method).

ACTIVITY SELECTION

It is necessary but not sufficient to identify the performance demands of an activity. If the client is to be engaged by the activity it must also be interesting, acceptable and of some value. Throughout the occupational therapy process described in Chapter 4 and earlier in this chapter, the therapist attempts to involve the client fully, engage his interest, elicit his co-operation and earn his trust. If she succeeds, there should be few problems in the implementation of therapeutic activities. Selecting activities that the client will find worthwhile and interesting, that will engage him, is the next step.

Engagement is 'the experience of involving oneself in an undertaking, occupying oneself in an activity or interest …When someone is engaged in an activity, his attention is focused on a goal and/ or on the experience, not on the skills and effort required' (Creek 2007). The factors that influence the extent to which someone engages in an activity are motivation, volition and autonomy.

Motivation

Motivation is 'a drive that directs a person's actions towards meeting needs' (ENOTHE 2006); it has been described as the energy source for action (du Toit 1974). Motivation can be extrinsic or intrinisic.

Extrinsic motivation is 'the drive to avoid harm and meet needs' (Creek 2007). For example, a woman's motivation for running three times a week is the desire to keep herself fit and maintain a healthy body weight. The circumstances that trigger extrinsic motivation can be external, such as cold weather prompting a man to wear warmer clothes, or internal, such as hunger causing him to eat. The therapist may use rewards to trigger extrinsic motivation, such as suggesting that the client chooses his favourite food to cook for lunch, or providing a cup of coffee during an interview.

Intrinsic motivation is 'the drive to act for the enjoyment of exercising one's capacities, for learning and for taking pleasure in activity' (Creek 2007). For example, a woman's motivation for rock climbing is intrinsic: she loves the challenge,

the exercise and the environment. Reilly (1974) proposed that playful behaviour is intrinsically motivated and driven by the exploratory drive of curiosity. This drive has three stages.

- **Exploratory stage**. This occurs when an event is new to the individual. Exploratory behaviour is focused on sensory experience and 'the pure pleasure of doing something for its own sake' (Reilly 1974, p146). The therapist can trigger exploratory behaviour by displaying a variety of interesting and attractive materials or offering a choice of new activities.
- **Competency stage.** This is characterised by a drive to have an active influence on the environment and, in turn, to be influenced by it. Competency behaviour is focused on practising a task until it has been mastered. Reilly suggested that persistence in a task is only elicited if the individual has 'trust in the environment and confidence in self'(Reilly 1974, p146). The therapist can maintain competency behaviour by setting tasks that have just the right degree of challenge to interest the client without seeming too difficult to attempt, and by creating a safe and accepting therapeutic ambience.
- **Achievement stage.** Motivation at this stage has moved from intrinsic to extrinsic because the individual measures his achievements against external standards of good or bad as well as against his personal sense of what is acceptable. Achievement behaviour is focused on performance and on competing with the self or with others. The therapist can support achievement behaviour by providing good-quality materials, giving sufficient support and allowing enough time for the client to reach a satisfactory standard.

Everyone has motivation, or a drive to be active, but people choose to do different things. The capacity to make choices about what to do is called volition.

Volition

Volition is 'the action of consciously willing or resolving something; the making of a definite choice or decision regarding a course of action' (New Shorter Oxford English Dictionary 1993). It has been defined for occupational therapists as 'the skill of being able to perceive and work towards a goal through choosing and performing activities that will achieve desired results' (Creek 2007).

Some of the factors that affect people's choices of action are as follows (Creek 2007).

- **Interests**: the 'individual's preferences for occupations based on the experience of pleasure and satisfaction in participating in those activities' (Kielhofner 1992, p157).
- **Personal goals**: the results that the individual wants to achieve by his actions.
- **Values**: the individual's 'personally held judgement of what is valuable and important in life' (Creek 2003, p60).
- **Awareness of own capacities**: the ability to predict one's own effectiveness in a given situation.
- **Meanings**: the significance or importance that an activity has for the person performing it (Creek 1998). These include the personal associations that it has for the individual and wider sociocultural meanings.
- **Nature of the choices available**: this will depend on what the environment can offer but also on the individual's ability to access an activity. For example, there may be a local cinema but a person cannot choose to watch a film if he does not have enough money.
- **Knowledge of what activities are available**: the individual can only choose activities that he is aware of.
- **Knowledge of how to access different activities**: it is not enough to know that an activity is available; the individual also has to know where it is, how to get there and the conditions for taking part.
- **Capacity to see opportunities for action**: some activities are not available all the time, so it may be necessary to know when they can be accessed. For example, it is usually necessary to enrol for adult education classes during a particular week of the year.
- **Information on which to base choices**: as can be seen from the last three points, a person needs information about what activities are available, how to access them and when they can be done.

The therapist can create conditions for the client to exercise volition by suggesting activities that have meaning and value for him, giving sufficient information about what is available and providing opportunities for him to practise making real choices. Some of the factors that the therapist might take into account when selecting or adapting activities to engage the client are shown in Table 6.3 and a sample extended activity analysis of hill walking is shown in Table 6.4.

Even if someone is highly motivated and able to choose a course of action, there will be times when he is unable to do what he wants due to circumstances. This means that his autonomy is compromised.

Autonomy

Autonomy is 'the capacity to think, decide and act on the basis of such thought and decision freely and independently and without … let or hindrance' (Gillon 1985/1986, p60). The ability to make and enact choices rests on three types of autonomy:

- **autonomy of thought**: being able to think for oneself, to have preferences and to make decisions
- **autonomy of will**: having the freedom to decide to do things on the basis of one's deliberations
- **autonomy of action**: the capacity to act on the basis of reasoning.

Autonomy is not an all-or-nothing condition; different people have varying levels of autonomy and it can vary for the same person at different times. For example, when I have a headache I find it more difficult to think clearly or to make decisions.

Conditions that may affect a person's autonomy include the following (Creek 2007).

- **Personal circumstances**: for example, poverty can block access to a range of activities.
- **Environmental barriers**: for example, lack of public transport can limit the choices available to someone who does not drive.
- **Social pressures**: for example, a young person may drink more alcohol than he wants in order to fit in with his peers.

Within the therapeutic environment, the therapist creates conditions that allow the client to exercise autonomy. However, it is also important

Table 6.3 Extended activity analysis format

Name of activity
Timing/length of time/number of sessions
Special features of the environment (space and setting)
Brief description of activity
Preparation (tools, equipment, materials, environment, participants, therapist)
Precautions

Performance requirements

Physical demands (e.g. sensation, co-ordination, fine motor skills, mobility)	Psychological demands (e.g. frustration, tolerance, trust, creativity, risk taking, autonomy)
Cognitive demands (e.g. attention, concentration, temporal awareness, abstract thinking, planning, knowledge)	Interpersonal demands (e.g. co-operation, compromise, sharing, competition)

Potential for engaging the client

Appropriateness	*Motivation*
Sex	Extrinsic
Age	Curiosity
Generation differences	Competence
Culture	Achievement
Religion	
Predictability	*Effect on identity*
Amount of structure	Personal identity
Certainty of the outcome	Social identity
Meaning	*Opportunities provided by the activity*
Actual and symbolic meaning in the components	To have an effect (e.g. on the self, on others, on the environment, on non-human objects)
Actual and symbolic meaning in the process	
Actual and symbolic meaning in the outcome	To develop (e.g. social identity, self-confidence, body image, managing emotions, perceiving others' feelings, construction of meaning)
Personal associations and inferences	
Social and cultural purpose and value	To gratify needs (e.g. create personal meaning, express feeling, exercise capacities, satisfy curiosity, identify with others, exercise choice, achieve)
	To learn (knowledge, skills, attitudes)
	To learn about the self (e.g. interests, abilities, limits)

Potential for grading

Materials and equipment
Environment – human and non-human
Method
Related activities (for sequencing)

to identify barriers within the client's own environments and to help him find ways of addressing them.

In this section, we have looked at some of the factors that the therapist takes into account when planning which activities to use to achieve therapeutic goals. Once the plan has been agreed with the client, it should be put in writing and copies given to the appropriate people, for example the client and the client's key worker. The next step in the occupational therapy process is treatment implementation or action.

Table 6.4   Sample extended activity analysis format

Name of activity: Hill walking

Timing/length of time/number of sessions Special features of the environment Brief description of activity Preparation Precautions	See Table 6.2

Performance requirements

See Table 6.2

Potential for engaging the client

Appropriateness

Suitable for both sexes.

Very young children may not be able to walk long distances.

In the UK, walking in an organised group tends to be seen as an activity for older people. Younger people may walk independently, often combining it with camping.

Motivation

Can be used to improve general fitness and stamina and to strengthen leg muscles. Walking in a group is a good way of meeting people. Can be combined with other interests such as bird watching or dog walking.

There are lots of footpaths in the UK, enabling exploration of different types of countryside and giving access to wonderful views.

Can be graded in length and difficulty to match different levels of fitness.

Different walking groups have their own preferred length of walk and pace so that a person can move on to more demanding walks as fitness improves. When walking in a group, it may be necessary for individuals to adjust their pace to match the others.

Predictability

Organised walks are planned and the length is advertised so that walkers know what to expect. However, weather conditions can vary and there may be unexpected changes to the route due to accident or changing circumstances.

Effect on identity

Climbing hills can increase self-esteem and confidence in own stamina.

Walking with a group of kindred spirits can give a sense of belonging; for example, the Metropolitan Walkers (20–30 age group) have 500 members.

Meaning

Walking is a good way of maintaining cardiovascular fitness.

Strenuous physical exercise improves mood and can be effective in relieving mild to moderate depression.

Climbing a steep hill can be physically demanding and may be perceived as a symbolic conquest. Putting on the correct clothing may be perceived as getting ready for the struggle.

An individual may want to overcome his own fears, such as fear of heights or of not keeping up with the group.

Eating lunch in the open air may be associated with childhood holidays and picnics.

Walking in open countryside can give a sense of freedom and self-sufficiency. It may symbolise the right of every person in the country to have access to the most beautiful areas of the UK.

Walking is not highly valued in British culture generally but is valued by some subgroups, such as the Ramblers (a campaigning walking organisation). To these groups, walking is important to keep footpaths open, check for any problems with footpaths and assert the right to roam in open countryside.

Table 6.4   Cont'd

Opportunities provided by the activity

Walking is a practical way of improving health and fitness. Dog owners can see the benefits to their pet. Walkers may see features of the countryside that need to be reported, e.g. unsafe trees, fences needing repair, blocked footpaths. Vigorous physical exercise can release feeling of stress or anger.
Joining a walking group can provide opportunities for social interaction. To gratify needs (e.g. create personal meaning. express feeling, exercise capacities, satisfy curiosity, identify with others, exercise choice, achieve).
A walker can become familiar with different parts of the country and with the footpath network. Following an experienced leader gives opportunities to learn about aspects of the countryside, such as the flora and fauna.
Walkers are expected to learn and abide by the Countryside Code and may also learn respect for the rural environment. Talking to others in a group while walking can be educational.
Regular walking allows a person to discover the extent and limits of his strength and stamina. Exploring different types of terrain can lead to other interests, such as wildlife, farming or archaeology.

Potential for grading

See Table 6.2

ACTION

This section considers the elements involved in putting the plan into action. These are the client, the therapist, the activity and the environment.

THE CLIENT

When a client sees an occupational therapist for the first time, he may already have been in contact with mental health services, perhaps for many months or years. His expectations of the type of help he will receive and of the behaviour expected of him will be coloured by that experience. It may take clients a while to adjust to the different approach that the occupational therapist uses, with its emphasis on active involvement and on sharing responsibility with the individual. Some people are unable to accept this type of intervention and prefer a more passive role while others are relieved to be encouraged to take control of their own lives and health.

The UK definition of occupational therapy as a complex intervention (Creek 2003) described occupational therapy as a client-centred process. Client-centred occupational therapy is a collaborative process in which the therapist, the client and relevant others negotiate and share choice and control. Occupational therapy interventions are most effective when the client is an active partner, fully involved in setting goals, taking decisions and engaging in activity. It has been argued that 'the therapist–client partnership is more than just an ideal to which we aspire; it is the essence of good occupational therapy practice' (Creek et al 2005, p283).

The College of Occupational Therapists' (2005) *Code of Ethics and Professional Conduct* states that 'the College is strongly committed to client-centred practice and the involvement of the client as a partner in all stages of the therapeutic process' (p5).

The principles of client-centred practice include (Creek 2003):

- respect for diversity
- recognition of the client's rights
- clear role expectations within the therapeutic relationship
- a collaborative therapist–client relationship
- a focus on the needs, problems and priorities of the client, rather than on the needs of the therapist or the service setting
- identification of problems and negotiation of goals with the client and/or carer
- consideration of the client's point of view at all stages of the intervention
- shared power and decision making between the therapist and the client and/or carer
- promotion of client autonomy and choice through sharing information
- interventions that are congruent with the client's life world context.

Sumsion (1999) stressed the importance of clarifying what we mean by 'the client' when we talk about client-centred practice. A client can be defined as 'a person who engages the professional services of another [who] has the right to demand information and is free to voice an opinion' (Sumsion 1999, p28). The client may not be an individual but could be a group of people, such as the family, carers or a community agency.

The concept of client-centred practice is idealistic and its implementation requires an acknowledgement of the unequal balance of power between therapist and client. This inequality is brought about by the client's need and vulnerability, contrasting with the therapist's knowledge and technical skills. Sumsion (1999) pointed out that language is an important vehicle for exercising power; using technical language that the client cannot understand allows the therapist to retain knowledge and control, whereas offering explanations in simple language and taking time to make sure they are understood enables the client to share in the therapeutic process.

THE THERAPIST

The occupational therapist can be her own most powerful therapeutic tool, using her personality, experience and skill to build an effective collaboration with the client. However, the success of an occupational therapy service also depends on the number and experience of the staff available.

Personality is important. The therapist who chooses to specialise in assertive outreach is likely to be a very different person from the one who works contentedly in a forensic learning disabilities service and they would not happily exchange positions. Personality also plays a part in determining the therapist's style of therapeutic interaction and the approach chosen. An understanding of her own needs, preferences and ways of relating to others will allow for more appropriate selection of roles in the therapist's relationship with the client.

The experience and skill of the therapist also influence which intervention techniques are used. Some techniques, such as psychodrama, require specialist postgraduate training. Basic occupational therapy education can only teach a limited number of activities, so the qualified therapist will add on new techniques to suit her interest and field of practice. Using a computer to encourage a child with learning disabilities to communicate, helping a group of adults to explore causes of anxiety with projective art and facilitating a drop-in creative activity group for primary school children all demand very different skills, although the same principles are used in selecting and applying the treatment media.

The more skills that the occupational therapist has in her repertoire and the more theories she is able to draw on, the better able she will be to work in a person-centred way and respond to individual needs and environmental demands.

When planning programmes to achieve both quantity and quality of intervention, the therapist takes account of several factors, including the number of staff available and their experience. Some activities cannot be used by a therapist working single-handed, either because of the nature of the activity or because of the degree of disability or disturbance of the clients. When working alone, it may be necessary to reduce either the intensity of treatment or the number of clients in order to ensure safety.

THE ACTIVITY

Activity is at the core of occupational therapy practice. If the therapist cannot engage the client in activity that has meaning and value for him, then there is no assessment and no intervention. Engagement is achieved by involving the client at all stages of the intervention process and by understanding the factors that will motivate the individual, as described on p119.

The process of analysing activities into their component parts and synthesising therapeutic activities was described in the previous section. Details of how various activities are used in practice can be found in Chapters 15 to 20.

The range of activities used by occupational therapists is very broad, from personal care and everyday tasks, through work-related activities, to creative activities and activities to promote personal growth. Almost any activity that a person would enact in support of his occupations comes within the remit of the occupational therapist. Carrying out everyday activities as part of therapy allows the client to develop or regain skills to a necessary level of competence. Learning new activities can change the way in which a person sees himself, build confidence and enhance personal and social identity. For example, learning computer skills can help a young person to find work, raise his self-esteem and command the respect of his peers.

Some activities, such as woodwork, centre on the materials and equipment used. Certain skills can be more easily assessed and developed using activities that are materials/tools orientated; for example, to develop hand–eye co-ordination it would be more appropriate to use woodwork than drama. The type of tools used can be varied to develop both physical and cognitive skills. Materials can be selected for their power to evoke feelings (e.g. wet clay may evoke the feelings of lack of control associated with the anal stage of development, as described by Freud). Materials can also influence the outcome of the activity (e.g. good-quality paints and paper will make it easier for a client to achieve a satisfactory painting than would poor-quality materials).

In other activities, such as drama, tools and materials are of secondary importance and the focus is on process and interaction. The main interaction may be between the client and therapist, between group members or between the client and family members, if the intervention involves them. The activities of everyday life tend to incorporate many elements: materials, people, environment and social context. For example, going shopping includes equipment (money, shopping bag), people (shop assistants, other shoppers), environment (route to the shops, shop interior and layout) and context (purpose of shopping, time of day, type of goods).

THE ENVIRONMENT

People cannot be considered in isolation from their usual environments and intervention cannot be considered separately from the environment in which it takes place. The therapeutic environment consists of human and non-human elements that can, to a greater or lesser extent, be manipulated by the therapist to facilitate engagement in tasks and the achievement of goals. Some

elements in the environment are physically or emotionally closer to the individual and some are further away.

The human environment consists of:

- the therapist
- other clients
- other staff
- relatives and friends
- neighbours
- peers.

The non-human environment consists of:

- the setting of the intervention (for example, hospital, community centre, clinic)
- the occupational therapy setting (for example, department, client's own home)
- the physical space where the intervention takes place
- the client's home
- the workplace
- the neighbourhood
- resources and facilities within the environment
- non-human objects within the environment, including aids to independent performance.

Hagedorn (2001) suggested that occupational therapists are concerned with two aspects of the environment: content, which is the features of the environment, and demand, which is the impact that environmental factors have on occupational performance. The physical and social features of the environment can be adapted to enhance performance or to provide therapy.

THE CONTEXT

During intervention, the therapist's actions are influenced not only by the wishes and needs of the client but also by external circumstances and requirements. These include:

- team working
- case management
- case review
- clinical governance
- evidence-based practice
- continuing professional development.

TEAM WORKING

Although some occupational therapists continue to work as members of an occupational therapy team, they are often part of a wider multidisciplinary (or multiprofessional) team, such as a community mental health team. If occupational therapists are shared between teams, their specialist skills are usually clearly targeted at specific client needs that the occupational therapist is best qualified to assist with.

Increasingly, however, occupational therapists are full-time members of the core team and, as such, they are required to complete generic work (tasks that all members of the team complete, such as Care Programme Approach/Care Co-ordination, initial assessments to the service and crisis work) where skills are shared and developed across all professional groups. Specific shared tasks may vary; however, the Department of Health has clearly identified 10 essential shared capabilities that the mental health workforce are expected to be trained in before they qualify (DoH 2004):

1. working in partnership
2. respecting diversity
3. practising ethically
4. challenging inequality
5. promoting recovery
6. identifying people's needs and strengths
7. providing service user-centred care
8. making a difference
9. promoting safety and positive risk taking
10. personal development and learning.

Each member of the team also brings specialist skills, which can be accessed when required by the client, and in this way the most appropriate assessment and treatment options can be chosen according to the client's needs. In order for an occupational therapist to work successfully as a member of a multidisciplinary team, she needs to be able to demonstrate the 10 essential shared capabilities in working practice, but also needs to be able to:

- gain an effective balance between the demands of generic working and offering specialist occupational therapy input where this is the most beneficial therapeutic input for the client at that time
- demonstrate the effectiveness of occupational therapy interventions through written and verbal communication of specific assessments, treatment planning and evaluation/outcome measurement, using the evidence base wherever possible
- understand and describe her generic and specific roles clearly to all those involved and have a clear understanding of the roles of others in order to promote mutual respect, support and understanding
- pass on skills and knowledge for use by others wherever possible.

Learning how to work in a team begins as an occupational therapy student on placement, where students are encouraged to spend time with other team members as well as with occupational therapy staff, identifying specialist roles and areas of overlap in practice.

CASE MANAGEMENT

Care Programme Approach/Care Co-ordination (CPA) is currently the most prevalent form of case management within specialist mental health services in the NHS. It involves close working between health and social care services and involves service users and carers as central to the assessment and planning of services to meet their needs. It has four main components (DoH 2006).

1. Systematic arrangements for assessing the health and social care needs of people accepted into specialist mental health services.
2. The formation of a care plan which identifies the health and social care requirements from a variety of providers.
3. The appointment of a key worker (care co-ordinator) to keep in close touch with the service user and to monitor and co-ordinate care.
4. Regular review and, where necessary, agreed changes to the care plan.

Care Programme Approach/Care Co-ordination, or case management, and the occupational therapist's specific input are not mutually exclusive: the two can work well together. It does, however, require skill to focus on specific occupational therapy assessments and interventions whilst simultaneously co-ordinating and monitoring input from others (as discussed with and required by the client). Occupational therapists often complain of losing their focus on occupational therapy-specific intervention due to the demands of the CPA/Care Co-ordination role. This is not unusual and other professions also experience similar difficulties; for example, a psychologist providing 12 sessions of cognitive analytical therapy may struggle to also co-ordinate their client's care. Clinical supervision can be used very effectively to help maintain focus where specific occupational therapy interventions are being completed alongside care co-ordination.

Skill is also required when occupational therapists are using shared care plans or treatment plans if they are to follow a team approach without compromising the requirements of professional standards for practice.

More information about the Care Programme Approach can be found in Chapter 7.

CASE REVIEW

Case review is one of the core components of CPA/Care Co-ordination and care management and also of clinical/professional supervision.

In relation to CPA/Care Co-ordination, review takes place at regular planned intervals but also takes place at key times such as:

- admission to and discharge from hospital
- incarceration and release from prison
- during significant life events, e.g. moving home, bereavement, experience of trauma, pregnancy/birth, divorce.

Consideration should be given to calling a review when a person is recovering well, as a way of affirming positive progress.

The service user and all those involved in the person's care should be included in any such review, where possible, and all domains of the person's life – mental, physical and social – are reflected upon. Outcomes of such a review may include:

- continuation of current treatment/care
- improved and more timely information sharing
- further negotiation in specific areas and/or with specific people
- identification of need for reassessment or additional assessment in particular areas
- minor or major changes to current treatment/care
- improved continuity of care and clearer, more fluid journey through services for all concerned
- up-to-date risk assessment and decisions about positive or therapeutic risk taking
- change of care co-ordinator
- improved therapeutic relationships
- increased service user involvement, decision making and choice
- identification of need for referral to other agencies or services
- discharge.

Occupational therapy case review

This takes place when any occupational therapy-specific goals that have been negotiated with a service user are due for review. An occupational therapy review usually involves the service user and the therapist only, although it may also include, for example, the client's family or carer. Results of this review can be fed into the wider multidisciplinary review process. Reflection upon progress is done with the service user and includes thinking about the reasons for progress or lack of it. Subsequent action and treatment are negotiated, with new short-term and/or long-term goals being set. A clear endpoint is identified where possible.

Occupational therapy case review should also take place within clinical and professional supervision. This supervision should be given by one or several occupational therapists with a greater level of knowledge and expertise in order for learning and development to take place through, for example, information sharing, advice, recommendations for further action and alternative perspectives. This also includes a quality assurance component in terms of maintenance of professional standards and adherence to current legislation and guidance. A small number of cases can be discussed during each supervision session and content may include:

- exploration of the therapeutic relationship with the service user and/or carers
- discussion of occupational therapy assessments that have been used and those that may be of future benefit
- clarification in identification of occupational performance strengths and deficits
- impact of environment on functioning and recovery
- influence of theory and its use in practice
- treatment choices and options
- roles engaged in by the service user and their influence on progress
- equipment issues and choices
- evaluation of progress, including methods used
- smart goal setting
- problem solving
- ethical implications of occupational therapy interventions (see Chapter 11)
- social inclusion opportunities
- relevant evidence base and examples of good practice
- training/development needs arising from this specific case
- discussion of risks.

CLINICAL GOVERNANCE

Clinical governance is 'a framework ... through which organisations are accountable for continuously improving the quality of their services and safeguarding high standards of care' (Creek 2003, p50). Clinical governance is concerned with the quality of services, the effectiveness of services and standards of safety (College of Occupational Therapists 2006). It encompasses a range of quality initiatives, such as:

- continuing professional development and performance management
- supervision
- setting, implementing and monitoring standards
- disseminating and building on good practice

- creating and utilising an evidence base through research and development
- clinical audit
- minimising and managing risk
- clarifying clinical and financial responsibility and accountability
- data protection.

Health and social care organisations are responsible for having in place policies and procedures to ensure that services are delivered in the most clinically effective, cost-effective and efficient ways possible. The performance of health services in England and Wales is monitored by the Healthcare Commission and social care organisations in England are monitored by the Commission for Social Care Inspection.

Individual therapists also 'have a duty to provide an occupational therapy service of the highest competence, safety, quality and value' (College of Occupational Therapists 2003, p41). Occupational therapists in the UK have to be registered with the Health Professions Council (HPC), which sets standards of proficiency for safe and effective practice (Health Professions Council 2003). Any therapist who fails to meet these standards is subject to a number of actions by the HPC, which include cautioning, suspending and removing the practitioner from the register. Occupational therapy is a protected title in the UK, so no-one can practise as an occupational therapist unless they are registered with the HPC. This also applies to occupational therapists working in the independent and voluntary sector as it is a guarantee of sound practice to both the general public and employers.

Professional supervision is an essential component of individual accountability. The College of Occupational Therapists (2005, p16) requires that all occupational therapy personnel 'shall be supported in their practice and development through regular professional supervision within an agreed structure or model'.

Further information about clinical governance can be found in Chapter 8.

EVIDENCE-BASED PRACTICE

Evidence-based practice is the process of seeking, appraising and implementing the most recent research findings to ensure that patients receive interventions that have been demonstrated to be effective. The term used to describe the use of interventions that are based on the best available evidence is *clinical effectiveness*. Clinical effectiveness 'is achieved by using interventions that are known to work and embedding these within an environment and systems that are of the highest possible quality' (Mead 1998, p27).

In areas where there has been a substantial body of research, it is not necessary for the therapist to do her own literature searches. Various critically appraised resources are available, such as reviews and guidelines. For example, the National Institute for Health and Clinical Excellence (NICE) produces guidelines for treatment that are based on reviews of the best available evidence.

There are several sources for finding systematic reviews of evidence and evidence-based guidelines. A selection is given in Table 6.5.

Not all areas of occupational therapy practice have been extensively researched, although the evidence base for the profession is growing all the time. At the present time, one of the key sources of evidence in the profession remains clinical expertise: 'from experience with patients, established practice, experts in the field, development of skills through continuing professional development' (Bury 1998, p6).

CONTINUING PROFESSIONAL DEVELOPMENT

Continuing professional development (CPD) is 'a range of learning activities through which health professionals maintain and develop throughout their career to ensure that they retain their capacity to practise safely, effectively and legally within their evolving scope of practice' (Health Professions Council 2006, p1). One of the principles set out in the College of Occupational Therapists' (2005, p16) *Code of Ethics and Professional Conduct* is that 'Occupational therapy personnel shall be personally responsible for actively maintaining and developing their personal development and professional competence'.

All occupational therapy personnel are expected to keep a record of their CPD and the HPC (2006, p2) requires that this record is 'continuous, up-to-date and accurate'. CPD activities must demonstrably contribute to the quality of the therapist's practice and service delivery and must

Table 6.5   Some sources of critically appraised evidence

Source	Type of resource
Bandolier www.ebandolier.com	An independent journal about evidence-based healthcare. Information about evidence of effectiveness (or lack of it), from systematic reviews, meta-analyses, randomised trials, and high-quality observational studies, is reviewed and the results are put forward as bullet points of those things that worked and those that did not
Cochrane Library Can be accessed through the National Electronic Library for Health (see below)	Produces and updates systematic and critically appraised reviews of evidence
Health Evidence Bulletins Wales http://hebw.uwcm.ac.uk	A series of bulletins signposting the best evidence across a broad range of evidence types and subject areas
National Institute for Health and Clinical Excellence (NICE) www.nice.org.uk	Produces treatment guidelines based on reviews of evidence
NHS Centre for Reviews and Dissemination www.york.ac.uk/inst/crd	Offers systematic reviews of research on selected topics, scoping reviews, which map the research literature, publications, reports and access to databases
National Electronic Library for Health (NeLH) http://nhs.uk/nelh/	This acts as a gateway to many resources, including databases, guidelines and systematic reviews

Table 6.6 Types of CPD activity (adapted from Health Professions Council 2005)

Type of activity	Examples
Work-based learning	Case studies
	Secondments
	Peer review
	Journal club
	Supervising students
Professional activity	Involvement with a professional body
	Supervising research
	Mentoring
	Organising journal club or other specialist group
	Giving conference presentations
Formal/educational	Attending courses
	Research
	Writing articles or papers
	Attending seminars
	Distance learning
Self-directed learning	Reading books or journals
	Reviewing books or articles
	Updating knowledge through the Internet or other media
Other	Public service
	Voluntary work
	Courses

be intended to benefit the service user. In other words, to count towards CPD, activities must be relevant to the therapist's practice. The HPC states that CPD must be a mixture of different kinds of activities. Some examples of the types of activity that would be acceptable are shown in Table 6.6.

SUMMARY

This chapter looked at four stages of the occupational therapy process: needs identification, goal setting, action planning and action. It also discussed some of the external factors that influence what the occupational therapist does and how she carries out her work.

Chapters 15–20 cover occupational therapy methods of intervention in more detail. The next chapter looks at record keeping in occupational therapy.

References

Bury T 1998 Evidence-based healthcare explained. Bury T, Mead J (eds) Evidence-based healthcare: a practical guide for therapists, Butterworth Heinemann, Oxford, pp3-25

College of Occupational Therapists 2003 Professional standards for occupational therapy practice. College of Occupational Therapists, London

College of Occupational Therapists 2005 Code of ethics and professional conduct. College of Occupational Therapists, London

College of Occupational Therapists 2006 COT/BAOT Briefing no. 41: quality briefing: governance in health and social care. College of Occupational Therapists, London

Creek J 1998 Purposeful activity. Creek J (ed) Occupational therapy: new perspectives. Whurr, London, pp16-28

Creek J 2003 Occupational therapy defined as a complex intervention. College of Occupational Therapists, London

Creek J 2007 Engaging the reluctant client. Creek J, Lawson-Porter A (eds) Contemporary issues in occupational therapy: reasoning and reflection. Wiley, Chichester

Creek J, Ilott I, Cook S et al 2005 Valuing occupational therapy as a complex intervention. British Journal of Occupational Therapy 68(6): 281-284

Department of Health 2004 The Ten Essential Shared Capabilities - A Framework for the Whole of the Mental Health Workforce. Available online at: www.dh.gov. uk/en/Publications/PublicationsPolicyAndGuidance/ DH_4087169

Department of Health 2006 Reviewing the Care Programme Approach: a consultation document. Care Services Improvement Partnership. Available online at: www. dh.gov.uk/assetRoot/04/14/05/45/04140545.pdf

du Toit V 1974 The background theory related to creative ability which leads to work capacity within the context of occupational therapy for the cerebral palsied. du Toit V (ed.) Patient volition and action in occupational therapy. Vona and Marie du Toit Foundation, Hillbrow, South Africa, pp47-54

ENOTHE 2006 www.enothe.hva.nl

Fidler GS, Fidler JW 1963 Occupational therapy: a communication process in psychiatry. Macmillan, New York

Gillon R 1985/1986 Philosophical medical ethics. Wiley, Chichester

Hagedorn R 2001 Foundations for practice in occupational therapy, 3rd edn. Churchill Livingstone, Edinburgh

Health Professions Council 2003 Standards of proficiency: occupational therapists. Health Professions Council, London

Health Professions Council 2006 Your guide to our standards for continuing professional development. Health Professions Council, London

Hopkins HL, Tiffany EG 1988 Assessment and evaluation: an overview. Hopkins HL, Smith HD (eds) Willard and Spackman's occupational therapy, 7th edn. JB Lippincott, Philadelphia

Katz N 1985 Occupational therapy's domain of concern: reconsidered. American Journal of Occupational Therapy 39(8): 518-524

Kielhofner G 1992 Conceptual foundations of occupational therapy. FA Davis, Philadelphia

Llorens LA 1976 Application of a development theory for health and rehabilitation. American Occupational Therapy Association, Maryland

Mead J 1998 Clinical effectiveness: another perspective to evidence-based healthcare. Bury T, Mead J (eds) Evidence-based healthcare: a practical guide for therapists. Butterworth Heinemann, Oxford, pp26-42

Mosey AC 1986 Psychosocial components of occupational therapy. Raven Press, New York

New Shorter Oxford English Dictionary 1993 Clarendon Press, Oxford

Reed KL, Sanderson SN 1992 Concepts of occupational therapy, 3rd edn. Williams and Wilkins, Baltimore

Reilly M 1974 An explanation of play. Reilly M (ed) Play as exploratory learning. Sage, Beverly Hills

Sumsion T 1994 The client-centred approach. Sumsion T (ed) Client-centred practice in occupational therapy: a guide to implementation. Churchill Livingstone, Edinburgh

Chapter 7

Record keeping

Mary Booth

INTRODUCTION

Health-care practitioners make records of their interactions with people to ensure that the identified health and social care problems and needs are documented, together with resulting interventions and outcomes. In addition to individual patient care records, systems will be in place to record anonymised information about care on a wider basis. It is essential that the occupational therapist understands, uses and contributes to these vital communication tools.

This chapter will discuss the different types of records traditionally made by different professionals. Each section is illustrated with examples of practice in the UK but the principles and practices of record keeping are relevant to all countries and practice settings. Occupational therapists will need to be able to work with traditional record-keeping systems, whether or not they are moving towards using a single integrated electronic care record. The chapter will discuss current methods of record keeping and outline some of the changes and challenges that practitioners of occupational therapy in the UK will be part of as the National Care Records Service evolves. Professional and legal implications of record keeping and the essential components for occupational therapy case notes will be discussed.

RECORDS ARE IMPORTANT

Good record keeping can be considered an essential foundation which underpins excellence in health-care planning and delivery. Accurately and adequately recording patient information, assessments, interventions such as phone calls, ordering equipment and consultation with other professionals and both direct and indirect treatments and outcomes is time consuming. In all areas of health and social care, but particularly in the mental health field, recording an activity can take as long as observing or performing it. However, it is vital to the provision of good-quality care that this time is both available and effectively used.

WHY RECORD?

- Patient records provide a detailed account of patients from the time they enter the care of a health facility until they are discharged. They can show whether the care has been appropriate, timely and effective.
- Recording is essential to individual health-care workers who should rely on the record, rather than on their own memories, with regard to the planning and progress of interventions with the patient.
- The existence of records means that all team members involved with the patient's care can, subject to confidentiality, immediately have an overview of the patient's and other care providers' aims, goals, progress and outcomes. As the National Care Records are implemented, this information will be available beyond the immediate team. For example, should a community mental health patient present at an accident and emergency department or be admitted to inpatient acute mental health services in another part of the country, his or her records will be immediately available.

- Occupational therapists have a statutory duty to maintain records, which is placed on their employing organisations. Currently, records for mentally disordered persons within the meaning of the Mental Health Act 1983 should be retained for 20 years after no further treatment is required or for 8 years if the client dies while still being treated. For children and young people, records should be retained until the client's 25th or 26th birthday if the young person was 17 at the conclusion of treatment; or for 8 years after death if death occurred before the 18th birthday.
- As occupational therapists, our *Code of Ethics and Professional Conduct* requires that 'Accurate, legible, factual, contemporaneous and attributed records and reports of occupational therapy intervention must be kept in order to provide information for professional colleagues and for legal purposes, such as client access and court reports' (College of Occupational Therapists 2005, p10). The College of Occupational Therapists has also published a booklet which explains the rationale that underpins some of the professional record-keeping requirements (College of Occupational Therapists 2006).
- Records can be useful tools in audit and research, leading to effective practice based on evidence.
- Good record keeping safeguards the patient as it gives a visual record of the quality of care provided. It also safeguards the occupational therapist and the employing organisation, in situations where complaints are made or litigation becomes an issue.
- If the government and primary care trust commissioners cannot obtain statistical reports, which include occupational therapy, they will not see the need to fund future occupational therapy services.
- Payment by results in NHS services in the UK, which should be fully introduced by 2008, means funding will be linked to activity in a fair and equitable way.

WHAT IS RECORDED?

Occupational therapists, like other health and social care professionals, are required to keep a range of records relating to patient activity. These can generally be considered to fall into three main categories:

- statistical information
- patient records
- staff records.

Much of the legislation that controls patient records, such as the Data Protection Act (1998) and the Human Rights Act (1998), will also apply to staff records. Staff records will not be discussed in detail here as they are best considered as part of management. It is important that occupational therapists consider and comply with their employing organisation's human resource department policies and procedures relating to staffing records.

In the UK, traditional methods of record keeping are in the process of being phased out between 2004 and 2010, as the new national electronic NHS care record is introduced.

National Care Records Service

Within the NHS in the UK, we are beginning a fundamental change to the way in which care is delivered. The way in which records are created, maintained and shared through the use of modern information systems has long been recognised as essential to this change, but this has been difficult to achieve. Information systems have too often been viewed as just an information technology project, missing the way that information technology can be used as a key enabler to help deliver the *NHS Plan* and contribute to better ways of delivering care. It is now recognised that modernising care, including patient involvement and choice, will be difficult to achieve without a national integrated care record service that incorporates:

- electronic bookings for appointments and planned inpatient care
- electronic prescriptions transfer
- the new electronic NHS care record.

In England, the NHS Care Record Service will be supported by the largest investment in information technology seen to date (NHS Confederation 2003). There will be a national data spine for the National Care Records Service and the Electronic Booking Service. The country will then be divided into five geographical clusters in which local service providers have the responsibility for delivering a full range of information technology services to meet the national demands and local requirements. Information will be held locally, where most care is delivered, but a summary patient record will be available nationally.

STATISTICAL RECORDS

Occupational therapists working in the health service are required by their employing organisations to keep statistical records. These records are demanded of the organisation for government information and by primary care trusts in England, local health boards in Wales and NHS boards in Scotland which are responsible for commissioning services. Currently, organisations have differing methods of recording the necessary information but all are increasingly likely to be linked to an organisation-wide information system. Input methods include:

- paper-based systems
- input into the computer system by data clerks
- direct input into the system by occupational therapists from networked personal computers
- regular downloads by occupational therapists from hand-held computers
- wireless technology, which can immediately transfer data, which is developing rapidly.

For the allied health professions, the statistics currently required in England are a minimum data set relating to:

- number of new patient episodes
- professional group
- government office region
- strategic health authority area
- patient age group
- referral source.

Currently, statistical information is mainly collected separately from what is recorded in the patient case notes. The new NHS National Care Record system aims to collect the statistical information required by the Department of Health electronically and directly when the health-care professional electronically inputs into the patient record, thus saving time and reducing duplication. For example, it is envisaged that an occupational therapist entering details into an electronic patient record will select a code that recognises him or her as an occupational therapist and enables the automatic collection of statutory information demanded by government, such as the mental health minimum data set.

Most information systems can provide analysis of other information which is helpful to both clinicians and managers. Individual occupational therapists and the service can obtain useful information from such records, which will help them to plan and organise their work. This information can include:

- case lists
- frequency and type of contact with patients
- waiting list times
- average contacts per case
- length of time of intervention
- a range of other information, depending on the records collected.

Clinical terms

A major aspect of the strategy for information for the NHS in England has been the development of a common information infrastructure including a thesaurus of agreed clinical terms, originally the Read codes (NHS Executive 1986). The Read codes are being incorporated into and replaced by SNOMED, which provides the coded thesaurus that is used by electronic health records (EHR) for coding terms that are entered by users. In practice, this usually works by software developers being given lists of terms for use in specific fields within the EHR system. The user chooses from the drop-down list and the software records that choice together with the related SNOMED coding information.

The strategy for the new NHS Care Record Service is to use SNOMED Clinical Terms (CT) and it is hoped that locally and nationally required data will be extracted from the patient electronic record without the need for the clinician to enter separate data. While occupational therapists do not need to know the detail, they should be aware of the existence of SNOMED-CT to help them understand and co-operate when they are asked to code data in a certain way. Until this type of information can be extracted from the National Patient Record, a variety of stand-alone electronic and paper-based systems will continue to be used.

The SNOMED thesaurus includes terms that allow occupational therapists to record their work with clients. However, the terms have been scattered throughout a structured hierarchy, one not designed to reflect the occupational therapy view of health care. Consequently it is very difficult for designers and software developers to identify which terms should be included in drop-down lists that will be used by occupational therapists. At the time of writing, the College of Occupational Therapists is leading a national project to create an occupational therapy dictionary that will become part of SNOMED-CT.

PATIENT RECORDS – MOVING TOWARDS ELECTRONIC HEALTH RECORDS

Patient records are kept by all professionals who are working with the patient. Increasingly within mental health services, a single set of patient notes is maintained for a patient in a particular setting. For example, within a community mental health team or an inpatient setting, a client is much more likely to have one set of notes which includes entries from all professionals involved. The advantages are clear and all team members have access to all the information available. While these are, in the main, still paper based, the single patient record can be seen as a positive step towards the fuller integration and availability of notes that will be provided by the national NHS care record.

By 2010, every NHS patient in England will have an individual electronic care record. The NHS Care Record Service will connect more than 30,000 general practitioners and 270 acute, community and mental health NHS trusts in a single, secure national system. At the time of writing, in early 2007, while the development of the national care record is well under way, most patients have several different paper and electronic records. These are difficult to transfer quickly and a central record containing all of a patient's health and social care information is still in the project stage. In addition, hospitals hold millions of records that have to be retrieved manually when a patient presents for consultation or treatment, clearly not an efficient or effective system in the 21st century. In future, patient records will be available 24 hours a day, 7 days a week. The aim is for the information held on the central record to grow over time and patients will eventually be able to access their own electronic record from their home computer or one publicly available, for example in their local library or health centre (10 Downing Street 2003). Each patient will have the right to restrict access to specific parts, or all, of their EHR. Anonymised data will still be available nationally for secondary uses such as research, audit and performance management.

Confidentiality is vital at all levels of health provision and electronic systems, such as the one being developed in the UK, must be maintained by robust mechanisms. NHS staff will have access to EHR through authenticated log-on mechanisms. Health professionals will have complete access to the EHR of each patient being treated by the team(s) they work in. Other NHS staff (administrators, managers, finance departments, human resource departments, etc.) will have different profiles of access to each EHR, depending on their specific role. Details of how this will operate are still to be finalised. It is expected that they will have access to anonymised data but some clinical staff, such as receptionists, ward clerks and medical secretaries, will need access to personal health information.

The position with regard to students is currently under discussion at national level. For occupational therapists, it is anticipated they should have full access to EHR, under supervision of their health-care professional supervisor. Other issues relating to confidentiality are also being discussed at national level, including third party information such as carers' assessments.

Separate professional notes

Where it is still normal practice for patients to have several sets of notes in one setting, all relevant sets should receive information about the patient's occupational therapy intervention. Separate professional notes may include:

- **case notes**: these are generally the psychiatrist's notes which relate to both inpatient and outpatient episodes of care. Occupational therapy assessments and reports should be copied to these
- **general practitioner notes**: these are retained in the general practitioner's office. Depending on local policy and procedure, occupational therapy reports and assessments may be sent directly to the general practitioner or may be included in team reports
- **nursing notes**: these may be inpatient nursing notes or community psychiatric nursing notes. Again, it is essential that occupational therapy reports are copied to nursing colleagues.

In addition, mental health patients may have psychology notes, occupational therapy notes and notes from the other allied health professionals and may also have separate sets of notes relating to physical ailments. Remember, by 2010 the plan is to have a single national electronic record available 24 hours a day, every day, with every health professional and the patient having instant access. Electronic records will overcome the practical problem of several people, often in different locations, wanting to access the same notes. Meanwhile, occupational therapists should be aware of the policy on single case notes in their working area and follow this.

In the UK, to meet the demands of the Clinical Negligence Scheme for Trusts, organisations are likely to have record-keeping policies which occupational therapists must be familiar with. Increasingly we may see health organisations setting up record libraries. These will authorise the type of documentation that can be used in patient records, including ensuring that the standardised assessments used by occupational therapists comply with copyright laws.

Single assessment process for older people

The *National Service Framework for Older People* (DoH 2001) introduced the concept of a single assessment process across health and social care for older people. A commitment was made to introduce the process by April 2004 across all older people's services, including mental health. There is a variety of off-the-shelf paper and software packages available but the intention is that this should become an electronic package and link with the NHS care record. Occupational therapists working with older people within mental health services should ensure that they use the locally agreed package within both assessment and record keeping.

OCCUPATIONAL THERAPY PATIENT RECORDS

Occupational therapists must make themselves familiar with the record-keeping section in the *Professional Standards for Occupational Therapy Practice* (College of Occupational Therapists 2003) and with the operational policies and guidelines on documentation and record keeping of their own services and employing bodies. It is good practice for an agreed format of notes to be used throughout an occupational therapy service as this can aid consistency, standards and audit.

General information

The patient record should be well thought out and designed to keep general information, history, assessments, treatment plans, progress notes and evaluations in a logical and easy-to-follow order. The format, either stand-alone occupational therapy records or integrated paper or electronic records, should conform to local policies.

The patient record should include:

- general information about the patient, such as name, address, next of kin
- legal and care programme status
- referral information
- contact details for all professionals involved
- a history
- any precautions to be taken.

Occupational therapy assessments

A record should be kept of all occupational therapy assessments used, both standardised and observational, and of the assessment results.

Occupational therapy intervention plans

The intervention plan should be clearly identified; however, the structure of the record will depend on the occupational therapy model or approach followed, or on the CPA where the occupational therapist is the care co-ordinator. It should include a reference to the model or approach being used and the problems or issues identified for occupational therapy intervention. Patient and/or carer (if appropriate) aims should be recorded, together with the therapist's aims and actions. Recording discussion and agreement with the patient about the plan, or rationale for not agreeing this with the patient, is good practice and informs the requirements for consent and patient choice.

Evaluation of treatment plans

A section may be included to allow for recording any evaluation of the treatment plan, outcomes of the evaluation and further action required.

Progress notes

A section to record progress notes and actions taken is essential. Depending on local protocols in integrated notes, this may be within an occupational therapy section of the notes or sequential within the main progress notes.

RECORDING CARE PROGRAMME APPROACH AND SECTION 117 AFTERCARE

The Care Programme Approach, supervision registers and Section 117 of the Mental Health Act 1983 are strategies to ensure communication between agencies and services involved in the care and management of people with mental health needs.

Care Programme Approach

Mental health services in the UK are the joint responsibility of both health and social services. Initially, health services were responsible for co-ordinating care through the Care Programme Approach (CPA), which was introduced on 1 April 1991 to provide a framework for effective mental health care. Care Management (CM) was introduced through the Community Care Act 1990 as the means by which those in need of community care services should be helped. Since the introduction of these two care systems, it has been recognised that the most effective and efficient delivery of care within mental health services is through integrated care systems and services. Hence, there has been a move towards the integration and joint management of health and social teams in mental health.

The CPA is discussed here because there are significant recording issues and standard forms may be in use. From April 2001, there have been two levels of CPA.

- Standard CPA applies to people who have low support needs, are likely to remain stable and have limited disability or health-care needs arising from their mental health problems.
- Enhanced CPA applies to people who are identified as having more severe and enduring mental health problems, often with complex health and social needs that require multiple inputs from more than one agency or service.

This is under review and out to consultation at the time of writing (DoH 2006) and it is planned that there will be one level of CPA in future.

The CPA is care management for adults of working age (DoH 1999a). In 1999, the *National Service Framework for Mental Health* (DoH 1999b) formalised the integration of CPA and CM and this was implemented by April 2001. The integrated approach provides for:

- a single point of contact
- a unified health and social care assessment process
- co-ordination of the roles and responsibilities of each agency in the system
- access, through a single process, to the support and resources of both health and social care services.

While this chapter does not discuss this approach in detail, the recording of the CPA underpins the process.

CPA and occupational therapy

The CPA will apply to all occupational therapists working for health or social services within mental health settings. It is vital that occupational therapists know the CPA status of patients they are working with and occupational therapy records should identify both the patient's CPA status and the CPA co-ordinator. Occupational therapy intervention should form an integrated part of the care plan and will be recorded in this as well as in the occupational therapy records.

An occupational therapist may be the CPA co-ordinator, a role which holds specific responsibilities over and above the provision of occupational therapy intervention. The extent to which occupational therapists act as CPA co-ordinators varies with the teams they work within; however, occupational therapists increasingly carry this responsibility, particularly in community settings. Locally designed documentation for recording the CPA process will be in use and it is this that the occupational therapist must use. CPA documentation currently tends to be additional documentation which appears within individual patient records and, where appropriate in accordance with local policy, should be copied to the occupational therapy notes. There is also specific information that must be recorded on CPA registers and occupational therapists must be familiar with the way this is collected locally. As the single electronic record is developed, the CPA recording process is likely to be incorporated.

Section 117 aftercare

Section 117 of the Mental Health Act 1983 requires health and social services to provide aftercare for certain categories of detained patients. Patients subject to Section 117 aftercare will meet the CPA indicators and the implementation of the full CPA, including recording, will ensure that these statutory obligations are met.

GOOD RECORD KEEPING

The NHS issued a Health Service Circular which sets out the legal responsibilities of NHS bodies to keep proper records, provides good practice guidelines, explains the periods of retention of records and indicates where further information can be found (DoH 1999c). This circular outlines key issues to address from the 1995

Audit Commission report *Setting the Record Right*, such as:

- low priority given to record keeping
- lack of awareness of good record keeping
- lack of information sharing between professions and units
- lack of co-ordination between paper and electronic records
- need to maintain confidentiality while legitimately freeing information (Audit Commission 1995).

The *Caldicott Review of Patient Identifiable Information* (DoH 1997) also raised concerns about NHS management of records. Different work streams from this review have introduced further guidance which can be accessed via the Department of Health website. At the time of writing, the most up-to-date guidance is the NHS code of practice on confidentiality (DoH 2003).

Most NHS organisations will have a policy for care records as well as policies for other types of records. Occupational therapists should be familiar with these local guidelines. Below are some of the practical and policy aspects to be considered to ensure good record keeping.

STORAGE OF NOTES

Paper records, while current, will be stored in a secure place, usually within the working area of the health-care worker. This might be a ward, a department or an office and can be in a hospital or community-based setting. Once the record is no longer active, the hospital case notes and medical notes will generally be sent to the medical records department for storage. In a community setting, such as a community mental health team, and in departments such as occupational therapy, the records not actively in use may be stored at the base.

Health organisations have different practices and policies relating to the storage of records. Some will convert the paper file to microfiche, which lasts longer and takes up less storage space. However, the process of recording and retrieving such records can be time consuming. Many organisations today use outside companies which offer secure storage with a rapid retrieval time of the original paper record. In this case,

the record will be stored in a sealed, numbered box and it is the box which will be recalled, for reasons of confidentiality. Notes stored electronically will have safeguard procedures to ensure confidentiality.

Data Protection Act 1998

The Data Protection Act of 1984 has been revised and the new 1998 Act came into force on 1 March 2000. This Act changes definitions and broadens the scope of the original Act. The new Act has eight principles and differentiates between personal data and sensitive personal data. It now covers certain types of manual records, including health records, as well as electronic records. Data are defined within the Act as information which is processed automatically, recorded with the intention to process automatically, recorded as or with the intention to be part of a manual relevant system or contained in a health, educational or social services record. Therefore, with the exception of anonymised information, most records concerning patients will fall within the scope of the Act.

The Access to Health Records Act 1990 allowed access to manual health records made after the Act came into force, but the Data Protection Act 1998 allows patients access to most manual health records as well as to all electronic records. Health and social care organisations will have policies and procedures relating to patient access to records and occupational therapists should familiarise themselves with them and with the eight principles of the Act, which are outlined in Box 7.1.

Access to records/information sharing

Requests for access to records fall into six types:

- professional-to-professional sharing of information
- legal summons to produce records
- solicitor's request related to a court case
- Mental Health Act tribunals
- client's request for access to their health records under the Data Protection Act (1998)
- manager's hearing or legal representation for a Mental Health Act tribunal.

Occupational therapists dealing with requests for such access should familiarise themselves with their employing body's procedures and policies in relation to the Data Protection Act 1998.

RECORDING CONSENT TO EXAMINATION OR TREATMENT

Consent is a patient's agreement to care; it can be non-verbal, oral or in writing. It is not the intention to fully discuss consent issues in this chapter but rather to raise awareness of the requirement for recording consent. NHS organisations are likely to have both policies and training on consent to treatment, which occupational therapists should familiarise themselves with. The main advice is that for significant procedures health professionals should document the patient's agreement to the procedure and the discussions which lead up to it, remembering that a signature on a form is evidence of consent but not proof of informed consent.

Within the field of mental health care, written consent is required for electroconvulsive therapy (ECT), clinical photography and video recordings and for the use of unlicensed drugs. There are four consent forms for different scenarios.

Consent form 1: patient agreement to investigation or treatment – for adults and capable children
Consent form 2: parental agreement to investigation or treatment for a child or young person
Consent form 3: patient/parental agreement to investigation or treatment (procedures where consciousness is not impaired)
Consent form 4: form for adults who are unable to consent to investigation or treatment.

The Department of Health has issued significant guidance on consent which can be accessed from the website. There are exceptional situations in which consent does not have to be obtained and these are set out in Section V of the Mental Health Act 1983. The consent forms can be downloaded from the website or printed versions can be purchased.

In practical terms, for most occupational therapists working in mental health settings who have discussed and agreed their intervention plans with the patient and recorded this discussion, consent is likely to be implied if the patient then voluntarily enters into the procedure. It is important to be mindful of consent for all occupational therapy interventions and to be conversant with local policies and procedures.

Photographs and videotapes

Occupational therapists may wish to take photographs or videotapes to record patient changes and, while this is more usual in physical settings, it is sometimes used in mental health, for example to record body posture, eye contact or other social interaction. The occupational therapist must ensure that the patient gives consent both to the photograph and to the uses to which it will or may be put, using the relevant forms as outlined in the previous section. Explicit consent should always be gained before using photographs or videotapes of clients for staff training or for reproduction in a textbook.

CONFIDENTIALITY OF RECORDS

The confidentiality of all records is equally important, whether stored electronically, on paper, as videotapes or as photographs. Confidentiality issues specifically relating to electronic records have been addressed above. A key principle is that a patient's health records are held by the health service to support that patient's health care and therefore cannot be disclosed for other purposes without explicit consent from the patient, or where legal justification or robust public interest is concerned. The Department of Health has published a code of practice on confidentiality (DoH 2003) which covers:

- the concept of confidentiality
- what a confidential service should look like
- the main legal requirements
- a generic decision support tool for sharing or disclosing information
- examples of information disclosure scenarios.

Occupational therapists are ethically and legally obliged to safeguard confidential information relating to clients and disclosure of confidential information is normally only permissible where the client gives consent or there is legal justification.

The College of Occupational Therapists, *Code of Ethics and Professional Conduct* recognises that local and national policies on electronic notes should be adhered to regarding confidentiality issues and reference should be made to other national and local policies on access to personal health information. Occupational therapists should be familiar with their code of professional conduct, with the *NHS Code of Practice* and with their employing organisation's policies and procedures for record keeping, consent and confidentiality.

Access to the new electronic NHS care record will be limited to health-care professionals who have a relationship with the patient. Each health-care professional who is authorised to access the record will only be able to see information relevant to their role. The new record will be protected by the Data Protection Act 1998, the Human Rights Act 1998, the common-law duty of confidentiality and

professional ethics. To reassure patients that their personal medical information will be held securely, it is proposed that patients will be able to place particularly sensitive private information from their EHR into an electronic sealed envelope. This will only be able to be opened with the patient's consent, except in emergency situations and when required by law (see National Electronic Library for Health website for further information).

AUDIT OF RECORD KEEPING

It is good practice to audit records regularly to maintain quality and to provide a continued emphasis on the importance of good record keeping. Organisations will have formal audit procedures which will include the audit of records; however, occupational therapists are recommended also to adopt a regular peer review of records. NHS organisations will have guidelines on minimum standards for record keeping which occupational therapists must be aware of and follow in their daily practice. Occupational therapists will also find standard and service monitoring forms included in the record-keeping section of the *Professional Standards for Occupational Therapy Practice* (College of Occupational Therapists 2003).

It is important that occupational therapists, like other health-care workers, write all patient records in the knowledge and understanding that a treatment record is a crucial piece of evidence around which legal action can be based (Schulmeister 1987, cited by Bradshaw 1999). Health-care records should be completed as if every note will be examined in a court of law. If this seems unrealistic, it is important to understand that some claims are successful not because substandard care was proved but because there was no evidence in the record to show that any care had been given (Schulmeister 1987, cited by Bradshaw 1999).

SUMMARY

This chapter has addressed the importance attached to record keeping in the modern health service together with information about the proposed new single electronic record in the UK as an example of the modernisation of health records and its impact on record keeping. Throughout, the emphasis has been on occupational therapists working in the field of mental health being conversant with, and implementing, the record-keeping policies and procedures of the professional body and of their employing organisation. Accurate, defensible record keeping protects the patient from poor care and the occupational therapist from complaints and litigation. National policies and procedures discussed are summarised in Box 7.2 and good practice points are summarised in Box 7.3.

ACKNOWLEDGEMENT

Thanks are due to Chris Austin for reading and commenting on an earlier draft of this chapter.

Box 7.2 Summary of national policies and procedures relating to record keeping

- **Care Programme Approach.** In 1999, the *National Service Framework for Mental Health* (DoH 1999) formalised the integration of CPA and local authority Care Management, and this was implemented by April 2001.
- **Clinical Terms.** SNOMED Clinical Terms have been approved as the preferred clinical terminology for the NHS (NHS Information Authority 2003). They will be used as the basis for the National Care Record.
- **Confidentiality guidance.** *Confidentiality: NHS Code of Practice* (DoH 2003).
- **Legal responsibilities for records.** *For the record* (HSC 1999/053) sets out the legal responsibilities of NHS bodies to keep proper records, provides good practice guidelines and explains the periods of retention of records (DoH 1999c).
- **National care record.** In England, by 2010, every NHS patient in England will have an individual electronic care record (NHS Confederation 2003).
- **Summary statistics** on occupational therapy patient activity are collected nationally. In England these are the Körner K26 published by the Department of Health.

Box 7.3 Summary of good practice points

- **Access to patient records.** Occupational therapists dealing with requests for access to records should familiarise themselves with their employing body's procedures and policies in relation to the Data Protection Act 1998.
- **Auditing.** Records should be audited regularly in line with local policies and the *Professional Standards for Occupational Therapy Practice* (College of Occupational Therapists 2003). Records can be useful tools in audit and research, leading to effective practice based on evidence.
- **Care Programme Approach.** Occupational therapists should know the CPA status of patients they are working with and the name of the care co-ordinator.
- **Confidentiality.** Occupational therapists should be familiar with the *Code of Ethics and Professional Conduct*, the *NHS Code of Practice* and their employing organisation's policies and procedures for record keeping, consent and confidentiality.
- **Consent to treatment.** Occupational therapists should be aware of the national consent to treatment forms and their organisation's policies in relation to their use.
- **Multidisciplinary single patient records.** These are a positive step towards the fuller integration of mental health services and the availability of notes that will be provided by the national NHS care record.
- **Professional standards.** Occupational therapists should make themselves familiar with the record-keeping section in the *Professional Standards for Occupational Therapy Practice* (College of Occupational Therapists 2003) and their local record-keeping procedures.
- **Safeguarding.** Good record keeping gives a visual record of the quality of care, safeguarding the patient, the occupational therapist and the employing organisation.
- **Single assessment process for older people.** Occupational therapists working with older people within mental health services should ensure that they use the locally agreed single assessment package for both assessment and record keeping.

References

10 Downing Street 2003 Email update 08/12/2003 (accessed 14/07/2004). www.number-10.gov.uk/output/page4955. asp

Audit Commission 1995 Setting the record straight: a study of hospital medical records. Department of Health, London

Bradshaw T 1999 Clinical treatment recording practice: still a cause for concern. British Journal of Therapy and Rehabilitation 6(1): 627

College of Occupational Therapists 2003 Professional standards for occupational therapy practice. College of Occupational Therapists, London

College of Occupational Therapists 2005 Code of ethics and professional conduct. College of Occupational Therapists, London

College of Occupational Therapists 2006 Record keeping. College of Occupational Therapists, London

Data Protection Act 1998. www.hmso.gov.uk

Department of Health 1997 Caldicott review of patient identifiable information. Department of Health, London

Department of Health 1999a Effective care co-ordination in mental health services: modernizing the care programme approach: a policy booklet. Department of Health, London

Department of Health 1999b National service framework for mental health. Department of Health, London

Department of Health 1999c For the record. HSC 1999/053. Department of Health, Wetherby

Department of Health 2001 National service framework for older people. Department of Health, London

Department of Health 2003 Confidentiality. NHS Code of Practice. Department of Health, London

Department of Health 2006 Reviewing the Care Programme Approach: a consultation document. Care Services Improvement Partnership. www.dh.gov. uk/assetRoot/04/14/05/45/04140545.pdf (accessed 13/02/2007)

NHS Confederation 2003 Briefing No. 88. The national strategy for IT in the NHS. NHS Confederation Publications, London

NHS Executive 1986 An introduction to the NHS Centre for Coding and Classification. Department of Health, London

NHS Information Authority 2003 SNOMED Clinical Terms – programme update. NHS Information Agency Website. www.nhsia.nhs.uk

USEFUL WEBSITES

Consent to treatment: www.dh.gov/consent

Sealed envelopes: www.connectingforhealth.nhs.uk/crdb/sealed_envelopes_briefing_paper.pdf

NHS care record guarantee: www.connectingforhealth.nhs.uk/crdb/docs/crs_guarantee.pdf

Secondary Uses Service (SUS): www.connectingforhealth.nhs.uk/sus/reference/sus_vision.pdf

NHS Code of Practice: www.connectingforhealth.nhs.uk/publications/nhs_code_of_practice.pdf

Snomed-CT: www.connectingforhealth.nhs.uk/terminology/snomed

National Knowledge Service: www.nks.nhs.uk/

National Decision Support Service: www.nks.nhs.uk/nks_decision_support.asp

National Electronic Library for Health. NHS Care Records: http://libraries.nelh.nhs.uk/healthManagement/viewResource.asp?keywordID=13524

Scottish Health Statistics: www.isdscotland.org

SECTION 3

Ensuring Quality

SECTION CONTENTS

Chapter **8**

Clinical governance and clinical audit

Clare Beighton

INTRODUCTION

There is a 'responsibility upon every occupational therapist to scrutinise, and improve where necessary, the effectiveness and efficiency of the service she or he provides to service users and their carers' (College of Occupational Therapists 1999, point 5). Clinical governance and clinical audit are means by which occupational therapists can meet this responsibility.

Clinical governance is defined as 'a framework through which National Health Service organisations are accountable for continuously improving the quality of their services and safeguarding high standards of care by creating an environment in which excellence in clinical care will flourish' (DoH 1998).

Clinical audit is defined by the Healthcare Commission as 'a continuous process where healthcare professionals review patient care against agreed standards and make changes, where necessary, to meet those standards. The audit is then repeated to see if the changes have been made and the quality of patient care improved' (Healthcare Commission 2004).

In 1998, the British government published *A First Class Service: quality in the new NHS*. This strategy document outlined the government's plans to improve quality in the NHS and reduce regional variations in the treatment people receive. Clinical governance is seen to be a fundamental part of this strategy. The document described how standards would be:

- set via national service frameworks and National Institute for Clinical Excellence (NICE) guidance
- delivered via clinical governance, with support from lifelong learning and professional self-regulation
- monitored via the Commission for Health Improvement, a national patient/user survey and a national performance framework.

The Commission for Health Improvement (CHI) was established as a statutory body to demonstrate improvement in the quality of patient care in the NHS, and started operating on 1 April 2000. One of the Commission's roles was to carry out clinical governance reviews in order to identify areas of notable practice and those that required improvement. The CHI ceased to operate on 31 March 2004 and a new organisation, the Commission for Healthcare Audit and Inspection, commonly known as the Healthcare Commission, was formed. The Healthcare Commission became responsible for most of the CHI's functions in England, including mental health care reviews.

This chapter will explore clinical governance and its impact on occupational therapy in a mental health setting. The seven pillars of clinical governance used by the CHI when carrying out clinical governance reviews will be used to structure this.

- Patient, service user, carer and public involvement
- Risk management
- Clinical audit
- Clinical effectiveness
- Staffing and staff management
- Education, training and continuing personal and professional development
- Use of information to support clinical governance and health-care delivery

Each component will be explored and consideration will be given to its practical application to occupational therapy. Although the chapter is based on a legislative framework developed within the NHS in England and Wales, the principles of ensuring that services are of a high quality can be applied to any setting, including social care, in any country.

PATIENT, SERVICE USER, CARER AND PUBLIC INVOLVEMENT

The experiences that service users and their carers have of the quality and effectiveness of treatment, the attitudes of staff, the care environment, information given and choices available can act as catalysts for change. These experiences are, therefore, central to improving the quality of services (DoH 2001). However, the involvement of patients, service users, carers and the public means more than just a concern with individual experiences. Everybody is likely to need to use health and/or social care services at some point in their lives and so it is important to seek opinions from potential as well as current service users. Indeed, the Health and Social Care Act (Parliament 2001) in England has now made it compulsory for organisations to consult with service users, carers and the public on proposals to change the way that health and social care are delivered and on day-to-day service provision. Devolved governments within the UK have other arrangements in place to ensure that service user, carer and public involvement is at the heart of health and social care delivery. For example, in Wales the Signposts framework ensures that there are robust arrangements in place (Commission for Health Improvement 2004a).

It is clear, then, that professionals are expected to consult the users of their services and the public on all aspects of service delivery. Box 8.1 provides some examples of topics that occupational therapists may like to consult on.

There are several ways in which service users, carers and the public can be consulted and involved. Cusack & Sealey-Lapeš (2000) looked at this from an occupational therapy perspective and suggested:

- open days to seek ideas and standpoints from a wide range of people, including the general public
- focus groups to establish views about something specific, for example redecorating the unit or the programme of activities on offer
- patient panels, consisting of service users who want to have an effect on the service offered
- suggestion boxes
- surveys and questionnaires.

Box 8.1 Examples of issues on which occupational therapists may want to consult service users, their carers and the public

- Access to the service, which may include public transport, car parking, signposting and disabled access
- Waiting times
- Provision for minority populations
- Range and choice of services available
- Experience of assessment and treatment
- Access to information about treatment, e.g. copies of letters, treatment plans
- Privacy and confidentiality
- How service users want to be involved in their own care
- How service users want to be involved in promoting well-being
- Attitudes of staff
- Concerns, issues and compliments
- Information available, e.g. information leaflets, newsletters, websites
- Physical environment, e.g. comfort of waiting area

It is essential that when opinions have been sought, there are systems in place for improving the quality of services. One of the main findings within the CHI report on patient and public involvement was that, despite many activities being undertaken to involve patients, there were few changes to policy and practice as a result (Commission for Health Improvement 2004a).

CASE EXAMPLE 1: INVOLVING SERVICE USERS

A mental health NHS trust had, within its clinical governance action plan, a corporate aim to improve the written information available to service users and carers. The occupational therapy service, therefore, incorporated this aim into their action plan and each department was asked to review their written information.

The occupational therapists working in the acute day hospital had an information leaflet for service users on occupational therapy and the treatments they could access that was made available in the entrance to the day hospital. Service users were made aware that the occupational therapists wanted to review and update the information available to them and were invited, via the day hospital newsletter, to an initial meeting to discuss how to take it forward. Six service users attended the meeting and all agreed to form a focus group.

The group designed a questionnaire, with help from the audit department, to see what day hospital attendees thought of the information currently available and what they would like to see information on. Members of the focus group were given time within occupational therapy groups to distribute the questionnaires, without occupational therapy staff present so as to ensure that service users did not feel inhibited in completing them. To facilitate a high rate of return, they waited while the questionnaires were filled in and collected them immediately. The results were collated and analysed by the audit department.

The focus group then worked with a group of occupational therapists to write new information leaflets, based on the data gathered from the questionnaires. These included a description of what occupational therapy is and how it can help people with acute mental health problems. They also contained information on each of the groups on offer within the day hospital. The leaflets were written to comply with the trust's corporate image but the group also ensured that they were eye-catching and written in language that was easily understood. Since a significant proportion of day hospital service users were Chinese speakers, the leaflets were translated and made available to this population.

The leaflets were piloted for 2 months and alterations were made as a result of suggestions from a wider group of service users. The focus group agreed to be available for consultation about monitoring the use of the leaflets and writing new leaflets as the groups on offer changed.

RISK MANAGEMENT

Exposure to risk can adversely affect a service user's experience of health or social care and so it is important that risks are identified and reduced wherever possible. There are times when, despite attempts to manage risk, both service users and staff will be exposed to it. Therefore, systems need

Box. 8.2 Five practical steps in identifying and reducing risks to staff and service users (Derived from Clarke 2000)

Establish what could go wrong

↓

Rank the seriousness of the outcome on a three-point scale–very serious, moderately serious or minor

↓

Establish how probable it is that the incident will occur using a similar three-point scale of very probable, probable or not probable

↓

Identify what is being done to prevent the incident from happening

↓

Identify what action will be taken if the incident does occur

to be in place to monitor adverse events, look for trends and learn from mistakes.

Clarke (2000) identified five practical steps for identifying and reducing risks to staff and service users (Box 8.2). This method could be used to reduce both clinical risks, such as a service user deliberately harming herself in an occupational therapy session, or non-clinical risks, such as the spillage of a substance hazardous to health. Ranking the seriousness of the incident and the probability of it happening will help the team to prioritise any action that needs to be taken to prevent the incident from occurring. In other words, if the outcome is very serious and it is very probable that the incident will happen, it will need to be given high priority in terms of resources to prevent it occurring.

There are more comprehensive clinical risk management tools available for use in specific situations, such as *Clinical Risk Management: a clinical tool and practitioner manual* (Morgan 2000), obtainable from the Sainsbury Centre for Mental Health for use in community mental health settings. This tool encourages a positive approach to risk taking by identifying how the service user is at risk and how the problems can be tackled (Strong 2001).

Inevitably, things will go wrong at times and when they do, it is important that lessons are learned. Many organisations will have a system for recording incidents and near misses. Despite this, the CHI has found that regular reporting of incidents is patchy and that staff do not always know what constitutes a near miss (Commission for Health Improvement 2004b). It is important that occupational therapists know what systems are in place in their organisation, that they are clear what to report and when, and that they receive feedback so that trends can be identified, practice changed and lessons disseminated.

CASE EXAMPLE 2: REDUCING RISK

A group of occupational therapists working in mental health services for older people had participated in the organisation's incident reporting system since its inception. Whenever an incident or near miss occurred, they filled in a report and submitted it to the risk manager. Once a month they received information that summarised the incidents that had taken place. This was reviewed in the monthly occupational therapy meeting so that consideration could be given to how risks could be reduced, both for one-off incidents and for emerging trends.

Between February and April there was an increase in the number of incidents reported in the occupational therapy garden. There were four reports of near misses, describing how service users had stumbled on the way out to the greenhouse, and one report of an incident where a service user had fallen over in the same place. Further examination of the reports revealed that the reason for the falls was a patio slab that had become raised during the hard frost of the winter to create an uneven piece of ground.

As a result of this analysis, a requisition was put into the works department and the slab was relaid to make the ground even again. Consequently, there were fewer incident and near miss reports submitted in May, and no service users were reported to have stumbled or fallen on the patio. To ensure that this risk did not occur in other parts of the organisation, the risk management department circulated a memorandum highlighting the risk and asking managers to check patio areas.

CLINICAL AUDIT

Clinical audit enables practitioners to improve the quality of services to patients by providing a framework for reviewing care systematically against specific standards (Commission for Health Improvement 2003). Clinical audit is sometimes confused with other activities, such as surveys or research, and so it is important to be clear that the aim of audit is to measure whether written standards or guidelines have been achieved. For example, an occupational therapist may want to:

- survey colleagues to see which risk management tools are currently in use
- complete a research project to establish which risk management tool is most appropriate for use within their setting
- complete an audit to see whether the risk management tool is being used in accordance with specified standards.

It may be that there is an issue of concern to practitioners or service users where no standards have yet been set. According to the *Collins Concise Dictionary* (1995), a standard is 'an accepted or approved example of something against which others are judged or measured'. A standard in relation to practice, therefore, needs to be common practice or based on evidence, and clear enough to enable measurement.

Topics for audit may be identified in a variety of ways. The following are examples of issues that might be audited.

- How a service compares with national standards, such as those produced by the National Institute for Clinical Excellence or the College of Occupational Therapists (2003), for example, on consent to treatment.
- How a service compares with the standards they have set for specific interventions internally, for example, those relating to a group.
- How a service compares with standards that have been set following other clinical governance activity, for example, an audit of incident and near miss reporting in relation to risk management.

- How a service compares with standards that have been set by the organisation they work for, for example, record keeping.

Clinical audit is often referred to as a cyclical process that follows six stages (Kellett et al 2001, Sealey 1999).

1. Identify the issue to be audited.
2. Set the standard.
3. Measure activity against the set standard.
4. Identify any necessary changes to practice.
5. Implement change.
6. Monitor the effect of the change against the standard.

An audit checklist, which relates directly to the standards, can be a useful tool to enable measurement to take place. Figures 8.1 and 8.2 provide examples of audit checklists that relate to the standards in case example 3.

Although clinical audit is well established within health and social care services, it does not always lead to changes in service delivery (Commission for Health Improvement 2003, Kellett et al 2001, Sealey 1999). It is therefore important for occupational therapists to ensure that they complete the last three stages of the audit cycle by identifying what change needs to take place, implementing the change and re-auditing to monitor the effects of the change. Sealey (1999) considered this issue in considerable detail, identifying 10 reasons why the audit loop is not completed and offering possible solutions. For example, one of the reasons identified for not completing the loop is a lack of proficiency. Possible solutions are to:

- find and use people within the organisation who have audit skills
- arrange for training to take place
- develop a collection of good reference books on audit methods.

Occupational therapists have a responsibility to ensure that they disseminate the lessons learned from their audit activity so that practice can be improved across a wide spectrum of services.

Standard	Participant											
	1		2		3		4		5		6	
	Y	N	Y	N	Y	N	Y	N	Y	N	Y	N
All referrals will be seen for an interview prior to the commencement of the group to explain the reasons for referral to the group												
All referrals will be seen for an interview prior to the commencement of the group to establish when their anger is a problem to them												
All referrals will be seen for an interview prior to the commencement of the group to establish what they would like to achieve in relation to improving their anger management												
At the end of each session participants will be given an anger management strategy to practise over the following week												
Each session will include an opportunity for participants to report on how helpful they found the anger management strategy												
At the end of the six week course participants will be given the opportunity to evaluate the group in terms of its effectiveness in meeting their individual goal												

Figure 8.1 Audit checklist for examining case notes.

Standard	Session											
	1		2		3		4		5		6	
	Y	N	Y	N	Y	N	Y	N	Y	N	Y	N
The group will not exceed 10 people and will not run with less than 4 people												
The sessions will be planned to meet the needs of the participants												
The first session will set the ground rules for the group on the course												
The first session will outline what will be covered during the 6 week course												
The first session will give participants the opportunity to amend the course content												
Each session will last one hour												
The group will run over 6 consecutive weeks												
Each group will begin with a warm-up exercise												
At the end of the six week course participants will be given the opportunity to evaluate the group in terms of its delivery												

Figure 8.2 Audit checklist for examining planning notes and post-group reflections.

CASE EXAMPLE 3: AUDITING AN ANGER MANAGEMENT GROUP

The issue

A senior I occupational therapist had been running an anger management group for a year. She felt that the group was no longer functioning effectively because there had been several non-attendances during the last 6-week course.

The standards

Standards for the group were written when the group was set up, as follows.

- The group will not exceed 10 people and will not run with less than four people.
- All people referred will be seen for an initial interview prior to the commencement of the group to explain the reason why an anger management group has been recommended.
- All people referred will be seen for an initial interview prior to the commencement of the group to establish:
  - when their anger is a problem to them
  - what they would like to achieve in relation to improving their anger management.
- The sessions will be planned to meet the needs of the participants.
- Each session will last 1 hour.
- The group will run over 6 consecutive weeks.
- Each session will begin with a warm-up exercise.
- The first session will:
  - set the ground rules for the group on the course
  - outline what will be covered during the 6-week course
  - give participants the opportunity to amend the course content.
- At the end of each session participants will be given an anger management strategy to practise over the following week.
- Each session will include an opportunity for participants to report on how helpful they found the anger management strategy.
- At the end of the 6-week course, participants will be given the opportunity to evaluate the group in terms of:

- its delivery;
- its effectiveness in meeting their personal goals.

Measuring the activity

A retrospective audit was carried out using the case notes of those involved in the last anger management group, the planning notes and the post-group reflections.

Two audit checklists were devised, using the standards that were written when the group was set up. The case note audit checklist appears in Figure 8.1 and the audit checklist for examining the planning notes and post-group reflections in Figure 8.2.

Identifying and implementing changes

The audit showed the following.

- Not all participants were interviewed prior to the commencement of the group and were therefore unsure of the reason for their referral, and the group was not tailored to meet their specific needs.
- Demand for the group was such that 12 people had participated in the last presentation.
- Some sessions had run over an hour because too much was covered during the session.
- Over 6 consecutive weeks, the group was not run because the senior I occupational therapist had been off sick.

The following changes to practice were agreed and implemented.

- Each group would be limited to six people only. It would therefore be possible to interview all participants prior to the commencement of the group to ensure that they understood the reason for their referral and that the group could be tailored to their specific needs.
- The senior II occupational therapist and a nurse would be trained to run the anger management group so that:
  - extra groups could be put on when the demand arose
  - the group could still be run in the absence of the senior I occupational therapist.

- The group would run over 8 weeks to ensure there was enough time to cover all topics in sufficient detail.

Monitoring the effects of the changes

The standards and audit checklists were amended to reflect the agreed changes, and a re-audit was planned to take place in 6 months' time to monitor the effects of the changes.

CLINICAL EFFECTIVENESS

All service users want to be assured that the treatment they receive is effective and based on the best available evidence. Hence, clinical effectiveness forms another important pillar of clinical governance.

Since government reforms of health care were introduced in 1998, practitioners have been assisted to put best evidence into practice via nationally set and published standards and guidelines (DoH 1998). The National Institute for Health and Clinical Effectiveness, operating in England and Wales, and the Scottish Intercollegiate Guidelines Network (SIGN), operating in Scotland, disseminate several types of guidance including:

- technology appraisals of new and existing health technologies, such as methylphenidate (Ritalin/Equasym) for childhood ADHD (NICE 2000)
- clinical guidelines for the management of specific conditions, such as schizophrenia (NICE 2002).

National service frameworks (NSFs) are service models for specific services and care groups. They include performance measures and timescales, such as the *National Service Framework for Older People* (DoH 2001).

In October 2001, the Social Care Institute for Excellence (SCIE) was launched. By gathering and evaluating information about specific areas of social care, the SCIE disseminates key messages for good practice and ascertains where more research is needed (www.scie.org.uk/about/index.asp).

EVIDENCE-BASED PRACTICE

Occupational therapists must ensure that they comply with national recommendations and implement those that are relevant to the service they deliver. However, national guidance does not cover every intervention and occupational therapists have a professional responsibility to ensure that their work is based on the best available evidence (College of Occupational Therapists 2000). Some occupational therapists will want to contribute to the evidence base by carrying out research but all occupational therapists need to be able to search for the evidence, critically appraise it and, where appropriate, use it to change their practice.

Searching for the evidence demands that therapists are able to identify the area of practice they want to find evidence on, be it a new intervention or one that is already established. They then need to be able to define what exactly they want to know by writing a focused question that identifies the intervention, the population and the outcome. Evidence can be accessed from many places including, for example, the National electronic Library for Health (NeLH), which has an occupational therapy portal (www.nelh.nhs.uk/OT). This site can direct the user to online databases and high-quality electronic specialist resources, and is designed to be fast and efficient. For those working in social care the electronic Library for Social Care (eLSC) has been developed (www.elsc.org.uk/).

Not all published research is considered to be rigorous, and so occupational therapists need to be able to critically appraise the evidence that they find. Bannigan (2004, p4) stated that 'therapists who apply research that is not robust could mean they do more harm than good'. Critical appraisal is a skill in which many organisations provide training and support. If training and support are not available then a checklist, designed to assist the professional in evaluating specific types of research, is a useful starting point. For example, '10 questions to help you make sense of reviews' is available via the critical appraisal skills programme (www.phru.nhs.uk/casp/reviews.htm). Further information about critical appraisal skills can be found in Chapter 10.

Once robust evidence has been found it must be put into practice, which may mean changing established ways of working. It is not always easy to make changes and barriers are often identified. However, it is vital that evidence is used if patients are to receive the best service possible, and so solutions must be found. Successful change requires a clear, long-term aim that can be broken down into targets that demonstrate how progress is being made. It is also important that staff understand why change is necessary and that they are fully involved in the process (Alper 2002). Lastly, it is vital to have systems in place to monitor how effective the application of evidence-based practice has been.

Further information about evidence-based health care can be found in Chapters 6 and 10.

STAFFING AND STAFF MANAGEMENT

In order to ensure that service users receive the best possible care, it is important to make certain that there are systems in place for:

- recruiting and retaining a sufficient number of staff with the appropriate skills
- staff induction
- staff supervision and appraisal
- dealing with poor performance.

RECRUITMENT AND RETENTION

A shortage of occupational therapists in many countries, including the UK, means that many organisations have to address recruitment and retention issues. There are several innovative ways in which this can be done, for example, Therapy Award Days that reward staff for good practice (Therapy Weekly: January 29 2004). Other ways in which this can be tackled are through promoting the profession and ensuring that occupational therapy students are offered high-quality placements.

Occupational therapists' recruitment processes need to be fair and equitable, and sufficient checks need to be carried out to ensure that candidates are registered with the appropriate body, such as the Health Professions Council in the UK, and possess relevant skills and qualifications. Many organisations are now considering how they can involve service users in the selection of staff.

INDUCTION

New recruits need to be familiar with the policies and procedures of the organisations in which they work. Occupational therapists need to have systems in place to check that all staff, including those on temporary contracts, complete a comprehensive induction programme.

SUPERVISION AND APPRAISAL

Clinical supervision enables staff to discuss their caseload and to reflect on practice and any problems or issues they may have. Staff are often able to choose their clinical supervisor; if open and frank discussion is to take place, the relationship between these two people is critical. Supervision takes place on a regular basis throughout the year, dependent on the organisation's policy and the grade of the member of staff being supervised.

An appraisal takes place between a member of staff and their line manager once a year, with periodic reviews in between times. Usually, both the appraiser and the appraisee prepare for the discussion by thinking about: the appraisee's job within the context of the team and the wider organisation; their performance in it; their ideas for service improvement, and any development needs they have. The aim is for the appraisee to receive feedback on his work, to set objectives for the year and to outline a personal development plan. The objectives may relate to both the direction of the service and the direction which the occupational therapist wants to take in his professional career. For example, the service may have an objective to offer psychosocial interventions, which would create a need to train staff to use this approach. If the occupational therapist has an interest in this area, and would like to obtain a Master's degree, it will be possible to meet both service and personal development needs by enabling the occupational therapist to complete a Master's degree in psychosocial interventions.

For appraisal to be most valuable, the appraiser needs to be skilled in listening and giving feedback and the appraisee must be capable of receiving constructive criticism. Hence, many organisations provide training in appraisal.

DEALING WITH POOR PERFORMANCE

Whilst appraisal provides managers with a systematic way of dealing with poor performance, it is also necessary to have systems in place to enable staff to report any poor performance they witness. Many organisations have a policy in place to tackle this, which is often referred to as a 'whistle-blowing policy'. Students on placement should know how to access this policy and what to do if they come across poor practice, since it can go unrecognised by those who are accustomed to what they see on a day-to-day basis.

EDUCATION, TRAINING AND CONTINUING DEVELOPMENT

All education, training and development should enable occupational therapists to do their job better and, as a result, improve the service user's experience of treatment. Ongoing research and development in the field of occupational therapy in mental health means that practitioners need to keep abreast of progress and to develop their skills accordingly, in order to ensure that they are competent to practise. Organisations will also have mandatory training that staff need to do to keep them up to date. Mandatory training may include, for example, fire training, cardiopulmonary resuscitation and coping with service users who become aggressive.

PERSONAL DEVELOPMENT PORTFOLIOS

The Health Professions Council, which is responsible for registering occupational therapists in the UK, is moving towards requiring all allied health professionals to be able to evidence their continuing professional development activity (Health Professions Council 2004). This will mean that occupational therapists need to develop and maintain a personal portfolio. The Health Professions Council described this as 'a record and evidence of all continuing professional development undertaken, both personal and work related' (Health Professions Council 2004, p28).

The personal development portfolio should be more than just a collection of course certificates and achievements and should demonstrate how skills, knowledge, attitudes and understanding have changed. This will require that the occupational therapist is able to reflect on practice. Reflection involves therapists critically examining their work and should inform what is done in the future. The UK College of Occupational Therapists has produced a template for developing a reflective log that guides the user through a series of questions about facts, feelings, learning and conclusions (www.cot.co.uk/lifelong).

OTHER TYPES OF CONTINUING PROFESSIONAL DEVELOPMENT

When considering personal and professional development, it is important to be able to think creatively. Continuing professional development is much more than formal education. For example, an occupational therapist may be able to develop skills in running a group by shadowing a colleague or another member of the multidisciplinary team. The Health Professions Council gives many more examples of continuing professional development activity in Appendix 1 of their *Continuing Professional Development Consultation Paper* (Health Professions Council 2004).

Once an occupational therapist has completed a learning activity, he should consider how to disseminate his learning. This may benefit his professional development further since, for example, running an in-service training session can in itself be a professional development activity.

Further information about continuing professional development can be found in Chapter 6.

USE OF INFORMATION TO SUPPORT CLINICAL GOVERNANCE

Statistical information about waiting times, clinical interventions and how the therapist accounts for time at work has been collected by staff working within health and social care services for many years. More recently, the development of information technology has made collection and analysis easier. In terms of clinical governance, information only becomes useful when it is used to monitor, plan and improve the quality of patient care. The other important issue that occupational therapists need to be aware of and address is how they handle patient-identifiable information.

USING INFORMATION SYSTEMS

There are a number of information systems that occupational therapists use to collect information, such as the Patient Information Management System (PIMS). Systems such as this allow the therapist to register clients and record daily activity, including, for example:

- the group or individual treatment sessions that the service user attends
- time spent preparing for treatment sessions
- time spent on telephone calls in relation to individual service users
- time spent in case discussions.

Many organisations have information departments whose job is to input data and work with clinicians to interpret and use it to monitor, design and develop services. However, the Commission for Health Improvement found that in many mental health NHS trusts these systems are underdeveloped (Commission for Health Improvement 2004b). This can lead to a position where data are collected but not used. A no-win situation emerges because data are not accurate, so no effort is put into improving the information recorded and this justifies not using it (Bevan & Bawden 2001). In many cases, this also makes clinicians less inclined to collect data. This problem needs to be addressed because information can be a very useful tool for improving the quality of services.

Creighton & Nicholls (2001) offered some advice on dealing with clinical information.

- Involve the whole clinical team in deciding what to collect and aim to keep it simple.
- Ensure that clinicians are clear about why they are collecting information.

- Enable staff to understand how the information they collect can be used to help them improve their service so that they are more committed to collecting it.
- Aim to collect the same information over a long interval so that shifts over time can be observed.
- Become skilled at interpreting variations and understanding trends.
- Make clinical information available to service users.

HANDLING PATIENT–IDENTIFIABLE INFORMATION

The handling of personally identifiable information is exceptionally important, not only from a legal perspective but also in terms of the quality of service delivered. Occupational therapists need to be aware of what their responsibilities are with regard to confidentiality and sharing information. The basic principle is that information should not be disclosed without the consent of the individual concerned. However, there are exceptions to this rule and the issue can be complex (DoH 2003). In order to address this, all health and social care organisations appoint a Caldicott Guardian, who is responsible for safeguarding the confidentiality of patient information. The Guardian can offer advice if there is a concern regarding the handling of information.

SUMMARY

Ensuring that service users and their carers receive a high-quality service is fundamental to modern health and social services. The seven pillars of clinical governance provide a useful framework for occupational therapists to think about how to address this agenda within their own practice. Striving for excellence is a continuous process. Occupational therapists need to be able to plan their clinical governance activities in relation to what is most important to the people who use their services. This will entail setting clear aims and objectives, with realistic time scales, and involving the whole team in achieving them.

References

Alper H 2002 Management briefing: change management. National electronic Library for Health. Available online at: www.nelh.nhs.uk/management/mantop/0119change.doc

Bannigan K 2004 Opinion. Therapy Weekly February 26: 4

Bevan G, Bawden D 2001 Clinical data and information, and clinical governance. Clinical Governance Bulletin 2: 2-3

Clarke C 2000 Risk management: a user guide. British Journal of Occupational Therapy 63: 529-531

College of Occupational Therapists 1999 Position statement on clinical governance. College of Occupational Therapists, London

College of Occupational Therapists 2000 Code of ethics and professional conduct for occupational therapists. College of Occupational Therapists, London

College of Occupational Therapists 2003 Professional standards for occupational therapy practice. College of Occupational Therapists, London

Collins Concise Dictionary, revised 3rd edn 1995 Harper Collins, Glasgow

Commission for Health Improvement 2003 CHI clinical audit programme. Commission for Health Improvement, London

Commission for Health Improvement 2004a Sharing the learning on patient and public involvement from CHI's work. Commission for Health Improvement, London

Commission for Health Improvement 2004b What CHI has found in mental health trusts. Commission for Health Improvement London

Critical Appraisal Skills Programme 2002 10 questions to help you make sense of reviews. Available online at: www.phru.nhs.uk/casp/reviews.htm

Cusack L, Sealey-Lapeš C 2000 Clinical governance and user involvement. British Journal of Occupational Therapy 63: 539-546

Department of Health 1998 A first class service: quality in the new NHS. HMSO, London

Department of Health 2001 The national service framework for older people. HMSO, London

Department of Health 2001 Involving patients and the public in healthcare: response to listening exercise. HMSO, London

Department of Health 2003 Confidentiality: NHS code of practice. HMSO, London

Healthcare Commission 2004 What is clinical audit? Available online at: www.healthcarecommission.org.uk/InformationForServiceProviders

Health Professions Council 2004 Continuing professional development consultation paper. Health Professions Council, London

Kellett S, Newman D, Hawes A 2001 The elusive final stages of the audit cycle: do we put results into action? Journal of Clinical Governance 9: 187-191

Morgan S 2000 Clinical risk management: a clinical tool and practitioner manual. Sainsbury Centre for Mental Health, London

National Institute for Clinical Excellence 2000 Attention deficit hyperactivity disorder – methylphenidate. Number 13. National Institute for Clinical Excellence, London

National Institute for Clinical Excellence 2002 Schizophrenia. CG1. National Institute for Clinical Excellence, London

Parliament 2001 Health and Social Care Act 2001 HMSO, London

Sealey C 1999 Two common pitfalls in clinical audit: failing to complete the audit cycle and confusing audit with research. British Journal of Occupational Therapy 62: 238-243

Social Care Institute for Excellence (SCIE) 2005 About SCIE. Available online at. www.scie.org.uk/about/index.asp

Strong S 2001 The risk factor. Therapy Weekly January 11: 6

Chapter 9

Management

Lynne Barr

INTRODUCTION

This chapter will clarify what is meant by management, including budget and information management, and address its application and importance to the profession of occupational therapy. Various models and structures of management will be introduced, because the environments in which occupational therapists are employed are increasingly diverse. An understanding of different models is therefore more relevant than knowledge of historical structures in traditional institutions, such as the British National Health Service. The chapter will also differentiate between the key issues of management and leadership, as the terms are frequently confused.

There are many popular preconceptions about management. Most of them are negative, especially in respect of management in the public sector. The practising therapist will benefit from understanding concepts, styles and models of management in order to enhance her therapeutic role. However, leadership roles are held by therapy staff of all grades and these skills and behaviours are of paramount importance to the profession in the short and longer term; therefore this chapter is for everyone, not only for aspiring managers.

WHAT IS MANAGEMENT?

An early management theorist, Mary Parker Follet (cited in Steers et al 1985, p29), said that 'management is the art of getting things done through people'. This statement implies that more or better things can be achieved through working with others than by an individual working alone. However, those efforts need to be co-ordinated so that all the effort is directed towards a common goal. Hence, the role of the manager emerged.

Steers and colleagues (1985) updated this concept to one which occupational therapists will recognise more readily: 'Management is the process of planning, organising, directing and controlling the activities of employees in combination with other organisational resources to accomplish stated organisational goals'. This concept can be related to specific aspects of management that apply to professions in the modern health and social care agencies.

The key functions of a manager can be discussed within the four domains referred to above (Steers et al 1985):

1. planning
2. organising
3. directing
4. controlling.

PLANNING

Planning may be strategic, i.e. long-term, or operational.

Strategic planning

Strategic planning in modern management terms usually involves a 3–5 year plan. Planning for a longer period becomes too vague as the influencing factors are unknown and more difficult to predict. The strategic plan influences the annual planning cycle.

The external environment of political and financial influences has a major impact upon the vision of the strategic plan; therefore, the national government agenda has both a direct impact and an indirect influence on occupational therapy. This influence comes through its central funding policy, national priorities, such as the public health targets (DoH 1997) and social policy decisions, such as the national service frameworks for various care groups, for example older people. It is important that a strategic plan for occupational

therapy recognises the impact of the external environment and appropriately uses the opportunities that it creates. A successful manager will anticipate and prepare staff and senior colleagues for the future with this framework in mind. This preparation includes forecasting the workforce requirements to enable therapists to respond to demands and future expectations.

Operational planning

This is the planning and scheduling of workloads within the resources available. To some extent, every occupational therapist is a manager when planning her own schedule with that of colleagues and balancing what is required with who and what is available. The manager needs to address these issues across a whole service, ensuring that the urgent and important work is done and that preparation and investment in longer term needs are not ignored. This balancing act needs to take into account the workload and the complexity of the work, together with the development needs of staff.

Operational planning is frequently done uni-professionally, on a weekly or monthly basis, and reviewed as and when necessary or discussed with other professional colleagues in regular meetings.

ORGANISING

Organisational skills are required on a day-to-day basis. The operational manager needs to be able to respond to the daily demands and fluctuations of the service. The manager who knows the service and staff well is able to handle several situations at once, keep calm in stressful situations and consistently deliver what is required. She will communicate openly with all concerned so that staff respond positively to the changes required. Changes may be temporary or permanent and opportunities can arise from such events, if handled well.

DIRECTING

Directing is activity that enables managers to gain the participation of the workforce. It is necessary to understand the dynamics of workgroups, key individuals and how they respond to situations. There are different cultures within workplaces and professions and it is important to recognise the impact of these and how to handle each situation. Textbook solutions rarely exist in the workplace and a good manager will exhibit leadership skills in order to resolve or, better still, to prevent the occurrence of problems that disrupt work or dishearten the staff unnecessarily.

Directing involves setting and being able to implement the objectives of the organisation, involving staff in negotiating the direction and setting specific objectives, keeping the impetus to achieve them in the time scale proposed.

Occupational therapists are familiar with group dynamics with their client groups. Once the value of this knowledge is recognised, the transference of these skills into management is relatively straightforward.

CONTROLLING

The term *controlling* implies a rigid and constraining force in order to achieve the desired outcome of the service. This is not the case in management terms; controlling arises out of the availability, knowledge and interpretation of data required by the manager. Managers must now have skills in information technology (IT), budgets and audit to gain access to the information that they need.

Information is the means by which managers gain tangible evidence to explain service activities carried out by the staff over a period of time. This information, or management reports, as they are frequently referred to, assists in communication with other management colleagues and helps managers to understand how the occupational therapy service is perceived by others. The types of reports that are usually generated are detailed in Table 9.1.

The emphasis of each report will, however, vary according to the project or employing organisation. Every organisation has to demonstrate its effectiveness and value for money and, in the case of public sector organisations, there are specific information reports engendered from the information required by, for example, the Department of Health.

Data must be interpreted by managers who understand the service they manage. Data should be used with caution and conclusions should only be drawn with full analysis of the situation. Data reports are best used over time, to identify trends and issues of concern or progress. Timely feedback to staff of the information gained is important so that they see the impact of their contributions on the service as a whole.

It is worth noting that some computer systems still have difficulty representing the activities of therapeutic professions. However, while data collection is costly in terms of staff resources and financial capital, the occupational therapy profession does need to continue in the quest for improvement if services are to be able to produce the required results in the future.

BUDGET CONTROL WITH MANAGEMENT

The diversity of management models and structures throughout the profession will be reflected in the financial and budgetary control systems that are in place. On the whole, the structure of an organisation will determine the level of budgetary devolution and the accountability of each manager. The flatter the management structure, the greater the devolution of responsibility for the service and the budget.

A budget is a useful planning and control tool. It is a financial statement of future expenditure and income (revenue) that helps a manager to plan the best use of resources. Resources can be people or machinery, equipment, basic materials or utilities, such as communication systems, heating or lighting.

Budgets serve several purposes. They:

- aid communication between managers about their commitment to the priorities of the organisation
- require a periodic review of the service objectives because of the fixed time scale related to the objectives
- contribute to the measurement of effectiveness of the use of resources.

Table 9.1 Types of management report

Report	Description/purpose	Frequency
Annual report	Summary of achievements and resources available within the year	Annual
Financial statement	Summary statements on expenditure and income	Monthly
	Predictions of the annual expenditure based on past performance	
	Explicit over- or underspend statement on the annual budget	
Activity report	Number of patients/clients received treatment	Monthly
	Subsection:	
	• by specialty/doctor or referrer	
	• by therapist	
	• by location of treatment	
	• by time spent in treatment	
	• by time spent on other duties	
	Ratio of new referrals to treatments	
	Number of non-attenders	
	Number waiting for treatment	
	Length of waiting times for appointment	
Staffing returns	Staff employed/leavers/hours worked	Monthly
	Sickness/absence rates	
Audit reports (internal and external)	Relevant to quality initiatives:	Quarterly or annual
	• Investors in People award	
	• evaluation of training	
	• clinical governance	
	• recruitment factors such as vacancy times, responses and number of applicants, turnover of staff by grade	

The occupational therapy budget will be constructed from one or more of the following:

- bid system
- financial planning system
- planning programme budget system
- zero based budget system.

These are all subject to best practice guidelines produced by the NHS Audit Commission, the National Audit Office and the professional accounting bodies (Wilson 1998).

THE ECONOMIC ENVIRONMENT IN THE UK

Public sector organisations include central and local government offices and public corporations. They exist to provide services on a not-for-profit basis and are funded by income raised from public taxes (84.5%), national insurance (11.3%), prescription charges and other sources. The size and efficiency of the organisation are measured by the public expenditure level rather than by the profit made, as would be the case in an independent agency or by an individual operating on a private basis.

The UK has what is known as a mixed economy and public sector organisations operate in that external environment.

New services or service developments are most likely to be resourced through:

- identifying national and local priorities, according to national priorities guidance
- confirming the resources available
- monitoring commissioned services against national targets and objectives for the NHS (DoH 1998, 1999).

The allocation of budgets against national and local priorities, focused through joint investment plans and partnership grants, is largely supportive of the type of investment in which occupational therapy services are involved. This means that the occupational therapy manager must work closely with other professional colleagues in order to take advantage of the opportunities that are available through this planning programme budget system. Funding is allocated to jointly commissioned ventures for specific client groups and targeted over a 3-year period to reshape services to address the needs identified.

The occupational therapy manager needs to understand how the NHS is funded in order to be able to recognise and address health priority targets for the locality. It is also important to be able to influence the primary care trusts as it is they who approve and support new developments for their localities.

SETTING THE BUDGET

Despite the above planning mechanism for service developments, the main public sector bodies are essentially constrained by central government's control of funding. Change can only be achieved by rethinking existing services. The costing exercise for the NHS is carried out on an activity-based costing and budgeting basis. The activity base is increasingly target orientated, with financial penalties for default. Targets are largely influenced by the political agenda of the day.

Close monitoring of the budgetary situation reflects activity towards targets and is used as an indicator throughout the year. Although it is possible to modify and influence activity as a result of analysis of the budget versus activity, there are only limited options available for action because of the political nature of the situation.

It is vital that the budget should be predicted as accurately as possible, as it will significantly affect the level of service that can be provided throughout the next year. Prediction is, however, not an exact science and the manager can only predict on the basis of the information that is available. The historical pattern of services can demonstrate trends over time but will not identify details.

Some of the management reports identified in Table 9.1 will help to inform the manager about changing trends in the service and where resources need to be directed.

THE OCCUPATIONAL THERAPY BUDGET

The occupational therapy budget is usually set once a year, several months ahead of the end of the financial year, that is, in January, basing costs on the fixed costs of the service, projected forward to the end of the financial year.

The occupational therapy budget can contain three elements.

1. **Pay costs.** These are related to the costs incurred by the employment and payment of staff.
2. **Non-pay costs.** These are related to the expenses incurred from running the service, such as materials used, stationery, training costs and travel.
3. **Income.** These accounts are established to monitor credits received by the department, usually in respect of services provided that are additional to the core or central services, income derived from providing training, or income from the sale of goods.

Financial statements about cashflow, month-on-month, are received monthly. These statements reflect the income and expenditure of the service for that specific month and are used to predict the financial situation at the end of the year. A sample financial statement is shown in Table 9.2 and a sample pay budget statement in Table 9.3.

BUDGET MANAGEMENT

Understanding how the budget management system operates enables the manager to maintain control. All expenditure goes through the accounts ledger and is charged to the appropriate account by a system of accounting codes. The coding of expenditure is therefore important if the correct budget is to be charged with the correct amount of expenditure.

Auditors oversee the financial management of the service. The main function of audit is to:

• prevent and check against fraud
• check that standing financial instructions are being followed
• check that the organisation's procedures are robust
• ensure that value for money is being achieved
• ensure that public money is being used appropriately.

Table 9. 2   Sample financial statement

Cost Centre = 1234	Occupational Therapy			Date:12 February 2000 Period: January 2000	
Staff expenditure	MPE budget	MPE actual	Annual budget	Current month	Variance month
Senior manager	1.00	1.00	28500	2500	125
OT grade 11	1.00	1.00	24600	2150	100
OT grade 10	5.60	6.55	157206	12025	(1075)
OT grade 9	4.53	4.00	72570	6748	(894)
OT grade 8	6.75	5.00	116346	5610	(1963)
Tech inst. 5	0.00	1.00	0	0	0
OT asst. 4	1.00	1.00	12500	1500	458
OT asst. 3	5.50	6.50	55000	5416	573

The figures in parentheses indicate an underspend. The variance for the month is an indicator. Predictions for the year end will be forecast by the variances and how much under or over the budget will be, depending on how long the variances occur. Variances may occur because the budget-setting exercise was not done well. In the case of this example, by the month of January the forecast should be quite clear and there would be another column indicating the forecast situation for the end of the financial year.

Table 9.3   Therapy budget statement: pay

Cost centre = 1234	Occupational therapy		Date: 12 Feb 2000 Period: January 2000	
Non-staff expenditure	Annual budget	Monthly budget	Actual	Variance
Therapy mats and equipment	2000	166	250	84
Provisions	300	50	25	(25)
Printing and stationary	1000	84	150	66
Lease car	2000	166	800	634
Uniforms	0	0	120	120

Some non-staff expenditure may not be funded although there are accounts open, such as uniforms in this example. In this instance, the total figure for non-staff expenditure will be the one that is taken into account. However, in the case demonstrated above, the whole of the non-staff expenditure can be predicted to be in a grossly overspent situation by the end of the financial year unless some additional action is taken. The monthly budget totals £465. The monthly expenditure is £1345, therefore the overspend would be 12 × the difference between the two, that is £880 × 12 = £10,560. However, this may have been an unusual month and a forecast based on one month could be grossly inaccurate. The trend over the whole year needs to be taken into account.

There are usually two main audit departments in contact with occupational therapy departments: the financial audit department and the NHS Audit Commission.

Financial audit department

The financial audit department will be in contact once a year to examine the accounting system for items for resale and for the sale of any goods produced by the department. This requires that all items are counted, if still in stock, or accounted for and appropriately charged for if sold. This task, known as the stock take, needs to be carried out at the end of each financial year, as close to 31 March as possible.

NHS Audit Commission

The NHS Audit Commission reports to Parliament on the economy and efficiency of services. It usually carries out the audits by visiting departments at prearranged times but at relatively short notice. Frequently, the same services across the country will be audited for a 6- or 12-month period. This allows the Commission to benchmark the audited services and gain an overview of the situation, at that time, across the country. This type of audit will happen only very infrequently for the same services and includes wider issues than financial audit.

MANAGEMENT ROLES

Other models of management will become familiar to therapists as they progress in their careers. These are based on management roles rather than tasks. Henry Mintzberg (1973) described a model, based on his research of the 1970s, in which he examined how different managers at all levels spent their time. It is more than the series of tasks, as the first, functional approaches to management would have led us to believe. From this research emerged the following constellation of roles (Lessen 1990):

- decisional roles
- informational roles
- interpersonal roles.

DECISIONAL ROLES

These can be subdivided into four types of role. Each is involved with decision making from a different angle or context.

1. **Entrepreneur.** The proactive decision maker, initiator of change.
2. **Disturbance handler.** Instant decision maker, responding to situations beyond her control.
3. **Resource allocator.** Pre-planned decisions about resource management.
4. **Negotiator.** Decision making in the context of negotiations involving both pre-planned and improvised responses, depending on the circumstances.

INFORMATIONAL ROLES

Mintzberg (1973) considered that the receipt and communication of information is the central issue for the manager. This includes both informal and formal aspects of communication. Informational roles are of three types.

1. **The monitor** seeks information, from formal or informal sources, to be used to best advantage, such as the management reports referred to in Table 9.1.
2. **The disseminator** distributes information that would not be otherwise available to those senior and junior to her. This information is usually passed on by personal contact.
3. **The spokesperson** takes formal responsibility for communicating information up and down the organisation, or even outside the organisation. This is a key role that frequently reflects the function of the organisation and the individual style of the manager.

INTERPERSONAL ROLES

Interpersonal relationships help to keep the service running smoothly at all times. The interpersonal role has three facets.

1. **Liaison.** The liaison person deals with people outside her immediate span of control. Success depends upon the interpersonal skills of the individual rather than pure decision-making skills.
2. **Figurehead.** This role is that of a formal representative at important functions.
3. **Leader.** The leadership role is by far the most important and involves projecting values and creating a sense of direction, empathising with others according to their needs and inspiring or motivating.

Leadership issues will be dealt with more thoroughly later in this chapter.

MANAGEMENT STRUCTURES

Management structures are formal frameworks of accountability and responsibility within an organisation. The framework will indicate the levels and type of management required to fulfil the goals of the organisation. These are outlined briefly below.

LEVELS OF MANAGEMENT

Levels of management are frequently referred to as tiers, as shown in Table 9.4.

While the manager has a complex role that involves many dimensions and numerous tasks, the tier of management will determine the major skills required for the fulfilment of the job. That is to say, the first-line manager will direct and monitor day-to-day issues, making sure that tasks are completed as well as possible and bringing problems to the attention of the middle manager. The senior manager will be more involved in longer term issues that will affect the workforce, such as planning staffing and recruitment levels. The senior manager needs to be able to rely on the middle and first-line managers to organise and carry out the jobs that are required. Essentially, the senior manager needs to be in contact with the other tiers of management in order to be able to plan effectively so that the expectations of staff are realistic and that services are planned where and how they are needed. This interrelationship is paramount to the success of any management structure. Each tier is as important as the others

Table 9.4 Management tiers

Tier	Skills
Senior management	Conceptual and co-ordinating skills
	Sense of vision and direction
	Negotiating and planning
	Awareness of trends and influences
Middle management	Frequently uniprofessional
	Organisational and personnel/ staff management skills
	Attention to detail and monitoring of information
	Able to respond quickly to changes and demands
First-line management	Team leadership
	Specialised/limited scope of responsibility
	Knowledge and skills primarily related to specialist field
	Day-to-day responsibilities for the service

and the communication between them needs to be open, honest and supportive.

It is important to recognise that each manager, while at a recognised level of management within the service, will be a part of another, often wider management structure across the organisation. Therefore, relationships and skills will need to be adaptable for the complex nature of this position. For example, the most senior manager of an occupational therapy service could be at the top of the career ladder within the professional structure but would be considered as a middle or first-line manager within the management structure of the organisation as a whole.

ORGANISATIONAL STRUCTURES

The lines of communication and number of tiers in an organisation will reflect the management style and structure. There are wide variations in the style and manner of communication depending upon the culture and historical patterns of behaviour within each organisation. These may be based on the type of work and responsibilities of the organisation or on the type and level of technical skills, knowledge base and working patterns of the workforce. Whatever the format of the organisation, it is essential not to underestimate the impact that this will have on the responses of the workforce, particularly during periods of change. Different management structures affect the scope of influence and/or responsibility of the managers of the service. Most organisations operate in a hierarchical structure within themselves. The structure resembles a family tree and the number of branches between the chief executive or management board and the manager demonstrates the lines of communication and, therefore, the level of authority of the manager within the organisation.

Structure can group different aspects of the organisation according to:

- division of work
- span of control and responsibility
- the nature of the work; that is, level of formality required
- preferred number of levels of management.

Familiar groupings include the following.

- **Functional.** Such as specialist areas, usually in small organisations.
- **General.** Full span of control over the whole process for particular population or client groups, such as a disability resource team.
- **Divisional.** These structures become efficient in dealing with their own area but largely operate as autonomous entities within the organisation. Duplication of resources can occur, for example within clinical divisions in a hospital setting.
- **Geographical.** These structures allow the service to be as close to the action as possible. This can be seen in community-based services, for example in community mental health teams.
- **Matrix.** These are mixed structures that attempt to be flexible and responsive to complex, changing environments. These are more common in the current public service arena where integrated approaches are being sought to resolve some of the increasing and chronic health and social care needs of the clients with whom occupational therapists work.

THE OCCUPATIONAL THERAPY MANAGER

The manager of an occupational therapy service may or may not be an experienced occupational therapist. If he is an occupational therapist, he may be regarded as a skilled technical/professional manager and may be required to be a practising therapist with modern skills in a particular field that are relevant to the employing organisation. More frequently now, occupational therapists are managed by general managers or managers from other professional groups, particularly in community settings where the team structure is truly multiprofessional. This may also be a feature for occupational therapists working in a partnership situation where a matrix management structure exists between the organisations involved. In this instance there should be a lead occupational therapist recognised by the organisation, who would advise both individual therapists and the organisation on any professional issues that arise. This role can include professional supervision of individual therapists.

The important additional element required, if the manager of the service is not an occupational therapist, is communication skills. It is vital that the manager listens well to staff about the service and its requirements but, equally essentially, that the occupational therapists themselves learn to articulate their needs, aspirations and achievements in a manner that is heard by their manager.

The role of the occupational therapy manager is diverse as the actual tasks of the manager will vary according to the organisation that they are working for. The profession needs to promote and support the development of eloquent and competent managers. The role of manager needs self-discipline and organisation. However, this can be more readily achieved and maintained if some leadership qualities and attitudes are already present.

LEADERSHIP

This part of the chapter attempts to demonstrate the differences between leadership and management and the importance of leadership to the profession of occupational therapy as a whole and to each individual occupational therapist.

Leadership is a complex activity of social interaction involving:

- processes of influence
- people who are both leaders and followers
- the commitment of individuals to common goals and the enhancement of group cohesiveness (Saddler 1999).

Management is concerned with the achievement of plans through tasks and processes, whereas leadership is about aligning people and gaining their commitment to the vision and direction of the service. Individuals in organisations can rarely be successful on their own; they must influence, lead and co-ordinate efforts to achieve their goals. The success of leadership rests on the ability to influence different groups in the organisation.

Leaders are people in a position of influence either by their status, which can be as a specialist or expert, or by their particular personal qualities, popularity or sense of judgement. Therefore, leaders are not always managers, although some managers are leaders. Some of the best known managers have become famous because of their leadership qualities. This explains why management and leadership can become confused.

LEADERSHIP IN OCCUPATIONAL THERAPY

Occupational therapists of any grade can find themselves in a position of influence and leadership, possibly much more frequently than some of their other working colleagues, because of the relatively low numbers of staff in each working situation. There will regularly be only one occupational therapist in a rehabilitation team compared, for example, with physiotherapists or nurses. The individual occupational therapist will therefore have a significant personal and professional influence on that team, acting as a role model for the profession, even at a relatively junior grade. Some people are natural leaders, for example the person who can organise a successful social evening for a staff group or someone who gathers people around them in order to resolve issues successfully.

Good leaders are consistent in their values and commitment and people respond willingly to them. 'Personal leadership is not an event, it is an ongoing process of clarifying (your) vision, values and aligning yourself with timeless principles' (Covey 1992).

Leadership is consistent with the ethos and values of occupational therapy and is therefore compatible with the role of the committed and inspired occupational therapist. It is important, when trying to understand the dimensions of leadership, to recognise and understand the subsets of motivation that are essential tools of the occupational therapist:

- goal setting and ownership
- energy and agreed action plan
- intrinsic reward system.

The occupational therapist will link the three subsets to the needs and rehabilitation goals of the patient or client, whereas the organisational leader will use the same skills with individual staff or colleagues. By linking goals, energy and rewards (often intrinsic), the effective leader can use the valuable skill of motivation to empower people to perform effectively.

In work-based teams, motivation and rewards for the individual need to be compatible with the ethos and objectives of the team and the organisation or project. The occupational therapist or manager working in an interagency or multidisciplinary team needs to be able to recognise the leadership role and the challenges that arise. The therapist should be able to respond constructively to, and operate within, the dynamics and motivational factors that affect the team. An effective team is much more than a group getting on well and it requires leadership to recognise the team's requirements and strengths. A successful leader will encourage and value openness and reflexivity which, in turn, will allow the team to challenge, learn and grow together to increase their effectiveness as a whole.

LEADERSHIP TRAITS AND BEHAVIOURS

The elements of leadership can be observed as attitudes and behaviours, succinctly described by Sundstrom et al (1990, cited in Leadership Effectiveness Analysis™ 1998) as 'Management is doing things right … leadership is doing the right thing'. These behaviours or traits are easily recognisable but are often difficult to describe, particularly in an objective manner within the work situation. Table 9.5 lists the traits of a leader and is taken from the Leadership Effectiveness Analysis™ (1998). This leadership model can be employed to clarify the terminology we use to identify the spectrum of behaviours we recognise in our leaders and in some of our managers.

A good leader will be able to select and use the above skills and behaviours appropriately to the best effect, in context. The skill of the leader is in being able to adapt, knowing when to use some traits and hold back on others. The therapy leader will use these skills alongside clinical or technical skills and make decisions with a balance of judgement, positive acknowledgement and a proactive stance.

The leadership element of management is now a requirement of the modern manager. However, it can be a beneficial and highly effective trait in all grades of staff, such as a co-ordinator of a graduate therapist group, a lead therapist in research or a health and safety representative. Individual therapists could find themselves in specific projects, clinical audits or trail-blazing ventures, where the approach that they take could

Table 9.5 Leadership traits and behaviours (reproduced with permission from the Leadership Research Group)

Leadership trait	Behaviour demonstrated
Creating a vision	
Traditional	Studying problems in the light of past practice, to ensure predictability and reduce risk
Innovative	Feeling comfortable in fast-changing environments; being willing to take risks and to consider new approaches
Technical	Acquiring and maintaining in-depth knowledge in a particular field, using the expert knowledge to draw conclusions
Self	Recognising the need for independent decision making
Strategic	Taking a long-range, broad-based approach to problem solving, thinking ahead and planning
Developing followers	
Persuasiveness	Building commitment by convincing others, winning others over to the point of view
Outgoing	A capacity to quickly establish easy relationships, a friendly and informal manner
Excitement	Operating with a good deal of energy and expression, keeping others involved and enthusiastic
Restraint	Maintaining a low-key interpersonal demeanour by working to control emotional expression
Implementing the vision	
Structuring	Developing and utilising guidelines; an organised approach
Tactical	Emphasising production of results; practical strategies
Communication	Clear expression of what is expected and needed; maintaining flow of information
Delegation	Enlisting the talents of others by giving them important jobs and autonomy to do it
Following through	
Control	Setting deadlines for actions and ensuring progression to completion
Feedback	Letting people know in a straightforward manner how well they are performing against the expectations
Achieving results	
Management focus	Seeking to exert influence over others
Dominant	Pushing to achieve results
Production	A strong orientation towards achievement, with high expectations of self and others
Team playing	
Co-operation	Accommodating the needs of others in order to assist with the achievement of their objectives
Consensual	Collecting and valuing the contributions of others in decision-making processes
Authority	Showing loyalty and respecting the opinions of people in authority
Empathy	Demonstrating an active concern for the needs of others through relationships

have a minimal impact or could make a radical difference. Most occupational therapists want to make a difference. The behaviours of the leader display skills and qualities that would help them to do just that, whether or not they have the title of manager.

SUMMARY

This chapter has addressed the management tasks and roles and the leadership qualities required by the modern occupational therapy manager. It is essential that the management of occupational therapists is in competent hands. The concept that this chapter hoped to convey is one of budget and financial management as information tools for the occupational therapy manager. Skills and a sense of purpose are fundamental to the successful use of these tools, as with any others. Once the monthly financial statement becomes a useful source of information for the manager, it holds few areas for concern. The information it conveys includes levels of activity, who is doing what and how much it is costing to do it. The statement should only reflect what the manager already knows about the service and, if there are any surprises, they are quickly investigated with the help of the financial advisor.

It may be that the manager of the team within which the individual works is not an occupational therapist. Whilst this may not be the preferred model of management, it is not necessarily a problem as long as the professions within the team are well respected and represented at senior levels through a professional lead person. The structure of the organisation and fairness of the manager will determine if this can be achieved successfully. Management tasks can well be achieved by a sensitive and empathetic manager with good leadership skills. However, the profession does need occupational therapists to be leaders. The long-term future of the profession, in its many and diverse roles and functions, needs individuals to do the right thing, whatever their status and place of work.

The relevance of strategic planning mechanisms and financial models is included to aid the manager in recognising opportunities that exist for the development of client-focused services. It is only by relating services to these strategic objectives and submitting bids through these routes that service developments will be recognised. These are more likely to be achieved if they are submitted through shared approaches with our colleagues. However, whatever the planning mechanism, the financial models that apply should be recognised and utilised to resource adequately the service developments required.

References

Covey S 1992 Seven habits of highly effective people: restoring the character ethic. Simon and Schuster, London

Department of Health 1997 Our healthier nation. HMSO, London

Department of Health 1998 The new NHS. HMSO, London

Department of Health 1999 Planning for health and health care. HSC1999/244. Department of Health, London

Leadership Effectiveness Analysis™ 1998 Management Research Group GabHm, Munich

Lessen R 1990 Global management principles. Prentice Hall, Hertfordshire

Mintzberg H 1973 The nature of managerial work. Harper and Row, New York

Saddler P 1999 Leadership in tomorrow's company. Centre for Tomorrow's Company, London

Steers RM, Ungson GR, Mowday RT 1985 Managing effective organisations. Boston Publishing, Kent

Wilson J 1998 Financial management for the public services. Open University Press, Buckingham

Chapter **10**

Research, evidence-based practice and professional effectiveness

Irene Ilott

INTRODUCTION

This chapter concentrates upon empirical knowledge derived from research. However, this does not mean that other sources of knowledge are of lesser value; each offers a distinct and equally valuable contribution to our understanding of occupation. Remember:

> Research is tremendously important, but it is a horse to be ridden and not a deity to be worshipped. At its best it can propel us into a more effective and assured future but, at its worst, it erodes the courage to say what we think without feeling obliged to prove that three other people have already said it. (Willson 2002, p312)

In this chapter, research is considered as one form of knowledge that underpins practice. Primary and secondary studies are introduced to highlight the connection between research and evidence-based occupational therapy. Evidence-based practice means incorporating the best available research into the clinical reasoning process to enhance the effectiveness of interventions. Criteria for judging research, and other information such as policy community knowledge, are presented. This is because it is essential to adopt a challenging approach to all sources and types of knowledge.

The aim is to highlight research principles and how they can be used to help fulfil the professional obligation to keep up to date. Resources are signposted in the boxes in the text and further reading is suggested in the bibliography. The chapter ends with some tips about where to start looking for relevant, high-quality evidence.

DEFINITIONS

There is a cyclical relationship between theory, research and evaluative practice, all of which are evolving. This means that new research should influence theory and change practice while practice informs both theory and research topics. In this way, there is an iterative increase in the knowledge base of the profession, as well as in the understanding of individual practitioners.

This section defines some of the terms used throughout the chapter. These terms are research, development, evidence-based practice, effectiveness, audit, evaluation, theory and knowledge. Research is defined first because research generates the evidence for evidence-based practice. Research can provide the service standards that are then audited as part of a quality assurance process.

Research and development

The Research Governance Framework for Health and Social Care defines research as 'the attempt to derive generalisable new knowledge by addressing clearly defined questions with systematic and rigorous methods' (DoH 2005, p3). Research is usually coupled with development – research provides a framework for exploring and offering explanation, whilst development refers to communicating and using the findings to enhance the payback from investment in research (Buxton et al 2000). Development also encompasses research utilisation, which means incorporating the evidence generated from research studies into decision making (Craik & Rappolt 2006).

In this section, three types of research are defined, namely primary, secondary and emancipatory studies. Primary research refers to original studies that address a question or test a hypothesis, whilst secondary research involves drawing together the results of similar primary research in a systematic way. The distinctive feature of emancipatory research is that it is controlled by service users.

Primary research

Primary research is multifaceted. There is a host of methods such as interviews, focus groups, randomised controlled trials, observations, case–control studies, questionnaire surveys and diary studies. The focus may be upon a specific place or person, as in case studies, or on how a disease is distributed across geographical areas, as in epidemiological research. Time is a dimension that is integral to historical and longitudinal studies.

Outcome studies are critical in health care. This is because they are designed to identify interventions that work and can be applied (or the results are generalisable) to similar patients in similar situations. This means that outcome studies must be as free of errors and bias as possible, and that they evaluate the process and context of implementation, such as the acceptability to the patient of the health intervention being tested in a randomised controlled trial (Bonell et al 2006). Randomised controlled trials (RCTs) are recognised as the most appropriate method for answering questions about the main effects of an intervention (Glasziou et al 2004). In RCTs, participants are randomly allocated to groups that receive different interventions. The groups should be similar in all aspects apart from the treatment they receive during the study.

Secondary research

Secondary research entails collating what is already known about a specific topic from existing studies. The results from primary research addressing similar questions are summarised and analysed, and conclusions are drawn. This process means that it is possible to examine conflicting results and to establish the generalisability (or transferability) of findings, as well as identify gaps in knowledge and make recommendations about topics and methods for future research. Secondary research comprises systematic literature reviews and meta-analyses.

A systematic literature review is a 'method of making sense of large bodies of information' (Petticrew & Roberts 2006, p2) through a transparent process that can be replicated by others. The method involves a comprehensive trawl of published or unpublished sources, such as electronic databases and theses, using search terms and inclusion criteria about the relevance of the study to the research question and rigour of the research method. The findings may be summarised in a table or critically appraised in a narrative to showcase what is known about a topic.

Meta-analysis is a statistical technique used to aggregate the results of several primary studies into a single estimate. This is to correct for bias (an error or deviation in results or inferences) and lack of power in individual RCTs. Power is an important concept when planning and reporting research. Power connects the sample size (number of participants) with the ability to detect statistically significant differences due to the intervention. In meta-analyses, the outcome may be represented graphically to show size effects and confidence intervals. These indicate whether there is strong or weak evidence of effectiveness and if the benefit is clinically significant.

Emancipatory research

Emancipatory approaches mean that the recipients of services, rather than researchers, hold the power and control the research. This type of research seeks to 'reflect the experience, concerns and priorities of service users – bringing individual experiences together to draw conclusions and make recommendations' (Hanley 2005, p5). It can involve primary or secondary studies and quantitative or qualitative methods. Emancipatory research challenges the power differentials between researchers and service users, as well as tokenistic approaches to patient and public involvement in research.

Occupational therapy research

In 2001, the College of Occupational Therapists produced a broad definition of occupational therapy research using the terminology of the *International Classification of Functioning, Disability and Health* (World Health Organization 2001):

> occupational therapy research incorporates the process and outcomes of occupational therapy interventions, theory, education, management and service delivery ... occupational therapy personnel work with people of all ages with mental and physical impairments to promote independence, health and well-being through engagement in the everyday activities of life. By concentrating upon the performance of daily occupations, such as self-care, work and leisure, interventions are intended to enable participation in valued social roles. As a consequence, occupational therapy research encompasses impairment, activity and activity limitations, and participation and participation restriction as they are experienced across the life span in the person's physical, social and attitudinal environment. (Ilott & White 2001, p271)

Evidence-based practice

Evidence-based practice is an approach to decision making. It means that the best available research findings are taken into consideration when planning to use an intervention with an individual or a group of people or when designing a service for a local population. Research studies are appraised and, if appropriate, the findings are applied to a particular setting. In this way, research supplements the client–therapist relationship as research findings are discussed with the person in order to obtain their consent and ascertain their preferences about the choice of interventions.

Clinical and cost–effectiveness

Effectiveness has two components: clinical and cost-effectiveness. Effectiveness means using interventions that are known to work, whether for a particular patient or for a population, in the real-life situation so as to achieve the greatest possible health gain within available resources (NHS Executive 1996). Questions about effectiveness underpin research utilisation in each context (Dobrow et al 2006), especially 'does it work?' and, if so, is it 'practical or feasible?' or 'should we do it?' and 'how should we do it here?'

Audit and evaluation

Audit is part of a cyclical quality improvement process. Audit involves checking compliance with the benchmarks that have been set in clinical guidelines, service standards or care protocols. This can be done by scrutinising documentation or obtaining feedback from service users. The audit findings may then be used to review and change the service or the standards (see Chapter 8).

Evaluation may be done informally, through a process of reflection, or formally, in a systematic way. The purpose of evaluation is to assess the impact and review the effectiveness of services. Evaluation is an intrinsic part of accountability, especially for new projects or capital (building) schemes, and it is usually done from the perspective of different stakeholders.

Theory and professional knowledge

Theories are ideas or the 'principles and statements of relationships which permit prediction of phenomena under specified circumstances. Theories

are usually thought to be the product of scientific disciplines in their attempt to explain natural phenomena' (Christiansen & Baum 1991, p12).

One of the strengths of occupational therapy is that it draws upon many theories, ranging from genetics to occupational science. All these theories underpin the biopsychosocial perspective adopted by occupational therapists. Such a broad view is essential when seeking to understand the person–occupation–environment relationship and its relationship to health (Hocking & Ness 2002) (see Chapter 3).

Professional knowledge comprises different types of knowledge, including public and personal knowledge, 'knowing what' and 'knowing how'. 'Knowing what' is the formal knowledge base of the profession that is publicly stated in the pre-registration curriculum (College of Occupational Therapists 2004). This propositional or codified knowledge is derived from theory and research. In contrast, 'knowing how' is more practical. It is the ability to do something, for example, to do an initial assessment or facilitate a group. There is also personal, tacit or non-propositional knowledge, which is the informal knowledge derived primarily through practice in a specific context. Personal knowledge includes:

> personalised versions of public codified knowledge ... (and) everyday knowledge of people and situations, know-how in the form of skills and practices, memories of episodes and events, self-knowledge, attitudes and emotions. (Eraut 2004, p174)

Professional effectiveness is the ability to blend, tailor and negotiate these different types of knowledge in each therapeutic encounter.

This chapter uses a classification of knowledge that was developed for social care (Pawson et al 2003). The social care classification identifies five sources of knowledge: organisational knowledge, practitioner knowledge, user knowledge, research knowledge and policy community knowledge. This classification was chosen because it depicts the complexity of professional knowledge. The five sources of knowledge, plus a quality criterion for evaluating each one, are outlined in a later section (see p184). Figure 10.1 illustrates the connections between knowledge and the requirement

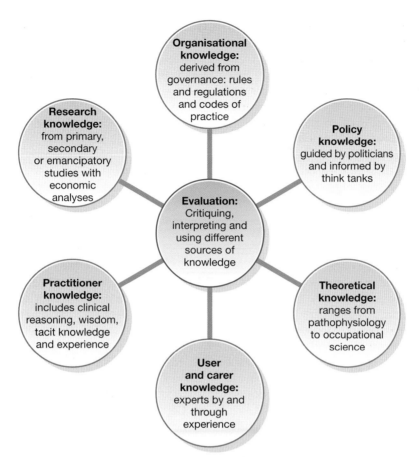

Figure 10.1 Evaluating different sources of knowledge is integral to being an effective practitioner (after Pawson R, Boag A, Grayson L et al (2003), with permission of Queen Mary University, London).

upon practitioners to think about what they are doing and then to evaluate whether their actions are really making a difference.

WHY RESEARCH IS INTEGRAL TO EFFECTIVE PRACTICE

The importance of evidence-based practice has made it imperative for all practitioners to strive to base their interventions and services upon the best available knowledge. This is for two reasons: to support the ethical responsibility to do no harm and to enhance the outcomes of health and social care. Research and development have much to offer occupational therapy. This section summarises some of the most important benefits for the profession as well as for individuals.

RESEARCH AND DEVELOPMENT ARE RELEVANT FOR EVERYONE

Research is a prerequisite for effective practice because it poses and answers some of the most challenging questions about occupational therapy, such as 'does occupational therapy work?' and, if so:

- what works for whom, when, in what circumstances and in what respects?
- how efficacious is occupational therapy in its entirety, as a complex intervention, and how effective are the most commonly used interventions?
- which outcome measures capture the measurable units of occupation (Bowman 2006)?
- how can occupational therapy personnel best contribute as part of a co-ordinated package of health and social care?

- what are the most efficient ways to organise and deliver occupational therapy services?

Service users, policy makers, commissioners and practitioners require answers to these fundamental questions. Effectiveness is of paramount concern to patients, their families and the public, who trust professionals to offer interventions that will do good and no harm. This is the prime reason why research and development are relevant to everyone.

Being an accountable professional

The right to practise independently, to exercise judgements for the benefit of others, is a privilege afforded to professions. The professional status of occupational therapy was formally acknowledged in the United Kingdom by Parliament in 1960, in the Professions Supplementary to Medicine Act (1960). The statutory framework for regulating the allied health professions was updated in the 1999 Health Act. This means that occupational therapy in the UK is regulated by the Health Professions Council (HPC), which was established on 1 April 2002.

Professional autonomy brings accountability. There is accountability to society via adherence to the standards of conduct, performance, ethics and proficiency for occupational therapists set by the Health Professions Council (2003a, 2003b). There is also accountability to the national and international community through the British Association/College of Occupational Therapists (BAOT/COT) and World Federation of Occupational Therapists. These are the professional bodies that set standards for life-long learning (College of Occupational Therapists 2002), education (College of Occupational Therapists 2003a, Hocking & Ness 2002), practice (College of Occupational Therapists 2003b) and research and development (College of Occupational Therapists 2003c, Ilott & White 2001, White & Creek 2007).

For a student or practitioner, accountability means respecting the ethical imperative to use interventions that work. This is why standards refer to research, evidence-based practice, audit and evaluation. For example, one of the Health Professions Council standards of proficiency states that registrant occupational therapists must:

- be able to use research, reasoning and problem-solving skills to determine appropriate actions
- recognise the value of research to the systematic evaluation of practice
- be able to conduct evidence-based practice, evaluate practice systematically, and participate in audit procedures
- be aware of methods commonly used in health-care research
- be able to evaluate research and other evidence to inform their own practice (Health Professions Council 2003b, p11).

Supporting the duty to be up-to-date

Professionals must keep their knowledge and skills up-to-date. This is not an expectation, it is a duty. The BAOT/COT enshrines this responsibility in its standards for ethical and effective practice. For example, the section on life-long learning of the *Code of Ethics and Professional Conduct* states that:

> Occupational therapy personnel shall be accountable for the quality of their work and base this on current guidance, research, reasoning and the best available evidence. (College of Occupational Therapists 2005, p16)

The Professional Standards for Occupational Therapy Practice (College of Occupational Therapists 2003b, p25) state that:

> Intervention should be in accordance with the best or evidence-based practice.
> Occupational therapists/occupational therapy services are required to:
>
> - develop an information and evidence resource to support clinical practice
> - seek evidence or descriptions of best practice to justify interventions or approaches
> - evaluate this evidence and incorporate findings within interventions.

Doing research is one of the best ways of keeping up to date. This means searching for, appraising and using only the best available evidence to inform decisions about any aspect of occupational therapy, whether practice, management, research or education. Using up-to-date knowledge demonstrates a commitment to continuing professional development. Exposure to new ideas garnered from the international literature is one of the pleasures of life-long learning. This is especially so when unexpected or counterintuitive results are found, necessitating a radical rethink and stopping the use of an intervention that does not give the desired outcomes.

Challenging the status quo

Research is a valuable tool for individuals as well as being a professional obligation. This is because the research process provides a systematic way of analysing and tackling problems. The research process, like the occupational therapy process (Creek 2003), comprises a sequence of stages. Figure 10.2 is a research process flow chart (Parker-Jones 2004) containing 10 stages, taken from RDDirect, part of RDInfo, an online resource funded by the Department of Health in England (see Box 10.1 for more details). On the website, there are links to a wealth of details about each stage of the research process.

The first two stages of the research process are relevant to many projects. In the first stage, transforming an idea into a clear, specific question that is feasible to investigate and will offer worthwhile findings demands clarity of thinking. The second stage is reviewing the literature. In this context, literature encompasses many forms, from textbooks to electronic journals. Starting from what is known, whether nationally or internationally, is essential to avoid wasting time by reinventing the wheel or, worse still, reinventing the broken wheel.

Perhaps the most important benefit of research is that it challenges custom and practice, received wisdom and the vagaries of fads, fashion or gurus (also known as eminence-based practice). This is because questioning is at the heart of research. Questioning demands the ability to scrutinise and evaluate. Researchers (meaning those who use research as well as those who conduct studies) need a mix of humility and

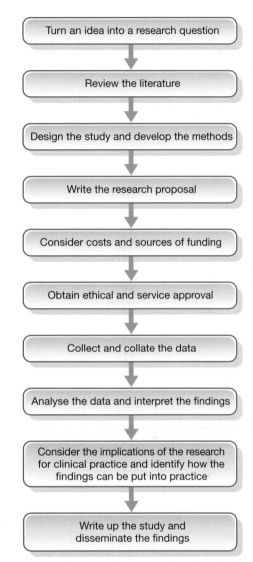

Figure 10.2   The research process flow chart (after Parker-Jones (2004) Research Process Flow Chart on the RD Direct website, with the permission of RDDirect).

Box 10.1 RDInfo: online resources about the research process, funding and training

This is an information service funded by the UK Department of Health. There are three resources: RDDirect is a signposting and advice service for researchers working in health and social care; RDLearning contains information about research training opportunities, and RDFunding is a database of funding for health-related research.
www.rdinfo.org.uk/

arrogance to challenge the status quo and to ask basic questions such as 'is there such a concept as a healthy balance of work, rest and play?' In the same way, practitioners and students need to be sceptical, to question the quality of the research and the applicability of findings to their context. No study is perfect, which is why researchers always report the limitations of their work. The appraisal, interpretation and application of research in practice are the core of evidence-based practice.

EVIDENCE-BASED HEALTH CARE

The 1990s was the decade of the evidence-based movement in health care. In 1992, there was one citation for evidence-based medicine on Medline and by 2004, there were 13,000 citations (Straus 2004). The movement started with evidence-based medicine and has spread around the world, encompassing evidence-based health and social care as well as occupational therapy (Canadian Journal of Occupational Therapy 1999). Evidence-based medicine originated as a way of addressing the gap between research and practice, particularly the time lags and inconsistent ways in which research is consolidated into routine practice.

The key features of evidence-based practice remain the same whether the term is applied to policy making, education or management. These key features are encapsulated in an early definition: evidence-based medicine is 'the conscientious, explicit, and judicious use of the current best evidence in making decisions about the care of individual patients' (Sackett et al 1996, p71).

Evidence-based practice provides:

> the opportunity to harness lifelong learning skills, developing a critical and systematic approach to incorporating evidence into decision making. By decreasing the emphasis upon opinion-led practice, it does not marginalise or negate experience derived from years of practice and what is learnt from educators and colleagues, but incorporates it into the decision-making process. (Bury & Mead 1998, p24)

FIVE STEPS TO EVIDENCE-BASED PRACTICE

Individual practitioners are expected to take a linear approach to evidence-based practice. Five steps are usually described (Bury & Mead 1998, Hammell 2001).

1. **Defining the question** from the perspective of the patient or overall service delivery. Question formulation involves specifying the problem, the intervention and the desired outcome.
2. **Searching the literature** for the most robust, current and relevant research.
3. **Critically appraising** the validity and usefulness of the evidence.
4. **Applying the research findings** by integrating this evidence with clinical expertise whilst respecting the wishes of the patient and their carers.
5. **Evaluating the impact** upon the service in relation to indicators such as value for money, effectiveness in meeting the health needs of the patient and the performance of the practitioner.

RESOURCES FOR EVIDENCE-BASED PRACTICE

There is a plethora of resources on the Internet to help people tackle the challenge of becoming an evidence-based practitioner. Many focus upon the first, easier steps of finding and appraising the quality of research. Box 10.2 contains information about three gateways, a critical appraisal training resource and Occupational Therapy Critically Appraised Topics. A gateway is an information portal where relevant resources have been grouped together.

BARRIERS TO AN INDIVIDUAL APPROACH

Although there are many resources to help practitioners find and appraise research studies, there are considerable obstacles to this individual approach to evidence-based practice. The barriers encountered at the first stages include lack of time to search during a busy working day, difficulty accessing the latest evidence via the Internet and problems understanding the statistics in research papers (Curtin & Jaramazovic 2001, Humphris

---

Box 10.2 Internet gateways about evidence-based practice and critical appraisal

Evidence-Based Occupational Therapy
This information portal, launched in 2006, is funded by the Canadian Association of Occupational Therapists and McMaster University and is endorsed by the World Federation of Occupational Therapists. The gateway contains a wealth of information, presentations and links to other sites as well as a discussion forum.
   www.otevidence.info/

National Library for Health
This is a gateway to a diverse range of links and resources, which is funded by the Department of Health. There are links to MEDLINE/PubMed with journal abstracts and to INTUTE: Health & Life Sciences with quality-reviewed Internet resources. The search engine gives quick access to quality sources such as the Cochrane Library. There is a specialist library for mental health.
   www.library.nhs.uk/
   www.library.nhs.uk/mentalhealth/

Social Care Online and the Social Care Institute for Excellence (SCIE)
Social Care Online complements the National Library for Health. It is a database of social care information and is a product of the Social Care Institute for Excellence (SCIE). Mental health and mental health care is one of the core subject areas. A search done in October 2006, using the terms 'occupational therapy' and 'mental health', produced 344 records, including articles and books.
   SCIE produces a range of resources that are available online. In 2006, this included a practice guide about assessing the mental health needs of older people and a research briefing about therapies and approaches for helping children who deliberately self-harm.
   www.scie-socialcareonline.org.uk/
   www.scie.org.uk/

Critical Appraisal Skills Programme (CASP)
The CASP is a programme within Learning & Development at the Public Health Resource Unit, established in 1993. The website contains tools for appraising quantitative and qualitative research. There is an extensive list of evidence sources ranging from databases to clinical guidelines.
   www.phru.nhs.uk/casp/casp.htm

Occupational Therapy Critically Appraised Topics (OTCATS)
A critically appraised topic (or CAT) is a short summary of evidence that gives a clinical bottom line. Since June 2003 the *Australian Occupational Therapy Journal* has contained two critically appraised topics in each issue.
   OTCATs is supported by the University of Western Australia and funded by the Motor Accidents Authority of New South Wales, Australia. In October 2006 there were over 40 CATs about specific interventions, as well as a template for doing a critically appraised topic. The website also contains links to other evidence-based practice resources.
   www.otcats.com

---

et al 2000). Incorporating the evidence into routine practice is even more difficult, since implementation demands a change of attitude and behaviour as practitioners make the transition from custom and practice to research informed decision making (McCluskey 2004). This is one of the reasons why, in England and Wales, an organisational approach has been adopted to embed evidence-based practice into the structures for health and social care.

EVIDENCE-BASED HEALTH CARE AS PART OF A QUALITY FRAMEWORK

An organisational approach to delivering quality standards was introduced in England by the Department of Health in the late 1990s (DoH 1998) and consolidated in 2004 (DoH 2004a). The original quality framework comprised three areas: setting national standards, implementing the standards in local health communities and monitoring the

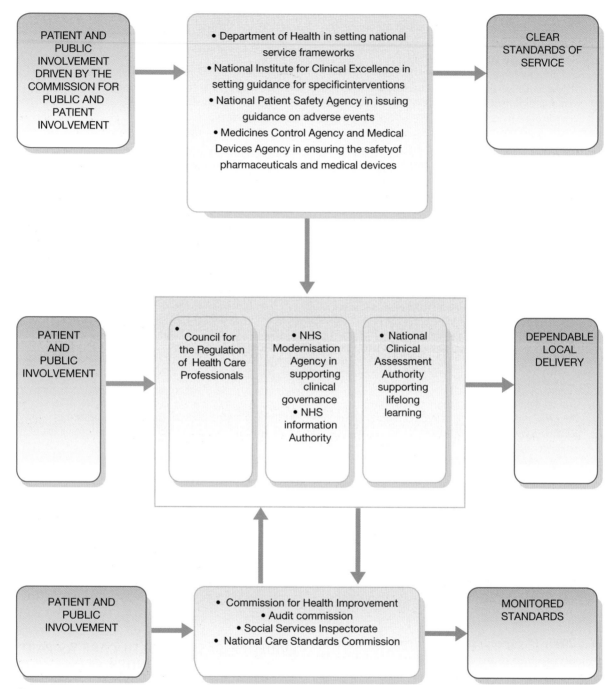

Figure 10.3 Framework for Quality in the NHS in England (from DoH (2002)) with permission of Her Majesty's Stationery Office.

delivery of standards nationally. Figure 10.3 shows the Framework for Quality in the NHS and the responsible organisations (DoH 2002, p54).

The quality framework is inclusive, in that it is multidisciplinary and multiagency. All personnel, whether employed by statutory, private or voluntary agencies, are expected to adhere to national, evidence-based quality standards that focus upon the experience of service users. This framework overcomes some of the challenges of the traditional, individual approach to evidence-based practice. Responsibility is shared in a top-down and bottom-up way as the organisational infrastructure supports the professional imperative to be effective.

Applying the quality framework

The National Institute for Health and Clinical Excellence (NICE) was established in April 1999 to issue guidance, based upon a rigorous appraisal of the evidence of clinical and cost-effectiveness, for the NHS in England and Wales. The guidance includes appraisals of drugs, interventional procedures and clinical guidelines. There is a variety of guidance about what NICE categorises as 'mental health and behavioural conditions', which is available from the NICE website at www.nice.org.uk.

In 1999, the *National Service Framework for Mental Health* was published, setting out values, standards and an implementation programme to improve the quality of local mental health services (DoH 1999). There is a section about mental health on the Department of Health website that contains a 5-year review of the National Service Framework (Appleby 2004). This website also contains the ongoing changes in the policy and legislative framework for mental health services in England (www.dh.gov.uk/ PolicyAndGuidance/HealthAndSocialCareTopics/ MentalHealth/fs/en).

Monitoring progress towards achieving the standards set in the national service frameworks or compliance with NICE guidance is the final part of the quality framework. This is through local clinical governance reviews and audits, national patient and staff surveys and the achievement of clinical quality and financial management criteria set by the Healthcare Commission

(www.healthcarecommission.org.uk/). For example, in December 2003, the Commission for Health Improvement (now known as the Healthcare Commission) produced a sector report about mental health services. The report drew upon 35 clinical governance reviews, including service users' perceptions of the care they received. There was a comment about inpatient activities:

> Service users commonly report feeling bored on inpatient wards. The availability of therapeutic programmes varies from trust to trust ... staff shortages in, for example, occupational therapy reduce therapeutic activity on the wards ... service users commonly report that the range and quality of activities is limited, with few activities to keep them occupied in the evening and at weekends.
> (Commission for Health Improvement 2003, p21)

The quality framework for mental health illustrates two of the sources of knowledge mentioned at the beginning of the chapter. While the framework provides knowledge derived from the policy community, the quotation about boredom reflects user knowledge. More details about a system of classification based upon the source of knowledge can be found on p184 (Pawson et al 2003).

HIERARCHIES OF EVIDENCE

One of the most controversial aspects of evidence-based practice relates to what comprises best evidence. The term *best evidence* usually refers to empirical evidence derived from outcome or intervention studies. Various hierarchies of the strength of evidence have been developed, which rank research methods according to the degree to which the observed results are likely to be attributable to the intervention rather than to chance. High-quality meta-analyses and systematic reviews of RCTs or RCTs with a very low risk of bias are usually ranked highest whilst expert opinion is usually ranked lowest (Harbour & Miller 2001). Different organisations use different hierarchies that grade and rank the evidence in different ways. There is some concern that 'the simplification involved in creating and applying hierarchies has also led to misconceptions and abuses' (Glasziou et al 2004, p39). Evidence hierarchies tend to devalue other research designs or sources of knowledge and ignore the fact that RCTs are not possible, ethical or appropriate for all health and social care research questions.

Ranking the quality of evidence presents particular problems for research-emergent professions such as occupational therapy (Higher Education Funding Council for England 2001). *Research emergent* means that a profession lacks a solid tradition of research and, thus, an infrastructure of research centres and a community of researchers. As a consequence, research questions have been neither asked nor answered in sufficiently robust ways to satisfy the formal hierarchy of empirical evidence. Much occupational therapy knowledge is derived from theoretical or practitioner sources rather than research studies. There is not even an explicit expert consensus (the lowest level of evidence for outcomes research) about what constitutes standard or routine or best practice in occupational therapy. However, this does not mean that quality criteria should not be applied to all sources of knowledge.

RESEARCH IN OCCUPATIONAL THERAPY

The paucity of empirical evidence applies to all professions working in the field of mental health, not just occupational therapy (Craik 1998, Craik et al 1998, Ilott & White 2001, Mairs 2003). In 1998, the College of Occupational Therapists produced a position statement on the way ahead for research, education and practice in mental health (Craik et al 1998). This noted:

> a lack of information on the scope, profile and evaluation of practice ... there is not only a lack of published evidence on which occupational therapists can base their practice but also little published from which others can understand the profession. (Craik et al 1998, p391)

Interestingly, research into mental health has a rich tradition. In 1960, Fransella, an occupational therapist, published one of the first intervention trials of occupational therapy. Two groups of patients with chronic schizophrenia received a 12-week, intensive programme of craft, recreational and social activities without the drug chlorpromazine. They then received 12 weeks of routine occupational therapy classes but continued with chlorpromazine. The results were promising. Fransella (1960) commented that:

> an intensive programme of occupational therapy is capable of producing a considerable behavioural improvement in a small group of chronic schizophrenic patients. (p34)

This example shows the need to go through back issues of journals by hand, rather than relying upon electronic databases such as CINHAL or AMED, because most databases started in the mid-1980s. Also, knowledge should be evaluated in context. The mental health services provided in the UK in the 1950s do not resemble current ones. It is a truism to say that the world is a very different place.

Unfortunately, most research studies in occupational therapy in mental health have continued to be small scale and self-funded. Many studies are done for a postgraduate programme (for example, Hvalsøe & Josephsson 2003, Le Granse et al 2006, Mee et al 2004, Pieris & Craik 2004) rather than projects being undertaken as part of a coherent, properly funded programme of research that adds new empirical, theoretical and methodological knowledge. The good news is that the situation is changing. Priorities for mental health research have been set and updated (Fowler Davis & Hyde 2002), more studies are being funded (for example, Bejerholm et al 2006, Fossey et al 2006) and many relevant studies are being done by other disciplines (see Box 10.7) so it is important to read widely.

TYPES OF KNOWLEDGE

There are many different types of knowledge, such as theoretical knowledge, ethical perspectives, empirical evidence, practical experience and wisdom. All contribute to our ability to understand, predict and explain events. Occupational therapy is a diverse profession that draws upon a range of scientific and applied disciplines in an attempt to comprehend the complexity of humans as occupational beings.

This section contains an overview of five different types of knowledge that have been used throughout the chapter. The aim is to put research into context, so that it is not seen as supreme but as one way of knowing that needs to be fit for purpose. The five types of knowledge are taken from a knowledge review produced for the Social Care Institute for Excellence (Pawson et al 2003).

ORGANISATIONAL KNOWLEDGE

Organisational knowledge refers to the regulatory framework that shapes the operation and accountability of organisations. It includes governance, which spans corporate, clinical and research governance, so that financial probity and quality standards, as well as ethical guidelines, are taken into account. The codes of conduct set by the Health Professions Council (Health Professions Council 2003a) and the College of Occupational Therapists (2005) are examples of organisational knowledge.

In England, the NHS Service Delivery and Organisation (SDO) Programme focuses upon research into the organisation, management and delivery of health-care services. The SDO website is a source of organisational knowledge (www.lshtm.ac.uk/hsru/sdo/briefingpapers.html for publications and briefing papers). Recent titles include 'Sharing mental health information with carers: pointers to good practice for service providers' and 'Continuity of care for people with severe mental illness'.

PRACTITIONER KNOWLEDGE

Much practitioner knowledge is tacit, non-propositional knowledge. It is based on experience, so it tends to be context specific and personal. It is:

> acquired directly through practice ... and the distillation of collective wisdom at many points through media such as education and training, requesting and receiving advice, attending team meetings and case conferences, and comparing notes. (Pawson et al 2003, p49)

Practitioner knowledge is captured in a variety of ways, such as studies of clinical reasoning and

---

Box 10.3 eGuidelines: a database about clinical guidelines and audit

eGuidelines is a one-stop shop for information about clinical guidelines and audit. It includes the clinical improvement projects (CLIP) database, which contains summaries of completed and ongoing clinical effectiveness initiatives within the UK. In October 2006 there were 77 occupational therapy audits, including an audit of the immediate psychological effects of creative and practical activities in a mental health setting and service users' perceptions of the value of horticulture.
http://eguidelines.co.uk

---

person-centred practice (Unsworth 2004). Audit and practice evaluations give insights into current interventions. These may be published or accessible via online databases, such as eGuidelines (Box 10.3).

The contextual nature of practitioner knowledge means considering factors impacting upon the local health community. These factors can range from the demographic profile of the community to facilities available for employment and leisure. Sensitivity to subcultural, cultural and ethnic differences is a vital part of local knowledge (Chiang & Carlson 2003).

POLICY COMMUNITY KNOWLEDGE

This is knowledge gained from the wider political, socio-economic and policy context, all of which impact upon the delivery of health and social care. The policy community includes think tanks and policy groups, plus voluntary organisations, such as the Sainsbury Centre for Mental Health (www.scmh.org.uk), that influence policy.

Evidence-based policy making should underpin evidence-based practice (Macintyre et al 2001). In 2003, the National Audit Office published a report entitled 'Getting the evidence: using research in policy making'. One of the key conclusions was that the 'early involvement of potential users of research will increase the likelihood that research results will be utilised' (National Audit Office 2003, p7). This finding reinforces one of the central messages of this chapter – that research and development are everyone's business.

SERVICE USER AND CARER KNOWLEDGE

This is knowledge gained from first-hand experience of, and reflection on, service use. It is premised upon respect for recipients as experts by and through their experience, so that service users and carers work in partnership with experts by profession. This participative approach should extend from influencing service design right through to individual care programmes. Charities, such as the Mental Health Foundation (www.mental-health.org.uk), provide a starting point for finding user and carer knowledge.

Some organisations are dedicated to promoting patient and public involvement in research at national and local levels. For example, INVOLVE (www.invo.org.uk) was established in 1996 as The Consumers in NHS Research Group. It is now funded by the National Institute for Health Research and continues to promote wider involvement in health and social care research.

EMPIRICAL KNOWLEDGE

Empirical knowledge is derived from research. There are many different methods of collecting information. Some of the key terms are introduced in this section but the reader is advised to consult other sources, such as the references given in the further reading list, for more details.

Research involves an investigation that is designed to gain knowledge or understanding. The research may be new and original or it may replicate other studies to test whether the same results are produced in different contexts with similar participants. Most research is a collaborative venture, comprising a complex network of partnerships between researchers, participants, organisations that commission, sponsor and fund research, policy makers and practitioners who want to use the results to improve the quality of health and social care.

Although there is a variety of ways to gather, collate, analyse and interpret research data, all should be fit for purpose. This means that the methods used should give the best answers to the research questions. Quantitative, qualitative or mixed methods may be used. In quantitative research, the data collected usually take the form

Box 10.4 Bandolier: an electronic journal and resource about evidence-based medicine

This journal was published between 1994–2007 and is available online. Secondary and primary research is summarised in a lively way. There is a section on mental health, an extensive glossary about evidence-based medicine and the knowledge zone explains the intricacies of topics such as the number needed to treat (NNT) and number needed to harm (NNH).
www.jr2.ox.ac.uk/bandolier

of measurements that are amenable to statistical analysis. Quantitative research follows precise, standard procedures that are intended to make the outcomes more objective and to reduce the risks of bias skewing the results. In qualitative research, words rather than numbers are used to elicit insights into the worldview of the participants. Each approach has strengths and weaknesses, which is why many researchers prefer to use both – a mixed methodology – to give a more rounded understanding of the processes and outcomes of health care.

Empirical knowledge is jam-packed with jargon but many of the resources highlighted in the boxes contain glossaries. For example, the glossary on Bandolier is particularly helpful for quantitative research and evidence-based practice (Box 10.4).

CHALLENGING THE POWER OF KNOWLEDGE

In the last edition of this textbook, Stewart used the phrase 'don't take anybody's word for it' (Stewart 2002, p51). All sources of evidence should be scrutinised and judged against quality criteria, regardless of whether the results are going to be ranked in a hierarchy of evidence. Such criteria are powerful democratic tools because they allow individuals to test the quality of knowledge, and knowledge is power. This section contains six quality standards that were developed to complement the five sources of knowledge (Pawson et al 2003). There are also references to critical appraisal tools.

GENERIC QUALITY STANDARDS

The following standards are taken from the Social Care Institute for Excellence Knowledge Review (Pawson et al 2003). There are six types of questions that should be asked by anyone generating or using knowledge, as they can help judge the trustworthiness of the information.

- **Transparency:** is the process of developing knowledge open to outside scrutiny?
- **Accuracy:** is the knowledge well grounded? Is it supported by and faithful to the events, experiences, participants and sources used in its production?
- **Purposivity:** are the approaches and methods used to gain knowledge appropriate to the task in hand? Is it fit for purpose?
- **Utility:** is the knowledge fit for use? Do the answers match the questions asked?
- **Propriety:** is the knowledge legal and ethical? Knowledge should be created and managed legally, ethically and with care for all relevant stakeholders.
- **Accessibility:** is the knowledge intelligible to all potential users?

CRITICAL APPRAISAL TOOLS

There are criteria for judging primary and secondary research, as well as guidelines for critically appraising practice guidelines and user studies. Guidance and critical appraisal forms can be found in standard texts, such as Herbert et al (2005), and on many evidence-based practice websites. For example, the CASP website (see Box 10.2) has appraisal tools for systematic reviews, RCTs, qualitative research studies, cohort studies, case–control studies, diagnostic tests and economic evaluations.

Critical appraisal checklists focus upon whether the study results are valid, reliable and applicable. This focus generates questions on the following topics.

- **Validity**: to what extent is the study a close representation of the truth? Are the conclusions justified by the description of the methods and findings?

- **Reliability:** are the results credible, repeatable and free from bias? Have the limitations of the study been acknowledged?
- **Applicability:** are the findings transferable to a wider population and other settings? What are the implications of the results? Can they be applied to, and used to inform, my practice?

OTHER TOOLS FOR SETTING STANDARDS

Specific tools for reporting research and developing clinical guidelines have been developed, for example, CONSORT and AGREE. CONSORT (Consolidated Standards of Reporting Trials) comprises a checklist and flow diagram that may be used by researchers, readers and practitioners to check the quality of RCTs (Nelson & Mathiowetz 2004). CONSORT can be found at www.consort-statement.org.

AGREE (Appraisal of Guidelines Research and Evaluation) is an internationally recognised framework for developing, reporting and assessing clinical guidelines. Clinical guidelines, like patient information systems, are mechanisms by which the best available evidence can be incorporated into routine practice. This is because they are systematically developed recommendations about specific interventions that are intended to assist decision making. Consult the website www.agreecollaboration.org for further information.

Generic standards, critical appraisal tools, CONSORT and AGREE are all mechanisms for challenging published or spoken wisdom. Adopting a questioning, evaluative approach stimulates life-long learning. As such, it is a vital part of professional effectiveness.

LEARNING TO BE A RESEARCH-INFORMED PRACTITIONER

Research and evidence-based practice should be core themes within pre-registration and postgraduate courses because both are intrinsic to professional reasoning and behaviour. The pre-registration student will gain a good understanding of the research process through studying primary and secondary research. There will be opportunities to explore the variety of qualitative, quantitative and mixed methods and to acquire the critical appraisal skills needed to assess the rigour and relevance of different types of evidence.

This section highlights the importance of research governance. There are also some tips about where, and how, to start looking for research evidence.

RESEARCH GOVERNANCE AND ETHICS

Research governance and ethics complement effective practice because they give primacy to the interests of participants, not researchers or practitioners. Research governance refers to a culture of quality that includes the setting, monitoring and reporting of standards (DoH 2005). Standards relate to five domains.

- **Ethics**: protecting the dignity, rights, safety and well-being of the participants is paramount. The principles and practice of ethical occupational therapy research are stated in the *Research Ethics Guidelines* (College of Occupational Therapists 2003c) and the *Professional Standards for Occupational Therapy Practice* (College of Occupational Therapists 2003b).
- **Science:** refers to the quality of research as judged by independent peer review. It is important to remember that 'Research that duplicates other work unnecessarily or which is not of sufficient quality to contribute something useful to existing knowledge is in itself unethical' (DoH 2005, p13).
- **Information**: encompasses free access to research as it is being conducted and also to the final results. Box 10.5 contains information about the National Research Register, a database of health-care projects. A National Research Register for Social Care is being developed on Social Care Online (see Box 10.2).
- **Health and safety:** relates to adherence to appropriate laws and regulations in order to protect all participants and researchers.
- **Finance:** refers to financial probity, liability and the management of intellectual property rights.

Box 10.5 The National Research Register (NRR)

This is a database funded by the Department of Health. It contains ongoing and recently completed projects that are funded by, or of interest to, the NHS. It is possible to search across multiple databases, including the Medical Research Council Clinical Trials Directory and the NHS Centre for Reviews and Dissemination Register of Reviews. A search using the terms 'occupational therapy' and 'mental health' produced 140 hits in October 2006. There are also links to other sites, such as the metaRegister of Controlled Trials (mRCT) and the Department of Health Research Findings Register (ReFeR).
www.nrr.nhs.uk

Box 10.6 PubMed: an online resource of journal abstracts

This service, provided by the US National Library of Medicine, gives free online access to abstracts from the MEDLINE database. It includes over 16 million citations from biomedical articles published since the 1950s. These articles have been subject to the peer review process of the original journal.
www.ncbi.nlh.nih.gov/entrez/

TRUSTWORTHY SOURCES OF KNOWLEDGE

When searching for evidence it is essential to use trustworthy sources. This means that the content has been subject to a quality assurance process or the source is authoritative. For example, academic and professional journals use a peer review system. Peer review means that all articles or reports are screened by at least two subject experts who judge the quality of the research prior to publication. Many journals are available online, via the Internet. Some are free whilst others allow access to abstracts but charge a fee for the full article. Box 10.6 contains a starting point for finding quality-assured information.

The credibility of the source is critical when selecting information from the Internet. Selectivity must be employed to deal with the overwhelming mass of information that is so easily available. Only the websites of government bodies, academic institutions

---

Box 10.7 Systematic reviews accessible via the Internet

The Cochrane Library
The Cochrane Library is an international online resource that consists of a regularly updated collection of evidence-based databases. These include the Cochrane Database of Systematic Reviews, the Cochrane Central Register of Controlled Trials, the Health Technology Assessment Database and the NHS Economic Evaluation Database. Many topics are relevant to occupational therapy, for example, family interventions for schizophrenia and life skills programmes for chronic mental illnesses. The Cochrane Library is published by Wiley Interscience and can be accessed via the National Library for Health (see Box 10.2).
    www3.interscience.wiley.com/cgi-bin/mrwhome/106568753/HOME

NHS Centre for Reviews and Dissemination (CRD)
The NHS Centre for Reviews and Dissemination (CRD) was established in 1994. It produces systematic reviews about health and social care interventions and maintains databases, such as the Database of Abstracts of Reviews of Effects (DARE) which contains over 4000 abstracts of quality assessed and critically appraised systematic reviews.
    www.york.ac.uk/inst/crd/

Occupational Therapy Systematic Evaluation of Evidence (OTSeeker)
OTSeeker was launched in 2003 with support from the Cochrane Collaboration and sponsors in Australia. This site is a one-stop shop with abstracts for systematic reviews and quality-rated RCTs that are relevant for occupational therapy. In October 2006, there were 218 records about mental health.
    www.otseeker.com

---

and registered charities have been used in this chapter, as they are credible sources and the resources are free. The organisations are also likely to be in existence for the immediate future, even though the web addresses given within the text may change.

Starting with secondary studies

Secondary studies are the best starting point for anyone seeking answers to questions about the effectiveness of their practice. This is because they synthesise primary research and present recommendations. The reader may follow up references to primary studies cited in secondary studies. Box 10.7 contains details about three sources of high-quality systematic reviews. Two hold a broad range of information, whilst OTseeker concentrates upon systematic reviews and RCTs that are relevant to occupational therapy (Bennett et al 2003).

SUMMARY

The newly qualified occupational therapist should be an informed consumer of research. This means being ready to tackle the organisational and individual challenges associated with using research to inform practice. One of the greatest challenges is the absence of easy answers. Whilst this may be attributed to a paucity of empirical evidence, it is really due to the complexity of humans as occupational beings. Research can help because it offers a methodical framework for challenging the status quo and for continually evaluating the process and outcomes of your practice. This requires the ability to draw upon all sources of knowledge and have the confidence to make judgements in partnership with others, whether service users or managers.

The new practitioner should also be enthused about research and development. The therapist who is 'fundamentally nosy ... tenacious ... (and) someone who wants to know what the "real" truth is' (Walker 2003, p339) may also consider becoming a career researcher and contributing to the transformation of occupational therapy from a research-emergent to a research-established profession. Only then will we be able to offer robust replies to those questions about whether occupational therapy works. It is salutary to remember that the benefits of moving from a research-emergent to a research-established profession, articulated nearly 50 years ago, are yet to be realised.

> A serious study of our practice as occupational therapists is long overdue ... Only by so doing can we justify our professional claims and stabilise our position ... (because) such research will make for wiser professional practice and for more efficient service to the patient. (ACO 1964 pp1–2)

This quotation highlights the interdependence of research, evidence-based practice and professional effectiveness. Research is not an end in itself. Research is about challenge, change and improvement. This is why research and development are at the heart of effective practice

References

ACO 1964 Editorial. Occupational Therapy 27(2): 1-2

Appleby L 2004 The national service framework for mental health–five years on. Department of Health, London

Bejerholm U, Hansson L, Eklund M 2006 Profiles of occupational engagement in people with schizophrenia (POES): the development of a new instrument based on time-use diaries. British Journal of Occupational Therapy 69(2): 58-68

Bennett S, Hoffmann T, McCluskey A et al 2003 Evidence based practice forum. Introducing OTseeker (Occupational Therapy Systematic Evaluation of Evidence): a new evidence database for occupational therapists. American Journal of Occupational Therapy 57(6): 635-638

Bonell C, Oakley A, Hargreaves J et al 2006 Assessment of generalisability in trials of health interventions: suggested framework and systematic review. BMJ 333: 346-349

Bowman J 2006 Challenges to measuring outcomes in occupational therapy: a qualitative focus group study. British Journal of Occupational Therapy 69(10): 464-472

Bury T, Mead J (eds) 1998 Evidence-based healthcare: a practical guide for therapists. Butterworth Heinemann, Oxford

Buxton M, Hanney S, Packwood T et al 2000 Assessing benefits from Department of Health and National Health Service research and development. Public Money and Management 20(4): 29-34

Canadian Journal of Occupational Therapy 1999 Joint position statement on evidence-based occupational therapy. December 267-269

Chiang M, Carlson G 2003 Occupational therapy in multicultural contexts: issues and strategies. British Journal of Occupational Therapy 66(12): 559-567

Christiansen C, Baum C (eds) 1991 Occupational therapy: overcoming human performance deficits. Slack, New Jersey

College of Occupational Therapists 2002 Position statement on lifelong learning. British Journal of Occupational Therapy 65(5): 198-200

College of Occupational Therapists 2003a Standards for education: pre registration education standards. College of Occupational Therapists, London

College of Occupational Therapists 2003b Professional standards for occupational therapy practice. College of Occupational Therapists, London

College of Occupational Therapists 2003c Research ethics guidelines. College of Occupational Therapists, London

College of Occupational Therapists 2004 Curriculum framework for pre-registration education. College of Occupational Therapists, London

College of Occupational Therapists 2005 Code of ethics and professional conduct. College of Occupational Therapists, London

Commission for Health Improvement 2003 What CHI has found in mental health trusts: sector report. Available online at. www.healthcarecommission.org.uk/_db/_documents/04000051.pdf

Craik C 1998 Occupational therapy in mental health: a review of the literature. British Journal of Occupational Therapy 61(5): 185-192

Craik C, Austin C, Chacksfield J et al 1998 College of Occupational Therapists: position paper on the way ahead for research, education and practice in mental health. British Journal of Occupational Therapy 61(9): 390-392

Craik J, Rappolt S 2006 Enhancing professional utilization capacity through multifaceted professional development. American Journal of Occupational Therapy 60(2): 155-164

Creek J 2003 Occupational therapy defined as a complex intervention. College of Occupational Therapists, London

Curtin M, Jaramazovic E 2001 Occupational therapists' views and perceptions of evidence-based practice. British Journal of Occupational Therapy 64(5): 214-222

Department of Health 1998 A first class service. Quality in the new NHS. HMSO, London

Department of Health 1999 National service framework for mental health. HMSO, London Available online at. www.dh.gov.uk/PublicationsAndStatistics/ Publications/PublicationsPolicyAndGuidance/ PublicationsPolicyAndGuidanceArticle/fs/ en?CONTENT_ID=4009598&chk=jmAMLk

Department of Health 2002 Learning from Bristol: the Department of Health's response to the report of the public inquiry into children's heart surgery at the Bristol Royal Infirmary 1984-1995. Available online at. www.publications.doh.gov.uk/bristolinquiryresponse/ bristolresponsefull.pdf

Department of Health 2004a Standards for better health. A consultation. Available online at: www. dh.gov.uk/Consultations/ClosedConsultations/ ClosedConsultationsArticle/fs/en?CONTENT_ ID=4082361&chk=hBbqBI

Department of Health 2004b Reconfiguring the Department of Health's arm's length bodies. Available online at: www.dh.gov.uk/PublicationsAndStatistics/ Publications2004. /PublicationsPolicyAndGuidance/ PublicationsPolicyAndGuidanceArticle/fs/ en?CONTENT_ID=4086081&chk=y4UIfP

Department of Health 2005 Research governance framework for health and social care. Available online at: www.dh.gov.uk/ PolicyAndGuidance/ResearchAndDevelopment/ ResearchAndDevelopmentAZ/ResearchGovernance/ ResearchGovernanceArticle/fs/en?CONTENT_ ID=4002112&chk=PJIaGg

Dobrow MJ, Goel V, Lemieux-Charles L et al 2006 The impact of context on evidence utilization: a framework for expert groups developing health policy recommendations. Social Science and Medicine 63(7): 1811-1824

Eraut M 2004 Editorial. Sharing practice: problems and possibilities. Learning in Health and Social Care 3(4): 171-178

Fossey E, Harvey C, Plant G et al 2006 Occupational performance of people diagnosed with schizophrenia in supported housing and outreach programmes in Australia. British Journal of Occupational Therapy 69(9): 409-419

Fowler Davis S, Hyde P 2002 Short report. Priorities in mental health research: an update. British Journal of Occupational Therapy 65(8): 387-389

Fransella F 1960 The treatment of chronic schizophrenia. Intensive occupational therapy with and without chlorpromazine. Occupational Therapy 23(9): 31-34

Glasziou P, Vandendroucke J, Chalmers I 2004 Education and debate. Assessing the quality of research. BMJ 328: 39-41

Hammell WK 2001 Using qualitative research to inform the client-centred evidence-based practice of occupational therapy. British Journal of Occupational Therapy 64(5): 228-234

Hanley B 2005 Research as empowerment? Report of a series of seminars organised by the Toronto Group. Joseph Rowntree Foundation, York. Available online at: www.jrf. org.uk/knowledge/findings/socialcare/0175.asp

Harbour R, Miller J 2001 A new system for grading recommendations in evidence based guidelines. BMJ 323: 334-336

Health Act 1999 HMSO, London Available online at: www. hmso.gov.uk/acts/acts1999/99008- -c.htm

Health Professions Council 2003a Standards of conduct, performance and ethics. Your duties as a registrant: 2003. Health Professions Council, London

Health Professions Council 2003b Standards of proficiency. Occupational therapists. Health Professions Council, London

Herbert R, Jamtvedt G, Mead J et al 2005 Practical evidence-based physiotherapy. Elsevier Butterworth Heinemann, London

Higher Education Funding Council for England 2001 Research in nursing and allied health professions. Report of the Task Group 3 to HEFCE and the Department of Health. 01/63 Bristol: HEFCE. Available online at: www. hefce.ac.uk/pubs/hefce/2001/01_63.htm

Hocking C, Ness NE 2002 Revised minimum standards for the education of occupational therapists. World Federation of Occupational Therapists, Perth

Humphris D, Littlejohns P, Victor C et al 2000 Implementing evidence-based practice: factors that influence the use of research evidence by occupational therapists. British Journal of Occupational Therapy 63(11): 516-522

Hvalsøe B, Josephsson S 2003 Characteristics of meaningful occupations from the perspective of mentally ill people. Scandinavian Journal of Occupational Therapy 10(2): 61-71

Ilott I, White E 2001 College of Occupational Therapists' research and development strategic vision and action plan. British Journal of Occupational Therapy 64(6): 270-277

Le Granse M, Kinébanian A, Josephsson S 2006 Promoting autonomy of the client with persistent mental illness: a challenge for occupational therapists from The Netherlands, Germany and Belgium. Occupational Therapy International 13(3): 142-159

Macintyre S, Chalmers I, Horton R et al 2001 Education and debate. Using evidence to inform health policy. BMJ 322: 222-225

Mairs H 2003 Evidence-based practice in mental health: a cause for concern for occupational therapists. British Journal of Occupational Therapy 66(4): 168-170

McCluskey A 2004 Increasing the use of research evidence by occupational therapists. Final report. School of Exercise and Health Sciences, University of Western Sydney, Penrith South, NSW. Available online at: www. otcats.com/summary/index.html

Mee J, Sumsion T, Craik C 2004 Mental health clients confirm the value of occupation in building competence and self-identity. British Journal of Occupational Therapy 67(5): 225-233

National Audit Office 2003 Getting the evidence: Using research in policy making. Stationery Office, London. Available online at: www.nao.org.uk/publications/nao_ reports/02-03/0203586-i.pdf

National Health Service Executive 1996 Promoting clinical effectiveness: a framework for action in and through the NHS. Department of Health, London

Nelson DL, Mathiowetz V 2004 Randomized controlled trials to investigate occupational therapy research questions. American Journal of Occupational Therapy 58(1): 24-34

Parker-Jones C 2004 Research process flow chart on RD Direct website. Your research project. How and where to start? Available online at: www.rdinfo.org.uk/newsletter/Handout.pdf

Pawson R, Boaz A, Grayson L et al 2003 Knowledge review 3. Types and quality of knowledge in social care. Social Care Institute for Excellence, The Policy Press and Queen Mary University, London

Petticrew M, Roberts H 2006 Systematic reviews in the social sciences. A practical guide. Blackwell Publishing, Oxford

Pieris Y, Craik C 2004 Factors enabling and hindering participation in leisure for people with mental health problems. British Journal of Occupational Therapy 67(6): 240-247

Professions Supplementary to Medicine Act 1960. HMSO, London

Sackett DL, Rosenberg WMC, May JAM et al 1996 Editorial. Evidence based medicine: what it is and what it isn't. BMJ 312: 71-72 Available online at: http: //bmj. bmjjournals.com/cgi/content/full/312/7023/71

Stewart A 2002 Research and professional effectiveness. In: Creek J (ed) Occupational therapy in mental health: principles, skills and practice, 3rd edn. Churchill Livingstone, Edinburgh, pp51-70

Straus SE 2004 Editorial. What's the E for EBM? BMJ 328: 535-536

Unsworth CA 2004 Clinical reasoning: how do pragmatic reasoning, worldview and client-centredness fit? British Journal of Occupational Therapy 67(1): 10-19

Walker MF 2003 The Casson Memorial Lecture 2003: past conditional, present indicative, future indefinite. British Journal of Occupational Therapy 68(8): 338-344

White E, Creek J 2007 College of Occupational Therapists' research and development strategic vision and action plan: 5-year review. British Journal of Occupational Therapy 70(3): 122-128

Willson M 2002 The Casson Memorial Lecture 2002: a culture to care for. British Journal of Occupational Therapy 65(7): 306-314

World Health Organization 2001 International classification of functioning, disability and health. World Health Organization, Geneva

FURTHER READING

Arksey H, Knight P 1999 Interviewing for social scientists. Sage Publications, London

Bell J 2000 Doing your research project: a guide for first-time researchers in education and social sciences. Open University Press, Buckingham

Bowers D 1996 Statistics from scratch: an introduction for health care professionals. John Wiley, Chichester

Bowling A 2002 Research methods in health. Investigating health and health services, 2nd edn. Open University Press, Buckingham

Bryman A 2001 Social research methods. Oxford University Press, Oxford

Drummond A 1996 Research methods for therapists. Chapman and Hall, London

Findlay L, Gough B (eds) 2003 Reflexivity a guide to researching self and others. Routledge, London

Gerrish K., Lacey A (eds) 2006 The research process in nursing, 5th edn. Blackwell Publishing, Oxford

Gomm R, Needham G, Bullman A (eds) 2000 Evaluating research in health and social care. Open University in association with Sage, London

Gorard S, Taylor 2004 Combining methods in educational and social research. Open University Press, London

Mays N, Pope C 1999 Quantitative research in health care. 2nd edn. BMJ Books, London

Petticrew M, Roberts H 2006 Systematic reviews in the social sciences. A practical guide. Blackwell Publishing, Oxford

Seale J, Barnard S 1998 Therapy research processes and practicalities. Reed Educational and Professional Publishing, Oxford

Thomas AB 2004 Research skills for management studies. Routledge, London

Willig C 2001 Introducing qualitative research in psychology. Adventure in theory and method. Open University Press, Maidenhead

Yin RK 2003 Case study research: design and methods, 3rd edn: Applied Social Research Methods Series, vol 5. Sage, Thousand Oaks, California

Service user commentary

This chapter is a very carefully constructed and well-informed account of research, evidence-based practice and professional effectiveness. It could be useful to service users insofar as it is well organised and could be a reference tool, with its definitions of research and development, evidence-based health care and types of knowledge. It also puts into perspective the reasons why research is integral to effective practice from the professional point of view and the value of this approach for the individual practitioner.

However, the language is very professional, the text imparting an immense amount of knowledge in a very short space so, while it fulfils the purpose of informing professionals, it falls into the trap of confirming all the lay person's perceptions of research: ivory towers, jargon, academia and so on. The inaccessibility of this world is probably no greater for anyone than for a mental health service user or their carer. A service user might prefer to start with a text that gives a more easily accessible introduction to research, set out from a lay person's perspective (for example, Pollard 2001), after which this chapter may be more digestible.

One of the issues that service users and carers have in relation to research is that the things that they consider relevant to them are often not the subject of research investigations. They want to be the ones to set the agenda, to see the outcomes of research improving their road to recovery and their quality of life. They want their experiences to be valued and harnessed within research projects. They want to be doing and/or contributing to research themselves. All of these aspirations, if achieved, can contribute to better social inclusion and empowerment for service users and carers.

The ways in which service users and carers can contribute to research vary enormously, from 'influencing service design right through to individual care programmes' (p186). The aim of all research projects should be to create a research culture which is meaningfully controlled or influenced by those who use, or care for those who use, services. Research and implementation will then be focused on the real concerns of ordinary people.

However good a book like this is and however many resources are available, such as those in Box 10.2 (p181), service users and carers, along with professionals, have many hurdles to overcome before any of these resources can be helpful. There are online databases to come to terms with, research ethics committees to satisfy, rejected proposals to live with and police checks, all likely to put a service user off research at the first acquaintance. Genuine help for service users and carers is needed in terms of practical support and positive attitudes. This has to begin with professionals understanding and supporting service user involvement in their everyday practice, and having a positive and proactive attitude towards such involvement (Walsh & Hostick 2005).

There are several agencies in the UK that support service user input to research, such as the Mental Health Research Network, which sees its role as broadening the scope and capacity of research and including the involvement of service users and carers. But service users need the right encouragement to become involved at the beginning of their journey of recovery, before a support network can kick in. Crucial factors in ensuring the success of service user and carer involvement include: a real commitment from all agencies, appropriate finance and resources, training, a culture of partnership and co-operation, involvement from the beginning, demonstrable change to services, good communications and sufficient time for service users to make their contribution (Barber 2002, Impact Research Team 2002).

As a research-emergent profession, occupational therapy might benefit from looking at the work on emancipatory and participatory research at Sheffield University, which involves people with intellectual disabilities participating in and undertaking research (Ramcharan et al 2004). This begins to break the traditional boundaries of research without relinquishing any of the standards. Perhaps a more liberated approach and the right support mechanisms will bring a service user to this chapter and make it come alive as part of a real process to assist service users to do their own research or contribute to a project.

Sarah King BSc(Hons) MSc

REFERENCES

Barber E 2002 Clinical guidelines for user involvement in occupational therapy. Mental Health OT 7(2): 27-30

Impact Research Team 2002 Patient involvement, a situation analysis. Paper delivered at National Clinical Audit Conference, Manchester, June 17

Pollard N 2001 A basic guide to research skills: beginning clinical research. Doncaster and South Humber Healthcare NHS Trust, Doncaster

Ramcharan P, Grant G, Flynn M 2004 Emancipatory and participatory research: how far have we come? In: Emerson E, Hatton C, Thompson T, Parmenter TR (eds) The international handbook of applied research in intellectual disabilities. Wiley, Chichester

Walsh M, Hostick T 2005 Improving healthcare through community OR. Journal of the Operational Research Society 56: 193-201

RESOURCES

National Institute for Mental Health in England (NIMHE): www.nihme.csip.org.uk

Mental Health Research Network: www.ukmhrn.info

Service User Research Group, England (SURGE): www.ukmhrn.info

SECTION 4

The Context of Occupational Therapy

Chapter **11**

Ethics

Jenny Butler, Jennifer Creek

A tale of two confidences: introduction

During the course of one day, an occupational therapist was confronted with two situations in which a client disclosed information that she subsequently asked the therapist not to pass on to others. One woman disclosed a history of sexual abuse when she was a child. The other woman feared that she might be HIV positive but did not want her partner to find out. In both cases, the therapist had to decide on the right course of action to take.

INTRODUCTION

In this chapter, we will be exploring how the therapist thinks when confronting difficult decisions, such as the ones in the tale of two confidences. We will start by explaining what ethics is and how the therapist might recognise when she is facing an ethical issue rather than a clinical one. We will then give a brief outline of human rights legislation, explaining how this makes it possible for vulnerable people to challenge abuses of power. This is followed by the two disclosures from the tale of two confidences, showing how the therapist might think about each one in order to decide on the best course of action. These analyses illustrate two approaches to ethical reasoning: applying ethical principles and thinking about the consequences of our actions. We then offer a framework of questions that you can use in thinking through ethical issues, with a story to practise on. We recommend that you try working through the framework for yourself before looking at our analysis. We give references so that the interested reader can find out more.

WHAT IS ETHICS?

Ethics is the branch of philosophy that is concerned with morals, or the distinction between right and wrong. Medical ethics, or occupational therapy ethics, is 'the analytical activity in which the concepts, assumptions, beliefs, attitudes, emotions, reasons and arguments underlying medicomoral decision making are examined critically' (Gillon 1985/1986, p2). Ethical decisions are 'those that concern norms or values, good and bad, and what ought and ought not to be done' (ibid.). Hence, professional documents that are intended to regulate the conduct of practitioners are called codes of ethics.

Such codes highlight the types of situation that the practitioner may encounter which have an ethical dimension. For example, the *Code of Ethics and Professional Conduct* of the UK College of Occupational Therapists (2005, p12) states that:

> Occupational therapists shall refer clients to, or consult with, other service providers when additional knowledge and expertise is required.

This suggests that knowing the limits of one's own competence is an ethical issue rather than simply a clinical one. In other words, it is not just ineffective but also morally wrong to provide treatment when you know that you do not have the necessary knowledge and expertise. Why might this be an ethical issue? Ask yourself what respect you are affording the person receiving your care, if that care is not based on expertise and knowledge. Might you be considered to be abusing that person's trust in you and your profession? Are your actions in any way good?

Thinking about the good of an action, or considering what action you might take in a situation to minimise harm, the question arises – whose good or whose harm? In any professional situation in which you are called upon to explain the reasons for your actions, you will be expected to have in the forefront of your mind a consideration of the good for another or others (rather than some good for yourself). Similarly, it should be evident that you are seeking to minimise harm for another or others, rather than for yourself. In such consideration of another, or others, as the recipient of good from your actions (or of the least harm), an understanding of and empathy with the other person's basic human rights should be fundamental to your thinking. The respect that you accord the other person's freedom, rights and dignity is the means through which your ethical thinking can be channelled.

HUMAN RIGHTS

Thinking about the fundamental freedoms and rights that humans are deemed to have will, in many ways, be context dependent. In the developing world, in areas of famine, disease or disaster, the Right to Life takes prime consideration. Other rights asserted by the Western and developed worlds become largely superfluous. It is clear that unless basic needs are met (for clean water, for food, for access to health care, for employment, for education) the rights and freedoms as laid out in the UK Human Rights Act (1998) cannot be neither aspired to nor demanded by the individuals concerned.

Consideration of human rights should be part of everyday practice. As much as anything, they are about respect for the person and her or his dignity.

You might like to think about whether an intervention or practice policy is likely to impact upon an individual's rights under the Act (whether patient/client or staff). Here are five questions that you could ask.

1. Is the person's mental or physical well-being affected?

The relevant sections of the Act are:

- Article 2 Right to life
- Article 3 Right to freedom from inhuman and degrading treatment
- Article 5 Right to liberty and security of the person.

Examples of interventions that might contravene these rights include: experimental interventions, interventions without evidence base and restraint practices.

2. Is there a risk of discrimination?

The relevant section of the Act is Article 14 Convention rights are secured without discrimination.

Some aspects of the person that might be the focus of discrimination include: religion, sex, race, colour, language, political views, social background and mental health.

3. Is the person's family or private life affected?

The relevant section of the Act is Article 8 Right to respect for private and family life.

Examples of policies and procedures that might contravene this right include: collection of data, consent to intervention, medical record keeping, parental involvement and attendance at a specialist facility.

4. Are you impacting on the individual's freedom of thought, expression or conscience?

The relevant sections of the Act are:

- Article 9 Freedom of expression
- Article 10 Freedom of assembly and association.

Issues that might impact on someone's freedom of thought, expression or conscience include: spoken language and access to interpreters, and the language used for pamphlets and information sheets.

5. Is a hearing or review involved?

The relevant sections of the Act are:

- Article 6 Right to a fair hearing
- Article 7 No punishment without law.

Examples of procedures that might contravene these rights include: grievance procedures, complaints procedures, formal detention of patients and the use of seclusion.

In the research context, the fundamental freedoms and rights of individuals have been considered by the Council of Europe Steering Committee on Bioethics (2001) to ensure that participation in research is freely undertaken by individuals, without coercion.

Occupational therapists would add to the list of human rights that people have a right to occupation. Further discussion of this idea can be found in Chapters 3 and 30 under the headings of occupational justice and occupational apartheid.

ISSUES OF POWER AND CONTROL

There is an inherent imbalance of power between those seeking and those giving health care. No matter how we, as health-care workers, try to redress that imbalance, by seeking to create an environment of equality and support, and to empower those seeking our services, service users need and want something from us. This need for current or continued health or social care places the health/social care worker in a position of power, and being in a position of power places upon us professional responsibilities (College of Occupational Therapists 2005).

Power in this context is not just about whether (or not) we provide a service or intervention, the length of that service provision and the timing of termination of services, although all of these are under the health/social care worker's control. Power is also about who holds the greatest knowledge and understanding (of a condition, illness or impairment; of legal requirements; of services available; of rationing criteria; of equipment available).

You should seek, at all times, to respect individuals, to engage in behaviours that enable the client to take power and to promote partnership working with clients in an atmosphere of trust and support.

There are considerations of power imbalance in research too (Council of Europe Steering Committee on Bioethics 2001). The relative positions of the clinician and the patient/client or the work colleague must be appreciated in terms of the power that one has in relation to the other. The consequent dependency of the potential participant in research who is also a patient/client (or a colleague) for their current or continued health or social care (or continuing professional work relationship) makes for particular vulnerability when the health/social care worker is also the researcher (Butler 2003). Research ethics guidelines advocate that researchers must seek to minimise the effects of the power imbalance wherever possible (College of Occupational Therapists 2003).

Why occupational therapists need to understand ethics

How do you start asking questions about the ethics of a situation you face? There is no *right* order or *right* way to ask the questions; you must find a way that suits you, using knowledge about ethical principles to help your thinking. In your work practice, it is necessary to find your own approach to identifying the key questions to ask. The next two sections aim to help you on your way and show you a possible process.

A TALE OF TWO CONFIDENCES

No occupational therapist should ever have to take difficult clinical or ethical decisions by herself; there should always be supervision in place. The inexperienced therapist may receive more structured supervision, with elements of training, and would be wise to give careful consideration to the opinion of the supervisor. The experienced therapist will have a more equal relationship with her supervisor; she may use the supervisor as a sounding board for exploring the options but will make her own decision. In either case, the supervisor would have the duty to contact the therapist's line manager, with the knowledge of the supervisee, if she felt that an unsafe decision had been made.

The service user should be made aware that there can be no absolute confidences in the therapeutic relationship and that any information may be shared with the therapist's supervisor or, potentially, with other staff.

ANALYSIS OF THE ETHICAL ISSUES RAISED IN RUTH'S DISCLOSURE

There are several ways to think about what action the therapist might take in response to what Ruth has told her. The therapist has informed Ruth about the specialist team and Ruth has stated that she does not want to be referred to them at the present time. There are now two possible courses of action for the therapist:

- to pass on to the specialist team what Ruth has told her about being sexually abused, or
- to withhold that information and carry on as though Ruth had not said anything.

One approach the therapist might try is to apply ethical principles to the situation. Ethical principles are moral rules that tell us whether our actions are right or wrong (Gillon 1985/1986); for example, respecting autonomy is an ethical principle. In Table 11.1, we suggest four principles that might be applied to the types of ethical

---

A tale of two confidences: Ruth's disclosure

Ruth was a woman in her 40s with a long history of severe depression. She was in hospital for a short admission to sort out her medication and stabilise her mood. She had established a warm, trusting relationship with the therapist and was excited about learning new ways of managing her depression. During an individual session one morning, Ruth mentioned that she had been sexually abused by her father when she was a young child. He was no longer alive at this time.

There was a specialist team attached to the unit that worked with the sequelae of childhood abuse, so the therapist asked if Ruth would like to be referred to them. She said 'No', that she was finding her occupational therapy helpful and did not need to do anything about events that had happened years ago. The therapist knew that if she told the team about Ruth's disclosure, her client would be interviewed by one of the specialists and perhaps persuaded to undergo psychotherapy. If Ruth agreed to this, she would be expected not to continue with occupational therapy.

The therapist's reasoning process was that Ruth felt safe disclosing painful memories within a trusting relationship but that this trust might be damaged if the information went any further. Ruth was making good progress towards the goals that had been set in occupational therapy and her achievements would form a foundation for setting further goals. If, at some time in the future, she decided that she would like to talk about her childhood experiences, the therapist could refer her to the specialist team. The outcome of this train of reasoning was that the therapist did not pass on the information about Ruth having been sexually abused.

Table 11.1 Ethical principles applied to clinical practice

Minimising harm must always be a priority	Who might be harmed in this situation? What form might this harm take for each identified person or group? • The individuals • A group • Society as a whole • Yourself
Doing good is one of the duties of a therapist	Of any number of actions that I might take, which will lead to the greatest good? Who will receive the good, or the benefit, in this situation? What form will the good take for each person or group? • The individuals • A group • Society as a whole • Yourself
The occupational therapist is expected to accord equal respect to all	What actions will ensure that each person/group in this situation is respected equally?
Each person has the right to make her or his own choices	Are all the people in this situation afforded the opportunity to make their own informed decisions (are they autonomous)? Are they *able* to make unfettered decisions? Without pressure, coercion or undue influence? What actions by the therapist will ensure that their decisions are respected?

issues that an occupational therapist is likely to encounter. Each principle is accompanied by a question or set of questions that will help you to think about what would be the best (that is, most morally right) course of action to take.

In thinking about what to do about Ruth's disclosure, the therapist might start by weighing up the potential harm that could result from either action versus the potential benefits. She decides that passing on the information would harm Ruth by damaging her trust in the therapist and by disrupting an occupational therapy programme that she is finding useful. Not passing on the information demonstrates a lack of respect for her colleagues' professional integrity and skill. This makes her feel uncomfortable, and she knows that her relationship with them is likely to be weakened if they find out that she has withheld relevant clinical information. She sees that she is measuring a more likely harm – damage to a good therapeutic relationship and an effective programme – against a less likely harm – weakening her own relationship with her colleagues and making her feel uncomfortable about her relationship with them.

Passing on the information might lead to Ruth engaging with the specialist team, despite her initial refusal, and coming to terms with what appears to have been a very traumatic experience in her childhood. This could lead to a significant improvement in her depression. It could also strengthen the therapist's relationship with her colleagues. On the other hand, deciding not to refer Ruth to the specialist team would allow for continuation of the trusting relationship they have and demonstrate respect for her decision not to have psychotherapy at the present time. It would still leave open the possibility of a future referral to the specialist team when Ruth feels ready for it. The therapist believes that it is crucial to respect Ruth's decision in this situation, not only to maintain their positive relationship but also to give Ruth a sense of being in control of her own life.

Weighing up all these points, and considering that no vulnerable person other than Ruth would be affected by her decision, the occupational therapist decides not to disclose what Ruth has told her.

A tale of two confidences: Janet's disclosure

The same afternoon, the therapist saw a woman she had been working with as an outpatient for some months. Janet was in her early 30s and had a serious alcohol problem. She had asked for help because her sisters thought her drinking made her an unfit parent and she was afraid that her 8-year-old son might be taken into care. She lived with a man and, unknown to her partner, had a long-term relationship with another man. She was trying controlled drinking, alongside working on her self-confidence and assertiveness skills. She was making positive progress.

That day, Janet turned back as she was leaving the room at the end of the session. She asked the therapist if a woman could contract HIV by having unprotected sex with a man who had subsequently died of an AIDS-related illness. When questioned, she admitted that she had had sex with an acquaintance one night when drunk. She had recently heard about his death and was worried that she might have caught the virus. The therapist told Janet that she needed to have a blood test but Janet refused. She said that if the therapist put pressure on her she would stop coming for occupational therapy. She then left.

The therapist thought carefully about what she should do. If she passed on to the multidisciplinary team (MDT) what Janet had told her, Janet would be put under pressure to have a blood test. If she refused, both her partners would be informed of the risk of infection. Janet's live-in partner may move out, which would increase the likelihood of her son being taken into care. She would stop attending for treatment and probably go back to drinking heavily. The best clinical outcome would be gained by not disclosing the information Janet had given her. To maintain confidentiality seemed to be the right clinical decision. However, if the therapist did not pass on the information, both of Janet's partners, and the wife of the second man, may be at risk. The therapist had to make an ethical decision, not a clinical one; she had to decide what was morally the right course of action.

ANALYSIS OF THE ETHICAL ISSUES RAISED IN JANET'S DISCLOSURE

In response to Janet's disclosure, there are also two possible courses of action for the therapist:

- to inform the MDT that Janet is at risk of having contracted HIV, or
- to keep the information to herself and continue trying to persuade Janet to have a blood test.

An alternative approach to untangling the ethics of a situation would be to start by thinking about what might happen if certain actions are taken, that is, the *consequences* of any action. For example, the therapist could ask: What action will result in the greatest benefit in this situation? (see Table 11.2). This is a different kind of question from the one posed above, that asks: *Who* will receive the good or benefit? In thinking about the possible consequences of our actions, we are asking what will be the greatest benefit for each person in the situation and for the greatest number of people overall. The answers will then have to be considered, weighed and balanced.

The therapist begins by thinking about the potential harm that might be caused by either possible course of action. If she passes on what Janet has told her, Janet may not trust her again and may stop attending for occupational therapy. This could lead to an increase in drinking, which might damage her relationship with her partner and lead to her son being taken into care; all three would be hurt by this. If she does not tell the MDT what Janet has told her, Janet may continue to refuse to have a blood test. If she is HIV positive, there is the risk of Janet developing AIDS and of at least four other people becoming infected: her son, her partner, her lover and her lover's wife. The therapist realises that the potential for harm may be greater if she does not pass on the information, but only if Janet is HIV positive.

Table 11.2 Consequentialism applied to clinical practice

What action will result in the greatest benefit in this situation?	What will be the greatest benefit for each person or group? What will benefit the greatest number of people?

The therapist then thinks about which action might lead to the greatest benefit. If she tells the MDT what Janet has told her, Janet will be pressured into having a blood test. If the result is negative, no further action need be taken. If it is positive, action can be taken to protect all the individuals involved. If she does not inform the team, Janet will continue to benefit from attending occupational therapy and her family is likely to stay together. She may, at some point, decide to have a blood test. The therapist sees that there are likely benefits to everyone in this course of action.

The therapist realises that she cannot take a decision on the best course of action because she does not have enough information on which to base that decision. If Janet is HIV positive, then the MDT must be informed so that potential harm to many people can be avoided. If Janet is HIV negative, the greatest benefit to the greatest number of people would derive from keeping the incident a confidence. The therapist decides to share her reasoning with Janet, explaining that if she does not go for a blood test the therapist will have to disclose the situation to the MDT.

These case examples illustrate how, when thinking about the ethical dimension of our clinical decisions, we have to weigh and balance many points, considering the harm, the benefit and the autonomy of individuals.

A FRAMEWORK FOR DEALING WITH ETHICAL ISSUES

There are a number of approaches to the exploration of ethical dilemmas (see, for example, Seedhouse 1988) which enable a systematic process of asking the questions you need to ask in such difficult situations. No system will *give* you the answers – you have to think these out for yourself – but it will give you a framework for your thinking. We suggest that in these situations, as always, it is a given that you will be honest. Personal morality and integrity are the cornerstones of professional practice and demand more than just adhering to a code of professional conduct.

In the tale of two confidences, we introduced you to two theories that might help you to think about ethical issues: ethical principles and consequentialism. We will now identify two sets of factors that need to be taken into account: external considerations and patient rights. For each of these areas, we suggest questions that you might ask to clarify your thoughts.

EXTERNAL CONSIDERATIONS

All the ethical decisions we make in the course of our work are taken within a social context that includes the wider society, our professional background and the working environment. This context is made up of constraints and considerations such as duties, expectations, codes, policies, laws and resources. In Table 11.3, we suggest some questions that you might ask to ensure that you take these external constraints and considerations into account when making an ethical decision.

PATIENT RIGHTS AND THE DUTIES OF HEALTH-CARE PROFESSIONALS

Earlier in the chapter we talked about the Human Rights Act and how, in considering the good of our actions as professionals, we must respect another's freedom and dignity. We also gave examples of areas in practice that could contravene the different Articles of the Act. Let us now expand a little on this area and consider some of the rights of people under our care and the consequent duties placed upon us (see Table 11.4).

At the end of the 20th century, there was an increased interest in and discussion of human rights, stimulated by the publication of the *European Convention on Human Rights* (Council of Europe Steering Committee on Bioethics 2001). However, not everyone understands exactly what the concept of a *right* implies or entails.

Rights are 'justified claims that require action or restraint from others – that is, impose positive or negative duties on others' (Gillon 1985/1986, p54). Such claims may be justified by 'law, morals, rules, or other norms' (Audi 1999, p796). An example of a legal right in the UK is the right of all children to a free education. An example of a moral right is the right to choose whether or not

Table 11.3   External constraints and considerations

Context	Questions to ask
Professional duties	Does my professional code of conduct steer me in a particular way, or towards a certain action or approach?
The law	Would a certain action be against the law?
Risks	What are the risks associated with certain actions in this situation?
Resources	Are there enough resources for certain actions in this situation?
Evidence base	What is the known effectiveness of the actions that I might take in this situation? Are there any facts or evidence in this situation that are unclear, uncertain or unreliable? Is the evidence reliable?
Work setting	Are there opinions of others that I should consider in my actions in this situation?

Table 11.4   Patient rights and health professional duties

Issue	Questions to ask
A person with mental health problems has the same basic human rights as every other citizen	Are the patient's basic human rights being upheld or compromised?
A right may be justified by law, morals, rules or other norms	Is this a legal or a moral right? Do I have a legal duty in this situation? Is there a rule in my working environment that imposes a duty on me to uphold a particular right?
Rights impose positive or negative duties on others	Do I have a legal or moral duty to act to uphold the patient's rights? Do I have a legal or moral duty to refrain from action to avoid compromising the patient's rights?
A person receiving mental health care has specific legal and moral rights related to her or his mental health needs	Does this person have any specific rights related to her or his mental health needs? Do I have any specific duties in relation to this patient's mental health needs?

to accept treatment for a physical ailment, without coercion.

The definition of rights given above incorporates the idea that a right imposes a concomitant duty on others. So, if every child has the right to an education, someone must have the duty to provide that education (a positive duty). If everyone has the right to choose, without coercion, whether or not to accept medical treatment, this implies a duty for everyone else to refrain from applying coercion (a negative duty).

When we think about patient rights, we can recognise that people with mental health problems have the same legal and moral rights as every other citizen. However, someone who is experiencing mental distress will be especially vulnerable to having his rights compromised. Carers, whether paid or unpaid, have a duty to uphold the basic human rights of those people for whom they have responsibility.

In addition, people receiving mental health care have specific legal and moral rights related to their mental health needs. Perhaps the most obvious of these is the right to receive the best available care and treatment (Thompson 2002). This means that health-care staff have a duty to give their patients the best available care and treatment within the constraints of finite resources.

While you must understand what your duties are in relation to your patients or clients, this understanding alone will not show you how to address ethical issues. The rights of the patient and the duties of the health-care professional are only two of the many factors to be taken into account when thinking about the ethics of a situation.

THINKING ABOUT THE ETHICS OF A SITUATION

When facing any ethical decision, you can start untangling the issues that are the constituent competing parts of the situation in a number of ways. Start where you feel most able to tease out the answer. The areas for consideration that have been identified in this section are summarised in Table 11.5.

You might begin by identifying the consideration that seems most pertinent to the situation you are thinking about. For example, in Ruth's story, the therapist begins by thinking about two ethical principles: minimising harm must always be a priority and doing good is one of the duties of a therapist.

When you have thought carefully through the situation from this first perspective, you can select another consideration to apply to the situation you are analysing. For example, in Janet's story the therapist, having thought about the consequences of her two possible courses of action, turns to thinking about external considerations: that is, the risks inherent in this situation and the lack of evidence on which to base her actions.

Continue working through the sections in Table 11.5 until you feel that you have addressed all the important considerations. It is unlikely that you will need to think about all 17 sections.

We will now present a case study, The story of Frank, that requires you to think about ethical issues in order to make a decision about the best course of action. Use the sections in Table 11.5 to help you identify all the important issues that must be considered.

ANALYSIS OF ETHICAL ISSUES IN FRANK'S STORY

On thinking about the story of Frank, you may have identified two possible courses of action:

- to decide not to intervene
- to work with Frank to change his activity patterns.

There are four perspectives that you might have adopted in order to decide which course of action

Table 11.5 Summary of ethical considerations

Ethical principles	Consequences	External constraints	Patient rights
Minimising harm must always be a priority	What action will result in the greatest benefit in this situation?	Professional duties	A person with mental health problems has the same human rights as all other people
Doing good is one of the duties of a therapist	What will be the greatest benefit for each person or group?	The law	A right may be justified by law, morals, rules or other norms
The occupational therapist is expected to accord equal respect to all	What will benefit the greatest number of people?	Risks involved	Rights impose positive or negative duties on others
Each person has the right to make her or his own choices		Resources available	A person receiving mental health care has specific rights related to her or his mental health needs
		The evidence base	
		The work setting	

would be the right one, as shown in Table 11.5: thinking about the principles of ethical behaviour; identifying the potential consequences of your actions; taking into account any external factors that might impact on your decision; and considering Frank's rights in this situation.

The story of Frank

An occupational therapist was asked by the support staff of a group home to visit a man with Down's syndrome, Frank, for a domestic assessment. Frank was in his late 30s and had spent most of his life in an institution before being rehomed with three other men. He had gout but was independent in self-care and independently mobile. He was mute but understood what others were saying.

The support staff, who had moved from the institution with the residents when it closed down, were concerned that Frank did not take part in the domestic activities of the house, allowing his housemates to do the cooking and cleaning, with help from staff. They requested an assessment of what Frank could do, followed by some skills training to enable him to take a share of the household chores.

The occupational therapist asked Frank to make a snack meal and set the table. She observed that he was very slow, possibly due to stiffness and pain caused by his gout, and that he had difficulty sequencing tasks in order to complete activities. Because of these problems, he needed constant prompting in order to be able to co-ordinate making toast, brewing tea and setting the table at the same time. The therapist also observed that Frank was not interested in the activities he was carrying out. His attention kept returning to the sitting room, where he had been watching a television programme. After the meal, he helped to clear the table but was too tired to wash up.

When the other residents of the house returned from an outing, the therapist told them that she and Frank had been cooking. They said that he could not cook and they liked looking after him. It was apparent that he was a popular member of the household.

QUESTION: What are the ethical issues that the therapist should consider in deciding how to proceed? Work through them and reach a decision on the best course of action before you go on to read the analysis of ethical issues.

You may have started by thinking about the ethical principles that are relevant in this case. Minimising harm should always be a priority, so you think about what harm might arise from either course of action.

If you decide not to intervene, there is the potential for various forms of harm, both to Frank and to the other people in the house. For example, Frank might lose skills and abilities by not carrying out domestic activities, or his housemates may resent Frank not contributing now they know that he can do some things. Already the support staff feel a sense of unfairness because of Frank not contributing. This may be counterproductive to the atmosphere in the home.

If, on the other hand, you decide to intervene to change Frank's activity patterns, there are also several possibilities for harm. A change in Frank's perceived role by his housemates could alter their relationships detrimentally. For example, the other residents could lose their roles in relation to Frank: being helpers, cooks, enablers. Frank may feel coerced into doing what he does not like, leading to a sense of powerlessness, or higher activity levels could cause him pain and discomfort and might be of some detriment to his health.

Having thought through the possible harm arising from your actions and identified that both courses of action have the potential to cause harm to the different people involved, you might then have considered which course of action would bring about the greatest good. For example, if you decide not to intervene, some existing advantages of the present situation will be maintained. These are that Frank feels comfortable in his dependent role and enjoys watching television, and that his housemates like looking after him. This role enhances their self-esteem.

However, there are also several potential benefits that could accrue to all the people in the story, if you decide to intervene to change Frank's activity patterns. Frank could find greater self-worth in making a more active contribution to the household. Higher activity levels, rather than causing problems, might lead to greater mobility and improved health status for Frank. He may discover an interest in cooking or in other activities, leading to increased engagement and participation. Finally, the support staff could feel that they have made a difference by enabling more equality within the household.

Another ethical principle that you might have decided is relevant to this case is that of according equal respect to all. If you decide not to intervene, you will be respecting Frank's preference for watching television rather than helping with the cooking and cleaning. You will also be respecting his housemates' roles in looking after him. If, on the other hand, you decide to intervene, this could be seen as allowing the staff to make decisions for the residents and not listening to them. If all are to be respected equally, Frank and the other housemates would have to agree to a different way of living and working to the betterment of all.

A fourth ethical principle is that each person has the right to make informed choices about her or his life. Carrying out an assessment with Frank has already changed the situation in the house, because the housemates now know more about his abilities and difficulties in carrying out household tasks, so any decision that they and Frank make about his future participation is better informed.

Having thought about four principles of ethical behaviour, you may then have gone on to consider the possible consequences of your actions, including the consequences of having carried out an assessment. Frank and his housemates now know what he might be able to contribute, which could lead to relationship consequences. Frank may feel embarrassed that the household know that he could do more to help. The support staff may feel aggrieved if you do not now implement a domestic skills training programme.

If you decide to intervene with Frank, new patterns of working and household tasks would have to be employed. It is possible that the whole group, including the staff, could grow and develop in relationships and participation. Frank may also grow in self-esteem and abilities. Alternatively, Frank may resent being told to change, and his housemates could be upset at not having someone to take care of.

So far, you may be thinking that both courses of action look equally viable. However, the context of your involvement with Frank could offer constraints or opportunities that change the picture. In thinking about this context, you may have decided that the issue of resources is a key one.

What resources, including your time, would be required to carry out a plan of intervention for Frank in order to increase his skills, stamina and contributions? Are those resources available? You will also have considered what resources might be needed to support the whole household to manage the change.

Another factor that you may have considered is whether or not there is evidence to support either course of action. You may have wondered why Frank does not appear to want to contribute to the work of the household, and why his housemates seem to want someone to care for. You may have realised that you do not have enough information to judge what the consequences could be of changing the balance of relationships in the household.

The last area for consideration is the rights of the people involved in this situation. You might think that Frank has the right to enjoy his life as it is, and that his housemates have the right to be his carers, thus enhancing their own sense of being useful. Or you may think that Frank has the right to be enabled towards greater participation, and his housemates can rightfully expect everyone to do their share for the good of the household.

Deciding on the right course of action

Having thought carefully through all these ethical considerations, you will have identified a range of reasons for and against intervening in Frank's situation or not intervening. It may have become clear, from your analysis, that you need more information in order to be able to reach a decision. In this case, you might decide to talk to Frank and to the other members of the household in order to elicit their views.

It may be that there are more possibilities in addition to the two courses of action you identified to start with. You could decide to explore the possibilities for Frank contributing just a little more, by identifying tasks that he could enjoy doing. You could look for other ways for the housemates to feel that they are taking care of Frank.

After examining the situation from four ethical perspectives, you may well decide that the right course of action is to enable the whole household to make a decision about how they would like to live their lives. Your job will then be to enable that decision to come to fruition. This may require increased resources to support a change of living practice or it may require further assessment to see if Frank could find other activities which he could enjoy and which would enable him to retain mobility.

SUMMARY

In this chapter, we have explored an aspect of the therapist's thinking that is used to determine the most moral course of action in a given situation: ethical reasoning. We began with a brief discussion of human rights legislation and issues of power. We then suggested how you might recognise when the issue you are dealing with requires ethical reasoning rather than clinical reasoning, and offered a framework of questions that might help you to think through a problem. The aspects of the situation that might have a bearing on your deliberations include: ethical principles; the possible consequences of your actions or inactions; external considerations, and patient rights and the duties of health-care professionals.

Occupational therapists have a professional duty to act in a responsible and ethical way towards their clients. In order to fulfil this requirement, they need to be skilled in ethical reasoning. Like other skills, ethical reasoning becomes easier with practice, and we recommend that you take every opportunity to develop this important way of thinking.

References

Audi R (ed) 1999 The Cambridge dictionary of philosophy, 2nd edn. Cambridge University Press, Cambridge

Butler JA 2003 Research in the place where you work – some ethical issues. Bulletin of Medical Ethics 185:21–23

College of Occupational Therapists 2003 Research ethics guidelines. College of Occupational Therapists, London

College of Occupational Therapists 2005 Code of ethics and professional conduct. College of Occupational Therapists, London

Council of Europe Steering Committee on Bioethics 2001 Draft additional protocol to the Convention on Human Rights and Biomedicine, on biomedical research. Department of Health, London

Gillon R 1985/1986 Philosophical medical ethics. Wiley, Chichester

Human Rights Act 1998 HMSO, London

Seedhouse D 1988 Ethics: the heart of health care. Wiley, Chichester

Thompson IE 2002 Ethics. In: Creek J (ed) Occupational therapy and mental health, 3rd edn. Churchill Livingstone, Edinburgh, pp191–206

Chapter 12

Roles and settings

Cathy Ormston

INTRODUCTION

The past decade has seen immense changes in mental health services in the United Kingdom. Attention has in recent times been on the implementation and consolidation of the reforms initiated by the the National Health Service and Community Care Act 1991 (DoH 1990), that firmly shifted the focus from hospital-oriented mental health service provision to care in the community, and continued with *Modernising Mental Health Services* (DoH 1998) and the development of the *National Service Framework for Mental Health* (NSFMH) (DoH 1999). These UK national initiatives have gone some way to address earlier problems of inequity of service provision across the country, define appropriate inpatient care and develop community services that can deliver more consistent standards.

The NSFMH continues to determine service models and standards for mental health and sets the context behind the more detailed mental health service commissioning guidelines, providing a united vision of modern mental health care for all key members of the multidisciplinary team. With its emphasis on multiprofessional and multiagency partnership and on engaging service users through respectful collaboration, it has, since its inception, impacted on the roles of all mental health service providers.

Crucially for occupational therapists in the UK, the impact of national policy has meant that mental health services now embrace a wide perspective in which attention to social outcomes and addressing peoples' everyday lives has moved higher up the agenda (Office of the Deputy Prime Minister 2004a,b, National Social Inclusion Programme 2006), thus making the role of occupational therapists within the various settings potentially more important.

Alongside these developments, there has been expansion in the roles of other established disciplines (for example, mental health nurses working with service users to develop healthy lifestyles, looking at diet and exercise; Social Services colleagues working as employment specialists within mental health teams), as well as the introduction of new workers, for example support, time and recovery (STaR) workers (DoH 2003) and graduate primary mental health workers. High-profile reports outlining the importance and scarcity of talking therapies have looked to mental health professionals from nursing and occupational therapy to take up specialist training in cognitive therapy, for example, as an antidote to the restricted access and long waiting times for psychological therapies. Layard (2006, p10), for example, recommended that '5,000 "psychological therapists" could be trained from among the 60,000 nurses, social workers, occupational therapists and counsellors already working on mental health in the NHS' and that 'to make them into fully professional therapists they should be re-employed as trainee "psychological therapists" in the new mental health teams and given one- or two-year part-time off-the-job courses in therapy'.

The growing awareness of the potential shortfall in trained mental health professionals is a theme repeatedly reflected in UK health policy. A further example of this is the recognition of the need to remedy the current and increasing shortage in approved social workers (ASWs) where the numbers of practitioners approaching retirement are not being matched by those undertaking ASW training (Huxley et al 2005). This trend serves as a driver behind some of the planned amendments to the Mental Health Act (1983) and recruits from a broader range of mental health professionals will be encouraged to train and act as approved mental health professionals, taking up the role and function previously performed by social workers in the implementation of the Mental Health Act (DoH 2004a, 2006, Jones et al 2006).

So occupational therapists might be said to face competition from other groups for those roles and functions that were once their unique priority, whilst at the same time feeling pressure to move into areas of practice that are outwith the occupational therapy traditional domains of concern (Royal College of Psychiatrists 2005).

The desire to achieve a robust body of mental health workers united by competences, common to all regardless of professional group, is also evident in the numerous workforce development initiatives that have been introduced (Hope 2004, NIMHE 2004, Sainsbury Centre for Mental Health 2001). These impact on all stages of workers' professional lives both before and after qualification. Shared learning with other health professionals at undergraduate level has been a feature for a number of years. Further to this, the publication of the *Ten Essential Shared Capabilities* document (Hope 2004) clarifies the generic competencies expected of all mental health professionals and is providing the foundation upon which other workforce competency frameworks are developing; for example, the National Social Inclusion Programme (NSIP) commissioned the identification of socially inclusive ways of working, using the framework of the *Ten Essential Shared Capabilities* as an underpinning structure.

Moves to develop more consistency across health professions are further evident in Agenda for Change – the restructuring of pay, terms and conditions for all staff groups in the NHS. All posts have been assimilated onto a single pay spine, jobs being graded according to the competencies required and the specification of knowledge, skills and experience. Job profiles are constructed from nationally recognised descriptions, termed 'dimensions', and definitions of performance within these dimensions are again nationally agreed. None of these dimensions is profession specific; rather, each professional group has profiles constructed around a baseline of descriptors that apply to all NHS jobs, with the addition of specific dimensions that describe competencies as they relate to a specific post (Agenda for Change Project Team, DoH 2004).

With all the overt moves towards shared competencies and the breakdown of professional boundaries, what is left for an occupational therapist to offer? Interestingly, whilst there continues to be marked pressure towards generic practice, there is an equal force compelling occupational therapists to ensure that their particular expertise is appropriately targeted to address occupational need and bring added value to the multidisciplinary team by contributing their distinct perspective. Occupational therapists are being urged to reassert the profession's central tenet regarding the relationship between occupation and health, to champion occupation as a human right and expose occupational deprivation as being a violation of these rights. They need to ensure that occupational therapists are the acknowledged experts in working with the occupational needs of people with mental health problems (College of Occupational Therapists 2006). The primary role remains: that is, of occupational therapists promoting good mental health and assisting recovery through engagement in activity. The centrality of occupation in the thinking of occupational therapists and their consequent strengths-based orientation continue to represent the added value they bring to a multidisciplinary team.

Modern mental health services provide a comprehensive range of services in the community and focus on the individual's needs specific to their own home context. NSFMH standards demand local, timely and consistent service provision and practice that is based on the best available evidence. Intervention goals are as much about helping people achieve optimal function within their community setting and providing practical support as about treatment of symptoms. As priority is given to service user involvement, outreach, ensuring people have opportunities for meaningful daytime activities and home-based support and the elevation of quality of life and functional ability as priorities for care, the role of the occupational therapist has never been so germane.

The extended development of a community focus to health has, in turn, impacted on the roles and functions of hospital-based care. People for whom even a comprehensive range of home treatments, long-term supports, crisis interventions and home outreach still cannot prevent relapse that is severe enough to warrant hospital admission are, by default, likely to be an increasingly disturbed, distressed and vulnerable population.

Acute admission stays are shortening and the proportion of inpatients who are compulsorily detained is rising (Dratcu 2006, Sainsbury Centre for Mental Health 1999). Similarly, longer-term inpatient services have to address the needs of a much more disabled and challenging group than before, not because mental illnesses have become worse but because many of those who previously faced years of hospitalisation are now rightly perceived as being able to succeed at, and having a right to, participative community living. The remaining very small group of people with needs that still make community living unrealistic may continue to need specialist care, sometimes in NHS hospitals or more often in specialist hospitals or units provided by private companies or the voluntary sector. Occupational therapists based in inpatient settings and longer term treatment/care settings have to continue to adapt to the changing needs of this population.

Now there is a wider acceptance of the need to address people's ability to function in their home environment, other professionals are embracing roles traditionally seen as particular to the occupational therapist. If the occupational therapist's role and identity are defined by goals and purpose, then it should be acknowledged that this is shared with a wide number of professionals who all aim to enhance independence and function, assist meaningful engagement in community settings and improve quality of life, as well as decrease people's distress and vulnerability to symptoms. Defined this way, the occupational therapist adopts a number of roles generic to any mental health worker in a contemporary service context. However, if occupational therapists' roles are defined by the specific part they play, that is, what they contribute to the team as a whole, then it is easier to distinguish their profession-specific roles.

Occupational therapists working in multidisciplinary teams, in widely dispersed settings, have to respond flexibly to a client-centred approach in which a number of generic skills are needed. This chapter therefore aims to explore the balance of generic and specialist, core, acquired and required roles of occupational therapists, in various mental health settings. It focuses on the occupational therapist as an individual professional and on the interface with other team members.

INFLUENCES ON THE OCCUPATIONAL THERAPIST'S ROLE

As we view each service user as a unique individual with a wide repertoire of roles, so every occupational therapist has a unique part to play in her distinct setting with a similar diversity of roles and functions, influenced by a complex interplay of intrinsic and extrinsic factors. Some roles are inherently accepted as core to occupational therapy, others are aspired to and achieved through growing competence and credibility and some are thrust upon the therapist by colleagues, employers and service users.

EXTRINSIC FACTORS

National policy and local implementation

The contexts in which occupational therapists operate influence both the roles available to them and those demanded of them (Creek 2003). The priorities of each service are determined by both national and local health and social strategies. For example, when national mental health policy focused on improving community responses to people with severe, long-term mental health problems who do not traditionally engage with services, the Sainsbury Centre for Mental Health's influential report *Keys to Engagement* (Sainsbury Centre for Mental Health 1998) reviewed care for this client group. They made recommendations targeted at central and local government and the NHS, regarding the developments needed to achieve the right mix of day-to-day engagement and active health care and rehabilitation. The *National Service Framework for Mental Health* (DoH 1999) supported the recommendations and included the availability, in all localities, of services based on an assertive outreach model, as a milestone in monitoring progress towards delivering elements of standards 4 and 5 of the framework (the standards relating to developing effective services for people with severe mental illness).

These teams have a definitive model of operation (Sainsbury Centre for Mental Health 1998, Stein & Test 1980) based on evidence of effective practice for work with people with psychoses (Lehman et al 1997, Marshall & Lockwood 1998, National Institute for Clinical Excellence 2002a). The model includes the use of biopsychosocial interventions, cognitive therapy, family psychoeducational interventions, team responsibility rather than key worker relationships, extended hours of availability, intensive contact over months or years and rights for direct hospital admission. The development of the Department of Health's Policy Implementation Guide for Assertive Outreach consolidated the model further (DoH 2002b).

Thus the shaping of the role of an occupational therapist employed in such an environment can be demonstrably linked to central government policy, local priorities and strategic planning within health and/or social services, research evidence, as well as the strategic planning of the employing NHS trust.

The other major area concerning mental health policy development is in the attention paid to addressing the risks of social exclusion faced by people living with mental health problems in the UK. The report of the Social Exclusion Unit (Office of the Deputy Prime Minister 2004b) and numerous subsequent guidance and progress report documents have a direct impact on the commissioning, provision and evaluation of services, as well as influencing the skill mix and competencies required of staff in these services (National Social Inclusion Programme 2007). With occupational therapy's long-standing attention to a person's fullest participation in the life of his community, the developments can clearly benefit from occupational therapists' contributions. Drives to combat exclusion (that would be evidenced through increased presence of people with mental health problems in mainstream social settings and involvement in activities typically available to all) and specific efforts to improve people's opportunities to obtain paid work, indicate that this external influence on roles provides an excellent context for occupational therapists to do as the College of Occupational Therapists' 10-year mental strategy, *Recovering Ordinary Lives*, urges, namely 'move the client in the direction of fuller participation in society through the performance of occupations that are appropriate to her or his age, social and cultural background, interests and aspirations' and to 'support adults in attaining, maintaining or regaining a work role'

(College of Occupational Therapists 2006, pp4–5). In this instance the congruence between national policy and stated professional strategic intent is plain.

Roles and the impact of particular work settings

There is an ever-growing range of settings where occupational therapists may work, all of which are subject to the same complex array of defining influences as that cited above. Though service patterns and configurations vary, the following are some common examples.

Inpatient services

- Acute admission wards
- Psychiatric intensive care units (PICU)
- Rehabilitation units
- Services for people with 'challenging behaviour'
- Specialist services, e.g. forensic/high/medium/ low secure settings; drug and alcohol; mother and baby units; eating disorders; child and adolescent units
- Elderly services: assessment and short-term/ intermediate/continuing care

Inpatient services may be provided by NHS trusts or by non-statutory or private service providers.

Day services

- Day hospitals/partial hospitalisation programmes (NHS)
- Non-building based 'bridge-builder' type services
- Day centres/day services (Social Services/independent and voluntary sector)
- Employment and training projects

Community services

- Community mental health teams (CMHT)
- Assertive outreach teams
- Early intervention services
- Crisis and home treatment teams
- Specialist services, e.g. drug and alcohol; homeless services; dual diagnosis; child and adolescent mental health services
- Primary care teams

- Hostels, supported housing and group homes
- Residential care homes (social services)

The particular constellation of roles the occupational therapist will fulfil in each of these will be influenced by a wide range of factors that may include:

- the client group at whom the service is targeted and the purpose for which the team exists
- the skill mix of the particular team: the personal qualities and skills of the team member and the mix of professionals
- team resources: roles may need to be more flexible in a team with few resources, or where a specialist team covers a broad geographic patch
- time constraints
- the clarity (or otherwise) of the team's individual job descriptions and the effective use of performance management to craft the team roles to meet shared service objectives
- particular service philosophies, operational models and the dominance of a specific treatment or intervention framework
- the management style and background of the team leader
- whether the practitioner works single-handed or as part of a larger occupational therapy team
- the status afforded to the occupational therapist and degree of resultant autonomy assumed by, or afforded to, the therapist
- cultural norms and historical expectations that predetermine accepted roles within a pre-existing team
- pressures to fill gaps by taking on roles not adequately covered within the team and the extent to which occupational therapy is understood and valued by team members and managers (Fortune 2000).

While the Mental Health NSF described the blueprint for mental health service provision in an overall sense, the detail regarding how the various teams should be configured, their priorities, the roles their staff should collectively undertake and the service's recommended outputs have been described in a series of Department of Health policy implementation guides (PIGs) developed to cover the key mental health services, for example the Mental Health

PIG (DoH 2001); PIG for Acute admissions (DoH 2002a); PIG for Community Mental Health Teams (DoH 2002b). As they are targeted also to inform commissioners of services, who have the ultimate say in what is financed, they can be regarded as key influences over the roles of all workers, including occupational therapists. Commissioners of mental health services may or may not have a useful understanding of the potential for occupational therapy to impact on positive outcomes within services and it therefore becomes incumbent upon occupational therapists to assert their contribution clearly. They need to attain, and sustain, sufficient visibility at all levels of the health and social care system to ensure that service agreements include attending to people's occupational needs and measuring occupational outcomes. Through engaging in and utilising available research, service commissioners can be helped to recognise the pertinent role of occupational therapy in delivering positive outcomes for mental health service users.

These extrinsic factors indicate a clear need for occupational therapists to take up a strategic role within policy development, thus influencing what are published as guidelines in the first instance: occupational therapists have a role and a responsibility in championing the occupational needs of service users; challenging occupational injustice (Townsend & Whiteford 2005) and asserting occupation as a human right; exposing its deprivation as a violation of human rights and ensuring that occupation is prioritised as worthy of intervention (College of Occupational Therapists 2006).

Embracing a role as researcher into the effectiveness of occupational therapy interventions and its added value as a component of a multidisciplinary approach within mental health is also key in securing a place in the future strategic planning for and provision of effective modern mental health services (White & Creek 2007).

INTRINSIC FACTORS

Though the tangible roles and functions of an occupational therapist will be outlined in a job description, many issues individual to each therapist will influence role performance. These include essential personality traits, professional philosophy and internal schema regarding her role as an occupational therapist working in mental health as well as individual interest. Creek (2003) summarises what the therapist brings to the therapeutic encounter, illustrating that all impact on what she does:

> Some of the intrinsic factors include: professional experience; professional beliefs and values; understanding of and commitment to client-centred practice; and thinking skills.

Creek adds that 'all these factors change both qualitatively and quantitatively, consequent on the length and quality of the therapist's experience' (Creek 2003, p27).

Experience

The scope and depth of the therapist's previous experience will have a direct bearing on the roles she comfortably undertakes. Clearly, an occupational therapist with several years' experience is more likely to seek out – or be offered –.opportunities to act as project leader, supervisor or chair of a management group than someone new to a field or recently qualified. However, the literature around clinical reasoning suggests that it is not the experience alone that enhances practice (and thus enables the therapist to respond flexibly to a variety of situations and roles) but the reasoning and reflection exercised during and after the experiences. The importance of active clinical reasoning is highlighted by Gamble et al (2001) who describe it as the necessary process ' by which an experience is brought into consideration, while it is happening or subsequently; and secondly, the creation of meaning and conceptualisation from experience'. According to Creek, this process is essential to fulfilling one's role as an occupational therapist, describing clinical reasoning as 'involving a range of mental strategies and high level cognitive processes which enable the therapist to reach decisions about the best course of action'. She continues, 'Clinical reasoning ensures that the occupational therapist practises occupational therapy and not some other form of intervention' (Creek 2003, p39).

As individuals amass a greater body of knowledge, based on a widening body of experience, the complexity of their clinical reasoning develops and will have consequent impact on their occupational therapy role. Schön suggests that 'as a practitioner experiences many variations of a small number of types of case, he is able to "practise" his practice. He develops a repertoire of expectations, images and techniques. He learns what to look for and how to respond to what he finds' (Schön 1991, p60). Hagedorn (1995) refers to the 'value of experience in building the therapist's mental "database"', leading to the development of a sound cognitive construct of occupational therapy and an ability to visualise a possible sequence of events leading to actions based on multiple hypotheses. Proficient practitioners with this advanced repertoire of expectation demonstrate greater flexibility, creativity and an increased ability to consider wider issues when finding solutions than their less experienced colleagues, whether other occupational therapists or members of the multidisciplinary team. These personal characteristics of therapists will affect the roles and status afforded them.

Personal traits

In addition to the roles described within the occupational therapist's job description, the therapist's personality and preferred working roles will influence the contributions she makes within a team. An example is Belbin's (1981) work on teams which characterises members' preferred behaviours and roles, demonstrating the very different strengths people bring to the overall functioning of the team. He postulates that effective teams need a wide range of personality types and advocates the use of team role analysis in recruitment, selection and development. A team needs innovators, lateral thinkers and people to generate enthusiasm and creativity, but must also have a body of people able to focus on a task, seek out resources and complete projects. The individual occupational therapist's own preferred work style will undoubtedly affect the role she undertakes within her team.

Another example of actively recruiting particular people with particular attitudes and personal attributes for the role they may then contribute is in selecting staff who can sustain low levels of expressed emotion (EE) in their relationships with service users into teams working with people with severe mental illness. Work by Kuipers (Kuipers & Moore 1995) suggests that relapse rates in people

with psychosis are positively influenced by family or care groups who demonstrate low EE; it is suggested that this knowledge be utilised when recruiting and training staff for this client group so as to maximise the likelihood that staff will not become frustrated in the face of repeated failure and will not generally blame service users for their difficulties (Ball et al 1992, Shepherd 1998).

The person's level of professional autonomy will also be a key factor influencing the occupational therapist's role. Many occupational therapists work single-handedly in a multidisciplinary team. The expectations of their colleagues and demands from managers of different professional backgrounds can lead to the therapist's role moving away from their core competencies and priorities as an occupational therapist (Peck & Norman 1999). Therapists may embrace generic roles that are seen as valuable to the team as a means of gaining acceptance within the group, providing the same interventions as their colleagues regardless of whether this makes best use of their occupational therapy skills.

Sometimes occupational therapists take on roles because the other team members are reluctant to take them on, without analysis of whether this is appropriate (Fortune 2000). Individuals need sufficient professional autonomy with the scope to define their occupational therapy priorities and a robust internal schema of their occupational therapy role (Creek 2003). Although the College of Occupational Therapists has recommended that the majority of casework should be focused on specialist occupational therapy interventions (Craik et al 1998) and in its 10-year strategy has stressed the need for occupational therapists to reassert the relationship between occupation and health (College of Occupational Therapists 2006), in a study of 40 community mental occupational therapists, Harries & Gilhooley (2003) found that most of the participants were not meeting this recommendation in spite of some therapists aspiring to being more specialist. The pressures to work generically may have been affecting referral policies.

Individual values and interests

Therapists' personal and professional interests will contribute to their assumed role. For example, one occupational therapist may believe strongly in preventive work and the contributions occupational therapy can make in promoting healthy lifestyles with a broad range of clients, offering an open door policy for referrals; another believes it important to target services for people whose illness has a severe impact on function. Meeson's (1998) study of the factors influencing the practice of a group of community occupational therapists demonstrated that the therapist's personal interest in a specific area (for example, anxiety management, creative therapies, supportive counselling and problem solving) was a key factor influencing her choice of intervention with an individual and hence the team role she assumed. Meeson noted that personal preferences seemed to be linked also with familiarity, knowledge and previous experience (and therefore confidence) rather than with a particular theoretical perspective.

Occupational therapists who have undertaken postgraduate training in a specialist area are likely to use it to develop the role they play within a team, perhaps acting as researcher, family worker or advisor/supervisor for a specific approach, for example cognitive therapy or family therapy.

INTRINSIC AND EXTERNAL INFLUENCES ON ROLE – IN PRACTICE

Other chapters describe in detail the contribution occupational therapy makes in many work settings but it is interesting to take an overview of the similarities and differences in the potential roles of occupational therapists doing very different jobs. The influences discussed above interact to shape the roles of four individual therapists presented here. A summary of their work is followed by an examination of some of the contextual influences on the therapist's role.

Case studies

Anna: working as part of an urban community mental health team

Anna is a senior occupational therapist working from an office base in a busy town centre. Having been part of the team for the past 5 years, she is perceived by her colleagues as highly skilled and her advice is often sought by those working with clients with complex needs.

Her mixed caseload includes clients with a range of problems, but more than half have a long-standing diagnosis of psychosis. Much of her work is with individuals and their families in their homes. Her work often involves problem-solving issues concerned with people's day-to-day activities, reflecting on achievements and talking through plans for the days ahead. She may visit people several times a week if it is felt they are at risk of relapse and uses part of her visit to help an individual construct coping strategies to deal with triggers that seem to increase their symptoms. However, most clients are seen on a weekly, fortnightly or monthly basis, depending on the stage of intervention and their degree of recovery. A few attend one of Anna's groups aimed at promoting healthy lifestyles, or the hearing voices group she and a service user facilitate together.

Anna makes use of local shops and cafés, the market, pub and YMCA with individuals and groups of clients who are socially isolated, anxious about public spaces or who are wanting to develop new interests and skills, or for whom simply getting the rent paid and the shopping done is an ordeal. Anna is keen to help people begin to see themselves as competent and encourages them to be optimistic about their prospects for employment. She has a good knowledge of local opportunities for volunteering and has regular meetings with the Jobcentre-plus staff, linking up particularly with the disability employment advisor based there.

Anna works as a single-handed occupational therapist, but regularly takes students for fieldwork placements. She meets with the head occupational therapist, who manages a number of dispersed community-based staff, on a monthly basis and is currently working with her on a proposal for an additional therapist to relieve the strain of increasing referrals.

Discussion

Without the facilities available in a day centre or occupational therapy department, Anna's work relies less heavily on creative and expressive activities than that of hospital-based colleagues and more on the productive, leisure or self-care activities connected with people's everyday lives. The urban community setting gives Anna opportunities for activities to occur in ordinary, valued settings and the chance to work towards her clients feeling increasingly included in community life as ordinary citizens. Anna feels her work is thus consistent with the values and targets expressed in the Social Exclusion Unit's report on social inclusion and mental health (Office of the Deputy Prime Minister 2004a).

Anna's groupwork reflects two major themes that have become an important focus for CMHT in general and occupational therapy in particular - addressing physical health and promotion of healthy lifestyles, and the move towards user-led, self-help approaches. Anna and a colleague run a weekly lifestyles workshop that seeks to address the wider health needs of people with severe mental illness, including promoting healthy eating, developing practical cooking skills and helping people become more physically active, thus addressing the serious weight problems experienced by some (Bradshaw et al 2005). Secondly, the establishment of the hearing voices group reflects Anna's interest in and respect for user-led, self-help approaches (Romme & Escher 1996). Indeed, Anna's co-facilitator role in this group is becoming peripheral as it gains its own direction and momentum and now that the group has secured a small budget to pay for the venue and some expenses.

Anna's focus on helping people explore employment options reflects the return of vocational issues high onto the agenda of occupational therapists and is consistent with the policy guidance based on what service users want for themselves and what is recognised to contribute to assisting recovery and maintaining positive mental health (Perkins & Rinaldi 2005, Secker et al 2006). Anna's role in helping the team recognise and address people's employment needs is well recognised and colleagues will regularly consult her either for advice or to refer an individual for assessment and specific intervention.

Anna's work as enabler and facilitator of people's wider recovery is a shared role; other multidisciplinary colleagues also assist people to participate as full citizens as this is a key objective within the team's operational philosophy and reflective of the PIG for CMHTs (DoH 2002b). Her role in using psychosocial interventions and

relapse prevention strategies is also generic to the team, who all operate within a similar theoretical framework. Her specialist occupational therapy role is more evident in her attention to her clients' needs for meaningful daily occupations, her concern in developing people's life skills, the manner in which she assesses and explores people's occupational goals and the graded application of activities that are relevant to each person's lifestyle.

Anna's focus on working with people with psychosis can be directly connected to her role as an occupational therapist; the head occupational therapist believes that people with the most severe mental health problems experience the greatest interruption in their role performance and a significant deterioration in their quality of life. As these are key concerns for occupational therapy, Anna's work, like that of the other community occupational therapists under the head occupational therapist's supervision, is directed towards this priority group.

As an established team with a stable staff group, members are comfortable with role overlap and respect individual skills and experience. Thus Anna's role is autonomous, accepted and advisory to colleagues working with clients with challenging needs.

Additional important roles for Anna include supervisor, fieldwork educator, counsellor and family supporter, researcher (preparing information supporting the need for additional resources and gaining information on effective practice), manager (of her own time and workload) and administrator.

Tony: working in a rural community mental health centre

Tony is a senior therapist working in a CMHT in a rural market town. Tony sees a number of people in small groups, particularly those with depression and anxiety problems. He supervises two StaR workers, who work with people in and from their homes facilitating self-care activities and acting as bridge-builders with local community groups, leisure facilities, churches and other resources scattered around the local towns and villages.

Tony has a particular interest in cognitive therapy and has undertaken specialist training in this area. He regularly leads anxiety management and relaxation courses in response to the large numbers of referrals he receives from colleagues and believes that this is a highly valuable skill he can contribute to the work of the team. Tony has a small caseload of individual clients whom he sees for individual cognitive therapy sessions; their needs fall outside the referral criteria for the psychology service, but they have been assessed as needing a psychological approach.

Once every fortnight, Tony acts as a duty worker for the team, responding to requests for emergency assessments and queries from GPs and other referrers. He holds care co-ordinator responsibilities within the Care Programme Approach (CPA) for the small number of clients he sees who have more severe and long-term needs, co-ordinating input from other workers and services and convening case reviews.

Tony and a community psychiatric nurse (CPN) colleague have been assisting the primary mental health team that work into a number of GP practices, developing stress clinics and supervising graduate mental health workers. As the primary mental health team develops, there is debate over whether there should be a specific occupational therapy post within the team or whether Tony should continue with sessional input.

Tony is managed by the CMHT manager, with access to the head occupational therapist for advice. He meets with other community occupational therapists throughout his area and receives specialist supervision from a psychologist for his cognitive therapy work.

Discussion

Tony's caseload mix is very typical of many occupational therapists working in community mental health teams. The high demand for work addressing problems connected with anxiety and/or depression is reflective of its high incidence within the spectrum of mental health problems and echoes the experiences of many community-based occupational therapists reported by Meeson (1998) and Harries (1998) (Harries & Gilhooley 2003). His embracing a broad spread of generic roles in addition to his occupational therapy-specific role is consistent with the study undertaken by Lloyd (2004) which sought to identify the roles

undertaken by mental health occupational therapists in Australia and clarify whether there was discrepancy between occupational therapists' actual and preferred roles. This study unsurprisingly demonstrated that occupational therapists had roles that were both specialist and generic; perhaps more surprising was that it illustrated that, in this sample at least, therapists would have liked to increase both their profession-specific activities and their generic roles. Fortune's (Fortune 2000) findings about gap filling also resonate with Tony's experience of needing to take on duties that fall to him rather than being a direct match, because of a lack of alternatives.

People in rural communities are statistically less likely to suffer from severe mental illness (DoH 1995) and Tony's close contact with primary care has also been significant in shaping his role. General practitioners are pressured by the high number of consultations by people with depression and anxiety-related problems and hence demand that mental health services provide for this group. Recent developments have seen new primary mental health teams and the introduction of graduate workers (DoH 2004b). The role of occupational therapy in primary mental health care has not so far been fully demonstrated in that Tony's work reflected more of his generic interests and skills. Many of Tony's roles are generic to his community team, for example care manager, group leader, duty worker, assessor. The duty worker role arose from a team decision that all senior staff would provide duty cover as all were perceived to have the core skills and sufficient experience to respond to urgent queries, provide an initial assessment and co-ordinate an appropriate first-line response. Whilst Tony was concerned that this further took away time from providing occupational therapy, he did not feel able to decline the role as it would have placed increased strain on other team members and appeared as though he was withdrawing an element of his expertise. Hughes (2001) described the dynamics experienced by many occupational therapists in CMHT in relation to role theories and outlined the options individuals can face in resolving role strain, proposing that often the occupational therapist accepts the role set of the CMHT and offsets the experience of role stress by choosing to identify more strongly with the CMHT than their professional group.

Tony is valued for his specialist knowledge within cognitive therapy and his work is noted for being evidence based (Roth & Fonagy 1996, National Institute for Health and Clinical Excellence 2004). The team has a pragmatic approach to client allocation: staff take on new referrals according to space within their caseload and to match client need with specific skills (for example, expertise in family work, eating disorders, cognitive behavioural therapy), rather than directing clients towards a particular professional.

Tony's role as an occupational therapist is made particular use of when he acts as co-worker with a colleague, sharing the care of someone with complex needs who, in addition to CPN support, can particularly benefit from an exploration of their occupational performance and needs and provision of activity-based interventions. As supervisor for the STaR workers, he can delegate some of this work, extending the number of people he can co-ordinate care for and enabling him to develop his other roles. The StaR workers have embraced some of the roles advocated in current policy in helping people become more socially integrated and included in the ordinary activities and life of their community. One of the key features the team looked for in appointing the StaR workers was evidence of their broad personal network of contacts across the villages.

One of the workers had long been a keen participant in a number of community groups himself and this helped his developing bridge-builder role (Office of the Deputy Prime Minister 2004b). Both use their local knowledge, network of contacts and useful relationships and confidence in negotiating transport links to facilitate introductions between service users and their local facilities, community groups and settings. By supporting them in their early engagement in community activities, then gradually withdrawing as the service users establish themselves in, for example, the pub quiz team, the local choir or the college outreach classes, more service users are enjoying increased inclusion in their local communities.

The CPA ensures that people with severe or enduring problems receive a high-quality care plan and a co-ordinated service, organised by an identified professional with an ongoing responsibility to assess and review ongoing needs and broker a range of services on the client's behalf (DoH 2000). While acting as care co-ordinator is a role undertaken by all the professionally qualified team members, Tony most often undertakes this function for people who have clear problems in daily living skills or who want to develop their work skills, two areas that remain identified with occupational therapy (Peck & Norman 1999). Thus he combines a generic role (co-ordinating care, linking with families and carers, initiating the review process, monitoring progress over an extended period) with that of a specialist assessor and provider of occupational therapy.

CMHTs are typically managed by one person, to whom all staff, regardless of profession, are accountable (Ovretveit 1993). Their effectiveness as a multidisciplinary resource has been the focus of much debate (Norman & Peck 1999, Onyett & Ford 1996, Shepherd 1998). There is clearly a balance to be struck: on the one hand, ensuring the sensible co-operation of a group of professionals towards common priorities and ensuring appropriate core generic skills are available in the team as a whole, while on the other hand maintaining a healthy tension between the differing approaches and varied theoretical frameworks contributed by the professions, enabling the distinct professional skills to remain available to clients who really need them (Sainsbury Centre for Mental Health 1997). The professional isolation of occupational therapists within CMHTs makes them vulnerable to group pressure to absorb generic tasks, provide interventions for people whose occupational needs are less pressing than their broader care needs and accept the values of the dominant group; pressure from CMHT managers can direct occupational therapists towards generic working (Lankshear 2003, Peck & Norman 1999). The need to be accepted by the team and a readiness to undertake those tasks seen as valued rather than retaining professional distinctness can result in roles becoming so merged as to be indistinguishable. This may not be in the interests of clients who, consequently, have access to a reduced range of potential responses to a given problem - in this team, as in many CMHTs, reduced access to distinct occupational therapy time because of competing roles and team pressures (Cooke and Birrell 2007, Reeves and Mann 2004). In this instance, Tony clearly identifies with the benefits of being fully integrated within the team, though he often debates with his colleagues the relative merits of specialist versus generic worker.

The head occupational therapist contributes to this debate and gives guidance to his developing role, but ultimately has to defer to the CMHT manager who has the final say on Tony's day-to-day work priorities and team function. The introduction of *Recovering Ordinary Lives* (College of Occupational Therapists 2006), with its emphasis on refocusing on occupational performance and a confident articulation of occupational therapy's added value, is providing them with food for thought.

Sally: working in an acute inpatient setting

Sally is a basic-grade occupational therapist working in an acute admission unit of a psychiatric hospital with a countywide catchment area. Often the clients she sees are in hospital only for a week or two, though some stay for longer, especially those who have been formally detained. The development of increasingly robust community services has meant that some of the work she had expected to do when she took up the post is in fact now dealt with by community teams (the Crisis and Home Treatment team, for example). When patients are becoming well enough to begin home visits and activities in preparation for discharge become a possibility, staff who will be continuing community support start to undertake this work. Sally has worked with her senior therapist to develop a screening tool that highlights which patients have occupational needs that would benefit from a specialist approach and which simply need support to re-establish home routines and daily functioning. She works with her community colleagues to ensure that they are not duplicating work and that areas of particular occupational dysfunction are not being overlooked.

Making use of the unit's newly refurbished activity and group rooms, Sally's work may include creative, expressive or domestic activities. There are clients whose distress is such that Sally needs to see them for very short periods,

two or three times throughout the day. They work on small, achievable tasks that help rebuild a sense of competence during this very confusing and disempowering period. Others take part in groups targeted at shared problems and issues, or work steadily on plans connected to their goals following discharge. Sally uses the Canadian Occupational Performance Measure (Law et al 1994) to identify priorities for intervention and to monitor progress towards the goals clients set. Sometimes the goals her clients see as the most important do not coincide with what the multidisciplinary team views as priority. Sally sometimes faces pressure from her colleagues who want her to work to change a person's daily routines.

Team members recognise that, seeing clients in a different context, Sally witnesses different behaviours, emotional responses, strengths and emerging vulnerabilities. She reports how symptoms affect an individual's roles, volition, routines and skills and describes the progress she sees as people become less symptomatic or develop ways of coping with residual illness or problems.

Sally shares an office with the team of three occupational therapists and receives fortnightly formal supervision from the senior therapist, who guides her work and provides support, development and training. She supervises the work of an occupational therapy support worker.

Discussion

Sally's role is most influenced by the speed at which people move through the acute admission unit and by the degree of distress and disturbance people face during this period. She has to focus on short-term goals, yet needs to keep a view to the person's home context and the longer-term goals as prioritised by the client and identified by the wider team. Sally's role may be catalytic in that she may provoke the beginning of a change in the person's coping strategies and self-esteem and the development of more successful and satisfying roles that she herself never sees to completion but hands over as an ongoing package of care on discharge.

Sally's role is clearly differentiated as an occupational therapist, providing a range of graded, personally tailored activities and using group processes to achieve occupational goals. The environment in which she works can offer access to many different types of creative, domestic, expressive and work-based activities and her use of these activities seems to reflect practice elsewhere (Griffiths & Corr 2007). She often acts as a motivator when acute illness or distress has directly affected people's volition, habits and routines and skills. Sally believes that the distinct contribution occupational therapy provides within an acute admission setting is offering an environment in which people can achieve or retain a sense of mastery (for example, over materials, media, the purpose and scope of their occupational therapy sessions) when so much else seems out of their personal control.

Sally is perceived as having an important contribution to assessments of strengths and interests and her approach can be more oriented towards solutions than problems (Cade & O'Hanlon 1993, de Shazer 1991). The team is particularly interested to hear feedback on changes in levels of performance in the various activities and interactive settings which may be a significant indicator of the person's overall response to interventions and treatments or, alternatively, represent relapse indicators (Birchwood et al 1998a). Sally similarly needs to glean as much information as possible from her nurse colleagues, who spend a much more intense period of time with the clients, to keep abreast of significant changes, responses to treatment and safety issues.

Sally's nursing colleagues have to exercise differing roles with inpatients, particularly those who are formally detained. Sally has, like any other member of the team, to work towards agreed team objectives expressed in each individual's care plan and pay close attention to safety and risk, but does not have to cope with the complexities that nursing, medical and social work staff face when they are directly involved in detaining someone without their consent or giving treatment that is not wanted by the client. This facilitates her collaborative role in working with her clients and supports her preference for client-centred practice. Sally wonders how this might change for her should she at a later point in her career feel pressured to train for and take on the Approved Mental Health Professional, an extended role being proposed through amendments to the Mental Health Act (DoH 2004a, 2006) or, alternatively, whether this might be a role she would be happy to enact.

Having an insight into the primary motivations for individual clients and exploring their preferred roles, personal performance goals and typical daily routines, Sally sometimes acts as an advocate for clients if the team sets priorities that do not reflect the client's personal drives. This is a difficult role and she has to be ready to recognise the difference between those times when the team can and should be urged to review their plans and when issues of safety, or a client's unrealistic expectations, require her own view to be revised. As Sally does not have a long history with the team or extensive personal experience, she has to work carefully to sustain and develop their confidence in her while not unduly compromising her position or her professional viewpoint.

As Sally's clients often experience distressing symptoms (for example, hallucinatory voices or destructive and compulsive thoughts) that can be alleviated by becoming absorbed in an activity, she often finds herself being asked to 'occupy the clients with something'. At first she worried that her role could be seen as diversional and was reluctant to fulfil this element of the team's expectations of her (Simpson et al 2005). Over time, however, she has begun to identify those occasions when specific activities can be graded and applied as a powerful coping mechanism, with the potential for it to become integrated into the person's repertoire of skills for managing residual problems.

Her position as a junior member of a broader occupational therapy team helps Sally consolidate her skills and build on her knowledge. Work requiring greater expertise and development work can be taken on by the senior therapist or she works alongside her supervisor as a co-therapist. Regular supervision and the identification of an appropriate role model or mentor is key to sustaining the morale and confidence of staff at all grades (Allan & Ledwith 1998, Blair 1998) but has particular pertinence for Sally as a newly qualified occupational therapist (Rugg 1996).

Karen: working in sectorised elderly services

Karen is a head occupational therapist in a sectorised service for older people in an inner city. She has a small caseload of people with functional illnesses but specialises in working with people with dementia, particularly in its early stages.

Some of her time is spent within an assessment ward in the local hospital; her base is a shared office with her nursing and social work colleagues.

Much of her clinical work is around supporting people during the difficult time when they are first diagnosed as having dementia. Karen plans with individuals how they can maintain as much independence as possible, especially in the areas they place as highest priority, and teaches memory retraining techniques. A lot of time is spent supporting carers and providing them with information to aid their understanding of dementia, as well as working together with families and carers building up portfolios of photographs, personal stories and memories and information connected to the person's past and current interests and important life events. Karen sometimes assesses for simple adaptive equipment and advises on physical problems that are impeding the person's independence in daily living skills.

Karen leads a team of four occupational therapists and an occupational therapy technical instructor, provides supervision for two generic support staff and regularly takes students for clinical placements. She is a visiting lecturer for the local occupational therapy course. She feels passionate about the value of working with older people and wants to influence new graduates' attitudes to this area of work.

Karen is recognised as having considerable experience in her field and is a member of the trust's elderly services strategy team. She is working on a current research project with the consultant psychogeriatrician and nurse specialist, looking at practice within the inpatient assessment ward.

Discussion

Karen's complex range of roles stems from her position of seniority and the combination of managerial responsibilities with those of an expert clinician. Karen's leadership role requires her to plan, support or review the work of others, develop their skills and potential, ensure the quality of the occupational therapy she and her staff provide, lead the development of occupational therapy within elderly mental health services and champion occupational therapy's

contribution within this field among her multidisciplinary colleagues.

Karen's colleagues' expectations of the broad contributions she can offer are based on their respect for the level of experience she has gathered. As a clinician, she has reached the degree of mastery where she can tackle complex and challenging work with a minimum of support and with insightful awareness and autonomy (Stoltenberg & Delworth 1987). Her practice has matured to the level where she can focus on specialist issues for occupational therapy and is shaped by theory, for example early interventions in dementia, based on theories of well-being and the maintenance of personhood (Kitwood & Bredin 1992).

Karen's work context also permits her to develop her role as a teacher and mentor, both in the workplace and, specifically, within the local university. This satisfies her own interest in passing on knowledge and is supported as a role seen to provide a useful academic link and promote the organisation's credibility as a centre of excellence.

Karen's organisational position, her research interests and the opportunities for multiprofessional initiatives lead to her inclusion within strategic planning groups and roles that extend beyond her core team, into the organisation as a whole. Her role as an agent of change within the elderly services is heavily relied on.

COMPLEMENTARY TEAM ROLES

Having looked at the ways in which the roles of *individual* occupational therapists may develop, the following case vignette demonstrates the effective use of the *complementary* roles and skills of a multidisciplinary team:

Case study

Carl's story

Carl's first psychotic episode occurred when he was 21 and in the final year of his university mathematics degree. Although this was the first time he had been seen by a psychiatrist, his parents had been worried about him since he was in his last year at school, preparing for A-levels when his behaviour had, to them at least, appeared strange.

He had at that time become increasingly distant from his family and friends, regarded attempts to draw him into family activities with suspicion and he had started to talk about complex conspiracy theories which were starting to overwhelm him so that he became alternately agitated and ready to fight society's ills or pessimistic and despairing of the future. At that time, Carl's parents were reassured by their family doctor that he was most likely just going through the anxieties associated with growing from teens to adulthood and that this was all part of preparing to move away from the family and develop his own independence. They continued to be worried about him, however. Sometimes they felt it best to leave Carl to work out things for himself but more often got drawn into arguments with him when his ideas seemed extreme and his schoolwork got behind as he spent increasing time 'researching' evidence for his theories regarding 'next evolution' humans who were developing 'ultra-sophisticated communication systems'. Carl's father was embarrassed whenever Carl sought discussion with him on the subject and felt more than a little guilt at the relief he experienced when Carl eventually left home for university.

Carl seemed to settle into his university course fairly easily initially and enjoyed his studies. Whilst not being a great socialiser, he developed a small group of friends and the year passed without any major upset. In his second year, Carl began to get behind with assignments, miss lectures and subsequently his grades began to suffer. When pursued by his personal tutor to urge him to improve his failing work as he began his third year, Carl took this as a signal that there were 'newly evolved humans' in the campus who were transferring his own thoughts to the university lecturers. Carl was terrified that he would be 'sacrificed' and had barricaded himself into his room in the house he shared with four other students. When he hadn't been seen for 4 days, his housemates, who had already become worried about Carl's health, contacted his parents who, after discussion with them about his recent behaviour, alerted his GP. The local crisis team was called but Carl remained in his room. Finally the police attended and Carl was removed from the house in a distressed and dishevelled state. He appeared to be responding to voices and was convinced that the police were acting on behalf of the 'super-evolved'. Carl was assessed by the crisis team and formally detained in the local acute admission unit and was immediately started on the antipsychotic medication olanzapine.

The medication had a swift and encouraging effect on Carl's symptoms. The hallucinations diminished over a period of days and within a couple of weeks his bizarre responses to his voices disappeared. Carl had initially avoided talking to any of the nursing team other than to insist that they were putting him at risk by keeping him in the ward where his 'ideas could be plundered and sold on for gain' but by the end of the first week he was prepared to discuss what he had been experiencing and seemed amenable to exploring what might be behind it all. In his third week he began work with a senior nurse who had undertaken specialist cognitive therapy training, to gently challenge the strength of his delusional beliefs and to educate him regarding why he had been prescribed the olanzapine, what the medication was meant to achieve and what the consequences might be in using it. Carl discussed the potential benefits and risks and agreed on how his responses to the medication would be monitored.

The occupational therapist who worked as part of the ward team introduced himself to Carl and began to form a tentative relationship with him. At first Carl was a bit suspicious as to why someone was so curious about his interests and did not want to disclose much about himself. Carl later became intrigued when he talked to a couple of fellow inpatients who had been working with the occupational therapist on some digital photographs that had been taken in the hospital grounds and were being prepared for a display in the reception area. Carl came to understand that the occupational therapist worked with people who were trying out activities that made them feel more like themselves again and that helped them feel that they could concentrate, at least in short bursts, and feel proud of what they could achieve. Carl subsequently worked with the occupational therapist, sometimes on activities that he enjoyed and gave him some distraction from his worries about being on the ward (and noticed that afterwards he felt calmer and less troubled by voices) and then began to explore his previous interests, routines, the things he felt were stressing him and the things he felt were particular strengths. The occupational therapist began to understand the pressure Carl had felt in having to cope with studying when he was exhausted by the strain of being around people he felt were a threat, managing to contribute to the smooth running of his shared accommodation and that, prior to his illness he had lost any opportunity for activities that helped him relax and feel he could let off steam.

It was hoped that Carl's admission to hospital would be brief. Once Carl had begun to talk to the team, a member of the community-based early intervention team, an occupational therapist, came to introduce herself and start to try and engage with him, making it clear that she expected him to leave hospital without too much delay and that she and the team with whom she worked would be around to help him make sense of all he had been through and to recover the threads of his life. After 4 weeks, Carl's psychotic symptoms were now mostly under control: his thinking had become more lucid and his ability to function around other people had improved, as he no longer felt constantly under threat. He was therefore discharged to his parents' home and to the care of the early intervention team.

Carl's parents made arrangements for his belongings to be brought back from his rented room and believed that he would be fine now that he was back home and away from the pressures of university life. Though disappointed for Carl, they believed that his course had proved too stressful and that he should contact the university to give up his place there.

Although Carl appeared to be insightful into his experience, he was not entirely convinced that the voices he had heard weren't a sign that perhaps he too had some specially evolved senses and expressed some mixed feelings about them having been taken away by the medication. He wondered if he might be missing out on some opportunities to discover something important about the progression of the human race. His care co-ordinator from the early intervention team explored his beliefs about his illness with him in detail, continuing to encourage Carl to generate a number of possible explanations for his experiences before and during his time in hospital and helped him work out for himself whether or not regaining the symptoms (which was a risk of discontinuing his medication) was likely to carry more potential benefits or risks (Rollnick & Miller 1995). Carl further discussed his options with his consultant psychiatrist and explored the likely consequences of changing or discontinuing the olanzapine. Ultimately, though somewhat reluctantly, he felt he needed to continue with the olanzapine for now.

After a couple of months Carl began to appear markedly depressed, reacting to his growing sense that the life he had planned for himself, his hopes and dreams regarding his power to work, earn a good salary and settle into a successful career now seemed to have been replaced with a vision of himself as a failure, someone who messed up at university and would probably have to rely on his parents for the foreseeable future. He felt cheated and that he had missed out on friendships. He suffered huge guilt as he realised the extent to which his parents had been upset and worried by his behaviour yet found their apparent need to keep a close watch on him irritating. He found that if he started to discuss how he felt with them, it quickly turned into a row and his mother would say that he was just starting to be paranoid again. His care co-ordinator played an important role in supporting him through this period, giving him opportunities to express his sadness, confusion and anger and explore his future options. It was agreed that the occupational therapist in the team would work closely with him to help him redevelop his independence, build up some social contacts again and look at his options for further study or work. Carl's stated goal was 'to feel more like a capable adult and prove I'm not useless'.

It became quickly apparent that Carl still felt committed to completing his degree and that while it was not realistic to return to university just now, it seemed reasonable to presume that he might after some time to recover. Together the occupational therapist and Carl approached the university and negotiated an agreement to defer his third year and some examination retakes, at least till the following academic year. It then became important to help Carl regain confidence in his abilities and gradually return to some daytime routines. The illness and the impact of his medication left him feeling tired and he had developed a pattern of rising around noon each day. With little to get up for and having low energy, this was difficult to address. Carl and his occupational therapist developed a range of activity commitments that first needed him to be up and ready to go out by noon and gradually introduced activities where Carl had to arrive by 10am (for example, volunteering at a local conservation project). A further consequence of Carl's medication was a tendency to overeat and to put on weight. The activities were therefore also targeted at countering this, namely using sports facilities, starting to cycle (a previous interest) and, later on, the conservation work which was physically demanding.

He worked also on negotiating with his family a range of domestic activities for which he gradually took on responsibility. Over time Carl started to feel he could see a future again that was something approaching what he had hoped for himself, though he had to make some adjustments to his projected narrative. All of this took some intensive work, support from a STaR worker (activities agreed with the occupational therapist and his care co-ordinator) and careful grading so that Carl could feel gradually more competent without being overstressed.

His care co-ordinator met over several weeks with Carl and his family to work through issues arising from his illness, educating them about what some of Carl's difficulties might be, as well as challenging their assumptions that a serious diagnosis meant a poor future with drastically lowered expectations. They were introduced to the notion that interactions between life stresses and inherent personal vulnerabilities had a role in triggering illness and looked at how best to provide support without undermining Carl's adult role and need to retain personal independence.

Both Carl's care co-ordinator and the occupational therapist reinforced some of the cognitive techniques he had learned to cope with stress and with invasive thoughts. They all worked together on identifying which activities were stress provoking and which were restorative and absorbing. The occupational therapist looked particularly for opportunities to combine those that helped block symptoms with demanding tasks or to sandwich helpful activities around those he found more anxiety provoking. Carl created his own menu of effective additional coping techniques, for example studying favourite magazines, listening to the local pop radio station, cycling, taking digital photographs while out walking and later working on the computer with them. His sense that he was exerting control over his situation gave him enormous satisfaction and hope.

Carl has decided that he would be best supported at his parents' home for 6 months or so, but hopes to move back to his university town after that, resume an independent lifestyle there and rebuild his contacts in anticipation of resuming his studies. Work is ongoing with his team to help Carl and his family understand the various stressors he faced previously that did, and could again, compromise his health. Plans are in place to identify and act on any warning signs that might indicate relapse.

Discussion

The roles of the different members of the team can be clearly seen to work together to contribute to Carl's progress. There are *shared* team goals, for example, management of acute illness and ensuring his personal safety, relief from symptoms, increased level of function and independence, improved quality of life, challenging negative and limiting expectations regarding his potential for recovery, resolution of family conflicts and family education about psychosis and development of satisfying relationships within and external to his family. There are also shared treatment approaches/models, for example, psychosocial interventions and use of the Stress/Vulnerability model (Birchwood & Tarrier 1992, Fowler et al 1995) and organisation of care in line with the CPA. The team operates collectively within what has been defined as good practice in early intervention in psychosis, where engagement is paramount, the period (or duration) of untreated psychosis (DUP) is minimised and symptoms are quickly identified and relapse prevented or limited. The DUP is evidenced as influencing longer-term outcomes where the shorter the period, the better the recovery (Birchwood et al 1998b, 2000, Spencer et al 2001). They therefore also shared a collective responsibility to help Carl plan ahead and move to a point where he could identify his stressors and any signs of relapse, taking appropriate steps to manage this.

There are also clear areas where *individual* contributions are specifically targeted, sometimes specific to professional roles, for example:

- **the crisis team psychiatrist's** decision to admit Carl to hospital, establish an appropriate medical management plan and later review of the medication regime, prescribing medication as recommended within agreed treatment guidelines (National Institute for Clinical Excellence 2002a, b)
- **the senior ward nurse's** collaborative work to ensure that Carl understood the rationale behind prescribing the particular medication, ensuring any unwanted side-effects of the medication would be minimised; using cognitive approaches to question his delusional ideas and generate explanations for his experiences and to ensure that he felt listened to and active in decision making over his continued treatment using motivational interviewing techniques and psychosocial interventions (Birchwood & Tarrier 1992, Birchwood et al 1998a, Fowler et al 1995)
- **the ward-based occupational therapist** using his early sessions to simply introduce himself, observing Carl interacting (or not) with fellow patients, assessing the extent to which Carl's skills were impaired/intact and introducing the notion that Carl's lifestyle and how he organised, performed and balanced his range of occupations could impact on and reflect his health. Carl began to consider that he could have some influence over his health, in part through his experience and reflection on some of the activities he became involved in and their short-term impact, but also through discussion with the occupational therapist about his previous lifestyle and resultant stresses. When the early intervention team began to get involved, the occupational therapist was able to share his knowledge of Carl's strengths and limitations and the activities that Carl had already discovered were of particular value, as well as some of his aspirations related to returning home
- **the care co-ordinator's** responsibility to maintain an ongoing generic assessment of Carl's needs and co-ordinate plans for his care, liaising with the various personnel involved in his treatment, support and recovery. In this instance the care co-ordinator was a nurse and as such was able to continue some of the cognitive work initiated while Carl was in the hospital and because of the specialist training in psychosocial interventions undertaken by all members of the early intervention team, was able to use skills to engage with him, work with him and his family so they had a better understanding of psychosis and what might help/hinder recovery, reinforce and develop Carl's skills in stress management and identifying relapse signs and planning coping strategies. Issues connected with his compliance with continuing with medication were addressed and Carl was helped to feel that he was increasingly in control of managing his illness
- **the occupational therapist's** assessment of Carl's occupational performance, goals and personal priorities. By understanding the disruption to Carl's life-narrative trajectory and the consequent grief at his lost vision of himself, she was able instil some hope for recovery and help Carl reconstruct a changed but ultimately acceptable anticipated future (Gould et al 2005). The analysis of activities in terms of their stress/therapeutic effects, the regaining confidence in daily living skills through graded application of domestic and self-care activities and negotiating an adult role within the family home were important parts of Carl's recovery. The attention to developing routines, positive use of time and exploring healthy lifestyles were also key occupational therapy roles
- **the STaR workers** having excellent interpersonal skills to engage with Carl and a non-stigmatising bridge-building approach to helping him build up a range of mainstream activities using their extensive community knowledge and commitment to activity. They were able to support the plans developed by the occupational therapist by allotting sufficient time to help Carl participate in activities he had prioritised as important and introducing him to new resources.

The other key individuals who were involved in developing the care plan for Carl were of course Carl's parents and Carl himself. They were central to the process at all points and contributed their expert knowledge of Carl's particular situation, his goals, dreams and fears. They monitored what seemed helpful and reported when things did not seem to be working so well. Carl was happy to have his parents consulted throughout the process, although when it came to Carl's longer-term future – leaving home again and returning to university – they had differing views. While taking Carl's parents' concerns seriously, the team worked towards them carrying greater optimism and supported Carl in negotiating sufficient independence even whilst living in the family home to help him achieve an image as a competent adult in his parents' eyes as well as his own.

Individual team roles sometimes evolve due to personal interest and development.

- The nurse specialist in cognitive therapy had pursued particular training to be able to offer this approach to people with psychosis.
- The care co-ordinator in the early intervention team had particular interest and training in the provision of family-based psychosocial interventions and had an accepted role within the team as co-worker and supervisor for this style of work.
- The occupational therapist had elected to work in the team because of the young age group and their interest in what happens when people have to adapt their self-developed narrative regarding their projected future (Finlay 2004).

In this team, there is also evidence of co-working between the professions and others to maximise the chances of success; for example, the joint family work initiated by the nurse and supplemented by the occupational therapist, both team members working closely to ensure they were consistent in their approach and that family sessions related to issues identified by both of them. Further examples include the reinforcement of cognitive strategies taught by the nurse during occupational therapy sessions, the careful management of the medication's positive and negative effects by the medical and nursing team and the future planning for Carl's hoped-for return to university between the occupational therapist, the student welfare department and a personal tutor. The ward team had first to liaise with the crisis team who were first to respond and assess Carl's situation and the early intervention team became part of Carl's treatment team long before he was discharged. All the team members across the services worked closely together, in collaboration with Carl, in exploring future options and planning to meet his needs in order that he might be able to move on from the hospital as quickly as possible. In this instance the seamless service aspired to in the guidance documents was evident and Carl's experience followed an optimal pathway (Birchwood et al 2001).

The effectiveness of this team required them to have a degree of consensus over what generic roles were required of them and how to make best use of profession/person-specific roles. Evidence shows that this balance of comfort between generic and specialist function, together with role clarity, is best for service users in terms of effectiveness and best for staff in relation to morale and maintenance of lower levels of work stress (Hughes 2001, Onyett et al 1995, 1997, Peck & Norman 1999).

Carl's case demonstrates the results of effective team working but it might not always work like that. It is worth thinking about what the result might have been if:

- the occupational therapist did not know what cognitive therapy coping strategies had been successful with Carl and believed that cognitive therapy was only appropriate for people with neuroses?
- the nurse had used a collaborative approach and taken Carl's reporting of medication side-effects seriously, but the psychiatrist felt the side-effects were minor and it was not worth the risk of altering medication and ignored the request for review and failed to involve Carl fully in the decision making regarding his ongoing treatment?
- Carl's weight gain had gone unchecked and the team had not ensured he was aware of this as a possible outcome of using olanzapine?
- there was competition over who should design Carl's care plan and who was best placed to deliver family interventions?

- members of the team did not share a hopeful, non-stigmatising view of recovery from psychosis and failed to recognise Carl's potential as an able student and motivated individual?
- any part of the biopsychosocial approach to Carl's complex needs was neglected?

ROLE BALANCE AND ROLE CONFLICT

Much has been written regarding the balance of necessary roles required from mental health professions, noting both the great value in diversity (the need to match the broad spread of clients' needs with the diversity of professional backgrounds and skills) and the need to develop consistent core competencies and generic abilities and aptitudes. The Sainsbury Centre for Mental Health proposes core competencies for all staff working with people with severe mental illness spanning the areas of administration, assessment, treatment and care management and collaborative working, while also describing profession-specific issues connected with the changing roles of mental health staff groups (Sainsbury Centre for Mental Health 1997).

The role balance health professionals are expected to achieve is highly complex. It is possible to see how the network of roles surrounding the individual, described by Merton (1957) as role sets, can explode into an elaborate mosaic. For example, *occupational therapist* can be exploded into:

- **manager**: leader, monitor, developer, motivator
- **researcher:** developer, communicator, champion, advocate, educator
- **clinician:** therapist, researcher, advocate, advisor, administrator
- **colleague**: supporter, challenger, negotiator
- **generic mental health worker**: counsellor, care co-ordinator, carer, supporter/educator.

In turn each of these can be further exploded. Each of the other members of the multidisciplinary team carries a similarly wide range of roles. As modern mental health care becomes increasingly complex and all the professions across the health and social services are forced to adapt their roles to embrace new structures and practice developments, the opportunities for role rivalries increase. Indeed, the more roles one holds, the greater is the possibility for role conflict, overload or ambiguity. The loss of familiar roles brings its own stresses, requiring adaptive responses (Blair 1998, Hughes 2001) and supportive management.

SUMMARY

Occupational therapists are operating in a complex system of mental health provision that relies on collaboration between service users, health and social care staff and non-statutory agencies and charities. They have to be flexible in their responses to differing client groups, service settings, team skill mixes and management styles and lines of accountability. They must respond to priorities as they emerge from central and local health and social care policy, but can celebrate the fact that policy documents are full of references to meeting service users' occupational, social and leisure needs. They attend to issues of independence in daily living skills, achieving full and equitable participation in the range of social domains and communicate optimism regarding people's opportunities to return to employment, social inclusion and living ordinary but satisfying lives.

The actual roles occupational therapists perform depend on the interaction of external demands and intrinsic values, skills, experience, interest and training. Despite potential role strain, ambiguity and competing priorities arising from the wide variety of roles assumed by occupational therapists, the place of occupational therapy within the multidisciplinary team is well established and evolving. Occupational therapists are well placed to undertake the generic work necessary for a team to be effective, yet are urged not to do so at the cost of their specialist value: using occupation at the centre of their practice to enhance people's functioning and quality of life, facilitate their development of satisfying relationships and promote resilience to the effects of mental illness.

References

Agenda for Change Project Team, Department of Health 2004 The NHS Knowledge and Skills Framework (NHS KSF) and the Development Review Process. Stationery Office, London. Available online at: www.doh.gov.uk/thenhsksf/knowledgeandskills.pdf

Allan F, Ledwith F 1998 Levels of stress and perceived need for supervision in senior occupational therapy staff. British Journal of Occupational Therapy 61(8):346-350

Ball R, Moore E, Kuipers E 1992 Expressed emotion in community care staff. Social Psychiatry and Psychiatric Epidemiology 27:35-39

Belbin RM 1981 Management teams: why they succeed or fail. Butterworth Heinemann, Oxford

Birchwood M, Tarrier N (eds) 1992 Innovations in the psychological management of schizophrenia. Wiley, Chichester

Birchwood M, Smith J, Macmillan F, et al 1998a Early intervention in psychotic relapse. In: Brooker C, Repper J (eds) Serious mental health problems in the community: policy, practice and research. Baillière Tindall, London. Ch 10

Birchwood M, Todd P, Jackson C 1998b Early intervention in psychosis: the critical period hypothesis. British Journal of Psychiatry 172(suppl):53-59

Birchwood M, Fowler D, Jackson C 2000 Early intervention in psychosis: a guide to concepts, evidence and interventions. Wiley, Chichester

Blair S Role. In: Jones D, Blair S, Hartery T et al (eds) Sociology and occupational therapy: an integrated approach. Churchill Livingstone, Edinburgh Ch 5.,

Bradshaw T, Lovell K, Harris L 2005 Healthy living interventions and schizophrenia: a systematic review. Journal of Advanced Nursing 49(6):634-654

Cade B, O'Hanlon W 1993 A brief guide to brief therapy. Norton, New York

College of Occupational Therapists 2006 Recovering ordinary lives - the strategy for occupational therapy in mental health services 2007-2017. College of Occupational Therapists, London. Available online at: www.cot.org.uk/publications

Cooke S, Birrell M 2007 Defining an occupational therapy intervention for people with psychosis. British Journal of Occupational Therapy 70(3):96-106

Craik C, Austin C, Chacksfield JD et al 1998 College of Occupational Therapists: position paper on the way ahead for research, education and practice in mental health. British Journal of Occupational Therapy 61:390-392

Creek J 2003 Occupational therapy defined as a complex intervention. College of Occupational Therapists, London. Available online at: www.cot.org.uk publications

Department of Health 1990 National Health Service and Community Care Act 1991. HMSO, London

Department of Health 1995 Mental health in England: statistical bulletin. HMSO, London

Department of Health 1998 Modernising mental health services. HMSO, London

Department of Health 1999 National service framework for mental health. HMSO, London

Department of Health 2000 Effective care co-ordination in mental health services: modernising the Care Programme Approach: a policy booklet. HMSO, London

Department of Health 2001 The mental health policy implementation guide. Available online at: www.dh.gov.uk/en/Publicationsandstatistics/Publications/PublicationsPolicyAndGuidance/DH_4009350

Department of Health 2002a Mental health policy implementation guide: adult acute inpatient care provision. Available online at: www.dh.gov.uk/en/Publicationsandstatistics/Publications/PublicationsPolicyAndGuidance/DH_4009156

Department of Health 2002b Community mental health teams - mental health policy implementation guide. Available online at: www.dh.gov.uk/en/Publicationsandstatistics/Publications/PublicationsPolicyAndGuidance/DH_4085759

Department of Health 2003 Mental health policy implementation guide: support, time and recovery (STR) workers. DH Publications, London

Department of Health 2004a Draft Mental Health Bill and Draft Mental Health Bill explanatory notes. DH Publications, London

Department of Health 2004b Fast-forwarding primary care mental health: graduate primary care mental health workers - best practice guidance. DH Publications, London

Department of Health 2006 Next steps for the Mental Health Bill (press notice). Department of Health, London

de Shazer S 1991 Putting difference to work. Norton, New York

Dratcu L 2006 Acute in-patient psychiatry: the right time for a new speciality? Psychiatric Bulletin 30:401-402

Finlay L 2004 From 'gibbering idiot' to 'iceman', Kenny's story: a critical analysis of an occupational narrative. British Journal of Occupational Therapy 67(11):474-480

Fortune T 2000 Occupational therapists: is our therapy truly occupational or are we merely filling gaps? British Journal of Occupational Therapy 63:5

Fowler D, Garety P, Kuipers E 1995 Cognitive behaviour therapy of psychosis: theory and practice. Wiley, London

Gamble J, Chan P, Davey H 2001 Reflection as a tool for developing professional practice, knowledge and expertise. In: Higgs J, Titchen A 2001 Practice knowledge and expertise in the health professions. Butterworth Heinemann, Oxford

Gould A, DeSouza S, Rebeiro-Gruhl KL 2005 And then I lost that life: a shared narrative of four young men with schizophrenia. British Journal of Occupational Therapy 68(10):467-473

Griffiths S, Corr S 2007 The use of creative activities with people with mental health problems: a survey of occupational therapists. British Journal of Occupational Therapy 70(3):107-114

Hagedorn R 1995 Occupational therapy: perspectives and processes. Churchill Livingstone, Edinburgh, pp160-161

Harries P 1998 Community mental health teams: occupational therapists' changing role. British Journal of Occupational Therapy 61(5):219-220

Harries PA, Gilhooley K 2003 Generic and specialist occupational therapy casework in community mental health teams. British Journal of Occupational Therapy 66(3):101-109

Hope R for NIMHE 2004 The Ten Essential Shared Capabilities - a framework for the whole of the mental health workforce. Department of Health, London. Available online at: www.dh.gov.uk/publications

Hughes J 2001 Occupational therapy in community mental health teams: a continuing dilemma? Role theory offers an explanation. British Journal of Occupational Therapy 64(1):34-40

Huxley P, Evans S, Webber M et al 2005 Staff shortages in the mental health workforce: the case of the disappearing approved social worker. Health and Social Care in the Community 13(6):504-513

Jones S, Williams B, Bayliss M 2006 Whose job is it anyway? Mental Health Nursing 26(4):10-12

Kitwood T, Bredin K 1992 Towards a theory of dementia care: personhood and well-being. Ageing and Society 12:269-287

Kuipers E, Moore E 1995 Expressed emotion and staff-client relationships: implications for community care of the severely mentally ill. International Journal of Mental Health 24(3):3-26

Lankshear AJ 2003 Coping with conflict and confusing agendas in multidisciplinary community mental health teams. Journal of Psychiatric and Mental Health Nursing 10:457-464

Law M, Baptiste S, Carswell A et al 1994 Canadian Occupational Performance Measure, 2nd edn. CAOT Publications A E, Toronto

Layard R 2006 (chair) Centre for Economic Performance's Mental Health Policy Group. The depression report: a new deal for depression and anxiety disorders. London School of Economics and Political Science. Available online at: http://cep.lse.ac.uk/research/mentalhealth/

Lehman AF, Dixon LB, Kernan E et al 1997 A randomised trial of assertive community treatment for homeless persons with severe mental illness. Archives of General Psychiatry 54:1038-1043

Lloyd C 2004 Actual and preferred work activities of mental health occupational therapists: congruence or discrepancy? British Journal of Occupational Therapy 67:167-175

Marshall M, Lockwood A 1998 Assertive community treatment for people with severe mental disorders. Cochrane Library. Update Software, Oxford

Meeson B 1998 Occupational therapy in community mental health, part 2. Factors influencing intervention choice. British Journal of Occupational Therapy 61(2):57-62

Merton RK 1957 The role set: problems in sociological theory. British Journal of Sociology 8:106-120

National Institute for Health and Clinical Excellence 2002a Schizophrenia: core interventions in the treatment and management of schizophrenia in primary and secondary care. Available online at: www.nice.org.uk/42424

National Institute for Clinical Excellence 2002b Guidance on the use of newer (atypical) antipsychotics for the treatment of schizophrenia. Health Technology Appraisal No. 43. National Institute for Clinical Excellence, London

National Institute for Health and Clinical Excellence 2004 Depression: management of depression in primary and secondary care. Available online at: www.nice.org.uk/CG023NICEguideline

National Institute for Mental Health in England 2004 National Mental Health Workforce Strategy. Department of Health, London. Available online at: www.dh.gov.uk/publications

National Social Inclusion Programme 2006 Second annual report. Available online at: www.socialinclusion.org.uk

National Social Inclusion Programme 2007 The capabilities for socially inclusive practice. Available online at: www.socialinclusion.org.uk

Norman I, Peck E 1999 Working together in community mental health services: an inter-professional dialogue. Journal of Mental Health 8(3):217-230

Office of the Deputy Prime Minister 2004a Mental health and social exclusion: Social Exclusion Unit Report. Office of the Deputy Prime Minister, Wetherby

Office of the Deputy Prime Minister 2004b Action on mental health: a guide to promoting social inclusion. Office of the Deputy Prime Minister, Wetherby

Onyett S, Ford R 1996 Multidisciplinary community teams: where is the wreckage? Journal of Mental Health 5:47-55

Onyett S, Pillinger T, Muijen M 1995 Making community mental health teams work: CMHTs and the people who work in them. Sainsbury Centre for Mental Health, London

Onyett S, Pillinger T, Muijen M 1997 Job satisfaction and burnout among members of community mental health teams. Journal of Mental Health 6(1):55-66

Ovretveit J 1993 Co-ordinating community care: multi-disciplinary teams and care-management. Open University Press, Buckingham

Peck E, Norman IJ 1999 Working together in adult community mental health services: exploring inter-professional role relations. Journal of Mental Health 8(3):231-242

Perkins R, Rinaldi M A whole system approach. In: Grove B, Secker J, Seebohm P (eds) New thinking about mental health and employment. Radcliffe Publishing, Abingdon, pp85-86

Reeves S, Mann LS 2004 Overcoming problems with generic working for occupational therapists based in community mental health settings. British Journal of Occupational Therapy 67(6):265-268

Rollnick S, Miller WR 1995 What is motivational interviewing? Behavioural and Cognitive Psychotherapy 23:325-334

Romme M, Escher A 1996 Empowering people who hear voices. In: Haddock G, Slade PD (eds) Cognitive behavioural interventions with psychotic disorders. Routledge, London, pp137-150

Roth A, Fonagy P 1996 What works for whom? Guilford Press, New York

Royal College of Psychiatrists 2005 New ways of working for psychiatrists: enhancing effective, person-centred services through new ways of working in multidisciplinary and multi-agency contexts. Final report 'but not the end of the story'. Department of Health, London

Rugg S 1996 The transition of junior occupational therapists to clinical practice: report of a preliminary study. British Journal of Occupational Therapy 59(4):165-168

Sainsbury Centre for Mental Health 1997 Pulling together: the future roles and training of mental health staff. Sainsbury Centre for Mental Health, London

Sainsbury Centre for Mental Health 1998 Keys to engagement. Sainsbury Centre for Mental Health, London

Sainsbury Centre for Mental Health 1999 Acute problems: a survey of the quality of care in acute psychiatric wards. Sainsbury Centre for Mental Health, London

Sainsbury Centre for Mental Health 2001 The capable practitioner framework. Sainsbury Centre for Mental Health, London. Available online at: www.scmh.org.uk

Schön DA 1991 The reflective practitioner: how professionals think in action. Arena, England Ch 2, p. 60

Secker J, Grove B, Seebohm P 2006 What have we learnt about mental health and employment? Mental Health Review 11:8

Shepherd G 1998 Models of community care. Journal of Mental Health 7(2):165-177

Simpson A, Bowers L, Alexander J et al 2005 Occupational therapy and multidisciplinary working on acute psychiatric wards: the Tompkins acute ward study. British Journal of Occupational Therapy 68(12):545-552

Spencer E, Birchwood M, McGovern D 2001 Management of first episode psychosis. Advances in Psychiatric Treatment 7:133-142

Stein I, Test MA 1980 Alternative to mental hospital treatment: 1. A conceptual model, treatment program and clinical evaluation. Archives of General Psychiatry 37:392-397

Stoltenberg CD, Delworth U 1987 Supervising counsellors and therapists. Jossey-Bass, San Francisco

Townsend E, Whiteford G 2005 A participatory occupational justice framework: population-based processes of practice. In: Kronenberg F, Algado SS, Pollard N (eds) Occupational therapy without borders: learning from the spirit of survivors. Elsevier, London, pp110-126

White E, Creek J 2007 College of Occupational Therapists' research and development strategic vision and action plan: 5-year review. British Journal of Occupational Therapy 70(3):122-128

Chapter 13

The developing student practitioner

Marion Martin, Sue Wheatley

INTRODUCTION

Students approach their placements with a mixture of excitement and apprehension. Whereas this is probably going to be the most enjoyable part of the course, there are also many aspects of this type of learning experience which are unknown or uncertain. It is human nature that when faced with any new situation, especially one where our performance is going to be assessed, we will understandably experience some level of anxiety. In particular, placements in mental health may cause extra concern and every occupational therapy student will have to complete at least one mental health placement during their education (Hocking & Ness 2002). In preparation for writing this chapter, the authors met with a group of first-year occupational therapy students to ask them about their feelings both before and after their first mental health placements. This chapter addresses their most important concerns.

Mental health placements are often very different from those in other settings. If a student has only had previous experience of working with people with physical disabilities, she will find many differences in the pace of work, in the models and approaches being used for treatment, the terminology employed by staff, the roles of the different professionals and in the levels of motivation of service users. All these aspects of mental health services will be examined more carefully later in the chapter.

Students may be apprehensive about working with people who have a mental illness. Myths and stereotypes about such people abound and students will have been affected by views expressed in the media and elsewhere. These will be examined in this chapter and challenged, demonstrating that many assumptions about people with mental illness are unfounded. Indeed, working with those who have emotional problems can be an extremely positive and rewarding experience.

Perhaps one of the student's greatest concerns is about professional boundaries. In any setting there is always an issue of how much to reveal about oneself to clients. On the one hand, self-disclosure can be a way of developing rapport with another person, but students are unsure of how far they can go and when professional boundaries have been breached. Individual professionals' views on this subject may vary enormously. This part of the chapter will examine in some depth the topic of disclosure in mental health and issues around the formation of relationships with people who use mental health services. The therapeutic relationship requires some degree of self knowledge, enabling the mental health practitioner to work in an empathic, client-centred way.

Finally, this chapter will look at ways of addressing some of the student's concerns. This will involve the importance of using reflection and supervision to both develop understanding and gain support from the educator. However, the purpose of this chapter is not to cover topics such as student learning styles, learning contracts and assessment. These are important aspects of all placements and have been very well addressed elsewhere (Alsop & Ryan 1996, Cross et al 2006, Lorenzo et al 2006, Rose & Best 2005). The authors of this chapter are addressing occupational therapy students, but they also hope that educators will read it to gain more insight into the student perspective.

STUDENTS' PRIOR EXPERIENCE AND ASSUMPTIONS

The College of Occupational Therapists' *Standards for Pre-registration Education* specifies that students should gain experience working with a range of people of all ages, from different backgrounds, with both long-term and short-term needs and with health conditions that affect different aspects of function (Hocking & Ness 2002). This means that they will have to undertake at least one placement in a mental health setting.

When students embark on such a placement they are likely to have formed some expectations based on their previous contact with this client group. Some may be quite familiar with the mental health services, as they may have worked in this setting before starting the course. They may have friends or relatives who have had experiences of mental health services or they may even have used these services themselves. For those who have had little or no prior contact with mental health services, however, or for those who may have had some negative experiences, the prospect of spending several weeks on such a placement may appear to be extremely daunting. There are, however, many strategies which students can employ to decrease their anxiety, one of which is to read this chapter!

THE VALUE OF MENTAL HEALTH PLACEMENTS

In spite of some initial reservations that students might have about this type of placement, mental health settings can offer students many opportunities which would not be available elsewhere. Often students return to university saying that they gained more satisfaction from their mental health placements than other areas of practice. Amongst the reasons they give is the opportunity to spend more extended periods of time with the service users and get to know them more as individuals. This is often not possible in services where the occupational therapist is only referred clients with a view to rapid discharge. Students also report that they are able to observe and take part in occupational therapy interventions which usually do not exist in short-term services, such as using creative activities as therapy and therapeutic groupwork. With the current emphasis in the curriculum of occupational science, this can be very rewarding. Finally, on such placements, students have more of an opportunity to challenge their own assumptions about mental illness, confront their insecurities and, in so doing, develop as individuals.

It is essential that all occupational therapists have some understanding of mental health. Some students may believe that they will never want to work in this field of practice, but they will be required to recognise signs of mental illness wherever they are employed. Many people with physical dysfunction may have emotional issues raised by their disability. For instance, in Parkinson's disease depression may be a feature due to physiological changes. Unfortunately, physical dysfunction does not protect an individual from also experiencing an enduring mental health need and this will need to be taken into account by an occupational therapist working in any type of practice setting. Whenever a job requires interaction with other people, it is important to feel able to cope with challenging interpersonal situations. Mental health placements provide students with an opportunity to find out more about themselves and others.

ATTITUDES ABOUT MENTAL ILLNESS

Many students who have never worked in mental health fear their first placement in this type of setting (Granskar et al 2001, Lieberman 1998). This is especially so if the unit is a locked one, for example in the forensic services. These students will have been exposed to the media's portrayal of mental illness, which tends to focus on high-profile cases of murder, where 'a schizophrenic' has randomly attacked a member of the public. There is a lot of ignorance in the general population about mental illness; for example, in a recent survey of young people, a quarter thought that it was caused by a brain abnormality. This is not helped by misuse of words in the media. An extremely angry person might be described as 'psychotic', 'mental', 'bonkers' or simply 'mad' (Mind Information Unit 2006). All these images of mental illness build up a picture of a service where the clients are always unpredictable and aggressive, so the expectation is that working with them will be extremely dangerous. It is quite common for students to request self-defence classes in order to prepare them for their first mental health placement.

In fact, statistics show that people with mental illness are far more likely to take their own lives than someone else's, as suicide and self-harm are extremely common in this population. In 2004 more than 5500 people in the UK died by suicide (Mental Health Foundation 2006) and one study has shown that up to 90% of people who kill themselves have at least one mental illness when they die. Between 20–40% of people with a diagnosis of schizophrenia have a history of attempted suicide (Hatloy 2005).

Occupational therapy students could also reflect on the way they see themselves in relation to mental health service users. One in four people in the UK will experience some kind of mental health problem in the course of a year (Mental Health Foundation 2006), so it is very likely that students may have had direct experience of mental illness themselves, either personally or through close friends or family. In the present climate of social inclusion, this could be seen as an advantage, since a student with personal experience of mental illness will possibly be better able to help others with similar problems.

One way of preparing for placements in mental health or for developing an understanding of people with mental illness and finding out about how best to help them is to read personal accounts of their experiences. Examples of such literature are Suzy Johnston's (2004) experience of depression and Ruth Deane's (2005) account of acquiring and overcoming obsessive-compulsive disorder.

RISK MANAGEMENT AND SUPPORT

As in most areas of practice, therapists now have to carry out risk assessments, as they have a duty of care towards the people they are employed to help (College of Occupational Therapists 2005). In the mental health services, however, clients may not only be a danger to themselves, either through neglect or self-harm, but they might also pose a risk to others (Neeson & Kelly 2003). As has been mentioned earlier, they are more likely to harm themselves than be a threat to others (Royal College of Psychiatrists 1996) and the vast majority of people who use mental health services are not violent (Audit Commission 1994).

After a mental health placement on a secure unit, students will often say that they felt safer than they did in other settings, as there are so many mechanisms such as alarm bells and high levels of staffing to protect them (Neeson & Kelly 2003). However, there are occasionally incidents of aggression towards staff and even verbal abuse can be hurtful. Students may also find that they become extremely distressed by some of the self-abusive behaviour of service users, such as suicide and self-harm. The need for posttraumatic counselling and support for mental health staff is now acknowledged by management. Students can benefit from this too and should find practice educators to be sympathetic to their needs for debriefing and reassurance. It has also been found that students on 2:1 models of placement, where two students are on placement with a single educator, can benefit from the mutual support of their peers, especially in mental health settings (Martin & Edwards 1998, Martin et al 2004).

STUDENTS' IMPRESSIONS OF OCCUPATIONAL THERAPY IN MENTAL HEALTH

Students usually remark on the unexpected differences between placements in physical and mental health settings. One of these is the faster pace in the physical practice setting where patients can be assessed, treated and discharged within a week. Mental health placements seem much slower, with many long periods of time to prepare for and reflect on the clients' progress, especially when they do not attend planned sessions. Some students find this extra time for reflection frustrating and prefer the more structured experience of the physical approach. Other students, however, may appreciate having longer to reflect on practice and to discuss concepts with their supervisor and others.

Students may be surprised at the lack of clarity of many of the concepts used in mental health. Most occupational therapists avoid using the medical model but even if they do, psychiatric diagnosis is a relatively unscientific process and can be very controversial. Many of the disorders share the same symptoms and respond to the same medication. Sometimes the diagnosis can change during

the course of treatment, or patients will be given a dual diagnosis or a borderline diagnosis. Some diagnoses are very controversial, such as personality disorder, which many people would argue is not a mental illness, and until 1980 even homosexuality was considered to be a mental disorder.

Another difference that students may find surprising at first in different types of placement is the terminology which is used. Even within mental health they may notice that some staff use words found in psychiatric textbooks, usually associated with the more medical model of practice, whereas professionals who identify themselves with a social model of disability may be using everyday language. Students can learn a great deal from observing the ways in which different professions communicate with one another and the terminology they use to do so.

MODELS OF PRACTICE AND APPROACHES

Occupational therapists prefer to use the functional model of disability, in which the emphasis is on what the client can and cannot do, rather than any illness they may have (World Federation of Occupational Therapists 2006). The World Health Organization has now adopted the *International Classification of Function* (2006), in which it is the environment that is seen as disabling rather than the individual. In mental health settings this approach emphasises that participation is the marker of a healthy society, so barriers to work and involvement in social activity should be removed for all, including those with a mental illness. The aim of occupational therapists has always been to make the environment accessible to service users, so that they can participate as much as possible in the community.

Humanistic approach

Possibly the most common approach used by mental health occupational therapists is the humanistic, phenomenological one (Rogers 1961), which involves the therapist attempting to understand how clients feel and viewing their problems and the intervention used from their perspectives. Almost all the occupational therapy models of practice are based on this approach – for example, the Model of Human Occupation (Kielhofner 2002) and the Canadian Occupational Performance Model (Canadian Association of Occupational Therapists 2002).

Humanistic models of disability and client-centred approaches to intervention are seen as being preferable to the medical model by the majority of occupational therapists, as they are judged to be more empowering for the client and therefore more ethical to use. Such an approach might, however, have the disadvantage for the novice practitioner of lacking a prescription for intervention (Toal-Sullivan 2006). As it is the service user who has to be consulted at all stages of practice, there is inevitably an element of uncertainty about what the therapist does in each situation. The more medical approach can seem more straightforward, with its impressive use of signs, symptoms, diagnoses, prescriptions and prognoses.

Client–centred approach

The client-centred approach embraces the possibility that the client may have different beliefs and attitudes from the therapist. He may want to live alone where this is viewed as dangerous by the staff team; he may not want to take his medication or comply with treatment and may not believe that he is ill in the first place. The humanistic approach to intervention has the advantage, however, of being much more likely to engage clients in the whole process of change by allowing them to take more control of their lives. It can also allow the therapist–client partnership to be extremely creative in finding solutions to the most difficult problems.

ENGAGEMENT WITH SERVICE USERS

Students who undertake their first placement in mental health with trepidation are often surprised that, in fact, these service users do not appear to be at all threatening. Indeed, the clients may be feeling frightened themselves and consequently be rather withdrawn and difficult to engage in conversation. If it is a community setting where the clients have less obvious problems, students often feel confused about why these people need

help, as they do not seem remarkably different from everyone else.

Levels of motivation

In a more secure, inpatient setting where service users display more florid symptoms, the main difficulty that students often find with clients is what is perceived to be a lack of motivation to engage in therapy. This apparent indifference can be an outcome of many different causes. It could be due to a feeling of hopelessness and futility on the part of the service user or it may be a result of the medication they are taking. The origin of the problem could also lie in the relationship between client and therapist, or in the structure of the whole service.

Challenges to engagement in therapy

Engagement in therapy is one of the challenges of working in mental health to which the occupational therapist needs to find creative solutions. One of the most obvious differences that students will notice between physical and mental health services is that whereas people with physical disabilities have obvious symptoms such as paralysis or pain, are motivated to engage in therapy and (usually) show appreciation for all the help they are given, very often people who are offered assistance for mental illness may deny that they have a problem at all and when asked to engage in therapeutic occupation, they may not co-operate. In an outpatient setting clients may be very aware of their difficulties and want help, but for various reasons often related to their illness may not be able to attend the appointments they have made with their occupational therapist. This can be very frustrating both for therapists and for students who feel that they have missed a learning opportunity.

In such circumstances there is a dilemma for the occupational therapist. On the one hand she believes in client-centred practice (Sumsion 1999). It is the role of the therapist to listen to her clients and allow them to formulate their own goals and direct their own intervention. On the other hand, she has a duty of care towards her clients (College of Occupational Therapists 2005) and feels that she would be neglecting her duties as a professional if she did not use all her skills to engage them in the treatment process. There is a danger, however, that in trying to persuade clients to attend therapy sessions, the therapist can be abusing her powers over another person who is in a weaker position.

There may be many reasons for the apparent lack of motivation demonstrated by mental health service users. This is one of the biggest challenges of working in this area of practice, but it can also lead to some of the greatest rewards when a previously unresponsive person engages with a process of recovery. The relationship between therapist and client can be very productive, but it can also block the client's progress if it is not functioning well. In mental health practice, this aspect of intervention is very often the subject of discussion amongst staff, as it is seen as being of critical importance. Students are advised to examine their relationships with service users through personal reflection and may want to share their thoughts with placement educators during supervision (Fish & Twinn 1997, Johns 2002). The therapeutic relationship is examined further in the following section.

THE THERAPEUTIC RELATIONSHIP

During the initial stages of a placement the student may have some of her previous thoughts and beliefs about the nature of the client group, the service and the occupational therapy role challenged. For others there may be a sense of confirmation and familiarity with this environment.

Students on mental health placements report back to the college that it is often not the pathology or medical aspects of a person's diagnosis and treatment that they find challenging, but the more subtle aspects of the placement setting. It is often in the day-to-day social interaction with clients that students find a complex arena in which to operate. Terms such as role modelling, boundaries, therapeutic use of self and self-disclosure enter into the routine discussions and conversations that the student will be having or observing amongst the multidisciplinary team. The student may have some theoretical understanding of these terms but may find areas such as professional boundaries confusing in an environment where the staff wear no uniforms and these boundaries are less apparent than in a general medical setting.

Students are usually required to engage in different types of social interaction with the client group. This can range from sitting in a coffee shop to participating in a more structured group activity. Student occupational therapists are often anxious about saying the wrong thing. They are concerned that if they do so, it could have a negative effect on the service user's mental health even to the extent that they might self-harm or possibly commit suicide. Students frequently have an overdeveloped sense of responsibility for the service user and their mental health. They may need to develop an appreciation that there are many other aspects of a person's life which affect their well-being.

THERAPEUTIC USE OF SELF

The therapeutic use of self broadly refers to the process of the therapist evaluating the effect of her characteristics, values and practice in interactions with others and the extent to which this brings development and insight for the client (Freshwater 2002). Alternatively this could be termed conscious use of self, or the ability of the occupational therapist to deliberately react to and respond to the client and his environment in a way that is designed to elicit a positive therapeutic outcome. This does not mean that the therapist should appear unnatural or lack spontaneity in her reactions. Rather, the therapist recognises her professional responsibility towards the client and that her presentation of herself can impact on the therapeutic benefits of that relationship. Just as occupational therapists extensively analyse the benefits of engagement in different types of activity, it is also possible for the therapist to analyse the impact that her interactions have with clients (see also Chapter 4).

Self-awareness

Each student, and indeed each occupational therapist, will view service users according to her own underlying assumptions and attitudes. In order for students to progress from this subjective viewpoint, it becomes essential that they develop sufficient self-awareness to allow them to be conscious of their personal values as well as those of both the context in which treatment is offered and of our wider society.

When working with clients, an occupational therapy student will find it useful to consider the following.

- Who is this person and how must he or she be feeling?
- What event brings this person here and how has this affected his or her normal life?
- How does this person make me feel?
- How can I help this person and what support does he or she have and need?
- What is important to this person?
- How does this person view his or her future? (Kwaitek et al 2005, pp29-30)

There are different approaches which an educator may adopt when introducing the student to her clients. Sometimes the placement educator will deliberately ask a student to meet the service user before reading any of their background history. This will allow them to develop a posture of 'unknowing' close to that described by Munhall (1993, p125), which paradoxically can allow us to know both ourselves and the client better. This is because we are open and can 'unearth the other's world' by admitting: 'I don't know you. I do not know your subjective world' (Munhall, 1993 p125). Taking an 'unknowing' approach will reduce the opportunity for students to develop assumptions and expectations about the service user. Munhall (1993, p125) described that 'knowing' a client 'has inherent in it a state of closure', that further exploration becomes limited, thus reducing the potential to examine the subjective world of the client, believing something to be fact when it is not and closing off opportunities to test alternative beliefs and perceptions. To develop a stance of 'unknowing' we have to hold our own beliefs in abeyance and put our assumptions to one side. Instead, Munhall (1993) suggests that we should enable clients to tell their own stories and construct their own realities. One way for therapists to achieve this is to develop a skilful and empathic relationship with their clients.

Student and educator may find it an insightful exercise to experiment and adopt both approaches of 'knowing' and 'unknowing' when the student has initial contact with different service users. Students are encouraged to write reflective diaries during their placement education. What were thoughts before, during and after their contact with the service user? The same exercise could be performed with any of our social contacts. Student occupational therapists need to develop self-awareness and have the ability to recognise their own values, prejudices and assumptions if they are to develop their skills as a practitioner and therapeutic use of self.

The role of supervision on placement is vital in supporting the student through the complex process of developing not only as an occupational therapist but also as a mental health professional and adopting the therapeutic use of self in the therapy process

SELF-DISCLOSURE

Self-disclosure forms the basis of many of our everyday relationships and will inevitably become part of the relationship that develops between an occupational therapist and service users within the context of a mental health setting. Derlega et al (1993, pp1–2) observed that 'it is hard to imagine how a relationship might get started without such self-disclosure'. Sidney Jourard (1971) believed that disclosure from the therapist facilitated disclosure on the part of the service user. Rogers (1961) identified that disclosure could promote trust and genuineness which are considered essential in the formation of a therapeutic relationship. Self-disclosure by the mental health professional needs to be considered in the context of the client and should have the potential to offer the client insight and understanding to their own experiences. The student will find it beneficial to reflect on her types and frequency of self-disclosure during formal supervision time with their practice educator.

One of the dilemmas for occupational therapy students on placement is how to develop their therapeutic relationship with the service user through self-disclosure, yet at the same time maintain their professional status. Egan (1990) distinguished between over-, under- and appropriate disclosure.

Overdisclosers are people who ... 'talk too much about themselves (the quantity is too much) or they talk too personally about themselves in social situations that do not call for such personal talk (the quality is too much)'.

Underdisclosers are individuals who .... 'don't want others to know them deeply and say little about themselves ... even when the situation calls for it'.

Appropriate disclosure avoids the two extremes and means that it is fitting, suitable, the right amount at the right time. (Egan 1990, pp44–45)

The type of self-disclosure by both service user and therapist will be partially influenced by the stage of the developing therapeutic relationship and also the environmental context. Self-disclosure by an occupational therapist may take place in informal situations, individual treatment sessions, activity-based groups or within talking therapy groups such as assertiveness training. In the latter type of group a student will be required to make self-disclosures as part of her contribution. In this situation the student needs to consider the therapeutic value of her contribution. For experienced practitioners, this is a regular part of their work and so they may have prepared disclosures. It might be helpful for students to discuss with their educator some of the contributions that they could make to the group, both in terms of leading activities and the therapeutic value of their disclosures.

Williams (2001) found that patients were more likely to like and trust nurses when they self-disclosed, as it made them feel more at ease and accepted as a person. Ashmore & Banks (2002, p176) identified that there was a real possibility that 'the health professional who discloses few or no items to patients may find it difficult to engage them in therapeutic activities'. Occupational therapists will find that they need to constantly adopt a therapeutic or conscious use of self to engage their clients in therapeutic activities. This is particularly relevant when working with a client group who feel socially excluded and may have poor motivation and self-esteem.

Self-disclosure questionnaire

To appreciate the value and opportunities of self-disclosure as well as the importance of professional boundaries, student and educator may find it helpful to consider Jourard's (1961, 1971) Self-disclosure Questionnaire. This ranked questionnaire (Box 13.1) can assist the educator and student to begin to discuss and understand the value of disclosure. Reflection on the types of self-disclosures which can appropriately be used within the therapeutic relationship will assist the student to develop their professional skills and their 'therapeutic use of self'.

Usually the nature and amount of self-disclosure will be determined by the placement setting and client group. For example, it may be beneficial for students or therapists to self-disclose that if they become anxious about something, they might choose to talk to a friend or go for a walk. What can be more complex is to identify what types of things lead a student to feel anxious and which are appropriate to disclose within the context of a therapeutic relationship.

Self-disclosure progresses from superficial to intimate subjects, with individuals' deepening familiarity (Altman & Taylor 1973, Jourard 1971). This highlights the need for trust and familiarity as prerequisites to disclosure and has implications for time and resources. Placement education by its nature is a time-limited structure and students may find it challenging to develop a therapeutic relationship with clients within the constraints of the length of placement. However, on occasion the converse of this can happen. Clients may find a fresh face quite motivating or that the student is an easier person to confide in than other members of the multidisciplinary team. This may be because they are perceived as more genuine since they are less attached to the hospital or health-care setting.

BOUNDARIES

Self-disclosure enables trust and a deepening of the therapeutic relationship. The formation of boundaries enables that to happen in a mutually safe manner. The occupational therapist is responsible for maintaining boundaries within

Box 13.1 Self–disclosure questionnaire (Jourard 1961, 1971)

Indicate if you would disclose the following.

1. Whether or not you have any favourite spectator sports. If so, what these are, e.g. football, tennis.
2. The kind of music that you enjoy listening to most, e.g. popular, classical, folk music, opera, etc.
3. The places that you have travelled to or lived in during your life – other countries, towns, etc.
4. What you like to do most in your spare time at home, e.g. read, sport, go out, etc.
5. Whether or not you drink alcoholic beverages; if so, your favourite drinks – beer, wine, etc.
6. The sports you engage in most, if any, e.g. swimming, tennis, etc.
7. The food you like best and the ways you like your food prepared, e.g. rare steak.
8. Any skills that you have mastered, e.g. arts and crafts, painting, sculpture, etc.
9. Your usual and favourite reading material, e.g. novels, non-fiction, science fiction, poetry, etc.
10. Whether or not you know or play any card games, e.g. poker, bridge, etc.
11. The kind of party or social gathering that you enjoy most.
12. The kind of future you are aiming towards, working for, planning for – both personally and vocationally, e.g. marriage, family, professional status, etc.
13. Whether or not you belong to any church; if so, which one and the usual frequency of attending.
14. Whether or not you belong to any clubs; if so, the names of the clubs.
15. What your political sentiments are at present – your views on political parties and policies.
16. Your chief complaints about your work or course of studies, e.g. the things that bore you or annoy you and upset you, such as assignments, people, etc.
17. How you feel about the appearance of your body, your looks, figure, weight, what you dislike and what you accept in your appearance and how you wish you might change your looks to improve them.
18. The personal deficiencies that you would most like to improve or that you are struggling to do something about at present, e.g. appearance, lack of knowledge, loneliness, temper, etc.
19. An exact idea of your regular income (if a student, of your allowance and earnings if any).
20. Whether or not you have been seriously in love during your life before this year, with whom, what the details were and the outcome.
21. Your problems and worries about your personality; that is, what you dislike most about yourself, any guilt, inferiority feelings, etc.
22. The characteristics of the people that you dislike, that you wish people would change and improve.
23. Whether or not you presently owe any money; if so, how much and to whom.
24. The details of your sex life up to the present time, including whether or not you have had or are now having sexual relations

British version adapted by Burnard & Morrison (1992) ranked by Ashmore & Banks (2001)

---

this relationship to ensure that the focus of the relationship is to meet the client's needs rather than those of the therapist. Therapeutic boundaries are crossed if there is a personal, financial or social gain for the therapist (Stuart & Laraia 2001). Often if a therapist feels that she has a 'special' type of relationship with a client or that she is thinking about a client more frequently than usual, then she should consider whether therapeutic boundaries are being violated. For both qualified and student occupational therapists, this can be a challenging aspect of therapeutic practice which can be considered within supervision.

Self–expression

We all reveal aspects of our self through our appearance. However, this opportunity for self-expression may come into conflict with the professional self that the student is developing. Davys et al (2006) debate presentation of self in both learning disabilities and mental health settings. A student's appearance may have a profound impact on the service user and on the benefits of the therapeutic relationship. For example, when working with clients in the community the therapist's appearance may enable the client to integrate within the setting or conversely may further alienate or even increase the client's anxieties about being in different environments (Davys et al 2006). The student's appearance needs to take into consideration the cultural norms of both the client and the society in which the therapist is working. Although a therapist may choose to challenge those norms or have subjective views about her appearance, there is also a responsibility for her to maintain her professionalism and consider her duty to the client and her adherence to the *Code of Ethics and Professional Conduct* (College of Occupational Therapists 2005).

STRATEGIES FOR MENTAL HEALTH PLACEMENTS

There are many strategies that students can employ to make sure that they feel supported during all placements. These include keeping in touch with tutors at the university and fellow students who will be out on placement at the same time. However, perhaps the greatest source of support will be from the practice educator. In all settings it is this person whose role is to make sure that students are feeling secure in the learning environment (Alsop & Ryan 1996, Cross et al 2006, Rose & Best 2005). All students should have the opportunity for regular supervision scheduled into their weekly timetable, as well as more informal supervision which takes place as required throughout the placement (College of Occupational Therapists 2004).

SUPERVISION

Practice supervision has many purposes, including an opportunity for management of the learning programme, education, instruction, feedback on performance and support (Alsop & Ryan 1996, Cross et al 2006, Rose & Best 2005). However, on mental health placements there is, perhaps, a greater need for students to receive help and guidance with emotional issues. Therapists and students can sometimes suffer from hurtful comments by clients due to their disturbed behaviour associated with their illness or students may simply be affected by the troubled lives which such people have experienced (Hawkins & Shohet 2000). Supervision

in this environment can therefore be a source of reassurance, as it allows emotions to be expressed in a safe relationship. In this way, negative experiences can be survived, reflected upon and learnt from. During supervision the student, supervisor and client are in a therapeutic triad, where the student's relationship with the client can be explored in the student–therapist relationship (Hawkins & Shohet 2000). This process presents the student with a wonderful opportunity for self-knowledge and personal development.

Supervision usually takes place between a student and a practice educator but it can happen in many other ways. On some placements students may be supervised in pairs or in groups by an educator. This can have the added benefit of enhanced learning as ideas and understanding can be further developed through peer learning (Martin et al 2004). In some services group supervision is arranged and a group of professionals or students may share reflective practice with their peers, possibly within a particular profession or, alternatively, in a multiprofessional group. One member with particular expertise, such as a psychotherapist, may act as a facilitator or the group may facilitate itself.

REFLECTIVE PRACTICE

Supervision allows time for both student and therapist to reflect on their practice and share their mutual learning. This is an important reason why the most enthusiastic practitioners enjoy supervising students on placement. The reflective professional's view is that practice is a complex, dynamic social activity and that every situation is unique, determined by values, traditions and theoretical perspectives (Schön 1987). Reflective supervision requires both student and supervisor to have open minds, exploring beliefs and attitudes which are responsible for determining their responses to practice situations. Alternative responses can be considered and sometimes adopted and in this way professional practice is developed. Fish & Twinn (1997) remind us that continuing professional development (CPD) is now a requirement for registration to practise and an important component of this is reflective practice.

Box 13.2 Model of Structured Reflection (13th edition, adapted from Johns 2000)

- Bring the mind home.
- Write a description of an experience that seems significant in some way.
- What issues seem significant to pay attention to?
- How was I feeling and what made me feel that way?
- What was I trying to achieve?
- Did I respond effectively and in tune with my values?
- What were the consequences of my actions on the patient, others and myself?
- How were others feeling?
- What made them feel that way?
- What factors influenced the way I was feeling, thinking or responding?
- What knowledge did or might have informed me?
- To what extent did I act for the best?
- How does this experience connect with previous experiences?
- How might I respond more effectively given the situation again?
- What would be the consequences of alternative actions for the patient, others and myself?
- How do I *now* feel about this experience?
- Am I now more able to support myself and others better as a consequence?
- Am I more available to work with patients/families and staff to help them meet their needs?

Christopher Johns is from a nursing background and his model of guided reflection is popular with students and practitioners from many clinical professions. His assumption is that the practitioner is ultimately self-determining and seeks to facilitate growth, both for herself and for the clients she works with (Johns 2000). Guided reflection involves being and becoming. The practitioner reflects on her practice as it is now and where she wants it to be. Box 13.2 contains Johns' suggested Model of Structured Reflection (Johns 2002) which is based on Gibbs' (1988) Reflective Cycle.

SUMMARY

This chapter has highlighted some of the unique challenges as well as professional and personal opportunities that are offered to student occupational therapists when undertaking a placement in a mental health setting. Although many students look forward to such placements, some may feel apprehensive, perhaps due to the portrayal of mental illness in the media. Popular myths and assumptions about mental illness have been challenged and a balanced viewpoint provided. Mental health placements can provide students with many opportunities, such as working in a truly collaborative way to provide a holistic service and the implementation of creative activities. These placements are valuable in many ways, enabling students to develop insight and understanding of social interactions, abilities which are necessary in all settings.

Once students have started their mental health placements they may be surprised at some differences between these and other types of placement. These include having longer periods of unstructured time, which can be unsettling but can be used as an opportunity for reflection on practice. Students may also be somewhat confused about the lack of clarity in diagnosis and the different approaches used by members of the multidisciplinary team. Occupational therapists tend to use social models of disability and humanistic approaches.

Involvement with service users may be very different to students' expectations. Students may be surprised at how ordinary the clients seem, yet due to the nature of their illness could find them difficult to engage in therapeutic occupation. Whereas this is often interpreted as lack of motivation, students are encouraged to consider the possible reasons for this and seek creative solutions.

During a mental health placement a student practitioner will develop her skills in terms of her 'therapeutic self' and will begin to realise the complex nature of areas such as boundaries, modelling and self-disclosure. How therapists consciously present themselves to their client group can have a significant impact on the therapeutic relationship and the clients' motivation to engage in activities. Strategies for maximising the learning potential of a mental health placement include gaining support from the practice educator in supervision. Supervision is an ideal opportunity for reflection and learning.

The authors' intention was not to present the reader with a list of instructions for a mental health placement. Instead, some of the issues and dilemmas which occupational therapists face when working in this area have been presented. There are no correct answers to the questions raised in this chapter. It is hoped that the reader will be encouraged to engage in a process of discovery, working out their own solutions as they progress through the placement. Having been practitioners in mental health services themselves for many years, the authors wanted to share with you some of their enthusiasm for the privilege of working with other people's emotional lives and the rewards that this type of practice can bring.

References

Alsop A, Ryan S 1996 Making the most of fieldwork education. A practical approach. Chapman and Hall, London

Altman I, Taylor DA 1973 Social penetration: the development of interpersonal relationships. Holt, Rinehart and Winston, New York

Ashmore R, Banks D 2001 Patterns of self-disclosure among mental health nursing students. Nurse Education Today 21: 47-48

Ashmore R, Banks D 2002 Self-disclosure in adult and mental health nursing students. British Journal of Nursing 11(3): 172-177

Audit Commission 1994 Finding a place: a review of mental health services for adults. HMSO, London

Burnard P, Morrison P 1992 Self-disclosure: a contemporary analysis. Avebury, Aldershot

Canadian Association of Occupational Therapists 2002 Enabling occupation: an occupational therapy perspective. CAOT Publications ACE, Ottawa

College of Occupational Therapists 2004 Standards for pre-registration education. College of Occupational Therapists, London

College of Occupational Therapists 2005 Code of ethics and professional conduct. College of Occupational Therapists, London

Cross V, Moore A, Morris J et al 2006 The practice-based educator. A reflective tool for CPD and accreditation. John Wiley, Chichester

Davys D, Pope K, Taylor J 2006 Professionalism, prejudice and personal taste: does it matter what we wear? British Journal of Occupational Therapy 69(7): 339-341

Deane R 2005 Washing my life away. Surviving obsessive-compulsive disorder. Jessica Kingsley, London

Derlega VJ, Metts S, Pertonio S, Margulis ST 1993 Self-disclosure. Sage, Newbury Park

Egan G 1990 You and me: the skills of communicating and relating to others. Brooks/Cole, Menlo Park

Fish D, Twinn S 1997 Quality clinical supervision in the health care professions. Butterworth-Heinemann, Oxford

Freshwater D 2002 The therapeutic use of the nursing self. In: Freshwater D (ed) Therapeutic nursing. Sage, London

Gibbs G 1988 Learning by doing: a guide to teaching and learning methods. Further Education Unit, Oxford Polytechnic (now Oxford Brookes University)

Granskar M, Edberg AK, Fridlund B 2001 Nursing students' experience of their first professional encounter with people having mental disorders. Journal of Psychiatric and Mental Health Nursing 8: 249-256

Hatloy I 2005 Available online at: www.mind.org.uk/Mind/Templates/Content%20(RelatedTopics). aspx?NRMOD

Hawkins P, Shohet R 2000 Supervision in the helping professions, 2nd edn. Open University Press, Milton Keynes

Hocking C, Ness NE 2002 Revised minimum standards for the education of occupational therapists. WFOT, Perth

International Classification of Function. Available online at: www3.who.int/icf/onlinebrowser/icf.cf

Johns C 2000 Becoming a reflective practitioner. A reflective and holistic approach to clinical nursing, practice development and clinical supervision. Blackwell Science, Oxford

Johns C 2002 Guided reflection. Advancing practice. Blackwell Science, Oxford

Johnston S 2004 The naked bird watcher. The Cairn, London

Jourard S 1961 Self-disclosure patterns in British and American college females. Journal of Social Psychology 54: 315-320

Jourard S 1971 Self-disclosure and experimental analysis of the transparent self. Wiley, New York

Kielhofner G 2002 Model of human occupation, 3rd edn. Lippincott, Williams and Wilkins, Philadelphia

Kwaitek E, Mckenzie K, Loads D 2005 Self-awareness and reflection: exploring the 'therapeutic use of self': a pilot partnership course was set up to help social care staff to explore new therapeutic ways of working. Learning Disability Practice 8(3): 27-32

Lieberman SS 1998 Inspirational beginnings in an occupational therapy mental health setting. Occupational Therapy in Mental Health 14(1/2): 143-154

Lorenzo T, Duncan M, Buchanan H et al 2006 Practice and service learning in occupational therapy. Enhancing potential in context. John Wiley, Chichester

Martin M, Edwards L 1998 Peer learning on fieldwork placements. British Journal of Occupational Therapy 61(6): 249-252

Martin M, Morris J, Moore A et al 2004 Evaluating practice education models in occupational therapy: comparing 1:1, 2:1 and 3:1 placements. British Journal of Occupational Therapy 67(5): 192-200

Mental Health Foundation 2006 Available online at: www.mentalhealth.org.uk/information/mental-health-overview/statistics/

Mind Information Unit 2006 Available online at: www.mind.org.uk/Information/Factsheets/Public+attitudes/

Munhall PL 1993 'Unknowing'. Toward a pattern of knowing in nursing. Nursing Outlook 41(3): 125-128

Neeson A, Kelly R 2003 Security issues for occupational therapists working in a medium secure setting. In: Couldrick L, Alred D (eds) Forensic occupational therapy. Whurr, London

Rogers CR 1961 On becoming a person. Houghton Mifflin, Boston

Rose M, Best D 2005 Transforming practice through clinical education, professional supervision and mentoring. Elsevier Churchill Livingstone, Edinburgh

Royal College of Psychiatrists 1996 Report of the Confidential Enquiry into Homicides and Suicides by Mentally Ill People. Royal College of Psychiatrists, London

Schön D 1987 Educating the reflective practitioner. Jossey Bass, San Francisco

Stuart G, Laraia M 2001 The principles and practice of psychiatric nursing. Mosby, St Louis

Sumsion T 1999 Client-centred practice in occupational therapy: a guide to implementation. Churchill Livingstone, Edinburgh

Toal-Sullivan D 2006 New graduates' experiences of learning to practise occupational therapy. British Journal of Occupational Therapy 69(11): 513-524

Williams A 2001 A study of practicing nurses' perceptions and experiences of intimacy within the nurse–patient relationship. Journal of Advanced Nursing 35(2): 188-196

World Federation of Occupational Therapists 2006 Available online at: www.wfot.org.au/office_files/ABOUT%20OCCUPATIONAL%20THERAPY

Chapter **14**

Working in a transcultural context

Kee Hean Lim

INTRODUCTION

Increased globalisation has fostered the freedom for individuals to travel, work and live abroad and has promoted the consequential cross-cultural exchange of narratives, ideas, knowledge, perspectives and experiences. In the United Kingdom, this increase in population diversity, enhanced by the free movement of individuals across boundaries, has similarly contributed to the rich diversity and vibrancy of the multicultural society in which we live. This greater diversity has meant that, as occupational therapists, we are increasingly likely to encounter individuals from cultures and ethnic groups that are different from our own. How we interact with and respond to each individual becomes even more essential as we strive to be more culturally aware and sensitive to the needs of those we encounter within our own practice.

The College of Occupational Therapists sets out the duty of occupational therapists to take into account the diversity of needs and perspectives of their clients, patients or service users. Standard 3.2.1 of the *Code of Ethics and Professional Conduct* (College of Occupational Therapists 2000, p9) states that 'Occupational therapy personnel shall be aware of and sensitive to cultural and lifestyle diversity. They shall provide services that reflect and value these societal characteristics. Occupational therapy personnel shall not discriminate unlawfully and unjustifiably against clients or colleagues'.

It is crucial that, as occupational therapists working within a transcultural context, we recognise the individual's cultural and ethnic needs. This requires a commitment to ensuring that we assess, treat and provide services that are culturally sensitive and inclusive, and that address the specific needs and values of our clients, patients and service users.

This chapter explores conceptual and contextual factors that dictate the need for a more culturally sensitive and inclusive approach to health and social care provision within a transcultural context. It is divided into three sections.

- Section 1: The transcultural context. Definitions of key terms, UK demographics, statistics in mental health; national policies that support the cultural sensitivity agenda; issues of institutional racism and discrimination; myths about refugees and immigrants; cross-cultural psychiatry.
- Section 2: Promoting cultural awareness and competency. A selection of exercises is introduced to encourage awareness and examination of personal attitudes, preconceived ideas, assumptions and prejudices.
- Section 3: Culturally sensitive occupational therapy. This section examines transcultural approaches and models of practice, including the Kawa Model. Two tools for exploring or measuring transcultural issues are introduced and applied to a case study, in order to demonstrate how culturally sensitive and appropriate care can be effectively provided. A series of case examples and a comprehensive case study are also used to clarify the issues highlighted within the chapter.

Although the chapter focuses on the UK, the issues raised and strategies suggested to tackle issues of cultural sensitivity and competency are relevant beyond the UK context.

The terms *client* and *service user* are used interchangeably within the text.

THE TRANSCULTURAL CONTEXT

It is important to understand the terms used here and to have an awareness of the statistical data, so that informed debate leads to an examination of practice. This section also discusses discrimination and racism and how mental illness is a social construct.

DEFINITIONS OF KEY TERMS

It is beneficial to define some key terms that will be mentioned within this chapter in order to minimise the confusion, apprehension and anxiety associated with discussions around issues of culture, ethnicity and minority ethnic groups. One of the main difficulties in understanding such terms is the variety of ways in which culture, ethnicity, minority ethnic groups and cultural competency are defined (Awaad 2003, Dillard et al 1992, Fitzgerald et al 1997, MacDonald 1998). This lack of agreement contributes to confusion and creates inconsistencies when exploring and researching cultural and ethnic concepts in relation to cultural awareness and sensitivity.

For clarity within this chapter, the following definitions have been adopted.

Culture

'Culture refers to a set of values, beliefs, traditions, norms, artefacts and customs that is shared by a group or society' (Wells & Black 2000, p279). An occupational therapist, Hasselkus (2002, p42), defined *culture* as 'the patterns of values, beliefs, symbols, perceptions and learnt behaviours shared by members of a group and passed on from one generation to another'. Both these definitions highlight a common set of values, beliefs, views, perceptions and patterns of behaviour that members of a cultural group subscribe to and uphold as important, meaningful and of value.

What is seen as significant is specific to a particular cultural group and may not be shared by the majority population or the wider society in which they live. However, culture is not static but is evolving and dynamic, so that assumptions made about any cultural group, and about their responses and reactions to any given situation or set of circumstances, may change and alter with time (Awaad 2003, Chaing & Carlson 2003). Lim & Iwama (2006) further challenge us to look beyond the narrow definition of culture along lines of ethnicity and race, to consider that ethnically diverse individuals socialised within a common community or society may subscribe to an agreed set of values and principles despite racial differences. They warn us of the dangers of racial assumptions and stereotypes that arise as a consequence of viewing culture within narrow limits.

This fluidity of culture may reduce the accuracy of information we gather in preparation for meeting the client we are about to interview or assess. The initial information gathering, although valuable, must be verified and supplemented by information gained from the client, as he will provide the best reference point in terms of his cultural and ethnic beliefs, needs and preferences. The process of culturally sensitive care depends on an appreciation of the richness that defines each culture and contributes to each individual's identity; therefore, the ability to acknowledge and affirm the values and experiences of our clients is crucially important (Hocking & Whiteford 1995, Howarth & Jones 1999, Lim 2001).

Ethnicity

The term *ethnicity*, as adopted by the Commission for Race Equality and detailed within the Office for National Statistics census categories (Office for National Statistics 2001), views ethnicity as a cultural concept that is shared by a group which has a common religious belief, genealogy, language, culture or shared traditions. This term is used to refer to a group of individuals who have shared racial origins, cultural norms and language that are ethnically rooted but not governed by nationality.

The term *minority ethnic group* is defined by Wells & Black (2000, p282) as 'a group of persons who, because of their physical or cultural characteristics, are singled out from others in the society in which they live, for differential and unequal treatment and who regard themselves as objects of collective discrimination'. These minority individuals are distinct from the majority population due to their racial origin, cultural background and shared beliefs and, as such, are treated differently and with less regard.

Bhugra & Bahl (1999), in their examination of ethnicity, make the point of excluding national minorities such as the Scottish, Northern Irish and

Welsh who, despite their equal rights, have distinct cultural traditions and values. They argued that current provision of services in respect of these national minorities does take into account their specific needs and requirements. However, this view may not be universally shared by the respective Irish, Welsh and Scottish communities, who may feel that their cultural traditions and values are not catered for sufficiently (Leavey 1999).

A study of undergraduate occupational therapy students at Brunel University explored issues of ethnicity, race, culture, health and well-being. The majority of white English students mentioned that they felt uncomfortable with the concepts and struggled to identify their own ethnicity. In contrast, students belonging to minority ethnic groups (Asian, black Caribbean, African) did not experience the same difficulties. They mentioned that issues relating to their ethnicity, race and difference were frequently reinforced within their daily lives, through experiences of discrimination and prejudice.

The white English students, interestingly, mentioned that they had never thought about themselves in terms of their ethnicity and roots, and therefore found the task of identifying their ethnicity 'difficult' (Lim 2004). In fact, one of the key questions that arises from this exercise is whether experiencing racial discrimination and being a member of a minority ethnic group both reinforces and raises your consciousness of who you are, where you have come from and where you belong.

Cultural competence

Cultural competence involves 'an awareness of, sensitivity to, and knowledge of the meaning of culture, including a willingness to learn about cultural issues, including one's own bias' (Dillard et al 1992, p722). This definition highlights that there must be a willingness to undertake personal reflection of our own attitudes, biases and presumptions, as well as a desire to acquire knowledge and skills, if we are to be more culturally aware and sensitive. Cultural competence cannot be achieved by undertaking a course of study or an examination and then ticking a box that says we are now culturally competent. It requires a continuous and ongoing process that includes:

- developing self-awareness
- amassing a cultural knowledge base
- knowing how to access relevant information
- learning the skills to interact with others with sensitivity and respect
- actively developing appropriate practice
- incorporating sensitive strategies and negotiation skills to accommodate the needs of the individual
- evaluating performance and outcomes appropriately. (Lim 2001, Wells & Black 2000)

UK DEMOGRAPHICS

The UK is increasingly becoming more multicultural and diverse. The Office for National Statistics (Office for National Statistics 2001) indicates that 8%, or 4.7 million, of the population belongs to minority ethnic groups and predicts that this figure will continue to grow over the next decade. These statistics might not initially appear to be significant. However, over the whole of London, 29%, or over one in four, of the population are from minority ethnic groups. In some boroughs, such as Brent, Newham and Tower Hamlets, minority ethnic groups make up more than 50% of the population (King's Fund 2003). The trend towards increased diversity is not limited to London but is reflected in other regions around the country, such as Leicester, Manchester and Bradford where minority ethnic groups make up a significant proportion of the local population (Office for National Statistics 2001).

A common misconception amongst the general public is that recent immigrants are still arriving primarily from the Caribbean or from the Indian subcontinent. This perception is inaccurate, as the majority of immigrants over the last 10 years have come from areas of recent conflict or disaster. These include Eastern European countries such as Bosnia, Croatia and Albania, as well as Iraq, Sri Lanka, Afghanistan and Somalia (Office for National Statistics 2001). Indeed, the expansion of the European Union, to include an additional 10 member states from May 2004, has resulted in an increase of Polish, Lithuanian, Latvian, Czech and Slovak nationals working and residing in the UK (Office for National Statistics 2005).

A view of the UK as a country already overpopulated and now overwhelmed by immigrants from former colonies is perpetuated by provocative and sensational headlines in the media and the popular press (Trivedi 2002). These perspectives contribute further to the prejudice and discrimination that exist within UK society and result in increased friction and racial tension. Such myths are, however, challenged when we examine the available statistics from the Office for National Statistics (2005). These statistics indicate that approximately a thousand British citizens are migrating from the UK everyday (Office for National Statistics 2005), therefore discrediting the view that immigration is leading to overpopulation within the UK.

There is further evidence that the majority of people from minority ethnic groups, especially recent immigrants or refugees, have significant health and social care needs. They also experience difficulties in accessing all public services, including health, social care, housing and employment (Smith 2005). The situation can be further compounded by failure to understand the complexity of public services and by limited English language skills, which contribute to even greater isolation, exclusion and marginalisation (Mind 2002, Office for National Statistics 2001).

The challenge for occupational therapists working within a transcultural context is to make steps in crossing the cultural divide and to establish relationships and partnerships with all communities, especially those that are marginalised, socially excluded or occupationally deprived. Whiteford (2000) proposed that occupational therapists should become agents of change through adopting an occupational perspective that considers the occupational needs of individuals within society. We should be prepared to invest time and energy in influencing social and institutional structures and policies (Townsend 1999, Wilcock 2006). This process begins with a vision for radical change and an active commitment to making a difference for all groups within society, irrespective of their age, colour, gender or creed.

REFUGEES AND ASYLUM SEEKERS

The prejudicial and negative press around refugees and asylum seekers has the potential to colour our views and perceptions of both these groups. It is easy with such biased reporting to fall into the trap of assuming that those individuals who seek refuge in the UK are economic migrants, rather than genuine refugees with real concerns for their personal safety and welfare. Some of the key barriers identified that limit their ability to settle and integrate into society are the prejudice, discrimination and intolerance they have to face, as described in case examples 1 and 2.

Case example 1

A Bosnian man said: 'My neighbours question why I am here in the UK, they are angry that I am receiving benefits and a house to live in. What they don't realise is that I was brought to the UK for medical treatment. I have no family left, they were all murdered in the conflict, when our family home was burned down.'

Case example 2

An Iraqi woman lamented: 'Because my family in Iraq paid money so that I could escape with my children to the UK, people think that we must be rich and just here for a better life. I have to live daily with the memory that Saddam killed my husband and all his family. I chose the UK because everyone believes the British are tolerant, fair and kind but, now I am here, I am not so sure.'

Assimilation and integration into mainstream society are ways for migrants and refugees to become more involved with their local communities. This is made easier if and when the host country is willing to accept the immigrant as part of the wider community. To assimilate and feel fully included goes beyond merely existing within a community; it includes being able to live, work and contribute (Smith 2005). It implies having the freedom to be and to belong. This is impossible when migrants and asylum seekers are segregated from the rest of society, in deprived areas with other, similarly socially excluded groups.

Conflict arises when the majority population feel that their already limited resources are being siphoned away by immigrant groups. Issues of social and occupational injustice arise as economic deprivation, lack of opportunities, prejudice, intolerance and discrimination prevail, leading to further exclusion from the mainstream of society (Whiteford 2000, Wilcock 2006).

In the face of prejudice and injustice, it is unlikely that any form of social inclusion or integration can take place. This situation is made worse when an individual experiences a mental illness. She will now be excluded on account of being an immigrant and of the stigma and discrimination that come with having a mental illness. The Social Exclusion Unit Report (Office of the Deputy Prime Minister 2004) indicated that refugees and individuals with mental illness are the two most excluded of all groups within UK society. In these circumstances, it is easy to see how social inclusion, allowing all individuals to participate fully in society, enjoy the same opportunities and engage in daily activities of their choice, remains an impossible dream.

Irrespective of whether we consider that the people we are working with are genuine refugees in need of security, protection, support and refuge, as occupational therapists we must maintain a level of professionalism in upholding the principles of promoting equality, justice and respecting diversity (College of Occupational Therapists 2006).

MENTAL HEALTH STATISTICS AND ETHNICITY

The available statistics highlight serious causes for concern about admission rates to mental health services. Both governmental and non-statutory organisations, such as the Sainsbury Centre for Mental Health and Diverse Minds, have noted significant overrepresentation of certain minority ethnic groups within mental health services (Mind 2002, Sainsbury Centre for Mental Health 2000). Wilson & Francis (1997) noted that African, African Caribbean and Irish people were overrepresented in psychiatric hospitals, and there is an overrepresentation of Irish men and women in alcohol services in the UK.

Browne (1997) found that not only were black people (African-Caribbean and African) overrepresented in terms of those admitted to psychiatric hospitals but they were also more likely to be compulsorily detained under the Mental Health Act (DoH 2005a, Mind 2002) and hospitalised for mental distress than their white counterparts. Although black (African-Caribbean and African) men represent 1% of the population of the UK, they are 10 times more likely to be diagnosed with a mental health problem. This situation is even more concerning when we consider that black men make up 16% of those detained in Rampton High Secure Unit. Black men are also more likely to be detained under the Mental Health Act (Mind 2002, Sainsbury Centre for Mental Health 2000), receive physical treatments and be given atypical medication, and they are less likely to be referred for talking therapies (DoH 2005a, Mind 2002).

In contrast, there is an underrepresentation of some other ethnic groups within mental health services, including Chinese, Asian Indians and Sikhs. This raises the question of whether these groups are less susceptible to mental ill health or, conversely, whether they have difficulty in accessing help or simply avoid using mental health services (Lim 2001). The Delivering Race Equality in Mental Health (DRE) Action Plan (DOH 2005b) highlights the need for more community development work to be undertaken with underrepresented communities. Time and effort must be invested in understanding their particular concerns, reservations and in overcoming barriers they face in assessing mental health services, in the overall interest of promoting positive mental health.

The Sainsbury Centre for Mental Health (2000) echoes the same worrying findings and reports that, despite much effort over recent years to combat the issues of discrimination and lack of appropriate care, mental health services are still failing to address the cultural and ethnic needs of the people who use their services. Token measures, such as providing culturally appropriate food on wards, having posters and leaflets in different languages and giving access to interpretation services, are a start. However, they do not go far enough in addressing some of the real concerns, including intolerance of religious beliefs, customs, discrimination and inflexibility in making adjustments that would respect the needs of the individual (Lim 2001, Reynolds & Lim 2005).

The full extent of the problem is reinforced by negative findings reported within the recent Healthcare Commission Census (DoH 2005a) of acute psychiatric services. The census indicated that black and minority ethnic (BME) service users encountered greater involvement of the police in their referrals and higher rates of physical restraint as opposed to other patient groups. High-profile cases, like the Stephen Lawrence (Macpherson 1999) and David Bennett (Blofeld 2003) inquiries, have further highlighted issues of institutional racism, poor levels of care, excessive use of force and discriminatory treatments experienced by BME service users within mental health care.

National consciousness and recognition of the scale of the problem have led to a governmental commitment to take action and address the issues of race equality, discrimination and cultural competence within health and social care. Within mental health, moves toward addressing these issues have been indicated by specific targets and provisions, within such policy documents as the National Service Framework for Mental Health (DoH 1999), the NHS Plan (DoH 2000), Race and Equality in Mental Health Consultation (DoH 2003), and the Social Exclusion Unit Report (Office of the Deputy Prime Minister 2004). These government policies have all focused on issues of client-centred practice, involving service users and their carers in planning interventions, providing culturally sensitive care in ensuring that minority ethnic groups are provided with opportunities to access the services they need and when they need them.

The introduction of the DRE Action Plan (DoH 2005c) has been a direct consequence of the Bennett inquiry (Blofeld 2003) and previous reports (Mind 2002, Sainsbury Centre for Mental Health 2000), which have made public the extent of discrimination, stigma and racism that exist. The 5-year action plan, supported by the National Institute of Mental Health in England (NIMHE), aims to achieve equality and overcome stigma, racism and discrimination through indicating clear objectives, initiatives and targets that strategic health authorities (SHA) and mental health services need to achieve in meeting the required standards.

DISCRIMINATION AND INSTITUTIONAL RACISM

The death of Stephen Lawrence, a black teenager, in south east London in 1993 brought to public attention the underlying racism and discrimination that exist within UK society. The report from the public inquiry conducted by Lord Macpherson reached several damning conclusions, which included the fact that institutional racism exists within public services and institutions and that minority ethnic groups are discriminated against within UK society. A clarification of these terms will help in examining the issue further and in identifying the implications for occupational therapists and the wider health and social care professions in practice.

Discrimination

Discrimination is the 'attitude, policy, or practice that knowingly excludes a person or group of persons from full participation and benefits' (Wells & Black 2000, p279). This definition indicates that the discrimination is not only unjust and unacceptable, but motivated solely on the basis of difference, disability or prejudice.

Institutional racism

The Macpherson Report (1999, 4262-i) described institutional racism as 'a collective failure of an organisation to provide an appropriate and professional service to people because of their colour, culture or ethnic origins'. Institutional racism can be overt or covert and is detected within the attitudes, behaviours and processes of an organisation. Such discrimination is often unintentional and is demonstrated through unwitting prejudice, thoughtlessness and racial stereotyping, which disadvantage people of minority ethnic origin. The Macpherson Report raised several important and potentially provocative questions, including whether the NHS and the mental health-care system are institutionally racist and guilty of levels of discrimination and prejudice.

Studies by Greenwood et al (2000) and by Secker & Harding (2002) explored the inpatient experiences of service users from Asian, African and African-Caribbean backgrounds. It was noted that participants mentioned a loss of control, experiences of overt and implicit racism, unhelpful relationships with some professional staff and lack of activities as negative factors related to their inpatient admission and stay.

Addressing institutional racism

An independent inquiry into the death of David Bennett (Blofeld 2003) once again highlighted the failure of the NHS to tackle the serious issue of institutional racism and the excessive use of control and restraint techniques. One of the key recommendations identified within the Bennett Inquiry was that all staff working in mental health services should receive training in cultural awareness and sensitivity, and be trained to tackle overt and covert racism and institutional racism (Khanna 2004).

It is evident from these examples that institutional racism exists in many areas of the public sector, including health services, and that racial discrimination is deeply enshrined within many of our structures and systems. This makes it difficult at times to separate our behaviours and practices from the organisational and societal influences around us. How we tackle the issue of institutional racism, as current or future clinicians, is crucial if we are committed to providing an inclusive, culturally sensitive and non-discriminatory service to those who need our help.

The commitment and provision of specific training at all levels of an organisation are essential to equip staff with the knowledge and skills to be more culturally aware and sensitive within their clinical practice. Discussions around diversity and cultural differences must be encouraged in order to dispel any mysteries or racial stereotypes relating to all groups within society. Specific skills training around interacting, assessing and working with individuals from a range of backgrounds must also be included (Lim 2001). The desire not to upset or offend by attempting to treat everyone the same creates difficulties, as it is obvious that we are clearly not all the same and that our individuality and differences must be acknowledged, affirmed and respected.

MENTAL ILLNESS AS A SOCIAL CONSTRUCT

What is considered normal and acceptable behaviour is often subjective, and behaviour that may be perceived as deviant or inappropriate within one sociocultural context may be considered acceptable and normal behaviour within another. Becker (1963) suggested that each culture labels some forms of action and behaviour as deviant and, therefore, contrary to what is acceptable within that society. McGruder (2001) went further in suggesting that what a society values and fears is represented by how it views and interprets mental illness. These perspectives prompt us to consider whether the concept of mental illness is a socially constructed phenomenon upheld by society in order to ensure that all members of that society conform to what is acceptable and expected (Helman 2000).

Richardson (2004) suggested that culture determines what is *normal* and *abnormal*, and dictates what is or is not a mental illness within a social framework. The potential for misdiagnosis increases in such circumstances, as we attempt to understand the variety of appropriate sociocultural norms, presentations and behaviours. Cross-cultural and social psychiatry are concerned with the psychological, behavioural and sociocultural dimensions associated with mental illness. How we understand these influencing factors may have a significant impact on how we interpret, relate, assess, treat and respond to the individual service user (Lim 2001).

Cross–cultural psychiatry

The cross-cultural interpretation of mental illness may be different from Western conceptualisations of mental illness. The Western medical model seeks to isolate, frame and fit the individual's experience into neat categories of ill health. Making a diagnosis is of paramount importance, as the whole focus of treatment is centred on identifying and removing the offending intrusion or prescribing medication to counteract the problem (Lim 2001, Masi 1992).

This view contrasts significantly with a non-Western perspective, where mental ill health may be attributed to a failure to maintain an overall balance in one's life or perceived as a consequence of witchcraft or incurring a curse (Helman 2000). If one subscribes to this latter view then adherence to a medication regime becomes irrelevant. A visit to a religious or spiritual healer, or maintaining a balance through consuming traditional remedies or potions, may be seen as more effective in restoring health and well-being than taking prescribed medication (see case example 3).

Case example 3

A Nigerian woman commented: 'I don't know why I was brought into hospital; there is nothing wrong with me. These people on the ward, they need help not me. I want to see my pastor so that he can pray over me and my husband and exorcise away these evil spirits that are out to harm us.'

In the UK, we no longer live within a homogeneous culture or society. It is therefore important that the occupational therapist is aware of and sensitive to cultural interpretations of health, illness and well-being, and that she examines the various attitudes and interpretations of mental health that are commonly shared by different ethnic and cultural groups.

Reform of the mental health system within the UK, towards a more social model of psychiatry, has resulted in a shift in the balance of power from the medical profession to other professional groups. Occupational therapists, psychologists and nurses are increasingly involved in assessing, diagnosing, monitoring and co-ordinating individual packages of treatment and care.

PROMOTING CULTURAL AWARENESS AND COMPETENCY

The ability to be culturally aware and sensitive to the needs of those we serve is central to providing client-centred practice within multicultural contexts. This sensitivity begins with self-reflection: looking within ourselves and examining our own cultural and ethnic influences, which impact upon our values, beliefs and perceptions of self and others. Only through examining our own attitudes, values, assumptions and beliefs may we be able to identify our prejudices towards those we encounter in our practice (McGruder 2003, Reynolds & Lim 2005).

Personal values and social norms directly impact upon how we relate and respond to others. Gross (2001, p351) defined *value* as 'a sense of what is desirable, good and worthwhile'. What we consider to be important will not necessarily be of importance to the next person, and we need to beware of imposing our own values, beliefs and prejudices on to our clients and their carers. The danger of presuming that we know what is most beneficial for our clients becomes all too apparent when they become non-compliant, demotivated, disgruntled or simply absent from treatment (Lim 2001).

Assumptions, which are acts or instances of accepting without proof (Gross 2001), are often inherent in the attitudes that we hold towards others. For example, racist attitudes may be grounded in unexamined assumptions that members of a certain group are lazy, shy or violent. Henley & Schott (1999, p51) define attitude as 'a settled opinion or way of thinking, which is reflected in behaviour'. They argued that the way we think about or perceive others has a direct impact upon our actions and behaviours towards them.

Although making assumptions about others is unhelpful, one reason for doing so is that it provides a way to make sense of the huge variety of social information to which we are exposed (Wetherell 1996). Instead of processing information about each person individually, we categorise them as members of homogeneous social groups (e.g. female, black, estate agents) so that our thinking becomes simplified and manageable. The obvious drawback of doing this is that our assumptions about and perceptions of others may become accepted as true and reliable. Misrepresentations can be reinforced by the mass media, which often portray members of certain groups in highly stereotypical terms (Reynolds & Lim 2005).

There is a danger that stereotypes can become self-fulfilling prophecies. For example, if we perceive all older people as passive, inactive and needing help, we may inadvertently encourage the very behaviour that we have anticipated. One of the key characteristics of stereotyping is that a single piece of information about an individual (such as age, gender or race) generates inferences about all other aspects of that person, including personality, interests, aspirations and so on (Levy et al 1998). Unexamined assumptions about members of other groups may ultimately contribute to discriminatory practices, as well as perpetuating myths and simplified perceptions (Reynolds & Lim 2005).

It is evident that the accepted norms within the community and society in which we live have a significant influence in determining what attitudes and behaviours are considered to be acceptable and legitimate. However, the process of understanding how others view, understand and interpret their experiences can enhance cultural awareness and sensitivity (Lim & Iwama 2006). It is crucial for the health professional to acknowledge that different ethnic or cultural groups and communities may have different ideas and understanding of what contributes to health and well-being. We need to remain mindful of broad cultural differences in family structures and values while treating each client as an individual with specific needs and requirements. Only in this way can we effectively provide culturally sensitive and appropriate care for each client (Helman 2000, Lim 2001).

EDUCATION AND TRAINING

There is a clear need to incorporate programmes of cultural awareness and competency training within current occupational therapy curricula in the UK. Paniagua (1994) suggested that practitioners across all mental health disciplines need to learn and apply skills that indicate they are culturally competent in the assessment and treatment of clients from multicultural groups.

However, a study by the author discovered huge disparities in the amount of cultural awareness training provided on pre-registration occupational therapy programmes and after employment. Training ranged from a day on equal opportunities to a comprehensive cultural awareness programme spread throughout the 3-year course (Lim 2004). At Brunel University, for example, occupational therapy students are exposed to a wide variety of diverse case studies, undertake personal development and cultural competency skills training.

Cultural sensitivity within teams and departments can further be enhanced by the creation of a cultural resource file. This file contains relevant information about local and community services working with minority groups, contact details of local translation services, immigrant services, local religious leaders and places of worship. The establishment of partnerships with non-statutory and community services could also be a positive step towards promoting cultural sensitivity, respecting diversity and appropriate clinical care.

EXERCISES TO PROMOTE SELF-AWARENESS

The two exercises given here were designed to promote self-awareness in students. They can be undertaken individually, in pairs or within a large group.

Exercise 1: Personal values, perceptions and attitudes

This exercise provides an opportunity to begin to examine our own values, perceptions and attitudes. Please allow sufficient time so that you do not have to rush through it. Begin the exercise on your own and then, if possible, discuss your answers with a partner or group.

1. List some of your personal values and what you consider to be important.
2. List the first few things that come to mind when you think of a person with a mental illness.
3. What factors have influenced your perceptions or views of this individual?
4. Do you think that person would have different personal values to you?
5. Are you aware of any prejudicial views you may have of individuals with mental health problems?
6. How do you think these views may influence your attitude and working relationship with someone with a mental illness?

Were you surprised at what you discovered about yourself and your own values, assumptions, views and attitudes? What have you learned from doing this exercise?

Exercise 2: Ethnic and cultural perceptions of health and well-being

This exercise requires an exploration of issues around our own ethnicity, culture, beliefs and perceptions. Answer the questions on your own and then, if possible, discuss your responses with a partner or within a small group.

1. How would you describe yourself in terms of your ethnicity and culture?
2. Does this view or perception of yourself influence your sense of identity? If so, how?
3. What are the common views and perceptions within your own culture around the value and meaning of occupation?
4. What are the common views within your own culture around what factors contribute to an individual's health and well-being?
5. What habits, behaviours or rituals do you adopt when you are not feeling well and are trying to get better? Why have you adopted them?
6. How important to you are beliefs, customs, spirituality or religion when you are unwell or in need of help?
7. Do you recall any clinical situations when you felt that the client's beliefs, identity, culture or ethnicity impacted upon his behaviour, presentation, health and recovery?
8. Identify one belief, ethnic group, culture or custom that you are unfamiliar with. Research this in relation to health, illness and well-being. Examine the possible implications of your findings to clinical practice. Examples could include: Rastafarians, Christian healing, Indian perspectives on mental health, Seventh Day Adventist dietary patterns, Five pillars of Islam or African healing.

How did you find the exercise above? Did you experience any difficulty in identifying your own ethnic and cultural identity? If so, why do you think this was the case? What have you discovered about the group or culture you have selected?

TRANSCULTURAL OCCUPATIONAL THERAPY PRACTICE

The way in which occupational therapy is practised and delivered is dictated by the theories and models that are available. The majority of these have been developed in the West and therefore reflect a Western perspective and philosophy of life, occupation, health, illness and well-being. Although these models may be effective in helping us to understand and work with individuals within a Western context, their value in terms of cultural appropriateness and sensitivity is far more limited (Lim & Iwama 2005). The possibility of alternative, competing worldviews and self-constructs challenges the adequacy of existing theoretical models and frameworks to explain occupational phenomena for all. Chaing & Carlson (2003) and Watson (2006) suggested that current, prominent Western models are biased in providing a predominantly Western perspective to restoring health and recovery.

CULTURALLY SENSITIVE MODELS AND APPROACHES

Occupational therapy conceptual models are products of a particular dominant worldview and construction of self that resonate with Northern or Western cultures. These models, such as the Model of Human Occupation (Kielhofner 2002) and the Canadian Model of Occupational Performance (Law et al 1990), assume that the self is situated centrally and is separate from the environment, which must be occupied through rational, purposeful action or 'doing' (Iwama 2003). Well-being coincides with the privileged self being able to exploit and exercise control over perceived circumstances and environment. Concepts such as independence, autonomy, egalitarianism and self-determinism are celebrated and valued mainly within a Western context (Lim & Iwama 2005).

Client-centred practice is only achievable if we are truly committed to individualised care, fostered by a continuous process of engaging with our clients in understanding their perceptions of reality and responding to their needs (Sumsion 2004). This process begins with a commitment to listening to the individual's narrative, acknowledging his experience, understanding his concerns and attempting to meet his needs. An appreciation of the client's perspective and priorities is essential, as we strive towards enabling him to engage in activities that promote his recovery and enhance his health and well-being (Lim 2006).

Global perspectives

An examination of research and literature in several countries highlights the differences that exist in how an individual experiences and expresses his illness. Understanding such differences may be a first step towards ensuring effective and culturally sensitive health care transculturally. A brief range of studies will be included next, highlighting this diversity. Santana & Santana (2001), in their review of Mexican culture and disability, indicate the stereotypical views that some clinicians have of particular ethnic groups. They discuss the actual experience of one of the authors (Felipe) undergoing manipulative therapy and being told by the doctor that due to his macho Mexican culture he should be able to manage with the pain of treatment without anaesthesia. When Felipe did complain about the pain and discomfort, he was chastised for not being macho enough. This incident highlights the dangers of stereotypical attitudes and behaviours and the lack of cultural competency training that some health professionals may receive in training. The authors also discuss the view that for many Mexicans, illness and health, including mental illness, are considered the will of God and that when a person is ill, some form of folk healing may be necessary in restoring health and promoting recovery (Santana & Santana 2001).

De Silva (2002) highlights that the early system of medicine in Sri Lanka was based on Ayurveda, herbal medicine, astrology, folk practices and religion and that even now, certain mental illness and physical ailments are treated with herbal preparations, oils and ceremonies consisting of dancing and chanting (thovil). Although appearing less sophisticated than Western interventions, these treatments have a rich and historical tradition, intertwined with a complex system of reason and logic. The British colonisation of Sri Lanka has, however, led to the imposition of Western models of health care that are perceived to be more valid, effective and reliable. These imported ideas that influence mental health care, rehabilitation and service delivery reinforce the cultural gap between the Western rooted mental health system and the views and experiences of the local population. The superior stance in support of Western models of health care adopted by many health professionals, over traditional beliefs and illness models, has serious implications for the promotion of culturally sensitive care.

Watson (2006), in her keynote speech at the World Occupational Therapy Congress in Sydney 2006, highlighted the dangers faced by the occupational therapy profession in failing to fully embrace the role and value of culture within daily practice. She warned that despite common professional foundations, we must not assume universal uniformity in practice and need to be mindful of sociocultural contextual differences. She discussed the Afrocentric collectivist view and how it differs from an individualistic Eurocentric worldview, based on autonomy and personal rights. She explained that within the Afrocentric perspective, people are valued in terms of their contribution and role within their wider community and that they derived rights as a consequence of being part of and belonging to a larger familial or community structure.

Watson (2006) further raises the unique importance in the South African educational curricula of examining the sociopolitical journey and aftermath of apartheid in understanding the health, social, justice and occupational experiences of its people. She supports the view expressed by Lim & Iwama (2006) that the developing countries in which occupational therapy is growing must be encouraged and supported in arriving at their own inspirations and foundations of occupational ideology, knowledge, practice and not be forced into adopting existing Eurocentric knowledge and models of practice.

In non-Western societies, a state of wellness is experienced when all elements in their frame, including the self, co-exist in harmony. Disruption of this harmony hampers the collective life-flow or energy within the individual. Enhancing or restoring harmony replaces enabling control as the primary purpose for occupational therapy in many non-Western contexts (Iwama 2004, Lim & Iwama 2006). With such radically different ways of understanding and appreciating the sociocultural context and influences that shape each individual, how do we begin to abide by one of the central tenets of our profession in striving for client-centred practice?

The Kawa Model

The emergence of the Kawa River Model, the first occupational therapy model based on Eastern philosophy, provides a radically different perspective of how occupation and the self are conceptualised. The individual is visualised within the Kawa Model as part of a larger whole, inclusive of the individual's family, community, sociocultural, economic and political environments (Lim & Iwama 2006). The principles of client-centred practice are promoted within the conceptually distinct framework of this new model, which focuses attention on the wider contextual factors that impact on the individual (Iwama 2004).

The significance of the Kawa River Model is its position as the first non-Western occupational therapy model. The genesis and evolvement of the Kawa Model have been a direct consequence of the unsatisfactory experiences of Japanese occupational therapists in utilising existing Western occupational therapy models and measures within their practice (Iwama 2006). These therapists felt that current Western models did not resonate with their personal nor their clients' sociocultural experiences and circumstances. Importantly, the very existence of the Kawa Model indicates a radical change from the norm of merely adopting Western concepts and ideas, promoting the importance of discourse and validation of alternative perspectives (Lim & Iwama 2005). Distinctively, the Kawa Model is devoid of linear structures, line, boxes and technical jargon. In contrast, it is infused with a naturalistic and holistic perspective of life, health and well-being and adopts the popular Japanese metaphor of a river. The word *kawa* is the Japanese word for river.

Each individual is perceived to have his own unique *personal river* that symbolises his life

---

Box 14.1 Five key components within the Kawa River Model

Water
Water represents the client's life energy and health.
  Water is flexible and is shaped by its container (experience, circumstances).
  The river can flow fully, dry up, change directions.
  Water can be clear or in a muddy state.

Riversides and riverbed
Represents the client's physical and social environment and human resources.
  Family, healthcare professionals, school, workplace, culture, society can shape one's environment.

Rocks
Represent the client's life difficulties.
  They block and slow down the water flow.
  Disease, symptoms, daily life challenges are represented as rocks.

Driftwood
Represents the client's attributes, values, character, experiences that can work positively or negatively (assets and liabilities).
  Driftwood can either further block the water flow or bump the rocks away, enhancing the flow.

Spaces
Represents the client's natural healing power and potential and includes abilities and positive points.
  Enhancing the client's inner ability and maximising opportunities is one of the major aspects of occupational therapy.

---

journey, with the upstream of one's river representing the past and the downstream representing the future. Personal health and well-being are expressed by the free and unrestricted flow of one's river, whilst life difficulties, problems, barriers, environmental, financial and social constraints are symbolised by *rocks* and the restrictive *river bank* (Lim & Iwama 2005).

There are five key components within the Kawa River as described in Box 14.1. To demonstrate the application of the Kawa Model, a case study has been included.

Kawa case study: Krishna Muttaran

Krishna Muttaran, 34 years old, is a friendly, sociable, unmarried man who enjoys using computers. He has a 15-year history of schizophrenia, with several relapses but is currently compliant with his medication regime. Following an intermittent work history, he is in receipt of long-term sickness benefit but is keen to take up voluntary work. He has poor concentration and self-care skills. His supportive family with whom he lives are overly concerned at times but he has a strong network of friends. He regularly attends appointments with his occupational therapists and community psychiatric nurse.

A pictorial representation of his *River* at a cross-section in time is illustrated in Figure 14.1.

The occupational therapy intervention using the framework of the Kawa Model to help him overcome his difficulties is shown in Box 14.2.

One essential quality of the Kawa Model is its refreshing simplicity. The author's experience of utilising the Kawa Model with several clients/service users has reinforced the opinion that the metaphor and concept of a River, representing one's life journey, is a simple concept understood by many clients (Lim 2006). This is in contrast to the author's previous experience of utilising existing Western models of practice, which are infused with complex professional terminology, jargon and technical concepts that are rarely understood by many clinicians or their clients. Krishna was immediately able to comprehend, understand and relate his life journey as a *personal river*, whilst using the Kawa Model.

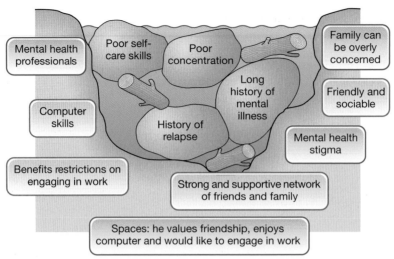

Figure 14.1 Pictorial cross-section of Krishna Muttaran's *River.*

Krishna gained awareness and understanding of how his personal river reflected his life journey and how the rocks in his river were symbolic representations of the difficulties he was experiencing. By focusing on his assets and strengths (driftwood and spaces) in terms of his friendly and sociable disposition, his previous computer skills and his desire to engage in work, he could utilise these positive aspects in overcoming his difficulties. During the process, Krishna identified the rocks within his river as representing his poor concentration, his history of mental illness and periods of relapse. His initial depiction of his river allowed for a process of discussion around what he considered to be his difficulties and what his family identified as an additional rock, his self-care needs, which he had not previously perceived to be an area of concern (Lim 2006).

The use of the Kawa Model further provided the opportunity to examine how Krishna's perspectives, priorities and concerns were different from those of his family. The pictorial representation of Krishna's river was useful as a visual catalyst for discussion within the family sessions. Krishna's parents were able to appreciate some of the issues that Krishna perceived as hurdles and barriers, which restricted him from achieving more and getting better. His family were also more able to understand how they might assist him in achieving his future goals.

The Kawa Model provides a framework and opportunity for the clinician and client to focus on the holistic interplay of strengths, difficulties, assets, circumstances and pressures that may impact on the individual. The representation of a pictorial image that includes not only the needs but also the strengths, assets and innate potential of the individual client to recover is unique to the Kawa Model. This visual element of the Kawa Model promotes greater understanding and clarity for the client on the purpose of occupational therapy. Clients with learning difficulties, children and those with limited literacy, who might otherwise struggle to understand existing occupational therapy concepts and technical terms, are able, through the visual qualities of the Kawa Model, to be more actively involved in determining their own care (Lim 2006)

Strengths of the Kawa Model

The Kawa Model operates within an open system that elicits the personal perspectives and experiences of each individual, situated within their wider sociocultural context (Iwama 2005, Lim 2006). It does not use a range of prescribed standardised measurements but ensures that the unique lived and narrative experience of the client is explored within a culturally sensitive, safe and appropriate framework (Iwama 2006). Through a process of individualised client

Box 14.2 Krishna's occupational therapy intervention

Water
- The aim of occupational therapy is to maximise Krishna's life-flow. This will involve reducing and removing elements that presently impede his river's flow and maximising existing channels or spaces where his water currently flows.

Rocks
- Identify the rocks, their relative size and location. Determine with Krishna (and his family) which obstacles are most troublesome to him.
- Krishna and his family report that he is not able to look after his self-care.

Manipulate the rocks
- Reduce the obstacles by providing help with self-care skills including personal grooming, laundry and meal preparation. Monitor his mental health status. Work on increasing his concentration skills (through participation in relevant/meaningful activities, such as computer skills training).

Spaces/Channels
- Identify current and potential spaces, and their location, paying attention to the context surrounding the flow. Determine which spaces are most important and meaningful to Krishna.

Maximising the spaces
- Promoting his inner strength, interests, abilities and skills. These may include: work preparation training, exploring voluntary work, attending the local sports centre to meet new friends and build stamina, and working on personal CV.

Riverbed and sides
- Widen the riversides and deepen the river bottom.
- Consult with benefits advisor to assess Krishna's benefit status in relation to paid voluntary work.
- Provide support for Krishna and his family in terms of regular family meetings to help the family understand Krishna's condition and his desire to engage in voluntary work, and to do more for himself.
- Facilitate a process to involve his whole professional team and family in supporting his engagement in voluntary work, his social interests and computer skills training.

Driftwood
- Identify aspects of character and attributes, and materials that may act as assets or liabilities in the Krishna's life-flow. Determine Krishna's cultural and social context, to aid an understanding of factors that will help or hinder his occupational well-being.

Utilise the driftwood
- Enhance the positive aspects of his character and attributes: friendliness, desire for voluntary work, build on his computer skills, etc. Getting his family to support his desire to get fit, socialise and engage in work, etc.

exploration, the most appropriate assessment or measure is then selected and adopted. It focuses on the strengths, assets, ability and innate potential of each client to recover and links well with the core concept of client recovery within mental health practice (Lim 2006). The principles of client-centred practice are also promoted through a commitment to explore the perspective and lived experience of the client, in the pursuit of collaborative planning and achievement of individual goals (Lim & Iwama 2005).

Evaluation of the model

Research into the use of the Kawa Model in Europe is limited at present but is beginning to gain momentum. In Japan where it first evolved, the Kawa Model has been used much more extensively, with over 800 case studies across the diverse spectrums of occupational therapy practice (Iwama 2006). Current research is focused on examining the utility and development of the model within the wider international and transcultural context.

An English language website and discussion forum has recently been established (www.kawamodel.com) to promote discussion on the relevance and appropriateness of the Kawa Model transculturally. Research is ongoing in several countries including Chile, Denmark, Holland, India, Australia, United States, Hong Kong, Sweden, Georgia, Canada, South Africa, Morocco, New Zealand, Japan and the United Kingdom (Iwama 2006). It has also been established as a part of the curriculum within the European Occupational Therapy Masters programme.

In conclusion, the philosophy and principles of the Kawa Model correspond well with the positive shift in mental health practice within the UK, away from paternalism and towards concepts of service user empowerment and involvement (Lim 2005). It further reinforces the importance of the client's narrative and lived experience and provides a framework to explore the diversity of contextual perspectives, situated meanings and recovery experiences of the individual client, within a collaborative structure that promotes culturally sensitive and safe care (Lim & Iwama 2006).

CULTURAL AWARENESS APPLIED TO THE OCCUPATIONAL THERAPY PROCESS

The occupational therapy process is often perceived to begin with the first contact we have with the client, and to proceed through the stages of interview, assessment, intervention, evaluation and, if appropriate, discharge, as shown in Chapter 5, Figure 5.1. In reality the process does not always flow along such smooth and predictable lines.

Assessment

When working with clients from a culture, race or ethnic background different from the therapist's own, it is particularly important to tailor the assessment, intervention and evaluation to the client's values and needs. The limitations of using culturally specific standardised assessments and outcome measures become apparent when the language used creates confusion. An example of this is reflected in a standardised assessment used within mother and baby units, which requires patients to indicate the last time they felt 'blue'. This term, understood by

British or American mothers, is incomprehensible to women from a different culture.

Referral and information gathering

The occupational therapy process begins well before the first face-to-face contact with the client. On receiving a referral, the therapist begins to gather relevant information about the individual, which will allow her to appreciate the situation and circumstances that the client is experiencing. This should include some awareness of ethnic background, language spoken and indicate whether translation/interpretation services are required.

Greetings and introductions

Preparation for meeting the client requires that we ensure that we address the client appropriately and pronounce his name correctly. This first contact provides a clear indication to the client of the value placed on him through the time and effort made to acknowledge him correctly and appropriately.

It is important to note that there are different naming systems in the world and that clients may be offended if not addressed appropriately. Checking the forename and surname, for example, and ensuring that pronunciation is correct is a small but significant gesture of respect. Names provide a sense of self and identity, and are crucial to the development of self-image, self-esteem and sense of belonging (Henley & Schott 1999). It should not be assumed that the individual would like to be addressed by his first name or that calling him by his surname would be too formal. The most effective way to get this right is to check with the client how he would like to be addressed.

Communication

Communicating with the client becomes more difficult when the therapist is unable to speak the same language. When booking interpreters, it should be ensured that they speak the right language or dialect. It would be naïve to assume that all individuals from a particular ethnic background, cultural group or country speak the same language. It would be presumptuous, for example, to assume that all people of Chinese origin speak Cantonese or that all Asian people speak Hindi or all those from Nigeria speak Yoruba.

Case example 4

Whilst working on an inpatient psychiatric unit, the author received a request from another ward to assist the staff with interviewing a Chinese man who did not speak English. When asked if the gentleman spoke Mandarin, the ward manager responded that, of course, all Chinese people speak Mandarin. Further clarification confirmed that the client only spoke Cantonese and therefore arrangements had to be made to get an alternative interpreter.

Trained professional interpreters who are also familiar with medical terminology should be used where possible. It is essential that the client's responses are translated accurately, rather than interpreted according to what the interpreter perceives the client is trying to say or what the interviewer wants to hear. Most health and social service departments will have access to a professional interpreting and translating service. It can be problematic when an interpreter cannot be found and a family member is required as a last resort to undertake the translation. The client's response to a question must be translated without compromise or editing, and this may be jeopardised if the family member decides to vet the answers in order to get a desired outcome (Lim 2001).

Not all health terms can be translated into the client's own language, and the process of phrasing questions accurately in order to get the desired information can be difficult. The term *stress*, for example, does not have a clear translation in any Chinese language so it would be difficult to find out from a Chinese speaker if he is experiencing stress. It may be easier to ask about the symptoms of stress, such as poor sleep, loss of appetite, headache or back pains. Within some cultures, a description of somatic symptoms may be a more acceptable way of presenting and communicating psychological distress.

Ting-Toomey (1999) suggested that communication is central to the therapist–client interaction and is necessary for the provision of appropriate services to any client. The occupational therapist needs to avoid the temptation of trying to complete the assessment form rigidly and instead adopt an attitude of interest, active listening, questioning, exploring, explaining and clarifying, leading eventually to negotiation and agreement with the client on the way to proceed.

Understanding the client

The client-centred values of the occupational therapy profession encourage an individualised client-focused practice that promotes an appreciation and understanding of each individual's experiences and circumstances. This process is enhanced through the use of exploratory models and assessment tools that assist in understanding the client's view of their circumstances and experiences, within a wider sociocultural and environmental context (Lim 2001).

One such tool is the Culturological Assessment of the Patient/Client Interview Schedule, devised by Berlin & Fowkes (1982). They proposed the five-stage LEARN Model to assist the process of understanding the client's perspective.

1. **L**isten to the client's perceptions and view of his problems.
2. **E**xplain your own perceptions, view point and understanding of why he may be experiencing these particular problems, whether they be physical, emotional or psychological.
3. **A**cknowledge and discuss the similarities and differences between your two perceptions of the presenting problems.
4. **R**ecommend measures to address and resolve the presenting difficulties or problems.
5. **N**egotiate and get agreement on the treatment plan proposed, incorporating specific aspects of the individual's culture where appropriate in providing the treatment and care.

The LEARN Model can be described as a transcultural assessment tool, appropriate for all client groups. Its use extends beyond clients from minority ethnic groups, who may have a different perspective of their situation and circumstances. It can also be easily adapted to assist the therapist in shifting the balance of power within the interview and assessment process. It promotes and facilitates the process of eliciting the client's perspective and encourages an active process of negotiation between both parties, thus enhancing the quality of the therapeutic relationship and the effectiveness of the assessment and treatment offered.

Detailed assessment

In mental health practice, many decisions are based on observations of the client's presenting behaviour. This could result in an inaccurate assessment due to a failure to appreciate sociocultural differences. It is important that any observations and assessments are examined with care in relation to sociocultural contextual influences and determinants.

Care must be taken to ensure that the assessment tools used are both clinically effective and culturally appropriate. The majority of assessment tools used by occupational therapists in their daily work have been created and developed in the West and were often designed in conjunction with Western models of occupational therapy practice (Iwama & Lim 2005). Their effectiveness when used with a culturally and ethnically different client group may be limited.

The language used within these assessments could also prove difficult for the individual to understand, due to the different sociocultural context. Steps must be taken to ensure that all questions are phrased appropriately, in order to elicit an accurate response from the client.

The Cultural Assessment Checklist (Lim 2002) in Box 14.3. can be used to check for inconsistencies in the mental health assessments made of an individual's behaviour which may lead to an inaccurate assessment being made (Lim 2001). This checklist highlights 20 areas to be considered when observing and assessing the client.

Treatment

Consideration must also be given to cultural and ethnic factors when planning interventions with clients. Specific areas of practice could be altered in order to accommodate the individual needs of the client. It is important to focus upon those smaller differences open to therapist control rather than trying to change systems, over which an individual practitioner may have little influence.

Efforts must be made to ensure that cultural sensitivity is promoted in all aspects of occupational therapy assessments and interventions, as listed in Box 14.4. For example, when faced with service users who are Muslims or Orthodox Jews within a cookery group, a first step is to ensure

---

Box 14.3 Cultural Assessment Checklist (Lim 2001)

Language barriers and communication
Eye contact
Physical contact
Decision-making abilities
Overall assertiveness
Behaviour and attitudes
Belief systems, religion and superstitions
Customs, traditions and practice
Task performance factors
Gender roles
Role of family and carers
Diet (food and drink)
Social contact
Structure of social networks
Community and support networks
Descriptive terms and language
Views on health and well-being
Attitudes to mental illness
Views on Western medicine and psychiatry
Views on alternative medicine

Box 14.4 Aspects of intervention to be considered for cultural appropriateness

Personal care: washing, dressing, grooming, hygiene
Domestic tasks: cooking, laundry, paying bills, shopping, housework
Diet: food, drink
Cognition: decision making, personal traits, mindset
Leisure and social interests: social networks, communities, social interaction
Productivity: work, gender roles, value
Life skills: stress management, assertiveness training, power dynamics/relationships
Group interventions and processes

---

that the food is halal or kosher. Care must also be taken to ensure that the equipment and utensils to be used have not been previously contaminated by having been used to prepare non-halal or kosher food. People from these religious groups will not be able to participate in cookery sessions if this adjustment is overlooked.

When undertaking activities of personal care, it is important to note, for example, that African, African-Caribbean and Asian individuals have a different hair texture and skin types, which require specific products. These may include coconut oil for hair maintenance or specific formulated skin moisturisers. Provision must be made for catering for these needs. It may also be appropriate for the occupational therapist to master the art of putting on a sari, shalwar kameez or hijab so that dressing practice for an Asian client is adapted to accommodate appropriate clothing.

Gender roles and cultural norms may also dictate what activities are appropriate and what the client can engage in. Interventions such as assertiveness training and goal setting may be limited in their effectiveness unless the dynamics within the family and social context of the individual are altered, as illustrated in case example 5.

Case example 5

A woman client from Somalia who attended an assertiveness training course said: 'All this is very interesting for me, but I don't think I will be able to use very much of what I have learned in the sessions. My family and community do not see a woman asserting her views and making independent choices as either desirable or acceptable.'

We need to continually demonstrate flexibility and resourcefulness in the delivery of occupational therapy interventions and services, when working with a diverse client group.

Case example 6

Kasmin was referred to a creative writing group, with the aim of helping him to interact socially and to promote self-expression. He mentioned a desire to write poetry, which was something he had previously found meaningful and enjoyable. To assist him in his self-expression, Kasmin was encouraged to express his thoughts and feelings through writing in Bosnian, rather than English, and to read his work to the rest of the group in his native language. Kasmin was immensely encouraged by being able to write in Bosnian and shared his work with the group both in his native tongue and in English.

Involving the family in discussions around interventions, may be appropriate within certain cultural groups.

Case example 7

A community psychiatric nurse who visited a Vietnamese family to see a 20-year-old male client was greeted on arrival by the entire extended family. After a period of 20 minutes of introductions and dialogue with all members of the family in hierarchical order, the nurse was finally able to speak to the client about his health and mental well-being. These customs and rituals play an important part within certain communities and must be respected, in order for the occupational therapist to work effectively with individuals within those communities.

Evaluation and outcome measurement

Outcome measurement has gained immense importance in light of the Department of Health's pursuit of clinical governance and evidence-based practice (DoH 2000). Much attention has been focused on evidencing occupational therapy practice in line with fulfilling the government's targets highlighted within the NHS plans and national service frameworks (Cusack & Sealey-Lapes 2000, DoH 2000).

In the relentless pursuit of evidence-based practice and outcome measurement, occupational therapists should not lose sight of whose outcomes they are actually measuring and whose health they are trying to promote. The client's outcomes can be left unmet while occupational therapists try to meet the competing demands to evaluate and evidence their interventions and approaches.

The current pressure to evidence practice and use standardised assessments to evaluate interventions raises several questions for those providing culturally sensitive care. This includes what measures are being used to ascertain outcomes and results. Have they been designed for a culturally different client group? Are these assessments and measures therefore culturally appropriate when applied to different groups of individuals?

Indeed, the extensive promotion of standardized assessments to achieve clinical effectiveness may be flawed if the measures selected are not chosen with due care. The majority of existing standardised assessments have been developed in conjunction with existing models of practice and largely constructed along Western sociocultural norms and may be limited in their appropriateness to clients from a different sociocultural context (Iwama 2005, Lim 2004, Wells & Black 2000). Such measures must be adapted appropriately when used with distinctly different clients and supplemented with additional qualitative reporting and narratives from the client. We must refrain from fitting the client into what we have already constructed but must be truly client focused in looking at their outcomes and tailoring our assessments in order to arrive at valid and reliable measures of the clients' occupational performance and functioning.

The following case study illustrates how the LEARN Model (Lim 2001) and the Cultural Assessment Checklist can be utilised in practice to promote cultural sensitivity.

Case study: Mrs Mohammed

Shireen Mohammed is a 23-year-old lady of Indian origin who is a Muslim. She grew up in Northern India and has lived in the UK since her arranged marriage 3 years ago. She lives in an extended family, which includes her parents-in-law, her husband and her sister-in-law. She does not have any children and is a housewife, with responsibilities for caring for the home and for her mother-in-law who has recently suffered a stroke.

Mrs Mohammed has been referred to the community mental health team by her GP. He has seen her several times over the last month, when she presented with stomach pains, loss of appetite, feeling tired, not sleeping and being tearful. The GP has done the necessary physical examinations, which have proved to be inconclusive, and he suspects that she may be depressed. Mrs Mohammed speaks some English and is nervous when attending the assessment at the clinic. She is to be assessed by the team leader and the occupational therapist in the team.

Assessment of Mrs Mohammed

Before seeing Mrs Mohammed, the staff team establish whether she will require an interpreter and whether she would like to bring a family member along with her. Mrs Mohammed decides to attend the assessment on her own and feels that she does not require an interpreter.

At the beginning of the initial interview, she is asked how she would like to be addressed and she states her preference for being addressed by her surname, Mrs Mohammed. The assessment is then carried out by two members of the team, using the LEARN Model as a framework and the Cultural Assessment Checklist as a guide.

Listen. The staff listen carefully to establish what Mrs Mohammed's perception is of her current situation, whether she feels there is a problem and if she feels that she needs help. Mrs Mohammed explains that she is constantly tired, not sleeping at night, feeling sad about her life and missing her family in India. She cannot stop crying at times. She is worried about her aches and pains and feels that she is physically unwell. She would like help to discover what is wrong.

Explain. One staff member explains to Mrs Mohammed the role of the CMHT and the purpose of the interview. They share with her their view of what they feel might be going on for her, and explain why and how they have come to this conclusion. After further questioning, they explain that she might be experiencing some stress and isolation, and that the physical symptoms of aches, pains and stiffness she is experiencing might be a consequence of this. They also explain that she may be feeling low or depressed, and that her tearfulness, tiredness, inability to sleep and missing her family might be symptoms of this.

Acknowledge. The staff acknowledge the differences between their views and those of Mrs Mohammed, and discuss with her what she feels about their assessment of her difficulties. They also clarify the meaning of terms that are unfamiliar to her, including stress and depression, and the effects these conditions may have on a person. She is keen to know how the CMHT can help. She agrees that she feels very isolated and that she is overwhelmed by doing all the housework and having to care for her mother-in-law. She explains that it is seen as the responsibility of the family and her duty to care for her mother-in-law, and that it is not their custom to seek help from those outside their home or community. She mentions that her husband is very supportive and loving but she is reluctant to tell him how she feels at present or about her worries and concerns.

Recommend and Negotiate. The staff members make recommendations and negotiate a plan of action, with her involvement and agreement. Mrs Mohammed agrees to the treatment plan and explains that she will have to consult her husband and family, as this is the way that decisions are made within her culture.

The treatment plan

- An appointment will be made for Mrs Mohammed to see the team psychiatrist to review her medication.
- The occupational therapist will see her individually to explore her needs. This will include exploring potential social networks, leisure interests and language courses, and establishing links with the local Muslim community to provide her with social contact and support. She will also be offered the opportunity to contact the imam (Muslim religious priest) who works with the trust.
- Both the team leader and the occupational therapist will offer Mrs Mohammed and her family a set of four family sessions, where mental health and treatment issues can be explored, subject to agreement from her whole family.
- The team leader will offer her some individual sessions to explore and work through her family concerns and personal worries, and to give her education about stress and depression. The team leader is the most appropriate person for this intervention as she is a woman and Mrs Mohammed has mentioned feeling more comfortable speaking to a woman.

Using the Cultural Assessment Checklist (Lim 2001) as a guide, the team now need to establish whether the non-verbal cues and presentations they observed are accurate reflections of the client's mental state. Working down the list, they established that:

- the limited eye contact they have observed from Mrs Mohammed is culturally appropriate rather than being due to lack of confidence
- the lack of decisiveness and assertiveness they perceived during the interview is culturally linked and appropriate to both her Indian and Muslim backgrounds, where all decisions of importance are discussed with elders and family

members before a decision is made, and where being assertive is considered undesirable
- within Mrs Mohammed's family and culture, gender roles and family responsibilities are clearly defined. Any attempts to explore the issue of fulfilling duties around the home, caring for her mother-in-law or accepting help from the CMHT need to be discussed with sensitivity. Cultural perspectives, beliefs, customs and traditions must all be examined when working with Mrs Mohammed and her family
- her reservations about being in contact with other service users must be respected and her request to be put in touch with services that meet her religious and ethnic needs pursued.

The Cultural Assessment Checklist will be used in subsequent assessments of Mrs Mohammed and her needs, and in revisions of the treatment plan.

SUMMARY

Acceptance that the client's interests are paramount is fundamental to working effectively within a transcultural context that promotes cultural sensitivity and competence. Clear lines of communication and a non-judgemental attitude are crucial if staff members are to be sensitive and respectful of the cultural and ethnic beliefs, perspectives, needs and preferences of their clients. Diversity and difference should be celebrated, not frowned upon, and professionals must be aware of their own attitudes, views and stereotypes when meeting with clients and carers whose personal views and life choices are radically different from their own.

The issue of cultural relativity must also be considered, in that any behaviour exhibited must be examined in relation to the cultural context in which it takes place. There are multiple ways of dealing with a situation and no one way is better than another. Ultimately, working successfully within a transcultural context requires a commitment to spending time to listen, acknowledge, respect, clarify, explain, negotiate and work in partnership with each client, carer and family member, to the betterment of their health and well-being.

References

Awaad T 2003 Culture, cultural competency and occupational therapy: a review of the literature. British Journal of Occupational Therapy 66(8): 356-362

Becker HS 1963 Outsiders: studies in the sociology of deviance. Free Press, New York

Berlin E, Fowkes W 1982 A teaching framework for cross-cultural health care. Western Journal of Medicine 139(6): 938-943

Bhugra D, Bahl V 1999 Ethnicity: an agenda for mental health. Royal College of Psychiatrists, London

Blofeld J 2003 Independent inquiry into the death of David Bennett. Suffolk & Cambridgeshire Strategic Health Authority, Norfolk, Norwich

Browne D 1997 Black people and sectioning. Little Rock Publishing, London

Chaing M, Carlson G 2003 Occupational therapy in multicultural contexts: issues and strategies. British Journal of Occupational Therapy 66(12): 559-566

College of Occupational Therapists 2000 Code of ethics and professional conduct for occupational therapists. College of Occupational Therapists, London

College of Occupational Therapists 2006 Recovering Ordinary Lives: the strategy for occupational therapy in mental health services 2007–2017. College of Occupational Therapists, London

Cusack L, Sealey-Lapes C 2000 Clinical governance and user involvement. British Journal of Occupational Therapy 63(11): 539-546

Department of Health 1999 National service framework for mental health. HMSO, London

Department of Health 2000 National Health Service plan. HMSO, London

Department of Health 2003 Race and equality in mental health consultation document. Stationery Office, London

Department of Health 2005a Healthcare Commission census. Stationery Office, London

Department of Health 2005b Delivering Race Equality in Mental Health Action Plan. Stationery Office, London

Department of Health 2005c Delivering race equality in mental health care: an action plan for reform inside and outside services and the Government's response to the independent inquiry into the death of David Bennett. Stationery Office, London

De Silva D 2002 Psychiatric service delivery in an Asian country: the experience of Sri Lanka. International Review of Psychiatry 14: 66-70

Dillard PA, Andonian L, Flores O et al 1992 Culturally competent occupational therapy in a diversely populated mental health setting. American Journal of Occupational Therapy 46(8): 721-726

Fair A, Barnitt R 1999 Making a cup of tea as part of a culturally sensitive service. British Journal of Occupational Therapy 62(5): 199-205

Fitzgerald MH, Mullavey-O'Byrne C, Clemson L 1997 Cultural issues from practice. American Journal of Occupational Therapy 44: 1-21

Greenwood N, Hussain F, Burns T et al 2000 Asian inpatient and carer views of mental health care. Journal of Mental Health 9(4): 397-408

Gross R 2001 Psychology: the science of mind and behaviour, 4th edn. Hodder & Stoughton, London

Hasselkus BR 2002 The meaning of everyday occupation. Slack, New Jersey

Helman CG 2000 Culture, difference and healthcare. Butterworth Scientific, Oxford

Henley A, Schott J 1999 Culture, religion and patient care in a multi-ethnic society. Age Concern Books, London

Hocking C, Whiteford G 1995 Multiculturalism in occupational therapy: a time of reflection on core values. Australian Occupational Therapy Journal 42: 172-175

Howarth A, Jones D 1999 Transcultural occupational therapy in the UK. British Journal of Occupational Therapy 62(10): 451-458

Iwama M 2003 Towards culturally relevant epistemology in occupational therapy. American Journal of Occupational Therapy 57(5)

Iwama M 2004 The Kawa (river) Model: nature, life flow and the power of culturally relevant occupational therapy. In: Kronenberg F, Algado SA, Pollard N (eds) Occupational therapy without borders - learning from the spirit of survivors. Churchill Livingstone, Edinburgh

Iwama M 2005 Occupation as a cross-cultural construct. In: Whiteford G, Wright-St Clair V (eds) Occupation and practice in context. Elsevier, Sydney

Iwama M 2006 The Kawa River Model: culturally relevant occupational therapy. Elsevier Churchill Livingstone, Philadelphia

Kielhofner G 2002 A model of human occupation: theory and application, 3rd edn. Lippincott Williams and Wilkins, Baltimore

Khanna T 2004 End of the road for NHS failures? Occupational Therapy News May: 28-29

King's Fund 2003 London's mental health. King's Fund, London

Law M, Baptiste S, McColl MA et al 1990 The Canadian Occupational Performance Measure: an outcome measure for occupational therapy. Canadian Journal of Occupational Therapy 57(2): 82-87

Leavey G 1999 Suicide and Irish migrants in Britain: identity and integration. International Review of Psychiatry 11(2/3): 168-172

Levy S, Stroessner S, Dweck C 1998 Stereotype formation and endorsement: the role of implicit theories. Journal of Personality and Social Psychology 74: 16-34

Lilja M, Bergh A, Johansson L et al 2003 Attitudes towards rehabilitation needs and support from assistive technology and social environment among elderly people with disability. Occupational Therapy International 10(1): 75-93

Lim KH 2001 A guide to providing culturally sensitive and appropriate occupational therapy assessments and interventions. Mental Health Occupational Therapy 6(2): 26-29

Lim KH 2003 Report on the King's Fund Mental Health Inquiry. Occupational Therapy News 11(3): 15

Lim KH 2004 Occupational therapy in multicultural contexts. British Journal of Occupational Therapy 67(1): 49-50

Lim KH 2005 Partnership, involvement and inclusion. Mental Health Occupational Therapy 10(1): 22-24

Lim KH 2006 Applying the Kawa Model. In: Iwama K (ed) The Kawa River Model: culturally relevant occupational therapy. Elsevier Churchill Livingstone, Philadelphia

Lim KH, Iwama M 2005 Emerging models – an Asian perspective:the Kawa River Model. In: Duncan E (ed) Hagedorn's foundations for practice in occupational therapy. Churchill Livingstone, Edinburgh

MacDonald R 1998 What is cultural competency? British Journal of Occupational Therapy 61(7): 325-328

Macpherson W 1999 The Macpherson Report. HMSO Command Paper No. 4262. HMSO, London

Masi R 1992 Communication: cross-cultural applications of the physician's art. Canadian Family Physician May: 1159-1165

Mattingly C, Garro LC 2000 Narrative and the cultural construction of illness and healing. University of California Press, Berkeley

McGruder J 2001 Life experience is not a disease or why medicalising madness is counterproductive to recovery. Occupational Therapy in Mental Health 17(3/4). 59–80

McGruder J 2003 Culture, race, ethnicity and human diversity. In: Crepeau EB, Cohn ES, Schell BAB (eds) Willard and Spackman's occupational therapy, 10th edn. Lippincott Williams and Wilkins, Baltimore

Mind 2002 Statistics on race, culture and mental health. Mind Publications, London

Office of the Deputy Prime Minister 2004 Social Exclusion and Mental Health Report. Social Exclusion Unit, HMSO, London

Office for National Statistics 2001 National census 2001. HMSO, London

Office for National Statistics 2005 International migration. Stationery Office, London

Paniagua F 1994 Assessing and teaching culturally diverse clients. Sage Publications, London

Reynolds F, Lim KH 2005 The social context of older people. In: McIntyre A, Atwal A (eds) Occupational therapy and older people. Blackwell, Oxford

Richardson P 2004 How cultural ideas help shape the conceptualization of mental illness. Mental Health Occupational Therapy 9(1): 5-8

Sainsbury Centre for Mental Health 2000 Breaking the circle of fear. Sainsbury Centre for Mental Health, London

Santana S, Santana F 2001 Mexican culture and disability. Centre for International Rehabilitation Research Information and Exchange, University of Buffalo, State University of New York, pp1–35

Servan-Schreiber D 2004 Healing without Freud or Prozac. Rodale, London

Secker J, Harding C 2002 African and African Caribbean users' perceptions of inpatient services. Journal of Psychiatric and Mental Health Nursing 9(2): 161-168

Smith HC 2005 'Feel the fear and do it anyway': meeting the occupational needs of refugees and people seeking asylum. British Journal of Occupational Therapy 68(10): 474-476

Sumsion T 2004 Pursuing the client's goals really paid off. British Journal of Occupational Therapy 67(1): 2-9.

Ting-Toomey S 1999 Communicating across cultures. Guilford Press, New York

Townsend E 1999 Enabling occupation in the 21st century: making good intentions a reality. Australian Occupational Therapy Journal 46(4): 147-159

Trivedi P 2002 Racism, social exclusion and mental health: a black user's perspective. In: Bhui K (ed) Racism and mental health. Jessica Kingsley, London, pp71-82

Watson RM 2006 WFOT Congress. Being before doing: the cultural identity (essence) of occupational therapy. Australian Occupational Therapy Journal 53(3): 151-158

Wells SA, Black RM 2000 Cultural competency for health professionals. American Occupational Therapy Association, New York

Wetherell M 1996 Group conflict and the social psychology of racism. In: Wetherell M (ed) Identities, groups and social issues. Sage, London, pp175-238

Whiteford G 2000 Occupational deprivation: global challenge in the new millennium. British Journal of Occupational Therapy 63(5): 200-204

Wilcock AA 2006 An occupational perspective of health. Slack, New Jersey

Wilson M, Francis J 1997 Raised voices. Mind Publications, London

SECTION 5

Occupations

Chapter 15

Mental health and physical activity: enabling participation

Fiona Cole

INTRODUCTION

Evidence for the health benefits of physical activity and the causal link that it protects against cardiovascular disease, obesity, diabetes, hypertension and musculoskeletal disorders has been well established (DoH 2004a). This ensured that regular physical activity has been promoted as a necessary and important component of physical disease prevention, health promotion and improved quality of life for at least the last two decades (Scully et al 1999). However, whilst there had been historical and intuitive knowledge of the mental health benefits of physical activity, research had been less rigorous and interventions using physical activity were not widespread or evidence based.

Fortunately this situation is now substantially changing with the mental health benefits well documented and commitment to increasing participation developing within the NHS (DoH 2004b) and voluntary agencies such as MIND (Grant 2004) and the Mental Health Foundation (2005). Consequently, although occupational therapists may have used exercise and other physical activities such as horticulture or dancing in the past (Wilcock 2001), this more recent evidence base for the mental health benefits, supported by developments in understanding the nature of occupation, provides occupational therapists with the *sine qua non* to include physical activity interventions within their professional domain.

This chapter aims to provide both newly qualified and practising occupational therapists with an understanding of the rationale for doing so in terms of potential benefits to the mental health service user; the role of occupational therapy and ways of implementing physical activity interventions into treatment programmes. It will explore the value of physical activity in the occupational lives of people with mental health problems, and the role of occupational therapy in enabling participation. It aims to demonstrate factors to consider when planning individual and group programmes utilising physical activity and the evidence base that underpins such occupational therapy interventions.

RATIONALE FOR DEVELOPING PHYSICAL ACTIVITY PARTICIPATION

This section will explore the wide-ranging evidence supporting the use of physical activity as a means of improving mental well-being, and justifying its inclusion within occupational therapy programmes.

THE NATURE OF PHYSICAL ACTIVITY

The emphasis on *physical activity* rather than *exercise* in this chapter reflects the evolution of guidelines and recommendations for promoting health (Box 15.1). Health promotion and exercise professionals in the United Kingdom traditionally adopted the guidelines issued by the American College of Sports Medicine in 1978, of a weekly minimum of at least three 20-minute sessions of vigorous intensity exercise (that is, 60% of maximum heart rate) to improve cardiorespiratory and muscular fitness (Dunn & Blair 1997). However, it was recognised that many people dislike vigorous exercise and/or were discouraged by the difficulty of adhering to such a programme, and participation rates in the general population were low.

Subsequent to these recommendations, an emerging consensus grew among epidemiologists, experts in exercise science and health professionals that physical activities need not be of vigorous intensity to improve health. Thus in 1996, the United States Surgeon General (US Department of Health and Human Services 1996) published a seminal report identifying that health benefits appeared to be proportional to the amount of physical activity; thus every increase in activity added some benefit. Through emphasising the *amount* rather than the *intensity* of physical activity, people are given more options for incorporating physical activity into their daily lives, for example through brisk walking or gardening. The promotion of moderate-intensity physical activity was found to offer considerable health gains, particularly to the least fit. These revised guidelines were also adopted by the UK Department of Health in its 1996 Strategy Statement on Physical Activity and are now widely utilised in health promotion fields. See Box 15.2 for physical activity recommendations.

Box 15.1 Physical activity terminology

Physical activity:

'Any force exerted by skeletal muscle that results in energy expenditure above resting level' (Health Education Authority 1994)

'Includes the full range of human movement, from competitive sport and exercise to active hobbies, walking, cycling, or activities of daily living' (DoH 2004a, p81)

Exercise

'Exercise is a subset of physical activity, which is volitional, planned, structured, repetitive and aimed at improvement or maintenance of any aspect of fitness or health' (Health Education Authority 1994)

Moderate intensity physical activities

Raise the heart rate sufficiently to the level where the pulse can be felt and the person feels slightly out of breath. A feeling of increased warmth, possibly accompanied by sweating on hot or humid days.

These include everyday activities such as brisk walking and climbing stairs, certain forms of household chores and occupational tasks, as well as active recreations like swimming and dancing. (DoH 2004a, p26)

Lifestyle activity

Activities that are performed as part of everyday life, such as climbing stairs, walking (for example to work, school or shops) and cycling. They are normally contrasted with 'programmed' activities such as attending a dance class or fitness training session (DoH 2004a, p80)

Box 15.2 Physical activity recommendations for general health benefit (DoH 2004a)

- Adults should achieve a total of at least 30 minutes a day of at least moderate intensity physical activity on 5 or more days of the week
- The recommended levels of activity can be achieved either by doing all the daily activity in one session, or through several shorter bouts of activity of 10 minutes or more. The activity can be lifestyle activity or structured exercise or sport, or a combination of these
- Children and young people should achieve a total of at least 60 minutes of at least moderate intensity physical activity each day
- The recommendations for adults are also appropriate for older adults. Older people should take particular care to keep moving and retain their mobility through daily activity

---

These guidelines, it should be noted, are for the positive impact that participating in physical activity has for the general population on psychological well-being, in addition to chronic physical diseases such as coronary heart disease, stroke, diabetes and some cancers (DoH 2004a). Research is emerging into the type and intensity of physical activity required to benefit mental health problems specifically and will be included later in this chapter.

THE MENTAL HEALTH BENEFITS OF PHYSICAL ACTIVITY

In response to the intuitive knowledge that exercise benefits mental well-being, sport and other physical recreations have been provided in psychiatric institutions since the 19th century. This approach is now supported by quality evidence worldwide. Outcome studies of physical activity interventions varied from demonstrating a statistically significant positive impact (Burbach 1997) to those concluding that links are inconclusive or equivocal (Lawler & Hopker 2001). In recognition of this diversity of research of varied quality, a 3-year project was commissioned in the UK to review the current scientific evidence available on physical activity and mental health, giving priority to evidence from randomised controlled trials, large-scale epidemiological studies and meta-analytic reviews. This culminated in an academic symposium, which agreed consensus statements on the position of current knowledge and was supported by professional and governing bodies such as the British Psychological Society, British Association of Sports and Exercise Sciences, and Exercise England (Grant 2000).

National consensus statements (Grant 2000)

These concluded that physical activity positively influences (to varying degrees) depression, anxiety, emotion and mood, self-esteem and cognitive dysfunction. Further evidence suggests that the most conclusive links are for reducing depression (Biddle & Mutrie 2001) to the extent that in its 2004 guidelines for treating depression, the National Institute for Clinical Excellence recommends exercise for the treatment of mild to moderate depression for patients in primary care settings.

Depression

- There is support for a causal link between exercise and decreased clinical depression.
- Physical activity is associated with a decreased risk of developing clinically defined depression.
- The antidepressant effect of exercise can be of a similar magnitude as that found for other psychotherapeutic interventions.

Anxiety and stress reactivity

- Exercise has a low to moderate anxiety-reducing effect.
- It can reduce long-term anxiety tendencies, and single exercise sessions can reduce short-term anxiety.
- Single sessions of moderate exercise can reduce short-term physiological reactivity to, and enhance recovery from, psychosocial stressors.

Emotion and mood

- Physical activity and exercise have consistently been associated with positive mood.
- Moderate-intensity exercise has a positive effect on psychological well-being.
- Aerobic exercise has a small-to-moderate effect on reducing tension, depression, fatigue and confusion, and improves vigour.

Self-esteem

- Exercise can be used to promote physical self-worth and other physical self-perceptions such as body image. This can be accompanied by improved self-esteem.
- Men and women of all age groups can experience the positive effects of exercise on self-perception. Evidence is greater for children and middle-aged adults.
- Positive effects are likely to be greater for those with initially low self-esteem.

Cognitive functioning

- Fit older adults display better cognitive performance than less fit older adults.
- Small but significant improvements in cognitive functioning occur in older adults who experience an increase in aerobic fitness.

Psychological dysfunction

- Many people with eating disorders undertake high levels of physical activity.
- Participation in physical activity will rarely lead to dependence on exercise. Generally physical activity is the symptom, rather than the cause, of psychological dysfunction.

Role of physical activity with other mental disorders

The most substantial evidence exists for the conditions outlined above, but exercise has also been suggested as an adjunct treatment for other serious illnesses, such as schizophrenia, and for conditions such as alcohol and drug dependence and more general mental malaise.

Schizophrenia

According to Faulkner (2005) evidence is limited and subject to methodological weaknesses (such as small samples of self-selected participants and lack of control groups) but he reports tentative support suggesting that physical activity has potential efficacy in controlling auditory hallucinations, and as a coping strategy for such positive symptoms. He also reviews evidence that cautiously indicates the influence of physical activity on negative symptoms such as depression, low self-esteem and social withdrawal. He suggests that alleviating these symptoms may improve overall quality of life and therefore contribute to relapse prevention. Many interventions for people with schizophrenia are provided by specialist mental health services, away from mainstream resources, yet taking part in everyday activities that people who are assumed to be without mental health problems might participate in is highly valued by some service users. One service user illustrated this by stating that 'the role of swimming is that I can jump in a pool and nobody knows me and I am just another swimmer' (Mental Health Foundation 2000, p79).

Alcohol and drug dependence

There is also some limited evidence for the benefits of physical activity for people with alcohol and illicit drug dependence. Biddle & Mutrie (2001) assert that it does not reduce drinking behaviour in problem drinkers but can be regarded as a lifestyle intervention to promote positive health behaviours and establish self-control and coping strategies. Donaghy & Ussher (2005) recognise the importance of interventions to enable participation in a range of new or previously enjoyed activities in order to contribute to the goal of alcohol rehabilitation of maintaining abstinence or controlled drinking. The small-scale research of Ussher et al (2000, p603) reported that a programme incorporating exercise had a positive impact on the lives of the participants and that 'the occupational therapist was shown to play a pivotal role in promoting fitness-oriented physical activity for those with substance misuse problems'.

Pope (2003) also cites the scarcity of published data concerning the benefits of physical activity amongst illicit drug users, although there is some

suggestion that the improved sleep patterns observed with exercise are of benefit in the withdrawal stage from drugs, and anecdotal evidence of the popularity of physical activity as a therapeutic intervention. Biddle & Mutrie (2001) also suggest that exercise may activate the opioid systems to produce similar pleasurable experiences to drugs. Finally, as noted above, the benefits of physical activity for depression, anxiety and low self-esteem are well accepted and these are also common features of alcohol and drug dependence

Subclinical levels of mental ill health

In addition, Fox et al (2000, p4) note the 'growing recognition of a widespread mental malaise in the general public that is expressed as mild depression, low self-esteem, high stress and anxiety and poor coping'. They suggest, therefore, that increasing physical activity participation may have a substantial impact on the incidence of subclinical levels of mental ill health among the general public. This would also concur with the healthy living messages currently promoted by the Department of Health (2004b).

EXPLANATORY MECHANISMS FOR MENTAL HEALTH BENEFITS OF PHYSICAL ACTIVITY

There is a considerable amount of literature concerning the physiological and psychological influences on psychological well-being, yet the underlying mechanisms that explain these positive effects are not well established (Biddle & Mutrie 2001). In fact, these may vary significantly between individuals as Biddle et al (2000) note, because the person just starting to participate may gain more from psychological mechanisms such as sense of achievement and social support, in contrast to the experienced runner, whose gains may be more physiological through increased levels of neurotransmitters such as endorphins.

Biochemical mechanisms

Examples of biochemical mechanisms include increased production of opioids such as endorphins which, although well reported in the media, has little supporting evidence and appears to require a high-intensity exercise which many people with mental health problems are initially unlikely to achieve (Carless & Faulkner 2003).

Hypotheses citing serotonin discharge with increased physical activity are interesting because the mechanism is comparable with commonly prescribed selective serotonin reuptake inhibitor (SSRI) antidepressant medication which also acts by preventing the reuptake of serotonin by neurons in the brain (Johnsgard 2004). Utilising physical activity may therefore be preferable as treatment because, as Crawford et al (2003) note, a substantial proportion of people with depression are reluctant or unwilling to consider pharmacological intervention, and between 30% and 50% fail to respond to initial treatment with medication.

Physiological mechanisms

The thermogenic hypothesis suggests that increased core body temperature with exercise decreases muscle tension and consequently anxiety, but again evidence is limited (Biddle & Mutrie 2001).

Improved cerebral blood flow and cerebrovascular health, and improved aerobic capacity and nutrient supply to the brain have been cited by Laurin et al (2005) as particular foci of emerging research. They regard them as plausible physiological explanations underlying the positive influence of physical activity on cognition and protection against dementia and Alzheimer's disease. They are optimistic about further research being able to demonstrate a more rigorous relationship.

A comprehensive summary of explanatory mechanisms is provided by Mutrie & Faulkner (2003) and Johnsgard (2004).

However, as Carless & Faulkner (2003) recognise, mental health is determined not just by biological or physiological mechanisms but also by the interaction of these with psychosocial factors. Therefore it would be unreasonable to focus exclusively on the former to explain the impact of physical activity on mental functioning.

Psychosocial benefits

Accumulated evidence into several aspects of mental health improvement asserts that it is factors associated with being physically active, rather than fitness itself, which are responsible for the benefits in short- and long-term mental well-being (Biddle 2000, Morgan 1997). Research evidence suggests that increases in aerobic fitness are not necessary, as people without physiological gains have psychological effects similar to those of subjects who have improved their fitness. Thus, individuals may choose activities that suit them and need not focus on the aerobic effect of training (Martinsen & Stephens 1994). Occupational therapists will understand this because we select 'activities for their potential to engage client interest, participation and enjoyment' (Creek 2003, p23).

The psychosocial mechanisms identified include experiencing a sense of achievement, mastery, self-determination and self-confidence in physical abilities (DoH 2004a). Again this concurs with occupational therapy theory and the *just right challenge* of occupational therapy in that for participation to be meaningful, there must be a feeling of choice or control over the activity, a focus on the task, a sense of challenge from the activity and a sense of mastery (Law 2002, p642). It is also suggested that benefits of physical activity are significantly enhanced by social influences. From research evidence, Carron et al (1999) identify that, because of the fundamental need for interpersonal attachment, exercising in groups or with a supportive family member or friend enhances positive attitudes and mood. This feature was recorded by Birch (2005) in his research into how a 'green gym' could meet occupational needs, as the participants particularly valued the social and teamwork aspects of the activity. He also noted the value of working in the natural environment for its impact on well-being.

Contact with green environments

Finally, intuition, practice experience and some research evidence support the notion that contact with green environments has a positive impact on psychological well-being. Many physical activities will be undertaken outdoors and Pretty et al (2005, p320) propose 'a synergistic benefit' in adopting physical activities whilst at the same time being directly exposed to nature, and refer to this as 'green exercise'. They also acknowledge that these natural settings need not be remote wilderness, but the everyday parks, gardens and open spaces within urban areas. Occupational therapists also are well aware of the importance of environment in the context of clients' occupational lives, for example when utilising the Canadian Model of Occupational Performance (Canadian Association of Occupational Therapists 2002) or the Model of Human Occupation (Kielhofner 2002). Pretty et al (2003) also note that the benefits of horticulture and healing gardens were recognised as early as the Middle Ages, and associated with the development of gardens around hospitals in the Victorian period.

Whilst these activities are clearly within the domain of occupational therapy, the authors still comment that health professionals have not widely adopted horticulture, nature or animal therapy. The exact explanatory mechanisms are still debateable, but one proposition by Kellert & Wilson (1997) is the *biophylia hypothesis* which suggests that there may be some primeval, instinctual preference for nature and natural landscapes. Therefore, closeness to nature increases well-being and can have restorative influences on mental health. Henwood (2003) reviewed research literature and concluded that evidence is extensive on how contact with and appreciation of nature can contribute to well-being and health. This suggests that engagement with nature occurs at multiple emotional and psychological levels, from clearing the head to reflecting upon personal goals and activities in life, through making sense of compatibilities between oneself and chosen respite environments.

HEALTH PROMOTION

Low levels of physical activity have become a major public health issue in most Western societies. In the UK, of particular concern are those who are sedentary or inactive as only 37% of men and 24% of women are sufficiently active to gain any health benefit. For children, accurate data are difficult to collect due to the need for self-report of activity levels, but data suggest that 30% of boys and 40% of girls are not meeting the recommended levels of physical activity, with particular concern regarding some groups such as teenage girls (DoH 2006a). In addition, there are many contemporary threats to children's overall activity levels including greater use of cars to transport children, increased perceptions of the dangers of outdoor play such as stranger danger or traffic, and more sedentary recreational alternatives such as computer games and television (DoH 2004a, p29).

Mortality rates are higher in psychiatric populations, even after excluding suicides and accidents (Cohen & Hove 2001, Osborn 2001). From a MEDLINE-based review, Osborn identified that people with depression have higher rates of cardiovascular disease, including myocardial infarction (MI), than the general population. Not only are people more at risk from depression after MI, but also depression itself increases the risk of infarction and is a predictor of poor prognosis after the event. The Department of Health's (2006b) review of data concluded that users of mental health services, particularly those with schizophrenia and bipolar disorder, are also at an increased risk of diabetes, infections, respiratory disease and obesity. The likelihood of dying from respiratory disease is four times that of the general population. Cohen & Hove's review also indicated that environmental and lifestyle factors contributing to physical ill health are more prevalent in people with severe and enduring mental illness. Unhealthy diet and lack of exercise are also commonplace in this population. Weight gain leading to obesity is also recognised as a significant side-effect of the atypical antipsychotic medications which are effective treatments for schizophrenia (Rethink 2004).

Thus mentally ill people may have poor physical health, but also the impact of their mental illnesses may make it more difficult for them to engage in physical activity. As Faulkner & Biddle (1999) noted, these factors reinforce the need for greater integration between the physical and psychiatric needs of mental health clients. Therefore, as a therapeutic intervention, physical activity is almost uniquely placed to address both the physical and mental health needs of service users.

Prevention of mental illness

As noted in the introduction, physical activity has positive influences on mental health, but it has also been identified as a means of preventing the onset of mental illness (Fox et al 2000). Physical activity can help to reduce the risk of specific conditions such as depression, which is important from a health promotion perspective because it is predicted to become the second most prevalent cause of disability worldwide by 2020 (DoH 2004c).

Promoting physically active behaviour

The psychological benefits of physical activity are also extremely important because these rewards can be critical determinants of people's motivation to be physically active, which is vital to the prevention of other diseases too (DoH 2004a). Reynolds (2001), however, states that health professionals need to be aware that many clients do not know about the levels and types of activity that are beneficial to health and that there are still misconceptions that physical activity needs to be exhausting and unpleasant to be beneficial. The Department of Health (2004b) expressed concern that NHS staff are also not aware of what the current physical activity messages are for both adults and children, which could inhibit the delivery of effective interventions. Reynolds cautions that simply presenting people with information about the health benefits of participating in exercise will rarely motivate a change in behaviour.

Marcus & Forsyth (2003) reinforce this opinion and discuss in detail how psychological theories of motivation can be utilised by physical activity promoters to develop positive changes in behaviour to initiate and maintain participation. They and many other researchers, such as Dunn & Blair (1997), have applied the Stages of Change Model developed by Prochaska & Marcus (1994) to understanding motivation for participation in physical activity. The model recognises the complexity of factors influencing the adoption and maintenance of exercise behaviour, and aims to identify readiness to change in order to select appropriate interventions matched to each stage. For example, those who are inactive may require a more educational approach to identify health benefits and ways of overcoming perceived barriers to participation, whereas those who are regularly active may need interventions designed to avoid relapse, such as dealing with unexpected stressful

events and transforming the new exercise behaviour into an habituated routine. Such research concentrated on sedentary but healthy populations, which may not account for the particular motivational problems of people with mental health problems.

However, for occupational therapists, the language of the model may resonate with Kielhofner's (2002) occupational change perspective within the Model of Human Occupation. This considers the complex processes of change in volition, habituation and performance capacity required to enable a continuum of change from exploration to competence to achievement in occupations (such as physical activity). This suggests that understanding of motivational theories may be useful for occupational therapists, to complement their own specialist knowledge and conceptualisations of clients' occupational needs. Thus, Reynolds (2001) recommends empowering clients to become more active 'through client-centred discussion that clarifies their health values, health fears, perceived barriers to exercise, activity preferences and goals' (p334). This is clearly an approach that occupational therapists will recognise as part of their professional interventions and models of practice.

Standard 1: *National Service Framework for Mental Health*

In the White Paper *Saving Lives: Our Healthier Nation* (DoH 1999a) and the *NHS Plan* (DoH 2000) mental health was targeted as a clinical priority for improving health outcomes. The actions and standards described in the *National Service Framework for Mental Health* (DoH 1999b), which were established in order to achieve these targets, have relevance to promoting physical activity. In particular, Standard 1 includes promoting mental health for all, working with individuals and communities, and recognises that people with physical illnesses have twice the rate of mental health problems compared to the general population. Standard 1 also aims to promote social inclusion and combat discrimination against individuals and groups, identifying a strong link between social exclusion and mental health problems.

Social exclusion and physical activity

This is also a contemporary issue for occupational therapists, especially those taking an occupational science perspective, such as Whiteford (2000) who envisaged that practice should achieve new relevance to both users of services and the unmet needs of society. Whiteford (2000) refers to social exclusion such as the marginalisation of certain groups, such as women, cultural minorities, people with disabilities or those who do not engage in paid work. She labelled it occupational deprivation because of 'preclusion from engagement in occupations of necessity and/or meaning due to factors that stand outside the immediate control of the individual such as poverty, lack of education or unemployment' (Whiteford 2000, p201). This is relevant to occupational therapists and physical activity participation because physical inactivity is associated with low social class, income and educational attainment. Additionally, a Health Education Authority survey (1999) of ethnic minorities found that South Asian and Chinese men and women in England had lower participation rates in physical activities, whether sport, exercise, walking or heavy housework and DIY. Bangladeshi men and women were almost twice as likely as the general population to be classified as sedentary, which clearly has health implications for these groups.

Health professionals need to be aware of such social factors and expectations when planning and delivering services, which requires a departure from the traditional treatment interventions that respond to illness and are delivered within a largely medical framework. A broader range of interventions will need to be provided such as within local health improvement programmes (DoH 1999b). Exercise referral systems offered in primary care are programmes recognised as having potential to promote social inclusion (NHS 2001) but according to research by the Mental Health Foundation (2005, p5), 'exercise therapy is very unlikely to be offered to patients who present to their GP with depression'. Thus, the development of occupational therapy services to promote participation in physical activity, particularly if integrated within community groups, has great potential to address these issues. Hayden (2004)

concurs with this, from an occupational perspective, and advocates the use of community-based occupations to address the social exclusion associated with severe and enduring mental health problems. The Mental Health Foundation (2005) is unequivocal in its assertion that exercise is a normalising and inclusive experience because it is regarded as an activity done by healthy people without the stigma associated with other treatments

PHYSICAL ACTIVITY AS A THERAPEUTIC INTERVENTION

The clinical potential of exercise as a treatment for mental disorders has been thoroughly researched and reviewed. Burbach (1997), in a non-systematic but extensive review, concluded that physical activity interventions may benefit a wide range of mental health problems. A Cochrane review (Crawford et al 2003, p1) stated that research 'without exception, reported positive effects' for exercise as a treatment for depression. The National Institute for Clinical Excellence guidelines for the treatment of depression (National Institute for Clinical Excellence 2004) detail this evidence and report that exercise has a clinically significant impact on mild-to-moderate depressive symptoms, and that structured and supervised programmes should be recommended for people of all ages with mild depression. Notably for occupational therapists who select individualised activities according to people's interests, NICE also report that there was no differential advantage between different types of exercise.

Physical activity may also serve as an effective adjunct treatment for schizophrenia (Faulkner & Biddle 1999) and for anxiety disorders including panic and agoraphobia, for example when combined with cognitive behavioural therapy (Cromarty et al 2004).

Fox et al (2000) identified that physical activity offers not only a treatment for mental illness, but also a means of coping and managing mental illness and of improving quality of life for the mentally ill. Whilst interventions are becoming more widespread (Clyne 2003) physical activity is not routinely considered as a treatment option across mental health services. Faulkner & Biddle (2002, p660) propose that 'the inclusion of physical activity in contemporary mental healthcare is most often as a result of the personal interests, beliefs and determination of either mental health practitioners, service managers or users of the service'. However, if participation in physical activity meets the clients' needs and goals, it can be provided within an occupational therapy context, but it also has the added flexibility that individuals can take on self-responsibility for their exercise routines outside therapeutic environments.

PARTICIPATION IN PHYSICAL ACTIVITY

As already noted, despite the health promotion messages from central government, schools, the media and other agencies, the majority of the UK population does insufficient physical activity to maintain or develop health. Riddoch et al (1998) identified that many individuals have very good intentions and try to become more active, but the general pattern is that the majority find insuperable barriers and eventually relapse into their previous sedentary lifestyle. Since the health benefits of activity are transient, no gain is achieved. An understanding of the nature of such barriers is important for occupational therapists in order to facilitate participation and enable clients/service users to achieve their individual goals (Cole 2003).

Barriers to participation

Occupational therapy intervention may initially need to be directed primarily at overcoming the barriers, prior to working on participation in physical activity itself. Barriers to participation as identified by systematic reviews of evidence are summarised in Table 15.1.

These barriers have been identified for non-clinical populations and there has been little research into the impact of mental health problems specifically on participation in physical activity. However, Table 15.1 suggests that while some

Table 15.1   Barriers to participation in physical activity – research evidence

Barriers	Authors
Poor physical health perceptions Lack of facilities Perceived time constraints Physical injury Lack of social support	Dishman & Buckworth (1997)
Cost Short-term nature of exercise schemes Access to facilities Anxiety	Riddoch et al (1998)
Negative experiences of health gains Personal safety Lack of follow-up at end of organised programmes	Hillsdon et al (1999)
Low self-efficacy Low motivational readiness to change Lack of social support Health perceptions Physical injury Family commitments Financial constraints Poor body image	Biddle & Mutrie (2001)

of these barriers are external to the person, such as access to facilities and cost, the majority are more intrinsic and related to personal attributions. These motivational, emotional and self-perception influences on participation could be significantly exacerbated by mental health problems. For example, with depression, symptoms of lack of energy, enjoyment, motivation and beliefs of hopelessness, lack of control and failure are commonplace. People with anxiety disorders may be preoccupied with apprehension, fear and danger, underestimate their ability to cope and characteristically avoid anxiety-provoking situations. For schizophrenia thought disturbance such as delusions, hallucinations, speech disturbance, difficulties in interpersonal functioning, inappropriate behaviours and emotional responses could significantly challenge the ability to participate in physical activities, particularly those of a social nature. Low self-esteem, which is a self-perception construct, not a formal clinical condition, is closely related to mental illness and frequently accompanies depression and anxiety disorders (Fox 2000). This rating of how well the self is doing, including both worthiness and competence, can therefore have a strong negative influence on the individual's motivation to test out these perceptions through activity. Low self-esteem can be maintained by unhelpful avoidant behaviour associated with negative predictions and anxiety about a situation, self-critical thoughts and depression (Fennell 1999). Thus, fear of failure, underestimation of abilities, and anxiety about undertaking physical activities or the social implications of joining an exercise class, for example, may strongly influence a person's ability to participate.

OCCUPATIONAL THERAPY AND PARTICIPATION IN PHYSICAL ACTIVITY

The therapeutic application of physical activities is of course not unique to occupational therapy, as it is a valued and fundamental part of, for example, physiotherapy (Chartered Society of Physiotherapy 2001) and is increasingly being recognised as relevant to mental health nursing (Faulkner & Biddle 2002). Nor are we the only profession to take a holistic perspective in

collaborating with the client in his care. Yerxa (1994, p588), however, observed that whilst people have been divided into minds and bodies to fit into specialist mental and physical health medical disciplines, occupational therapy education prepares students to 'look at persons as having not only muscles and joints but feelings, perceptions, families, communities and unique patterns of daily activity'. This is important because the traditional Cartesian mind–body dualism, which had been prevalent within the medical community and assumed that the mind and body were separate, may still influence the promotion of a physical activity within a mental health context.

Mutrie (2000) identified that this philosophical assumption leads to a lack of attention to psychological in comparison to physiological issues in research into, and the promotion of, physical activity and that this dualistic tendency still persists in mental and physical health interventions. Faulkner & Biddle (2001) also express concern that there is still a practical adherence to this mind–body dualism, whilst lip service is paid to holistic treatment. If this is the case, it is essential that occupational therapists are able to demonstrate the theoretical underpinning of interventions utilising physical activity because, as an element of occupational performance, it overlaps these physical and mental domains. The occupational therapist also needs an understanding of its utility as a treatment intervention for both physical and mental disorders, and a holistic perspective of the factors that affect a person's ability to participate in the context of their occupational lives.

A consideration of occupational therapy models of practice is appropriate in order to facilitate this understanding, and as an evidence base with which to distinguish the occupational therapy approach. This will be incorporated within the following vignettes of an individual with depression who wished to become more physically active, and also a group programme of walking facilitated by an occupational therapist.

SELECTING PHYSICAL ACTIVITIES

The initiation, maintenance and resumption of many health behaviours, including being physically active, are rarely easy, especially when compounded by the effects of mental illness. Complex psychological, social, environmental and biological factors influence participation (Biddle & Mutrie 2001) which highlight the difficulty of understanding each individual's support needs in order to enable them to undertake physical activities. Occupational therapy intervention with clients will be based upon thorough assessment of individual needs and within the context of the person's overall treatment programme within a mental health team, which should identify these factors. If, when interventions are planned and goals set, participation in physical activities is identified, then it is also necessary to ascertain the motivating factors for the person making these activity choices.

Motivating factors

This is important because the degree to which a person is intrinsically or extrinsically motivated could influence the type of intervention required to overcome participation difficulties. Biddle & Mutrie (2001) concluded that intrinsic motivation is key to sustaining involvement in exercise behaviours; that is, doing something for its own sake, in the absence of external (extrinsic) rewards or pressures. Fun, excitement, social contact and satisfaction are frequently involved and participation is often linked to feelings of self-control or self-determination. In contrast, extrinsic motivation is usually through pressures outside the person's control such as being 'told' to exercise because of being overweight or other health concerns, or 'because it's good for you'. From a psychologist's viewpoint, Biddle & Mutrie suggested that if these external pressures were removed, motivation would decline in the absence of any intrinsic interest. This is analogous to the occupational therapy perspective summarised by Creek (2003, p33) that 'the value that an individual ascribes to an activity influences her/his commitment to spend time on it'. The challenge for the occupational therapist is then to identify as far as possible intrinsically motivating factors to enable participation. This could involve considerable ingenuity because, for example, people with depression may not be able to experience the intrinsic motivator of enjoyment, because of a profound loss of pleasure in life (O'Neal et al 2000).

Valuing participation

Clients of occupational therapy services may wish to increase their participation in physical activity, because a particular form of exercise in itself meets their occupational needs and has value and meaning. As with any occupation, physical activity may fall into one or more of the three broad areas of self-care, productivity and leisure (Canadian Association of Occupational Therapists 2002). For example, a dancer may engage in yoga as a self-care activity to improve her flexibility and control; a postman may build up his walking tolerance in order to return to work; or a person may cycle in order to be able to go out with her friends for leisure and fun at the weekend. These occupations therefore have intrinsic value and also have social, cultural, symbolic and spiritual significance for the individuals (Creek 2003). Goals for occupational therapy intervention will therefore have direct relevance to overcoming the occupational performance deficits currently preventing the person engaging in these occupations.

Physical activity to enable other occupational goals

Physical activity, however, may not necessarily have value and meaning for individuals, yet they may still wish to engage in some form of exercise because they are aware of its mental and physical health benefits or to enable them to achieve other occupational goals. For example, a father may wish to improve his fitness in order to assist with coaching his son's football team or a person trying to remain drug or alcohol free may use exercise as a coping strategy or to improve sleep. These motivations are toward the extrinsic end of the continuum, and participation in physical activities may be more short term and require imaginative choice of activities in order to sustain commitment. For example, if improved fitness or weight loss is the main motivator rather than enjoyment of the activity per se, then the person will not immediately feel the benefit of his efforts. He may not gain immediate positive reinforcement of participating, compared to the person who does the same activity for fun and then experiences immediate reinforcement through enjoyment. The former may need to incorporate his physical activity into his lifestyle, for example through walking to work or to the shops rather than driving, experiencing immediate satisfaction through his achievement rather than the exercise itself. Alternatively, the rewards of a tidy garden, having expended an afternoon's energy digging and mowing the lawn, may be sufficient reinforcement to maintain participation.

These examples illustrate the need to collaborate with the client in order to comprehensively assess his occupational performance needs and plan effectively to achieve them. Occupational therapy models of practice such as the Canadian Model of Occupational Performance (Canadian Association of Occupational Performance 2002) and the Model of Human Occupation (MOHO; Kielhofner 2002) are widely utilised within mental health services to underpin such assessment and support intervention planning.

Types of physical activity

One of the advantages of improving health through physical activity is the wide range of options that are available, and consequently the choice and control that the individual is afforded. However, there is also some limited research that may influence any recommendations that the occupational therapist may negotiate with clients, depending on individuals' goals. Evidence suggests that rhythmic aerobic forms of exercise such as brisk walking, jogging, swimming, cycling or dancing are most effective for overall health gain. For those who are physically fit enough, it appears that competitive sports and vigorous forms of exercise are an important source of psychological well-being (DoH 2004a,b). Research is somewhat equivocal on the benefits of physical activity for particular psychological dysfunctions but may have some relevance here.

Improving self–esteem

There is increasing attention to studies investigating the potential of weight training and other resistance types of exercise to improving self-esteem. It seems that the increased muscle tone and body definition leads to improved physical self-perceptions and body image which are strongly associated with global self-esteem across the lifespan (Carless & Fox 2003).

However, since many people are initially inactive and sedentary, it is also encouraging to note that observable fitness change, as measured by standard tests of fitness, may not be necessary for enhanced self-esteem or improved physical self-perceptions. It is suggested that the feeling that the body is improving through exercise may be sufficient to generate increased perceptions of health, physical competence, fitness and body image (Fox 2000).

Fitness levels

Initial fitness levels need to be considered when choosing activities, as, for example, people with depression typically possess reduced levels of cardiorespiratory fitness compared to mentally healthy individuals (O'Neal et al 2000). They may also have difficulty initiating physical activity and tolerating discomfort during exercise, because of features of the depression. Therefore, it is imperative that the occupational therapist utilises skills of activity analysis and grading to initiate and sustain engagement in the activity. Side-effects of medication such as drowsiness, fatigue and dry mouth are further reasons why a gradual approach is required (Mutrie & Faulkner 2003).

Rhythmic exercises and hearing voices

Another example of exercise type and a particular mental health problem is the anecdotal evidence from service users with psychoses about the benefits of rhythmic activities to distract from hearing voices. As one person noted:

> ... because some of the exercises are repetitive they take over from the repetitive nature of the voices. And, you know, I can, if I'm say, rowing, I can count the number of strokes rather than listen to the voices saying 'dead, dead, dead, dead, dead!' (Mental Health Foundation 2000, p78)

This may, however, be highly individualised and is not yet substantiated by research evidence, but it does suggest that an occupational therapist can utilise the client's expertise in knowing his own illness to identify the types of activity that are most likely to be beneficial. This need for individualised and client-centred programmes will be illustrated in the following vignette of Lisa.

AN INDIVIDUAL PROGRAMME OF UTILISING PHYSICAL ACTIVITY

Lisa is a client of a community mental health team where she was referred by her GP who was becoming increasingly concerned about her deterioration in functioning and social withdrawal associated with depression. She was first diagnosed with this in her early 20s and was treated with antidepressants. Lisa's history showed that she had a difficult adolescence, which started when she was bullied at school. Her parents attended to her material needs, but she says that they never demonstrated any love to her and were very critical of her lack of achievement. She has intermittently experienced depressive symptoms since the first episode, but suspects that her depression started when she was still at school. She is now much improved but her mood is still low and she has not yet been able to fully resume her occupational roles and responsibilities. Lisa is on the Enhanced level of the Care Programme Approach (CPA) (DoH 1999c) and her care co-ordinator is an occupational therapist. She is 35 years old, married with two children aged 8 and 10. She has a part-time job working nights as a care assistant in a residential home but is currently off work due to depression.

Assessment

The occupational therapist had already gathered much information from Lisa about her mental health and how it impacted on her own and family life, for the purposes of assessment for the CPA. However, she still needed to assess Lisa's own perceptions of her occupational competence and the impact of her environments on her occupational adaptation. The therapist therefore chose to administer the Occupational Self-Assessment (OSA; Table 15.2), which is based on the Model of Human Occupation and is designed to 'give voice to the client's perspective and to give the client a role in determining the goals and strategies of therapy' (Kielhofner 2002, p221). This was felt to be important for Lisa who, when depressed, has feelings of being powerless to change and therefore needed *empowering* to take responsibility for herself. The starting point for this was within the supportive environment of a therapeutic relationship with the occupational therapist.

From Lisa's assessment it becomes clear that it is her volitional features, in combination with her environment, that are having most influence on her functioning and activity choices. The therapist was able to develop a conceptualisation of Lisa's difficulties, and then use her clinical reasoning to collaborate with Lisa to develop an intervention plan which would respond to her needs. The occupational therapist would also feed back her assessment to the multidisciplinary team, in order to inform Lisa's overall programme of care. Figure 15.1 is a representation of Lisa's volition.

Planning

As part of the OSA, Lisa selected her priorities for change relating to herself and to her environment. She decided that for herself, she wanted to introduce physical activity back into her lifestyle to enjoy it for its own sake, and also to help with restoring her health. She could clearly remember how much she enjoyed swimming and walking, and how good she felt mentally during and after exercise. Her environmental priority was to gradually increase her social contacts to reduce her sense of isolation.

As noted earlier in this chapter, physical activity has been shown to be an effective treatment for depression but for some people it may not be effective on its own, or other interventions may need to be initiated to lift mood sufficiently prior to engaging in exercise (Cole 2003). The Model of Human Occupation underpinning Lisa's OSA indicates the interrelatedness of factors involved in her occupational performance and suggests why it has been so difficult for her to participate in physical activity, despite her own awareness that she would almost certainly feel better for it. Therefore, for Lisa, physical activity could, at the outset, be regarded as an adjunct treatment, because of the complexity of her situation and her history. For these reasons, she was initially prescribed antidepressants; followed by referral to a cognitive therapist, to challenge her negative beliefs and assumptions about herself. The occupational therapist is responsible therefore for enabling Lisa to achieve her occupational goals within the context of the whole programme offered by the mental health team.

Table 15.2   Outcome of Lisa's Occupational Self-Assessment

MOHO concepts	Items identified by Lisa as being most difficult and most important to her	Comments
Skills/occupational performance	Concentrating on my tasks Taking care of myself Expressing myself to others	Lisa is able to use her skills to manage the household and children, with some help from her husband. However, she does not address her own needs. She has gained weight, and no longer cares about her appearance. She believes that her husband and friends are fed up of her and her depression, so she no longer talks to them about how she feels.
Habituation Roles Habits	Relaxing and enjoying myself Having a satisfying routine	Lisa used to love to go swimming and walking but no longer feels able to. Now she rarely even takes the dog out to the park across the road. She does not participate in any leisure or social activities, and is off work with depression. Once she has completed her household tasks, she 'sits in the chair all day doing nothing'.
Volition Personal causation Values Interests	Doing activities that I like Working towards my goals Accomplishing what I set out to do Effectively using my abilities	Lisa's self-esteem is very low and she believes that she does not deserve to enjoy herself. She is very self-critical and is frightened of setting goals because she fears she will not succeed in attaining them. She does not value herself or her physical appearance and will not therefore go to the swimming pool because of her weight. Her sense of capacity and self-efficacy are challenged, as she perceives that she is not capable of exercising and has 'given up' trying.
Environment Physical/Social	People who support and encourage me people who do things with me	Lisca's relationship with her husband is poor. They no longer go out together. She feels very alone, and avoids contacting her friends and work colleagues because she is ashamed of her depression and need for treatment.

Lisa's occupational therapy programme

It is important that Lisa experiences success to help with her motivation, and improve her sense of capacity and efficacy. Although what she really wanted to do was to go swimming, Lisa realistically knew that this initially would not be an attainable goal. She hoped that by working on her self-esteem with the cognitive therapist, and through practical activities within occupational therapy, longer term she would get to the swimming pool. It is recognised (Shaw & Henderson 2000) that poor physical self-perceptions and body image are common barriers to participation in physical activities such as swimming where one's body is publicly visible, particularly for women.

As a starting point, Lisa decided that one of the activities she wanted to resume, but had been unable to achieve, was gardening. She had in the past enjoyed it and valued having a tidy garden that she could also sit and relax in. The occupational therapist initially helped Lisa in the garden, starting together with some simple weeding and tidying that could be graded according to her energy levels and did not require any complex planning or decision making. Lisa progressed to gardening on her own and the occupational therapist assisted with planning tasks that gradually increased in complexity.

Physical activity was also used to facilitate Lisa's goal of increasing her social contacts. She wanted to meet up with an old friend again, but did not yet feel confident enough to invite her into her home. This friend also had a dog, therefore Lisa arranged to meet her in the park so they could walk together. This fulfilled a dual function

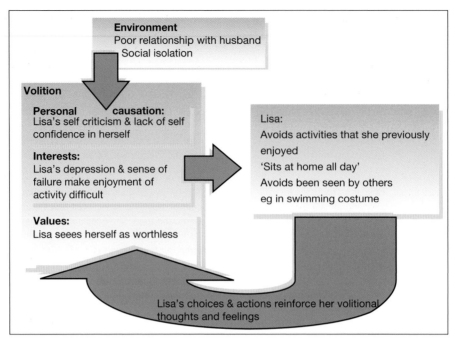

Figure 15.1   Conceptualisation of Lisa's volition based on the Model of Human Occupation. Adapted from Keithofner (2002 p 165)

of establishing regular social interactions, but also helped Lisa overcome her initial lack of motivation and anxiety about walking her dog on her own. As her therapy progressed and confidence in her abilities increased, Lisa achieved further goals and resumed habits such as walking the children to school. The occupational therapist and cognitive therapist liaised with each other and with Lisa in order to support each profession's individual plan and the overall treatment package. For example, Lisa was encouraged by both therapists to keep a diary, to record activity and mood, which thereby reinforced the links between activity and improved mood and gave Lisa positive feedback about the extent of her achievements.

Over time, Lisa felt ready to resume swimming, and initially she was accompanied by the occupational therapist to a women's only session at the local leisure centre. Although she had lost some weight, she had to work hard to overcome her fears about wearing a swimsuit in a public place. However, once she had attended and put her anxious predictions to the test, she found that she did not feel out of place and her anxieties subsided to

a level that allowed her to enjoy herself. As the occupational therapist gradually withdrew her support, Lisa arranged to meet her friend there as she felt that she would also enjoy the social contact in addition to the swimming.

Outcome

Lisa's programme took 6 months of regular sessions with the occupational therapist. Upon discharge, her physical activity had become habituated into her routine, and her depression had lifted significantly. Not surprisingly, in view of the long-term nature of her low self-esteem and depression, she still had issues relating to the personal causation component of volition when reassessed with the OSA, although this had greatly improved. Lisa was extremely pleased with the changes she had made incorporating physical activity into her lifestyle and the associated benefits to her social environment and overall sense of psychological well-being. She was optimistic that she would be able to habitually engage in physical activity as part of her lifestyle and everyday routine.

A PHYSICAL ACTIVITY GROUP

This is an example of a community-based walking group designed to empower mental health service users to participate in a physical activity for the duration of the group, and also to continue with their own programme of activity upon completion of the 12 sessions. It was designed to be facilitated by an occupational therapist and a co-facilitator, who could be from a voluntary organisation such as MIND or a former user of mental health services. Occupational therapists frequently use group-based therapeutic interventions and are aware of the rationale for these, but there is also research evidence (Carron et al 1999) that exercising in groups results in increased adherence and more positive attitudes, in addition to enhanced mood states.

Aims of the group

- To introduce and maintain regular participation in walking as a physical activity.
- To develop personal awareness of the effects of physical activity on the individual's mental and physical health.
- To develop strategies for utilising walking and/ or other activities, both to improve mental well-being and to cope with the effects of mental ill health.
- To enable participants to develop their own routine of regular physical activity outside of the group.
- To provide opportunities for social interaction and improved social confidence.

Objectives

The group met once per week over 12 sessions and included the following objectives for members to achieve:

- participate in weekly walks with the group, including the planning and organisation
- monitor feelings such as mood and anxiety levels before and after the sessions and for the duration of the group, through self-report
- contribute to discussions about incorporating physical activity into their lifestyles

- set individual goals for increasing the amount of physical activity in between sessions
- upon completion of the group, will have a personalised plan for continuation of physical activity as part of their lifestyle.

Venue

The meeting place was in a local community hall away from recognised mental health services, a facility that already included exercise classes such as yoga and badminton.

Evidence base

Walking is the most popular form of physical activity, and the one most likely to allow successful engagement and longer-term adherence (Hillsdon et al 1999). According to Johnsgard (2004, p257) 'nothing can compare to what walking has to offer those of us who are struggling to leave a sedentary life behind' and thus to develop better mental and physical health. Siegel et al (1995) also identify a unique epidemiological feature of walking which is relevant to the previous discussion of social inclusion. Whereas low socio-economic status is associated with decreased physical activity participation, walking for exercise has been shown to be as prevalent among people with low as with high family incomes. Walking is accessible, convenient, economical, easily graded and offers an ideal opportunity for socialising (Johnsgard 2004; Walking the Way to Health Initiative).

Type of walk

Motivation problems in *getting going* have been identified as barriers to participation in physical activity, therefore *doorstep walks* were chosen; that is, those that are within easy reach of people's homes and do not, for example, require complicated travel or other arrangements to be overcome (Walking the Way to Health Initiative). This type of walking is also accessible in terms of minimal financial expenditure; it does not require specialist equipment or skills, and it can be graded to allow people of initial low levels of fitness to commence participation and achieve success.

Group discussion

As noted earlier in the chapter, participation rates for physical activities for the general population are very low, and people with mental health problems have additional challenges to overcome. Therefore it is important to provide group activities that will facilitate both initial engagement and longer-term adherence to activity. From a randomised control trial in a socially and economically deprived community, Lowther et al (2002) concluded that those participants who received 'exercise consultations' had the best longer-term adherence, for those initially not regularly active. Within the group sessions, these consultations were in the form of discussions about exercise preferences to identify likes and dislikes; the advantages and disadvantages of change; barriers to change; social support available; goal-setting; and relapse prevention. The group also discussed developing support from both health professions and family and friends which has been widely identified in the literature as important to maintaining participation (Biddle & Mutrie 2001, Riddoch et al 1998).

Assessment of risks

As a starting point for the walking, a prerequisite for the group was that each individual could walk briskly for at least 15 minutes. Personal safety is also a consideration and because aims included members continuing to walk independently of the group, this was covered in group discussion, including suggestions to walk with a friend/companion wherever possible. This not only promoted safety, but also provided the additional social benefits and enjoyment of the walk identified by authors such as Carron et al (1999).

A risk assessment was carried out for the group following the NHS trust's health and safety guidelines. This particular group was considered to be low risk because of the type of walking, accessibility of support if necessary in the locality, and because the key worker for each client assessed him/her for clinical risk prior to referral to the group. All groups or individual programmes of activity will need assessing for the degree of risk, and for some this will include physical health screening and/or medical approval to participate. Clyne (2003) describes such requirements in detail including fitness testing, or screening tools such as the Physical Activity Readiness Questionnaire, which are important in risk assessment and management. The Chief Medical Officer (DoH 2004a, p73) identifies risks but states that the risks associated with taking part in physical activity at levels that promote health are low. However, his key points are important to recognise when planning programmes.

- Higher risks occur predominantly among those exercising at vigorous levels and those taking part in contact sports and high-volume fitness training.
- People with low levels of habitual physical activity, who are unfit or who have existing disease, should pay particular attention to increasing activity levels gradually.
- People with pre-existing musculoskeletal disease have a higher risk of injury caused by physical activity.
- Adolescents are generally prone to ligament and muscle injuries due to rapid changes in body composition during the growth spurt.
- People with eating disorders may use physical activity as a further means of weight control. The frequency and intensity of exercise are often excessive and likely to be counterproductive to health.
- Exercise addiction is extremely rare and is likely to be a consequence of persistent underlying psychological dysfunction.

The Chief Medical Officer concludes, however, that the health benefits of activity far outweigh the risks.

Format of the group

Each session included a discussion, followed by a walk. Topics included:

- understanding the benefits of physical activity, the amount and intensity required for health

- strategies for overcoming lethargy, motivational problems and other barriers to participation
- dealing with anxieties and other concerns
- setting personal goals, short and longer term
- self-monitoring of physical and mental health with exercise
- active living, how to incorporate physical activity into one's daily routine
- practical issues, clothing, safety, wet weather alternatives
- route planning
- planning for the end of the group, how to sustain participation and take part in other community resources.

The walk was planned with group members and graded from an initial 15 minutes, increasing by approximately 10 minutes duration each week, up to a maximum of 1 hour. This was an initial guideline and would of course need to be flexible, depending on the membership and fitness levels of the group. Walks included the local park and riverside which were accessible from the town centre. The definition of a *health walk* was followed; that is, a purposeful, brisk walk undertaken on a regular basis (Walking the Way to Health Initiative).

Self-monitoring: charts and diaries

Experiencing the mental health benefit of physical activity was a prime focus of the group so it was important for individuals to monitor their own feelings and moods during and after the walk. Therefore individuals kept a chart of the intensity and type of their feelings as shown in Table 15.3.

The group aimed to increase activity levels so this needed to be measured, in order to give feedback and reinforcement to the participant, and also serve as an outcome measure for the group's effectiveness. A diary of time spent on physical activities was kept on a weekly basis, and individuals were encouraged to include not only walking of any type, for example to the shops, but also other activities such as DIY, gardening or active leisure pursuits (Table 15.4). Personal goal-setting included identifying means of gradually increasing activity over the course of the group.

Preparing for discharge from the group

One aim of the group was that individuals would be able to continue exercising independently, incorporating it into their routines and lifestyles, so it was important to prepare for this. Members were encouraged to find out information on local activities and share them with the group, making individual arrangements to try them out together if they wanted to. In addition, there are certain nationwide initiatives to encourage participation in physical activity, such as Walking the Way to Health Initiative and green gyms (Reynolds 2002) (Box 15.3). Members collected weekly route plans drawn onto the local town map that they could keep on discharge for future reference, and to share with friends and family whom they may wish to encourage to walk with them.

The group was evaluated from the perspectives of the individual members by comparing records of psychological well-being when active (see Table 15.3) and by using the physical activity record to measure activity levels at the beginning and end of the programme (see Table 15.4). Evaluation of the group as a whole was through client feedback and self-report of their experiences, and their recommendations for future groups.

LIFESTYLE PHYSICAL ACTIVITY

Health-promoting agencies such as the former Health Development Agency (now within the National Institute for Health and Clinical Excellence – NICE) and the Health Education Board for Scotland have recognised the utility of advocating an active living or lifestyle approach to increasing participation in physical activity. Activity then becomes part of an everyday routine rather than something to be planned and arranged specifically for the purpose of gaining exercise, which many individuals may not regard as having sufficient value and meaning to justify the effort of participating. Active travel, for example, incorporates walking and cycling as part of everyday journeys to work, school and local services. Clients can gain further support in achieving participation via linking in with local programmes, for example the *walking buses* that are part of Safer Routes to School (Transport 2000 Trust 1999). The

Table 15.3   An example of self-monitoring psychological well-being and physical activity

	How do I feel? Before activity	Rate 1–10	How do I feel? After activity	Rate 1–10	Comments
Week 1	Anxious Frightened	8 8	Anxious Frightened	4 2	I was worried about meeting new people and about being left behind in the walk. I feel much better now, I enjoyed it
Week 2	Tired and lethargic	9	Refreshed	6	I really struggled to get out of bed this morning, and thought about not coming. I feel much more awake after the walk
Week 3					
Week 4					
Week 5					
Week 6					
Week 7					
Week 8					
Week 9					
Week 10					
Week 11					
Week 12					

Rate where 1 is as low as it could feel, and 10 is the highest intensity of feeling

UK government has identified that a health and social care system in which advice and support for physical activity are an integral part would help people lead healthier lives. The Activity Menu for Adults and Children has been devised to demonstrate ways in which physical activity can be incorporated into people's lifestyles (DoH 2004b, p6) (Table 15.5).

Of relevance in the Department of Health's consultation document (2004b) is the goal for health professionals to increase the provision of advice to patients on lifestyle, particularly on physical activity, both routinely and opportunistically. Occupational therapists have the credentials to meet this goal because this lifestyle activity approach resonates with the way we consider activities within the context of individuals'

occupational lives. One relevant theoretical perspective to support this is the Model of Human Occupation (Kielhofner 2002), in particular the habituation component. This is the taken-for-granted everyday routine of life, which Kielhofner (p22) defined as: 'an internalised readiness to exhibit consistent patterns of behaviour guided by our habits and roles and fitted to the characteristics of routine temporal, physical and social environments'.

Patterns of attitude and action develop as people repeatedly interact with the various characteristics of these contexts. Eventually the pattern becomes established and active choice is no longer required, thus potentially enabling routine participation in physical activity. Walking to work rather than driving, for example, could become routine so that the person

Table 15.4 Physical activity record

	Monday	Tuesday	Wednesday	Thursday	Friday	Saturday	Sunday	Total minutes this week
Week 1								
Week 2								
Week 3								
Week 4								
Week 5								
Week 6								
Week 7								
Week 8								
Week 9								
Week 10								
Week 11								
Week 12								

At the end of each day record the total amount of walking or other physical activity that you did. Make a note of anything of 10 minutes' duration or more.

Box 15.3 Examples of community resources utilising physical activity

Green gyms
Green gyms are run by the British Trust for Conservation Volunteers, a large conservation charity in the UK. The groups offer a way of keeping fit and engaging in physical activity in the open air through practical work such as clearing woodland, repairing walls, fences and footpaths, or building community or wildlife gardens. They have been established across the UK, in recognition of the potential of using the natural environment as a health resource, accessible to people who would not wish to attend traditional gym-based exercise schemes. The BTCV facilitates the formation of local green gyms, offering training and support, with the ultimate aim that they are sustained by local community groups, often in partnership with NHS primary care trusts or local authorities who can then refer clients to them for physical or mental health reasons (Reynolds 2002). There has been only limited research into their use within occupational therapy programmes, but Birch (2005) identified that participants valued the green gym as a means of enhancing mental well-being and that this mainstream form of volunteering can be utilised as a means of achieving occupational needs.

The Walking the Way to Health Initiative
The Walking the Way to Health Initiative aims to encourage more people to walk in their own communities, especially those who take little exercise or live in areas of poor health. Although supported by the British Heart Foundation and Natural England, it also advocates walking for its mental health benefits, and also aims to improve the quality of life for those most disadvantaged in society. Walks are accessible to where people live and aim to be achievable for those with low fitness levels; that is, they are usually flat and no more than 1.5–2 miles. Many are also designed to enable people with pushchairs, prams, etc. to bring their children, and are at a pace to allow socialisation between walkers (Walking the Way to Health Initiative). In a national evaluation of the first 5 years of the led walks of the programme (2000–2005), the researchers (Dawson et al 2006) identified vital functions of significantly contributing to physical activity levels, and increased opportunities for social contact. Of particular interest is their evidence suggesting that the walks can offer social-psychological support or an opportunity for rehabilitation (physical or mental health) without necessarily drawing attention to these features.

Table 15.5 Activity Menu for Adults and Children/ young people (adapted from DoH 2004b)

30 minutes on 5 days a week for adults	Organised activity in clubs such as football, badminton and judo
	Walking/cycling to work, school or social events
	Therapeutic exercise – referral by a health professional
	Weekend family activity, e.g. trips to the countryside and parks for walks
	Informal activity with friends, e.g. dancing, skateboarding, swimming
	Occupational (work-related) activity
	School breaks, lunchtime and after-school active playground time
	Quality PE and school sport
	Recreational walking, dancing, cycling
	Individual activity, e.g. jogging, swimming, aerobic
	Volunteering and leadership activities

(right side label: 60 minutes every day for young people)

can do it without consideration or concern and thereby achieve his daily 30 minutes of moderate activity. Occupational therapists can use their ingenuity to collaborate with clients to habituate them to more physically active lifestyles and thus achieve and sustain mental and physical health benefits.

SUMMARY

Increasing participation in physical activity is clearly high on the public health agenda in recognition of the benefits to mental and physical health. Providers of mental health services can also play a significant role incorporating physical activity into programmes both from a health promotion perspective and as a treatment. Overcoming the barriers to participation and sustaining an ongoing and active lifestyle can be extremely challenging for service users. However, occupational therapists are uniquely placed to utilise their theoretical knowledge and skills to work with individuals, groups and other members of the multidisciplinary team to enable successful engagement in physical activity.

References

Biddle SJH 2000 Emotion, mood and physical activity. In: Biddle SJH, Fox KR, Boutcher SH (eds) Physical activity and psychological well-being Routledge London, pp63–87

Biddle SJH, Mutrie N 2001 Psychology of physical activity. Determinants, well-being and interventions. Routledge, London

Biddle SJH, Fox KR, Boutcher SH, et al 2000 The way forward for physical activity and the promotion of psychological well-being. In: Biddle SJH, Fox KR, Boutcher SH (eds) Physical activity and psychological well-being. Routledge, London, pp154-168

Birch M 2005 Cultivating wildness: three conservation volunteers' experiences of participation in the Green Gym Scheme. British Journal of Occupational Therapy 68(6): 244-252

Burbach FR 1997 The efficacy of physical activity interventions within mental health services: anxiety and depressive disorders. Journal of Mental Health 6(6): 543-566

Canadian Association of Occupational Therapists 2002 Enabling occupation. An occupational therapy perspective. CAOT Publications, Ottawa

Carless D, Faulkner G 2003 Physical activity and mental health. In: McKenna J, Riddoch C (eds) Perspectives on health and exercise. Palgrave Macmillan, Basingstoke, pp 61-82

Carless D, Fox K 2003 The physical self. Everett T, Donaghy M, Feaver S (eds) Interventions for mental health. An evidence-based approach for physiotherapists and occupational therapists. Butterworth Heineman, Edinburgh, pp69-81

Carron AV, Hausenblas HA, In: Estabrooks PA 1999 Social influence and exercise involvement. In: Bull SJ (ed) Adherence issues in sport and exercise. John Wiley, Chichester, pp1-17

Chartered Society of Physiotherapy 2001 Exercise referral systems: a national quality assurance framework. CSP Policy Briefing Government Initiatives. Chartered Society of Physiotherapy, London

Clyne A 2003 Adoption of physical activity in hospital and community settings. In: Everett T, Donaghy M, Feaver S (eds) Interventions for mental health. An evidence-based approach for physiotherapists and occupational therapist. Butterworth Heinemann, Edinburgh, pp98–108

Cohen A, Hove M 2001 Physical health of the severe and enduring mentally ill. A training pack for GP educators. Sainsbury Centre for Mental Health, London

Cole F 2003 Physical activity for its mental health benefits: how can occupational therapists enable participation? Unpublished MSc Thesis, Lancaster University. Available from College of Occupational Therapists library

Crawford MJ, McGuire H, Moncrieff J et al 2003 Exercise therapy for depression and other neurotic disorders (protocol for a Cochrane Review). The Cochrane Library, Issue 1. Update Software, Oxford

Creek J 2003 Occupational therapy defined as a complex intervention. College of Occupational Therapists, London

Cromarty P, Robinson G, Callcott P 2004 Cognitive therapy and exercise for panic and agoraphobia in primary care: pilot study and service development. Behavioural and Cognitive Psychotherapy 32: 371-374

Dawson J, Boller I, Foster C, et al 2006 Evaluation of changes to physical activity amongst people who attend the Walking the Way to Health Initiative (WHI). Countryside Agency, Cheltenham

Department of Health 1999a Saving lives: our healthier nation. Department of Health, London

Department of Health 1999b National service framework for mental health. Department of Health, London

Department of Health 1999c Effective care coordination in mental health services: modernising the care programme approach – a policy booklet. Department of Health, London

Department of Health 2000 The NHS plan. Department of Health, London

Department of Health 2004a At least five a week. Evidence of the impact of physical activity and its relationship to health. A report from the Chief Medical Officer. Department of Health, London

Department of Health 2004b Choosing health? Choosing activity. A consultation on how to increase physical activity. Department of Health, London

Department of Health 2004c Health and personal social services statistics for England. Office for National Statistics, London

Department of Health 2006a Health Challenge England factsheets. Factsheet on physical activity. Department of Health, London

Department of Health 2006b Choosing health: supporting the physical health needs of people with severe mental illness. Commissioning framework. Department of Health, London

Dishman RK, Buckworth J 1997 Adherence to physical activity. Morgan WP (ed) Physical activity and mental health. Taylor and Francis, Washington

Donaghy M, Ussher M 2005 Exercise interventions in drug and alcohol rehabilitation. In: Faulkner GEJ, Taylor AH (eds) Exercise, health and mental health. Emerging relationships. Routledge London, pp48-69

Dunn AL, Blair SN 1997 Exercise prescription. In: Morgan WP (ed) Physical activity and mental health. Taylor and Francis Washington, pp49-62

Faulkner GEJ 2005 Exercise as an adjunct treatment for schizophrenia. In: Faulkner GEJ, Taylor AH (eds) Exercise, health and mental health. Emerging relationships. Routledge, London, pp27-47

Faulkner G, Biddle SJH 1999 Exercise as an adjunct treatment for schizophrenia: a review of the literature. Journal of Mental Health 8(5): 441-457

Faulkner G, Biddle S 2001 Exercise and mental health: it's just not psychology! Journal of Sports Sciences 19: 433-444

Faulkner G, Biddle S 2002 Mental health nursing and the promotion of physical activity. Journal of Psychiatric and Mental Health Nursing 9: 659-665

Fennell MJV 1999 Overcoming low self-esteem: a self-help guide using cognitive behavioural techniques. Constable and Robinson, London

Fox K 2000 The effects of exercise on self-perceptions and self-esteem. In: Biddle S, Fox K, Boutcher S (eds) Physical activity and psychological well-being. Routledge, London, pp88-117

Fox KR, Boutcher SH, Faulkner GE, et al 2000 The case for exercise in the promotion of mental health and psychological well-being. In: Biddle SJH, Fox KR, Boutcher SH (eds) Physical activity and psychological well-being. Routledge London, pp1-9

Grant T (ed) 2000 Physical activity and mental health: national consensus statements and guidelines for practice. Health Education Authority, London

Grant T 2004 The Mind guide to physical activity. Mind, London

Hayden R 2004 Social Inclusion through occupation in community mental health. In: Molineux M (ed) Occupation for occupational therapists. Blackwell, Oxford, pp122-136

Health Education Authority 1994 Moving on: international perspectives on promoting physical activity. Health Education Authority, London

Health Education Authority 1999 Active for life: promoting physical activity with black and ethnic minority groups (guidelines). Health Education Authority, London

Henwood K 2003 Environment and health: is there a role for environmental and countryside agencies in promoting benefits to health? NHS Health Development Agency, London

Hillsdon M, Thorogood M, Foster C 1999 A systematic review of strategies to promote physical activity. In: MacAuley D (ed) Benefits and hazards of exercise. BMJ Books London, pp25-4

Johnsgard K 2004 Conquering depression and anxiety through exercise. Prometheus Books, New York

Kellert SR, Wilson EO (eds) 1997 The biophylia hypothesis. Island Press, Washington DC

Kielhofner G 2007 Model of human occupation. Theory and application, 4th edn. Lippincott Williams and Wilkins, Baltimore

Laurin D, Verreault R, Lindsay J 2005 Physical activity and dementia. In: Faulkner GEJ, Taylor AH (eds) Exercise, health and mental health. Emerging relationships. Routledge London, pp11-26

Law M 2002 Participation in the occupations of everyday life. American Journal of Occupational Therapy 56(6): 640-649

Lawler DA, Hopker SW 2001 The effectiveness of exercise as an intervention in the management of depression: systematic review and meta-regression analysis of randomised controlled trials. BMJ 322: 1-8

Lowther M, Mutrie N, Scott E 2002 Promoting physical activity in a socially and economically deprived community: a 23 month randomised control trial of fitness assessment and exercise consultation, Journal of Sports Science 20(7): 577-588

Marcus BH, Forsyth LH 2003 Motivating people to be physically active. Physical Activity Intervention Series. Human Kinetics, Champaign, Illinois

Martinsen EW, Stephens T 1994 Exercise and mental health in clinical and free-living populations. In: Dishman RK (ed) Advances in exercise adherence. Human Kinetics, Champaign, Illinois, pp55–72

Mental Health Foundation 2000 Strategies for living. A report of user-led research into people's strategies for living with mental distress. Mental Health Foundation, London

Mental Health Foundation 2005 Up and running. Exercise therapy and the treatment of mild or moderate depression in primary care. Mental Health Foundation, London

Morgan WP 1997 (ed) Physical activity and mental health. Taylor and Francis, Washington

Mutrie N 2000 The relationship between physical activity and clinically defined depression. In: Biddle SJH, Fox KR, Boutcher SH (eds) Physical activity and psychological well-being. Routledge, London, pp46-62

Mutrie N, Faulkner G 2002 Physical activity and mental health.In: Everett T, Donaghy M, Feaver S (eds) Interventions for mental health. An evidence-based approach for physiotherapists and occupational therapists. Butterworth Heinemann Edinburgh, pp82-97

National Health Service 2001 Exercise referral systems: a national quality assurance framework. Department of Health, London

National Institute for Clinical Excellence 2004 Depression: management of depression in primary and secondary care. National Clinical Practice Guideline 23. NHS, London

O'Neal H, Dunn A, Martinsen E 2000 Depression and exercise. International Journal of Sport Psychology 31: 110-135

Osborn D 2001 The poor physical health of people with mental illness. Western Journal of Medicine 175: 329-332

Pope C 2003 Illicit drug misuse. In: Everett T, Donaghy M, Feaver S (eds) Interventions for mental health. An evidence-based approach for physiotherapists and occupational therapists. Butterworth Heinemann, Edinburgh, pp231-238

Pretty J, Griffin M, Sellens M et al 2003 Green exercise: complementary roles of nature, exercise and diet in physical and emotional well-being and implications for public health policy. University of Essex Centre for Environment and Society Colchester

Pretty J, Peacock J, Sellens M et al 2005 The mental and physical health outcomes of green exercise. International Journal of Environmental Health Research 15(5): 319-337

Prochaska JO, Marcus SH 1994 The transtheoretical model: applications to exercise. In: Dishman RK (ed) Advances in exercise adherence. Human Kinetics, Champaign, Illinois

Rethink 2004 Only the best. Rethink, London

Reynolds F 2001 Strategies for facilitating physical activity and well-being: a health promotion perspective. British Journal of Occupational Therapy 64(7): 330-336

Reynolds V 2002 Well-being comes naturally: an evaluation of the BTCV Green Gym at Portslade, East Sussex. Oxford Centre for Health Care Research and Development, Oxford

Riddoch C, Puig-Ribera A, Cooper A 1998 Effectiveness of physical activity promotion schemes in primary care: a review. Health Education Authority, London

Scully D, Kraemer J, Meade M et al 1999 Physical exercise and psychological well-being. MacAuley D (ed) Benefits and hazards of exercise. BMJ Books, London, pp200-225

Shaw S, Henderson K 2000 Physical activity, leisure and women's health. In: Sherr L, St Lawrence J (eds) Women, health and the mind. John Wiley, Chichester, pp339-354

Siegel PZ, Brackbill RM, Heath GW 1995 The epidemiology of walking for exercise: implications for promoting activity among sedentary groups. American Journal of Public Health 85(6): 706-710

Transport 2000 Trust 1999 A safer journey to school. Transport 2000 Trust, London

US Department of Health and Human Services 1996 Physical activity and health. A report of the Surgeon General (Executive Summary). Superintendent of Documents, Pittsburgh, PA

Ussher M, McCusker M, Morrow V et al 2000 A physical activity intervention in a community alcohol service. British Journal of Occupational Therapy 63(12): 598-604

Walking the Way to Health Initiative. Available online at: www.whi.org.uk

Whiteford G 2000 Occupational deprivation: global challenge in the new millennium. British Journal of Occupational Therapy 63(5): 200-204

Wilcock A 2001 Occupation for health, vol 1. A journey from self-health to prescription. British Association and College of Occupational Therapists, London

Yerxa E 1994 Dreams, dilemmas, and decisions for occupational therapy practice in a new millennium: an American perspective. American Journal of Occupational Therapy 48(7): 586-589

Chapter **16**

Cognition and cognitive approaches in occupational therapy

Edward A. S. Duncan

INTRODUCTION

Cognition (derived from the Latin *cognoscere* 'to know') focuses on the broad area of how people (and computers) process and understand information. The field of cognition is vast and has significant influence in a range of applications. These include, but are not restricted to, philosophy, pedagogy, linguistics and computer science. Another area in which cognition has had a significant impact – and one of direct relevance to this chapter – is psychology. Such has been the breadth and depth of developments within the field of cognition in psychology that it is understandably viewed as the current dominant model of understanding.

The breadth of research and information that exists regarding cognition can at times appear both abstract and overwhelming. This chapter aims to give a practical overview of the importance and position of cognition in occupational therapy in mental health. Specifically with regard to human beings and their inherent occupational nature, the role and impact of cognition are perhaps most easily understood by examining what happens when a person's cognitive functioning is impaired. Two areas where cognitive impairment can significantly affect an individual's occupational functioning are organic brain syndrome and psychiatric disorders.

ORGANIC BRAIN SYNDROME

Organic brain syndrome is a descriptive term used to categorise a range of predominantly physical disorders, all of which impact upon cognitive functioning. These include degenerative disorders (e.g. Creutzfeldt–Jakob disease or Huntington's chorea), cardiovascular disorders (e.g. cerebrovascular disease; strokes) and traumatic brain injury (e.g. subarachnoid or intracerebral haemorrhage) amongst other conditions. Due to the physical disorder focus of these conditions, this chapter does not consider their cognitive limitations in any greater depth. Interested readers are directed to other sources of information where these issues are considered further (Turner et al 2002).

PSYCHIATRIC DISORDERS

Three broad categories of psychiatric disorder all have cognitive impairments: dementia, psychosis and affective disorders.

Dementia

Dementia is a psychiatric disorder typified by the gradual decline in cognitive functioning. This occurs due to differing variations of dementia (see Chapter 24) which cause brain changes greater than would be expected through normal ageing. Specific changes that could be expected in a person with dementia include memory loss, attention deficits, problem-solving difficulties and later disorientation of time, place and person.

Psychoses

Psychoses is an umbrella term used to describe various forms of schizophrenia, manic depressive psychoses and psychoses not otherwise specified. People living with these conditions will frequently experience a range of functional cognitive deficits including attention deficits, memory problems, verbal functioning and abstract problem solving. Research into cognitive deficits in psychoses indicates that performance in a range of psychological assessments is predictive of an individual's ability to function in the community (Green 1996). Evidence also suggests that cognitive functioning

in people with psychosis declines significantly more over time than in people who do not have such illnesses (Morrison et al 2006). Given the direct connection between cognitive functioning and community living, the importance of maintaining cognitive functioning for this population cannot be overestimated. This has led to the development of a specific occupational therapy approach (discussed below) to help clients with psychosis to maintain and potentially improve their cognitive functioning.

Affective spectrum disorders

Affective spectrum disorder is an umbrella term for a wide range of psychiatric disorders. These include relatively common conditions such as general anxiety disorder and clinical depression, amongst others. Research into the cognitive deficits of people who experience anxiety suggests that their functional performance is limited due to attentional deficits, selective attentional hypervigilance and memory difficulties. Individuals who experience depression also experience cognitive dysfunction, including loss of concentration and memory problems, amongst others. A person's clinical depression or anxiety problems are thought to be closely linked to his cognitive thinking pattern and this hypothesis has proven fundamental to the development of cognitive behaviour therapy which is discussed below in greater depth.

OCCUPATIONAL THERAPY AND COGNITIVE FUNCTIONING

Within occupational therapy, therapists should always consider a client's cognitive functioning as part of their overall assessment of a person's needs. An assessment of a client's cognitive functioning is a central component of many therapists' observational assessments, either in hospital settings or in the client's natural environment. While such unstructured observational assessments may be sufficient for certain purposes, various standardised assessments also exist. These can be used if a therapist is looking for a detailed assessment of a client's cognitive abilities or if she wishes to measure the effect of an intervention on a client's cognitive functioning. Such tests include Doors and People (which tests memory) (Baddeley et al 1994), the Test of Everyday Attention (which does what it says in the title!) (Robertson et al 1994) and specific occupational therapy assessments such as the Assessment of Motor and Process Skills (Fisher 2003).

As well as unstructured and structured assessments of cognition in occupational therapy, therapists use two approaches which focus in a particular way on the impact of cognition on clients' functional performance. These are the cognitive behavioural approach and the Functional Information-Processing Model. An introduction to both approaches and their role in occupational therapy practice is given below. Interested readers are encouraged to use the reference list to broaden their reading should they be particularly interested in either approach as space limitations only enable a general overview to be given in this chapter.

THE COGNITIVE BEHAVIOURAL APPROACH

Background

Cognitive behavioural therapy (CBT) is a popular and evidence-based psychotherapeutic approach. Citing ancient Greek thought as providing its historical roots, current developments emanate from the modern theoretical frameworks of behavioural therapy and cognitive therapy (see Hawton et al 1996 for further discussion of the history of CBT). Contemporary cognitive behaviour therapy has developed significantly over three decades and now represents a broad church of theoretical developments, interventions and professional groupings (British Association of Behavioural and Cognitive Psychotherapies 2003). Whilst CBT is often associated with the work of psychologists it is, in fact, a theoretical approach shared by a variety of health professionals, including occupational therapists.

CBT's robust and developing evidence base has consistently drawn occupational therapists to use it in practice (see Duncan 2006 for an overview of the development of CBT in occupational therapy). Due to its strong evidence base in a variety of contexts (e.g. anxiety, depression and psychosis) (DoH 2001), CBT has become an increasingly popular method of intervention and has swiftly developed over the last 20 years. As well as having a strong evidence base for practice in the forenamed conditions, CBT is often associated with interventions to address alcohol abuse (e.g. Longabaugh & Morgenstern 1999), personality disorders (e.g. Young 1999), family therapy (e.g. Epstein 2003) and drug abuse (e.g. Beck et al 1993). As well as conditions traditionally found within the mental health spectrum of interventions, CBT has also been positively associated with various other conditions including chronic pain (Strong 1998) and chronic fatigue syndrome (Prins et al 2001).

However, whilst the strong evidence base has attracted occupational therapists to employ its techniques, this has led to the potential for therapists to become general mental health practitioners and not use their core occupational therapy skills. This has been cited as a professional concern and considerable debate has taken place and continues regarding the appropriateness of occupational therapists' use of CBT as a form of psychotherapy in practice (Duncan 1999, 2003a, b, Forsyth & Kielhofner 2005, Harrison 2003, Kaur et al 1996, Stewart 2003). Distancing from the occupational therapy role is, however, not essential in order to use a cognitive behavioural therapy approach in practice. This section focuses on the use of a cognitive behavioural frame of reference within an occupational therapy context. In order to discuss this meaningfully, however, it is necessary to first provide an outline of the theoretical basis of cognitive behavioural therapy.

AN INTRODUCTION TO THE THEORETICAL FRAMEWORK OF CBT

CBT has a problem-focused perspective of life and focuses on five key areas.

- Thoughts
- Behaviours
- Emotion/mood
- Physiological responses
- The environment (Greenberger & Padesky 1995)

Each aspect of life experience is influenced by the social and physical environment in which it

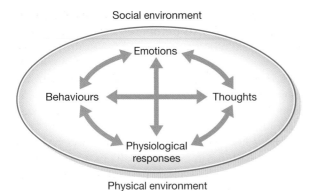

Figure 16.1 The influence of the social and physical environment on aspects of life experience.

is placed (Fig. 16.1). Cognitive behaviour therapy suggests that changes in any factor can lead to an improvement or deterioration in the other factors. For example, if we exercise (behaviour), we feel better (mood); if we feel nervous (mood), we may experience an increased heart rate or sweat more (physiological reaction); if we find large social gatherings difficult (social environment), we may avoid them (behaviour). One of the key theoretical components to understanding the theoretical basis of CBT is its hierarchical levels of cognition.

Levels of cognition

Beck et al (1979) outlined three levels of cognition that are amenable to therapeutic intervention. Key to this understanding is that, unlike other psychotherapeutic approaches (e.g. a psychodynamic approach), each of these levels is accessible by the client. The levels are hierarchical in nature with *automatic thoughts* being the most frequently occurring and easily accessible, *beliefs* being more constant but less obvious, and *core schema* representing the building blocks of all thought processes, less immediately accessible and more challenging to shift.

Automatic thoughts

Automatic thoughts are habitual and plausible. They are the uninvited thoughts that pop into your head (e.g. 'I'm bound to make a mistake in front of my practice educator'). Everyone has automatic thoughts. However, frequently clients' automatic thoughts are more unhelpful in nature. Another characteristic of automatic thoughts is

that they can be situation specific; for instance, a person may find themselves frequently having unhelpful automatic thoughts at work, due to stress, but not have these at home. Understanding that a client is experiencing unhelpful automatic thoughts is useful as they can have a direct impact on clients' presentation and ability to carry out daily life activities. Several techniques can be used to elicit automatic thoughts and these are described in greater detail in other texts (Beck et al 1979, Duncan 2006, Greenberger & Padesky 1995, Hawton et al 1996).

Where thoughts are recognised as being unhelpful, the therapist and client can work together to help the client to challenge the nature of their thinking, in the knowledge that this will help their behaviour. Importantly, changing thoughts is not the same as simply thinking more positively, which is unlikely in itself to lead to improved functioning (Greenberger & Padesky 1995). Challenging automatic thoughts is about gaining a sense of perspective on a situation, taking alternative perspectives and exploring new perspectives and solutions. A variety of techniques can be used to challenge automotive thoughts (Beck et al 1979, Duncan 2006, Greenberger & Padesky 1995, Hawton et al 1996).

Beliefs

These are conditional beliefs which we hold about ourselves and can also be unhelpful. Whilst automatic thoughts are often easily accessible, beliefs may be slightly less obvious. Beliefs lie beneath and shape the automatic thoughts that pop into our head. All our lives are governed by beliefs to a certain extent and these influence our behaviour. Some people, however, develop unhelpful beliefs about a range of issues and these can often significantly impact the way in which they lead their lives. Examples could include making sweeping statements such as 'Everything I do goes wrong' or thinking in extremes: 'If I can't get it right there's no point in doing it at all' (Duncan 2006).

Core schema

Our schemas provide the foundation of our cognitive constructs. They are absolute core beliefs which we hold about ourselves (e.g. 'I am worthless', 'I am bad' or 'I am good', ' I am important'). Current thinking suggests that schemas are formed during the early years of life and are influenced by childhood experiences and genetic composition. A useful analogy for understanding core schema is to consider them as the fundamental building blocks of cognition: from *core schema* develop *beliefs* and from *beliefs* come *automatic thoughts*. Changing a client's schema is very difficult, as these processes are deeply ingrained. This is a specialist skill and should be left to individuals with specialist cognitive behavioural training. Fortunately, it is not always necessary to address a person's core schema in order to help them. Most people who deliver or receive a CBT intervention focus purely on the more superficial levels of cognition and find that these are sufficient for symptomatic relief of the presenting problem.

A COGNITIVE BEHAVIOURAL FRAME OF REFERENCE

The terms *cognitive behavioural therapy* or *CBT* are used within occupational therapy in a variety of ways and this can at times lead to confusion. In order to lessen this, Duncan (2006) proposed that 'all forms of primarily didactic psychotherapy that use a CBT approach are referred to as CBT [or cognitive behavioural therapy], whilst the use of cognitive behavioural theory or practice within an occupational therapy is referred to as employing a cognitive behavioural frame of reference' (p225).

A theory of mind

Perhaps the most useful way of employing a cognitive behavioural frame of reference in occupational therapy is to use it as a *theory of mind*. A theory of mind is an understanding of the inner psychological workings of a person (Wellman & Lagattuta 2004). There are numerous conceptualisations of how people understand each other's interactions, behaviours, relationships and lives in general. Daily, we form opinions about the rationale of other people's actions, a process that has become known as *folk psychology* (Wellman & Lagattuta 2004). Some theories of mind are formalised, for example the psychodynamic frame of reference (see Blair & Daniel 2006) and the cognitive behavioural frame of reference. Rather

than relying on idiosyncratic folk psychology to guide a clinician in their interactions and conceptualisation of clients, it is proposed that they should develop the ability to use a more evidence-based theory of mind. The cognitive behavioural approach has undergone rigorous research to underpin its theoretical basis; its evidence base and pragmatic here-and-now philosophy suggests it as the theory of mind of choice for occupational therapists in practice (Duncan 2006). A case study illustrating an occupational therapist's use of the cognitive behavioural frame of reference as a theory of mind is presented in Duncan (2006).

Using a cognitive behavioural frame of reference with a conceptual model of practice

Whilst employing a cognitive behavioural frame of reference can be clinically useful, it does not give an occupational therapist a detailed understanding of a client's occupational performance and identity needs. However, it can be easily used in conjunction with a clinician's occupation-focused conceptual model of practice. Conversely, occupation-focused conceptual models of practice provide excellent theories and tools upon which an occupational therapist can conceptualise the occupational challenges facing a client but do not contain all the theoretical basis required for occupational therapists to practise effectively. The cognitive behavioural frame of reference assists occupational therapists to understand the client more comprehensively and work collaboratively with him in order to address their occupational performance challenges. However, this requires an explicit use of a cognitive behavioural frame of mind and judicious use of cognitive behavioural techniques in practice, in clear conjunction with the therapist's occupation-focused conceptual model of practice or alternative understanding of the client's occupational needs.

SUMMARY

A brief overview and summary of the theoretical framework of CBT has been presented. CBT's broad evidence base was acknowledged and the guiding principles of CBT (problem focused, working in the here and now, collaborative and time limited) were recognised as principles that resonated with occupational therapy theory and practice. Aaron Beck, often cited as a founding father of CBT, would certainly approve of the use of cognitive behavioural principles in occupational therapy as he views the principles discussed in this section as the basis of all good therapeutic relationships.

> ... I hope in 10 years it no longer exists as a school of therapy [he hoped that]... what we call cognitive therapy ... will be taken for granted as the basics of all good therapy, just as Carl Rogers's principles of warmth, empathy and genuine regard for patient were adopted as necessary basics for all therapy relationships' (cited in Salkovskis 1996).

Whilst the principles and characteristics of CBT appear congruent with occupational therapy, the method of its integration into practice has attracted criticism. This section and other publications (Duncan 2003a, 2006) have explored methods by which occupational therapists can effectively use a cognitive behavioural frame of reference in occupational therapy practice whilst remaining true to their professional role and identity. It is proposed that the cognitive behavioural frame of reference, with or without the concurrent use of an occupation-focused conceptual model of practice, enhances a clinician's therapeutic potential by increasing her understanding of a client and allowing appropriate and judicious use of cognitive behavioural and other techniques within an occupational context.

THE FUNCTIONAL INFORMATION-PROCESSING MODEL

The Functional Information-Processing Model (FIPM) developed from the work of Claudia Allen, an American occupational therapist whose earlier work focused on the cognitive disability model, from which the FIPM developed (Allen 1982). Heavily influenced by Piaget's theory of cognitive development (Piaget 1952), the FIPM is designed for use with clients who experience cognitive impairments, including those with acquired

brain injury and developmental delay, as well as psychiatric disorders such as depression and schizophrenia. Its predominant use in the UK is with older people who experience dementia (Pool 2006).

The model's early development originated in the 1970s when the Allen Cognitive Battery (which later developed into the Allen Cognitive Level Screen) was developed by Claudia Allen and a group of colleagues. Its original use was for patients experiencing mental health problems. Whilst earlier versions of the assessment were not standardised, later versions of the assessment battery have undergone reliability and validity evaluations and the model continues to evolve and develop.

Although in essence an occupational therapy tool, it has also been suggested that the assessments associated with the FIPM could be used by other health-care professionals who have an academic and clinical understanding of working with clients who have an information-processing impairment (Pool 2006). The FIPM is now widely used throughout the world, including the UK.

AN INTRODUCTION TO THE THEORETICAL FRAMEWORK OF THE FIPM

Allen's conception of cognition is that it was what affected an individual's motor and verbal responses, as well as determining what a person pays attention too; in other words, 'the processing capacity that determines how a person engages in everyday activities with their environment' (Pool 2006, p128). This conceptualisation is a continuum along two paths (motor and verbal) both linked by attention. Borrowing from the work of Piaget (1952), Allen & Betrand (1999) defined the structures of cognition in the FIPM in broad and general terms that were intended to be universal and free from gender and cultural bias. Allen's cognitive structures, listed below, guide the actions and activities of individuals (Allen & Bertrand 1999; Pool 2006).

- **Observations.** These include attention to cues or external stimuli and making sense of them.
- **Speed.** This refers to the rate at which the information-processing system operates.

- **Visual spatial.** These are the working memory processes that are applied to understanding objects and space, including: sensation, perception, topographical orientation and imagination.
- **Verbal propositional**. These are processes of working memory that are applied to understanding communication, social order and time. It includes non-verbal communication and verbal communication; cause-and-effect relationships where relationships are transferred into sounds; classifications of objects by perceptual properties, functional use or abstract concepts; and orientation to time and social rules.
- **Memory**. These processes are divided into declarative (explicit) intentions to learn and non-declarative (implicit) learning that occurs without being aware of storing or retrieving knowledge.

The FIPM outlines seven cognitive levels (each with three components: motor control, verbal performance and attention), which range from 0 (profound impairment) to 6 (normal functioning). Each level is defined as follows.

- **Level 0.** The individual is alive but in a coma or under general anaesthesia. No conscious control of movement is evident.
- **Level 1.** The individual responds to external stimuli. A general response (e.g. a change in heart rate) usually precedes a specific response to noxious stimuli (e.g. pain), followed by additional stimuli (e.g. bells, voices, familiar sounds and pictures).
- **Level 2.** An individual controls their gross body movements to sit, stand, walk and do push/pull exercises. Adaptive equipment that protects an individual from dangerous postural movements or that supports functional position is required.
- **Level 3.** At this level a person uses their hands to reach for and grasp objects. Repetitive manual actions are common, but the effect produced on the object is not judged by the person. A person continues to require constant supervision to protect themselves from harm.
- **Level 4.** At this level a person's actions are goal directed. Routine activities of daily living

can be completed independently. Assistance continues to be required to deal with unforeseen changes in the environment.
- **Level 5.** A person can learn new actions. Individuals appear to enjoy the novelty presented by new situations. Hazards are still not anticipated and supervision in dangerous situations is advised.
- **Level 6.** An individual anticipates the consequences of his or her actions and plans an effective and efficient course of action.

In order to further discriminate between the levels, Allen also presents five modes of performance within each cognitive level. These allow therapists to more precisely locate their clients' function level.

- **Point 0**. A client is likely to be functioning in only some of the described aspects.
- **Point 2**. A client is characteristically more likely to have problems of orientation in time and place.
- **Point 4**. A client at this point is consolidating their skills within the level.
- **Point 6**. A client is likely to be progressing to the next level.
- **Point 8**. A client is almost at the next level and may be incorporating some points from that level.

It is important to note that Allen's cognitive level scale is ordinal, not interval. In other words, there is not an equal distance between each level and mode. In the FIPM, there is a larger distance in ability between point 4 and point 6 of a mode, and between point 8 and point 0 of a mode, than between any of the others (Pool 2006). In order to use the scale in practice, it is necessary to conduct two assessments. First, the cognitive ability of a person must be measured (using the battery of assessments, designed by Allen and colleagues, outlined below) and second, the cognitive demands that a task or activity requires must be assessed by the therapist using her skills of task or activity analysis. Successful performance, it is postulated, occurs when the cognitive demands of an activity are matched or exceeded by the cognitive abilities of a client. The role of the occupational therapist, states Allen, is to predict likely performance in an activity and to facilitate a client to engage in the activity to the best of his abilities.

THE CLAUDIA ALLEN DIAGNOSTIC MODULE

As a part of the FIPM, a range of diagnostic tests have been developed that assist in the assessment of clients' cognitive performance. These assist therapists to predict clients' performance and function in daily living activities. Collectively these assessments are referred to as the Allen Diagnostic Module (ADM) (Earhart et al 1993). The ADM is composed of several separate assessments and kits.

The Allen Cognitive Level Screen (ACLS) and the Large Allen Cognitive Screen (LACLS) (Allen 1985, 1996, 1998)

This assessment analyses clients' problem-solving and new learning abilities. New learning situations are assessed as it is believed that such situations provide the therapist with a true understanding of a client's cognitive ability as opposed to assessing his ability to complete a familiar task. The ACLS and LACLS are designed to assess clients in the middle of the range of the FIPM as clients who are at the first two stages cannot work with objects and the higher stage (i.e. Level 6) is more concerned with attention to symbolic cues (Pool 2006).

The Routine Task Inventory (RTI)

The RTI is an assessment of a client's ability to carry out everyday tasks (Allen et al 1992, 1995). It particularly focuses on clients' self-awareness, situational awareness, occupational role and social role within each daily living task. A client's ability to perform a task is assessed by self-report, caregiver report or direct observation. This allows for interesting comparisons between observed and reported performance. And studies of observed cognitive performance using the ACLS and a caregiver's report using the RTI have revealed significant test–retest reliability and a positive correlation between RTI and ACL scores (Wilson et al 1989). Other studies have reported that the RTI has an acceptable degree of test–retest and interrater reliability (Bar-Yoseff et al 1999, Conroy 1996).

The Cognitive Performance Tests (CPT) (Allen et al 1992)

The CPT assess a client's working memory. Working memory processes new information in order to adapt to a new or changing environment (Pool 2006). This is important as clients must be able to process new information when they are moving into a new environment (such as moving into the community or entering sheltered housing). Initially, the CPT were used as a research tool for use in longitudinal studies which examined functional changes over time. More recently, they have also been used to measure changes over shorter periods of time in order to detect responses to pharmacological or environmental interventions.

In the CPT, the client is sequentially presented with a series of six tasks: shopping, using the telephone, getting dressed, travelling, making a piece of toast and washing hands. There are standardised instructions for each task (Burns 1992). In each task, the client is given a set of verbal instructions. Observing the client, the tester then responds to the client's behaviours by performing a series of standardised interactions that correspond to the specific behaviours of the client. By doing so, the tester changes the task demands of each activity in response to a client's observed deficit behaviours. This is achieved by controlling or simplifying the information-processing requirements of the task.

As with the ACLS and the LACLS, the CPT are not appropriate for all clients. The CPT focus on activities associated with Level 6 of the FIPM, though some tasks only require functioning above Level 5.3. A client's CPT score is reported to be a valid representation of global ability and the assessment's interrater and test–retest reliability; congruent, internal and predictive validity have all been established (Conroy 1998).

Allen Diagnostic Module projects (Earhart et al 1993)

The Allen Diagnostic Module (ADM) consists of 24 craft projects which are used to assess working memory. A lack of interest in using craft activities within occupational therapy in recent years has led to these projects being less used in the UK, though it has been noted that they are still highly regarded in the USA (Pool 2006). Each project is standardised to control the information presented to individuals. Projects are selected by therapists to match the client's ACLS score and are meant to have meaning and value to the individual and it is this that may limit their potential for use at times. Each craft project has extensive rating criteria and is sensitive to small degrees of change in client's ability to function (Pool 2006).

The Sensory–Motor Stimulation kits (Blue and Allen 1992)

The Sensory-Motor Stimulation (SMS) kits are designed for people with severe cognitive impairment. Two kits are available. The first is designed for people at the lower end of cognitive functioning (i.e. Level 1.0 to 2.2) and the second for people with slightly higher cognitive functioning (i.e. Level 2.2 to 3.2). Each kit contains materials which stimulate the five senses and encourage mobility. Therapists are encouraged to add to the existing materials with their own items. The kits contain a manual presenting the background to the SMS, guidelines for use and rating sheets for observed behaviour.

USING THE FIPM IN PRACTICE

The FIPM can provide useful information for therapists which they can use to support the design (in collaboration with the client, of course) of a meaningful and appropriately pitched therapeutic programme. Importantly, the FIPM does not answer all questions a therapist may have and it assumes that each therapist has excellent skills in task and activity analysis. Another important function of the FIPM is that it can be a useful method to gain information about a client's function which can then be relayed to carers, assisting them to understand their friend's/relative's abilities and difficulties and helping them to provide the least restrictive environment in which the client will be able to optimally function (Pool 1997). But the FIPM is not solely designed to maintain client functioning – it also has a rehabilitative element.

The FIPM can be used to inform intervention plans. Building on the assessment information from the ADM, therapists and clients can develop an intervention programme which introduces a range of activities, carefully selected to gradually increase the cognitive demands required for task completion. It must be remembered, however, that the FIPM is a purely cognitive model and does not take into account a client's physical, psychological or social functioning. These elements must be separately considered by the therapist when designing the programme. Moreover, the interaction between a client's cognitive, social, psychological and physical needs is often complex and unclear; for example, it has been suggested that as well as focusing on cognitive levels directly (using the FIPM), a client's cognitive functioning may improve indirectly through intervention directed to his social or psychological needs (Pool 2001). Further information regarding the implementation of the FIPM in practice can be found in a useful case study presented by Pool (2006).

Despite its uses, the FIPM and its associated assessments are not greatly accepted by clinicians in practice. The predominant criticism of the FIPM is its focus on craft activities. The ACLS is a leather lacing activity, which appears demeaning and irrelevant to everyday activity and perhaps may be perceived as reinforcing stereotypical images of the profession to colleagues (Pool 2006). Allen & Reyner (2002) defend its use, stating that the activity was selected as it was a new activity and was able to be standardised. Kielhofner (2004), however, further criticises the FIPM, stating that whilst its focus on cognitive factors is useful, it oversimplifies clients' functional deficits.

SUMMARY

The FIPM and associated tests provide a detailed assessment of a client's occupational functioning. Allen's focus, through the model, is on determining clients' current levels of ability and making maximum use of these whilst minimising their limitations through appropriate environmental and activity adaptation. Such an approach is significantly different from other occupational therapy models which focus on improving the function of clients primarily and only latterly give consideration to environmental adaptation (Keogh 1998). The FIPM is not widely used in practice settings in the UK. This may, in part, be due to its craft orientation and focus on activities, such as leather lacing, which appear to lack meaning and purpose. Further information regarding the FIPM can be found at the following websites:

- Allen Cognitive Network: www.allen-cognitive-network.org
- Jackie Pool Associates: www.jackie-pool-associates.co.uk

References

Allen CK 1982 Independence through activity: the practice of occupational therapy (psychiatry). American Journal of Occupational Therapy 36: 731-739

Allen CK 1985 Occupational therapy for psychiatric diseases: measurement and management of cognitive disabilities. Little Brown, Boston

Allen CK 1996 Large Allen cognitive level screen test manual. Allen Conferences, Florida

Allen CK 1998 Administering the Allen cognitive level screen (video). Allen Conferences, Florida

Allen CK, Bertrand J 1999 Structures of the cognitive performance modes. Allen Conferences, Florida

Allen CK, Reyner A 2002 How to start using the Allen diagnostic module. Allen Conferences, Florida

Allen CK, Earhart CA, Blue T 1992 Occupational therapy treatment goals for the physically and cognitively disabled. American Occupational Therapy Association, Bethesda, Maryland ·

Allen CK, Blue T, Earhart CA 1995 Understanding cognitive performance modes. Allen Conferences, Florida

Baddeley AD, Emslie H, Nimmo-Smith I 1994 The doors and people test: a test of visual and verbal recall and recognition. Thames Valley Test Company, Bury St Edmunds

Bar-Yoseff C, Weinblatt N, Katz N 1999 Reliability and validity of the cognitive performance test (CPT) in an elderly population in Israel. Physical and Occupational Therapy in Geriatrics 17(1): 65-79

Beck AT, Rush AJ, Shaw BF et al 1979 Cognitive therapy of depression. Guilford Press, New York

Beck AT, Wright FD, Newman CF et al 1993 Cognitive therapy of substance abuse. Guilford Press, New York

Blair SS, Daniel M 2006 An introduction to the psychodynamic frame of reference. In: Duncan EAS (ed) Foundations for practice in occupational therapy, 4th edn. Elsevier Churchill Livingstone, Edinburgh, pp233-254

Blue T, Allen CK 1992 Sensory Motor Stimulation kit I and II. Allen Conferences, Florida

British Association for Behavioural and Cognitive Psychotherapies 2003 BABCP away day. BABCP News 31(1): 2-3

Burns T 1992 Cognitive performance test in occupational therapy treatment goals for the physically and cognitively disabled. American Occupational Therapy Association, Bethesda, Maryland

Conroy MC 1996 Dementia care: keeping intact and in touch. Avebury, Aldershot, pp106-109

Conroy MC 1998 Allen's cognitive levels with people who are dementing. British Journal of Therapy and Rehabilitation 5(1): 21-26

Department of Health 2001 Treatment choice in psychological therapies and counselling. Department of Health, London

Duncan EAS 1999 Occupational therapy in mental health: it is time to recognise that it has come of age. British Journal of Occupational Therapy 62(11): 521-522

Duncan EAS 2003a Cognitive-behavioural therapy in physiotherapy and occupational therapy. In: Everett T, Donaghy M, Feaver S (eds) Interventions for mental health: an evidence based approach. Butterworth Heinemann, Oxford

Duncan EAS 2003b Cognitive behaviour therapy: seeking a common understanding. British Journal of Occupational Therapy 66(5): 231

Duncan EAS 2006 The cognitive-behavioural frame of reference. In: Duncan EAS (ed) Foundations for practice in occupational therapy, 4th edn. Elsevier Churchill Livingstone, Edinburgh

Earhart CA, Allen CK, Blue T 1993 The Allen diagnostic module instruction manual (ADMIM). Allen Conferences, Florida

Epstein N 2003 Cognitive-behavioural therapies for couples and families. In: Hecker LL, Wetchler JL (eds) An introduction to marriage and family therapy. Haworth Clinical Practice Press, Binghamton, NY

Fisher AG 2003 Assessment of motor and process skills, vol 2, 5th edn. Three Star Press, Fort Collins

Forsyth K, Kielhofner G 2005 The model of human occupation: embracing the complexity of occupation by integrating theory into practice and practice into theory. In: Duncan EAS (ed) Hagedorn's foundations for practice, 5th edn. Churchill Livingstone, Edinburgh,

Green MF 1996 What are the functional consequences of neurocognitive deficits in schizophrenia? American Journal of Psychiatry 153: 321-330

Greenberger D, Padesky CA 1995 Mind over mood. Change how you feel by changing how you think. Guilford Press, New York

Harrison D 2003 The case for generic work in community mental health. Occupational Therapy 66(3): 110-112

Hawton K, Salkovskis P, Kirk J et al (eds) 1996 Cognitive behaviour therapy for psychiatric problems: a practical guide. Oxford University Press, Oxford

Kaur D, Seager M, Orrell M 1996 Occupation or therapy? The attitudes of mental health professionals. British Journal of Occupational Therapy 59(7): 319-322

Keogh C 1998 Cognitive disability model: moving to an informed position. Irish Journal of Occupational Therapy 28(2): 2-7

Kielhofner G 2004 Conceptual foundations of occupational therapy. FA Davis, Philadelphia

Longabaugh R, Morgenstern J 1999 Cognitive-behavioural coping-skills therapy for alcohol dependence: current status and future directions. Alcohol Research and Health 23(2): 78-86

Morrison G, O'Carroll R, McCreadie R 2006 Long-term course of cognitive impairment in schizophrenia. British Journal of Psychiatry 189: 556-557

Piaget J 1952 The origins of intelligence in children. International Universities Press, New York, p311

Pool J 1997 Helping carers change their role. Journal of Dementia Care 5(3): 24-25

Pool J 2001 Making contact: an activity-based model of care. Journal of Dementia Care 9(4): 24-26

Pool J 2006 The functional information processing model. In: Duncan EAS (ed) Foundations for practice in occupational therapy, 4th edn. Elsevier Churchill Livingstone, Edinburgh, pp125-141

Prins JB, Bleijenberg G, Bazelmans E et al 2001 Cognitive behaviour therapy for chronic fatigue syndrome: a multicentre randomised controlled trial. Lancet 357: 841–847

Robertson IH, Ward T, Ridgeway V et al 1994 The test of everyday attention. Harcourt Assessment, Oxford

Salkovskis PM (ed)1996 Frontiers of cognitive therapy. Guilford Press, New York

Stewart A 2003 The case for generic working in mental health. British Journal of Occupational Therapy 66(4): 180

Strong J 1998 Incorporating cognitive-behavioural therapy with occupational therapy: a comparative study with patients with low back pain. Journal of Occupational Rehabilitation 8(1): 61-71

Turner A, Foster M, Johnson SE 2002 Occupational therapy and physical dysfunction. Principles, skills and practice, Churchill Livingstone, Edinburgh

Wellman HM, Lagattuta KH 2004 Theory of mind for learning and teaching: the nature and role of explanation. Cognitive Development 19: 479-497

Wilson DS, Allen CK, McCormack G et al 1989 Cognitive disability and routine task behaviours in a community based population with senile dementia. Occupational Therapy Practice 1(1): 58-66

Young JE 1999 Cognitive therapy for personality disorders: a schema-focused approach. Practitioner's Resource Series. Professional Resource Exchange, Sarasota, Florida

Chapter **17**

Client–centred groups

Marilyn B. Cole

INTRODUCTION

Participation in groups is essential to participation in life. We are born into families, neighbourhoods and communities. As children we interact in play groups, classrooms, sports teams, clubs and informal peer groups. As adults we join work groups or work teams, religious and political groups, charity organisations, informal social groups and extended family groups. As older adults, we find that group status sustains our integrity as others seek our input or advice. We depend on support from religious groups, friendship groups and family groups in times of sorrow or adversity. Mosey called these naturally occurring groups 'primary groups' (Donohue 2003, Mosey 1986). For people with mental illness, therapy groups become a part of this continuum.

Illness often isolates individuals by restricting their ability to participate in primary groups. There are several reasons for this.

- Mental or physical limitation inhibits the performance of occupations associated with group roles.
- Cognitive, emotional or spiritual reactions to illness interfere with a person's natural inclination to participate in groups.
- Negative social attitudes stigmatise people with disability, creating a social barrier to participation.

Whether these barriers to group participation are intrinsic (occurring within the self) or extrinsic (originating from the external environment), the exclusion of people with disability is inconsistent with today's health-care paradigm, which is holistic, client-centred and systems oriented (World Health Organization 2001).

Occupational therapists assist clients in recovering lost roles or developing new or adapted roles in society. They do so by facilitating engagement in occupations that support the client's participation in desired social/group roles. When clients understand the connection of occupational therapy group interventions with their own goals and priorities relative to social participation, they will be motivated to engage in therapeutic activities. This connection is central to the client-centred focus of groups in occupational therapy.

Client-centred groups follow the principles of client-centred practice defined by Law et al (1995), such as non-judgemental acceptance (empathy for clients with diverse viewpoints), contextual congruence (meaning and relevance of interventions) and client autonomy (giving priority to client goals). Creek (2003, p50) defined client-centred practice as:

> a partnership between therapist and client in which the client … actively participates in negotiating goals for intervention and making decisions [and] the therapist adapts the intervention to meet client needs.

When groups of potential members collaborate with the occupational therapy leader in setting goals and priorities, the client-centred therapeutic partnership is extended to the group as a whole.

HOW OCCUPATIONAL THERAPISTS USE GROUPS

Occupational therapists form client groups for both assessment and intervention. Their purpose is to:

- evaluate client problems with communication, interaction and relationships with others
- engage people with similar goals, problem areas or life roles in activities that address common issues
- capture the energy naturally generated by group interaction (including Yalom's therapeutic factors) and use it to maximise client effort in coping with adversity and to motivate positive change
- use the principles of the social microcosm in dealing with issues of inclusion or exclusion from desired roles in society
- develop self-awareness, self-understanding, self-efficacy and insight through consensual validation (group reality testing) and mutual group feedback
- enlist group support during the learning and practice of motor, process and/or communication/interaction skills required for the occupational performance that supports social participation.

None of these advantages of groups is specific to mental illness; they are equally important in all areas of occupational therapy practice.

A STRUCTURE FOR OCCUPATIONAL THERAPY GROUPS: COLE'S SEVEN STEPS

For the beginning student, a concrete structure for group leadership provides a logical starting place. The purpose of Cole's seven steps is to learn the basics of therapeutic group facilitation. This prototype can then be adapted as the student integrates higher level knowledge and experience with various health conditions, theoretical frames of reference, levels of human development (age groups) and health-care delivery settings. These seven steps address the needs of highly functional clients and, as such, are appropriate for students to practise with groups of their peers.

STEP 1: INTRODUCTION

The session begins with stating your name, the name of the group and your role as the occupational therapy group leader. To assist the group members in learning one another's names, in addition to **stating names** around the circle, members can tell the group something else about themselves that is unique, such as where they are from, what most concerns them about the group, even something as simple as their favourite colour. What is shared should match client factors such as cognitive level, disability area and age. Names should be repeated at the beginning of each session, not only as an introduction but as a way to acknowledge the importance of each member's presence, a gesture which builds self-identity and encourages participation.

For most groups, a **warm-up** activity is highly recommended. The warm-up is a short activity, 5 minutes or less, which precedes the main activity of the group. Warm-ups serve several important purposes. First, they capture the attention of the members, diverting their attention from whatever they came to the group thinking about. Second, the right warm-up prepares members for the activity to come. For example, members may choose picture cards with different facial expressions to express their mood as a warm-up for a group role play

to practise appropriate expression of emotions. A warm-up can energise or calm. For example, a series of stretches may wake up an early morning group, while a short relaxation exercise might counteract agitation. Another purpose is for the occupational therapy leader to observe the status of members prior to beginning an activity. Daily fluctuations in mood, energy level, cognitive level and other areas occur in most individuals. A skilled leader will be able to adapt and grade the activity along the way, according to changes in member status. Warm-ups may be formal or informal. When members know each other well, an informal chat about how they are feeling today may suffice.

Setting the mood is another function of the introduction. The occupational therapy leader conveys this in her facial expression, body language and tone of voice, as well as her words. The mood of the group should match the goals and content. If the activity of the day is light-hearted, the introduction can set an upbeat mood with humour, smiles and a playful warm-up such as balloon play. A more serious tone is needed for topics such as work readiness or coping with loss. The mood set in the introduction will also cue the members as to what may be expected of them during the activity to follow.

Explaining the purpose clearly is the most important component of any introduction. That is why it should occur after the initial greetings and warm-up, when members are alert and ready to listen. The purpose of the group includes both goals and methods and should clarify how the selected activity addresses the goals of members. The occupational therapy leader explains the purpose in everyday language that can be easily understood by members. When group members are severely disabled, the purpose may be communicated non-verbally, with a smile and a gentle touch that says, 'trust me, this activity will help you'. From a client-centred perspective, member goals are incorporated into group goals, while the occupational therapist's expertise guides activity selection to meet goals. When clients understand why they are being asked to take part in a group activity, they will actively participate and collaborate with the leader in meeting group goals.

In groups which focus on learning, sometimes **introductory educational concepts** are outlined. For example, a cultural awareness group may begin with a definition of culture and some exploration of the perceptions of members regarding different aspects of culture. When member discussion is included, introductory concepts usually replace the warm-up, since they serve a similar purpose.

The final component of the introduction is a **brief outline of the session**. Time may be used to further clarify each segment. For example, 'we will be drawing for 15 minutes, then for the next 30 minutes we will share our drawings and discuss their meaning with the group'. This brief outline conveys several important ideas. First, the 15-minute time limit gives members a guideline for how detailed and complex their drawings should be. Second, it tells them that what they draw will be discussed with the group, so that they should limit the content of their drawings to things they are willing to share. When clients have concerns about privacy, the occupational therapy leader might add, 'Your drawings will not be analysed by anyone other than yourself and you may take them with you when you leave'. Such reassurances also convey the expectation that clients should feel free to self-disclose without fear of unknowingly revealing some hidden conflict or character flaw. Third, the brief outline conveys to clients that the emphasis of the group will be on discussion, not drawing. They need not worry about their artistic ability or lack thereof. The point of the drawing is to clarify some aspect of the self and to communicate its meaning through discussion.

While the introduction may seem complex, it exerts a powerful influence on group outcomes. Recent research has shown that the initial guidelines, including purpose and structure set forth in the first meeting, have a lasting influence on subsequent sessions (Gersick 2003). The importance of this initial step in group facilitation cannot be overstated.

STEP 2: ACTIVITY

The activity provides the means or method for accomplishing group goals. In our prototype, this portion of the group lasts from 10 to 20 minutes. Within that short time, the group activity must generate enough raw material to sustain discussion for the next 30–40 minutes. Activity selection is a complex process based on the occupational therapist's knowledge of theory and research,

activity demand, client factors and health conditions. For the beginning student, a simplified method of selection is outlined here, with the expectation that students will build upon it as they gain more knowledge and experience. This process includes activity analysis and synthesis, timing, goals, physical and mental capacities of members, knowledge and skill of the leader.

Most activities will need to be adapted for use with groups. This is accomplished through activity analysis and synthesis. **Activity analysis** is 'a process of dissecting an activity into its component parts and task sequence in order to identify its inherent properties and the skills required for its performance, thus allowing the therapist to evaluate its therapeutic potential' (Creek 2003, p49). **Activity synthesis** is 'combining activity components and features of the environment to produce a new activity that will enable performance to be assessed or achieve a desired therapeutic outcome' (Creek 2003, p50). The outcome of this complex matching process between member abilities, skills and preferences and the components of a potential activity determines the group activity selection.

The **timing** of groups limits the range of activity from which to choose. Most group sessions last from 30 to 90 minutes, with an average of about an hour. If discussion is emphasised, the activity should take no more than one-third of the total session time. In addition, members of the group need to be able to work on the activity simultaneously within the same environment. Activities must be adapted to fit these time constraints.

Therapeutic **goals** guide the selection of activities. In client-centred practice, client occupational goals are given priority and groups are formed of clients with similar goals and priorities. Ideally, occupational therapists should hold a group discussion of goals, priorities and activity preferences before finalising the group design. Then, through activity analysis and synthesis and the application of appropriate theory, the occupational therapy leader determines a range of activities which incorporate techniques to address the most pressing therapeutic goals. Not all clients are capable of this level of collaboration and not all settings will afford its facilitation. In this case, the occupational therapy leader relies on pre-group interviews with individual members, caregivers and/or significant others to identify potential group member goals and priorities.

The **physical and mental capacities of members** are a primary consideration in selecting any activity. Formal or informal assessment of client occupational performance should precede client selection for group membership. Interventions work best with groups of clients having similar functional abilities. For example, Claudia Allen (Allen et al 1992, 1995) defined six cognitive levels and 52 modes of performance, giving occupational therapy one of its most well-researched and detailed assessments of client cognitive ability. Each whole level (especially 2–5) offers guidelines for task selection, analysis and adaptation, cueing (assisting) during task performance and adapting the environment to enable clients' best ability to function. Allen suggested grouping clients of similar Allen Cognitive Level (ACL).

The occupational therapy leader also considers her **own experience** and selects group activities based on familiarity, comfort level and past effectiveness.

STEP 3: SHARING

The activity step should have a definite end. At that point, materials used during the activity are removed from view and the product is shared. The occupational therapy leader may model sharing with her own example (e.g. drawing or writing) or may ask for a volunteer to start. The best way to make sure everyone gets a turn is to proceed around the circle, a norm which becomes automatic after the first few sessions. For activities which include group discussion as a component, the sharing step is unnecessary.

STEP 4: PROCESSING

Processing answers the question 'How did you feel about the activity, the leader and each other?'. Feelings are discussed first in order to prevent them from interfering with subsequent discussion. The occupational therapy leader generates the discussion of feelings by asking open-ended questions, which cannot be answered 'yes' or 'no' and which require some elaboration. For example,

asking 'What was hard about communicating non-verbally?' enables expression of feelings of frustration, inadequacy or objection to the activity requirements. 'Whose drawing most relates to you?' encourages group interaction and emotional feedback responses.

STEP 5: GENERALISING

This step answers the question 'What did you learn?'. Abstract reasoning is needed to derive a few general principles from the data of the group activity. Occupational therapy leaders facilitate generalising by asking open-ended questions such as 'What were some common triggers of stress we shared?' or 'Which coping strategies are good or bad?'. Ideally, the general principles discovered by the group will closely align with group goals. Some client groups need more help than others with this step.

STEP 6: APPLICATION

For learning to be effective, clients need to understand how what has been learned applies to their own lives. In this step, the occupational therapy leader asks discussion questions that enable this connection. For example, 'What part of today's activity will you take home with you?' or 'How can you use social skills in your life outside the group?'. With the client-centred approach, each member interprets the group experience in his or her own way. The application step offers each client an opportunity to verbalise the meaning of the group experience with respect to individual goals. For this reason, occupational therapy leaders need to make sure every member contributes to the discussion of application and, if possible, gives a specific example. Assigning homework or keeping journals can also reinforce application of learning in members' lives outside the group.

STEP 7: SUMMARY

A summary of the session reviews the highlights from each of the seven steps and reinforces the main principles learned. Members should be as involved as they are capable of being. Occupational therapy leaders should always end by thanking members for participating and by sharing their own positive feedback on the group experience. Plans for the next session and reminders for application can be added as a final note.

GROUP LEADERSHIP SKILLS

Most people think of leadership as a formal position that carries with it certain responsibilities. Occupational therapy leader responsibilities are to select members, set goals, design the group methods and structure and provide guidance during the session(s). This section on group leadership deals with leading the session; the other functions will be covered in a later section on designing group interventions. Leadership has been defined as 'the process of influencing group activities toward goal achievement' (Shaw 1981, p317). A half-century of research has concluded that there is no one best style of small group leadership. In the current view, ideal leadership changes to meet varying needs and circumstances (Barge 2003, Gouran 2003, Hersey & Blanchard 1969, Mosey 1986).

Mosey (1986) suggested a multilevel approach to the leadership of occupational therapy groups. She defined five developmental groups for the purpose of assisting clients in learning group interaction skills (see Table 17.1). Mosey's groups recapitulate (repeat) the normal sequence in which children learn to interact in groups. Recently, Donohue (1999, 2003) has validated Mosey's developmental group theory using structured observation with children's groups. Mosey's concept of the changing nature of leadership is consistent with current research findings.

THREE STYLES OF OCCUPATIONAL THERAPY LEADERSHIP

Leadership styles in occupational therapy may best be understood as a continuum: directive, facilitative and advisory. One is not better than the others, but rather each is preferred in different situations. Many factors should be considered in determining which leadership style to use for a given client group, such as client abilities and maturity, goals of the task and theoretical approach. Table 17.2 addresses how these factors influence occupational therapy leadership styles.

Table 17.1 Mosey's developmental group leadership

Group level	Occupational therapy leader role	Activity examples
Parallel (directive leadership)	Provide task, structure and emotional and social support for members	Imitative group exercises, painting or other creative tasks, simple crafts
Project/Associative (modified directive leadership)	Provide some choices of task, encourage member interaction around task issues and awareness of others. Leader continues to provide support	Structured learning groups, Allen's Level 3–4 craft groups
Basic co-operative (facilitative leadership)	Members choose task, occupational therapist facilitates interaction and assists members in meeting one another's social and emotional needs	Task-oriented groups, insight-oriented verbal groups, self-exploration and communication focus
Supportive co-operative (advisory leadership)	Relationships and socialisation take precedence over task accomplishment. Members provide social/emotional support for each other. Occupational therapist acts as advisor, provides resources as needed and assists with problem solving or conflict resolution	Playing beach volleyball, having a birthday party, group outings
Mature (participatory leadership)	Members self-lead, occupational therapist participates as a co-equal member, uses modelling, therapeutic self-disclosure and social learning to influence outcomes	Fund-raising events Self-help groups

Directive leadership

Directive leadership exerts the most influence over the group and is the best choice for clients functioning at a low cognitive level or lacking motivation. Groups focused on education, learning and practising skills may also require a directive approach. Groups using a sensory integrative approach require directive leadership in continually grading and adapting the activity according to member responses throughout the session. The term *directive* should not be confused with authoritative or autocratic. In simple terms, directive leadership should be used when clients require direction in order to benefit from the group activity.

Facilitative leadership

Facilitative leadership is sometimes compared to a democratic approach and as such may be the most familiar to occupational therapists. The word *facilitate* means 'to make easier'. Occupational therapy leaders use a variety of techniques to enable group participation, encourage communication and self-disclosure and reinforce positive group problem solving and social learning during group sessions. Facilitation is the preferred style when group members have the capacity for reasoning and when the goal is to develop self-awareness and insight. Sometimes facilitation involves shared leadership, allowing group members to take on leadership responsibilities. Shimanoff & Jenkins (2003) have called this a group-centred approach to leadership.

Advisory leadership

Occupational therapists use advisory leadership primarily with mature and highly motivated groups. An advisor intervenes only when members run into difficulty in solving a problem, require additional resources or expertise, or need assistance with conflict resolution. Advisory leadership is appropriately used in a consulting role when working with community groups. Certain tasks with mental health groups may require advisory leadership, especially when the goal involves learning social skills such as co-operation or compromise, or problem-solving skills such as making decisions and anticipating consequences. Occupational therapy advisory leadership exerts the least amount of authority over the group and is reserved for groups of clients who have the ability to structure and organise the group for themselves.

Table 17.2 Occupational therapy leadership continuum

Factors that influence leadership style	Directive leadership	Facilitative leadership	Advisory leadership
Power factors	Most influence, provide structure, task and support	Medium influence, encourage group participation in decisions and support for each other	Least influence, intervene on an as-needed basis only
Group maturity	Low, little connection between members	Medium, interrelationships are inconsistent	Highly cohesive
Client factors	Low cognitive level, psychological issues create barriers to group interaction	Medium cognitive level, capable of some reasoning and insight	High cognitive level, highly motivated
Task factors	Productivity oriented, non-verbal interaction, psychoeducational goals	Learning oriented, self-awareness or insight oriented	Socialisation oriented, problem oriented
Theoretical factors	Sensory motor and cognitive disabilities approaches	Psychodynamic and cognitive behavioural approaches	Developmental and systems-oriented approaches
Group focus	Task achievement, skill training	Interpersonal learning, communication or relationship goals	Problem solving, wellness or prevention goals

GROUP FACILITATION

Facilitating interaction

Group interaction is highly desirable in most groups. Occupational therapy leaders use several techniques for facilitating interaction among members. During the initial session, the leader initiates interaction by asking members to give opinions or contribute ideas and to respond to each other. When the group begins, members tend to look to the leader for direction and care must be taken not to set up a pattern of communicating only through the leader. When asked a direct question, the leader can defer to another member, asking 'What do you think?' or 'What would you do in Mary's situation?'. Observing who responds most often, the occupational therapy leader looks for ways to involve less verbal members and to make sure all have an equal opportunity to participate. Silence may raise anxiety levels in some members but jumping into every silent moment should be discouraged. Sometimes silence allows members to think about the topic being discussed and formulate their own contribution. When asking a discussion question, be sure that several if not all members have an opportunity to answer before moving on. Never assume that one or two members speak for the group as a whole. Only when every member has contributed can a true consensus on any issue be reached.

Directing

When members deviate from the group task or goal, the occupational therapy leader needs to redirect. This function of the leader in work groups was defined by Gouran (2003, p172) as the 'art of counteractive influence'. It refers to the appropriate leader intervention to assist the group with overcoming obstacles to reach goals. In therapy groups, we use various techniques to **set limits** on inappropriate behaviours that interfere with successful group outcomes. Setting limits is best accomplished using the least possible amount of authority. For example, when one overactive member monopolises the group, the occupational therapy leader can interrupt by asking the other members, 'How does it make you feel when John does all the talking?'. This invites group members to share the responsibility for setting limits. A good rule of thumb in adapting one's leadership during a group session is never to do for the group what the members can do for themselves.

Communicating empathy

Communicating empathy is another important aspect of group leadership. Empathy is an understanding of each client's emotions and unique point of view. The occupational therapy leader needs a broad feeling vocabulary to convey an accurate understanding of how clients feel about themselves, the task or each other during the session. For example, 'You must be terrified of crowds if you're going to so much trouble to avoid them' might be an empathetic response to a group member who has shared an episode of agoraphobia. Such statements serve a number of purposes. First, they acknowledge the client's feeling with non-judgemental acceptance, encouraging him or her to further self-disclosure. Second, they give other members permission to verbalise their own emotions. Third, they model for the group an empathetic way to respond to one another. Communicating empathy is one of the best ways to build trust among members, a necessary step in developing group cohesiveness.

In summary, according to Barge (2003, p200), 'effective leaders are complex information processors who are sensitive to the subtle qualities of individuals and the group environment'. Occupational therapy leaders should remain flexible and adjust their style according to the group's level of development, member psychological or cognitive maturity, the theoretical approach being used and the goal of the group activity.

UNDERSTANDING GROUP DYNAMICS

Finlay defined group dynamics as the 'forces, social structures, behaviours, relationships and processes which occur in groups' (Finlay 2002, p256). Researchers in many disciplines have studied group dynamics for nearly a century, producing a vast body of knowledge on the subject. This section will review therapeutic factors in groups, group process, norms, roles, group development and termination issues.

THERAPEUTIC FACTORS IN GROUPS

Yalom's (1995) therapeutic factors offer insight into the healing power of groups (see Table 17.3). They were derived from the summarisation of many research studies over several decades. Falk-Kessler et al (1991) found that group cohesiveness, hope and interpersonal learning were most highly valued within occupational therapy groups. Once learned, these factors can be easily recognised within occupational therapy group sessions.

GROUP PROCESS

Group process may be best understood by what it is not: it is not content. Content includes what is said and what is done by group members. Process refers to social structures, symbolic meanings, transference, countertransference, communication patterns, non-verbal communication and emotional responses that often lie beneath one's conscious awareness. Yalom (1995) described group process as a focus on reflection about the inter-relationships of members in the here and now; that is, during the session itself. He described a *self-reflective loop* with both an *experiencing* and a *reflection* component. In simple terms, the group participates in some type of shared experience and then reflects upon its meaning through group discussion. Cole's seven steps incorporate this concept using short, structured tasks upon which to reflect through processing, generalising and applying. Through reflection, group members have an opportunity to develop an awareness of how their own behaviours affect others and what must be changed in order to engage in meaningful relationships with others in their own lives.

Table 17.3 Yalom's therapeutic factors of groups

Therapeutic factor	Brief interpretation for occupational therapy groups
Instillation of hope	Even in anticipation of group membership, clients are inclined to believe that change is possible through the group experience
Universality	Through group sharing and interaction, members learn, often with great relief, that they are not alone
Altruism	With coaching and modelling from a skilled leader, members become aware that they have much to offer each other and that offering help to others can benefit themselves as well
Imparting information	Groups offer a practical means of educating those with similar issues but often the most useful information comes from group members sharing advice, ideas and solutions
Corrective recapitulation of the primary family group	Maladaptive learning from one's own imperfect family can be openly explored and modified within an emotionally safe group environment and through altered perceptions of reality
Development of socialising techniques	According to Bandura's (1977) social learning theory, people learn appropriate social behaviours through observation of others. Groups offer multiple opportunities to do this
Imitative behaviour	When group members observe that certain behaviours have positive consequences for others, they tend to imitate those behaviours
Interpersonal learning	Groups offer multiple opportunities for giving and receiving feedback from others. Through feedback, members develop a more accurate self-perception and reality orientation
Group cohesiveness	Cohesiveness is a preferred state in which group members accept and support one another and freely self-disclose
Catharsis	Emotional expression of previously hidden emotionally charged issues or experiences can, in itself, have a healing effect
Existential factors	Many spiritual concerns, such as the meaning of one's life, the acceptance of anxiety as a part of living and an awareness of one's own mortality, can be clarified through group interaction

Because of the subtle yet complex qualities of group process, occupational therapy leaders only become skilled at observing and facilitating through experience. For this reason, supervision is necessary for students to become fully aware of these very powerful but often invisible forces within their groups.

GROUP NORMS

Group norms are customary ways of doing things within a group. Explicit norms (or rules) are verbalised by the occupational therapy leader at the outset, such as the time and place of meeting, the expectation for participation and the importance of confidentiality and respect for each other. Non-explicit norms are not verbalised but assumed. For example, social conventions, such as 'If you don't have something good to say, don't say anything', may incline members to avoid conflict, resulting in the censorship of negative emotions or responses. Therapists should discourage social norms which inhibit the free expression of emotion, while preserving conventions of respect and genuineness. Occupational therapy leaders sometimes need to model the constructive expression of negative emotions or feedback. For example, 'Sometimes you come across as rude' can be stated more positively as 'When you use sarcasm it makes me (or others) feel defensive and I'm not sure that's the response you were looking for'. It is suggested that students practise doing this with each other before attempting to model it for clients.

Norms can be therapeutic or non-therapeutic. Members speaking only to the leader and not to each other is an example of a non-therapeutic norm. Once set, group norms are very persistent, therefore occupational therapy leaders should never hesitate to redirect the group at the first sign of trouble. Therapeutic norms lead the group toward a state of cohesiveness while non-therapeutic norms create barriers to group development. See Table 17.4 for some examples of therapeutic norms.

GROUP ROLES

Roles in groups may be assigned or voluntary. In work groups, managers supervise subordinates according to a predetermined organisational chart, with each role (or job description) specifically defined. Health-care teams include doctors, nurses, social workers and occupational therapists, for example. In the classic study by Benne & Sheats (1948), three types of non-explicit or voluntary roles were identified: task roles, group maintenance roles and individual roles. Task roles include initiator, information/opinion seeker and giver, elaborator, co-ordinator, orienter, evaluator, critic, energiser, recorder and procedural technician. These roles help the group to accomplish the task. Group maintenance roles influence the relationships among members: encourager, harmoniser, compromiser, gatekeeper/expediter, standard setter, group (process) observer and commentator and follower. Members of a mature group voluntarily take on a variety of roles; conversely, a member's comfort with a variety of roles is regarded as a sign of maturity. All the group maintenance roles facilitate a smooth running group, while the task roles enable goal accomplishment. Finlay (2002) suggested that occupational therapy leaders determine what roles are essential to meeting therapeutic goals and assist members in taking on those roles.

Group roles may be understood as shared leadership. When members take on task and maintenance roles, they can accomplish the goal with minimal intervention from the leader (advisory leadership). When members are unable or unwilling to play these roles, the leader steps in (directive leadership). Facilitative leadership falls somewhere in between these two extremes, as the occupational therapy leader enables members to take on some roles, while retaining others as leader according to the best interests of the group.

Problem group behaviours

The individual roles defined by Benne & Sheats (1948) tend to interfere with group functioning and thus may be equated with problem group behaviours. The primary responsibility of any occupational therapy group leader is to preserve the group's integrity; to do so she must discourage these problem behaviours. Attention-seeking roles, such as dominator, aggressor, recognition seeker, special interest pleader and self-confessor, will take up the group's time with non-relevant

Table 17.4   Therapeutic norms of occupational therapy groups

Group norm	Occupational therapy example
Open self-disclosure	Sharing person drawings with the group, including both positive and negative aspects of self-identity
Group interaction	Members ask each other questions about their drawings and offer empathy responses
Focus on process	Open discussion of feeling responses to the task after sharing, including what was hardest and easiest and why
Giving feedback to others	Members discuss what they like and do not like about each other's behaviour, stating dislikes constructively
Receiving feedback thoughtfully	Therapist uses empathy to help members explore both positive and negative responses to feedback
Verbalising concrete application of group learning for each member	Members use an 'ideal person' drawing to define qualities they admire in a friend. They agree that each will identify and have a conversation with one such friend during the coming week

issues unless redirected by the leader. Empathy and group member involvement are possible strategies for meeting the member's need for attention or recognition while allowing feedback to expose the effect of their individually centred behaviours. Likewise, the blocker, help-seeker and playboy use self-centred behaviours which meet their own emotional needs at the expense of the group. Blockers are often silent or stubbornly resistant to open self-disclosure, eventually causing other members to feel judged or criticised. Help-seekers actively seek help but reject it, angering advice-giving members. Playboys remain cynical and uninvolved, also provoking resentment among members. These difficult behaviours must be dealt with effectively by the occupational therapy leader in order to preserve the group's integrity. When one member's behaviour continues to block the group's development, that member should be removed from the group and treated individually. The occupational therapy leader should never sacrifice the group's well-being because of one member.

GROUP DEVELOPMENT

Theories of group development have undergone major changes in the past two decades. Until the mid-1980s, there was relative agreement that all groups evolve through predictable stages of development. Phase theorists, such as Tuckman (1965), Bion (1961), Schutz (1958) and Yalom (1995), all defined an initial phase marked by dependence on

the leader and a search for structure and purpose. Subsequently, the group encounters a conflict phase, during which the leader, the task and/or the group structure are challenged; all theorists concurred that conflict must be resolved in order for the group to reach cohesiveness. Yalom (1995) later redefined the final two stages, suggesting that groups tend to embrace a new-found harmony, following resolution of the conflict, during which members avoid the expression of negative affect. Continued growth involves the free expression of both positive and negative emotions, moving the group toward true cohesiveness, the final and ideal group stage. Yalom continues to defend this model, explaining deviations as the 'revisiting' of issues from earlier stages. See Table 17.5 for a summary of both traditional and current models of group development.

Two newer models are reviewed here as representative of current thinking about small group development. These systems-oriented models come from business management literature (just as some previous models have), but are helpful to our understanding of the dynamics of occupational therapy groups as they change and grow over time.

Poole's multiple sequence model

Poole (2003) challenged the validity of group development phase theory, focusing on decision making in work groups for his research. He suggested that group decision making generates

Table 17.5   Summary of traditional and current group development models (from Cole 2004, reprinted with permission from Slack Inc.)

Theorist	Year	Beginning of the group --- End of the group				
Bion	1961	Flight		Fight		Unite
Schutz	1958	Inclusion		Control		Affection
Tuckman	1977	Forming	Norming	Storming		Performing
Yalom	1985	Orientation		Conflict	Cohesiveness	Maturity
Poole	2003	Multiple sequences, cycles and breakpoints, multiple activity tracks				
Gersick	1988	First meeting	Phase 1	Midpoint transition	Phase 2	Conclusion

multiple clusters of associated behaviours along at least three activity tracks:

1. task process activities, which the group enacts to manage its task
2. relational activities, which reflect or manage relationships among the members (process)
3. topical focus, which includes issues and arguments of concern to the group (discussion, conflict resolution).

Central to Poole's developmental theory is the concept of **breakpoints**. Breakpoints are points of change or transition, of which Poole acknowledged three types: normal (changes in discussion topic, different parts of the task), delays (setbacks due to emerging problems, group problem solving) and disruptions (major conflicts, major changes required for the group to proceed). Poole suggested that no distinct phases occur in all groups but that different tasks, goals and group member characteristics produce unique patterns of content and process (Poole 2003).

Gersick's time and transition model of group development

Gersick studied eight diverse work teams to discover how their function changed over time (Gersick 2003). She changed the focus of group development from one of typical behaviours to one which attempts to explain the mechanisms of change and considers environmental contingencies. Gersick applied the theory of 'punctuated equilibrium' (Eldridge & Gould 1972) in which systems progress through periods of inertia 'punctuated by concentrated revolutionary periods of quantum change' (Gersick 2003, p62).

In **Phase 1,** the first half of the group's calendar time is an inertial movement, the direction of which is set during the first meeting. This places great importance on the initial meeting as a time when the group's process and content may be easily shaped. During the first meeting, Gersick speculated, member behaviours may be influenced by prior expectations, contexts relating to the sponsoring organisation (social, cultural contexts) and preferred behaviours or strategies characteristic of their personalities (client factors).

At the midpoint of the allotted calendar time, groups undergo a **midpoint transition** during which the direction of the group is revised. This transition is compared to Levinson's 'midlife crisis' in which, around age 40–45, an adult reappraises life so far and redefines what remains as 'time left to live' (Levinson 1978). At the midpoint transition, the group acknowledges earlier problems and faces the reality of limited time left to complete its task. The ideal outcome gives way to a more realistic one and both content and process change to accommodate this altered goal.

Phase 2 focuses on carrying out the plan formulated during the transition. Progress may spurt ahead in order to reach a markedly accelerated **conclusion**, in which the group finishes off the work generated during phase 2.

The **influence of context** on groups, not addressed by phase theorists, is significant in Gersick's model. Context impacts on the group's development at three critical periods: (1) design of the group, (2) the first meeting and (3) the midpoint transition. Translated into occupational therapy terms, the occupational therapist's selection of members for the group, structuring of the task and support for the group from outside sources greatly influence the group's functioning. During the group's first meeting, both content (the task and its purpose) and process (the norms for interaction and reflection) have a lasting impact on subsequent groups. During the phases of inertia, groups are less responsive to environmental influence. The next and final time the group opens itself to outside influence is the midpoint transition. At this time in the life of the group, members are familiar enough with the task to realise that outside resources, requirements and guidance are needed as a basis for rethinking their work, and the stress of a rapidly approaching deadline motivates them to pick up the pace while there is still time to produce a reasonably successful outcome.

In client-centred occupational therapy groups, when members take on more leadership responsibility, we are more likely to see the kind of dynamics reported in Gersick's study. Occupational therapy group leaders should acknowledge the importance of initial planning and of establishing therapeutic norms aggressively during the first meeting. With today's economic pressures in health care, more of our occupational therapy groups will be time limited. Subsequently, occupational therapy group leaders should anticipate the midpoint transition and use it as an opportunity to redirect and refine goals, correct non-therapeutic norms and provide needed resources to increase the likelihood of a positive outcome.

GROUP TERMINATION

Termination issues affect groups which have met over a period of time and need to be considered as the end approaches. Just as in life, when relationships end some people are better at letting go and moving on than others. Occupational therapy leaders need to be aware of both positive and negative coping as separation anxiety increases in the group. In an ongoing group of six or more sessions, **preparation** should begin 2 weeks ahead, with comments or questions during the session summary. This gives group members time to think about what needs to be done prior to the group's ending. **Unfinished business** from prior groups, such as intermember conflict, should be revisited and openly discussed.

Sometimes members withdraw emotionally from the group, causing a regression in development and a devaluation of the group's benefits. When the occupational therapy leader encourages **open expression of feelings**, the value of the group is preserved. Reviewing the group's activities from the beginning can help the group to **summarise** what was learned. Finally, the occupational therapy group leader shares her own perspective, **reinforcing positive outcomes**. For those members who typically cope negatively with loss (anger, depression, withdrawal, re-emergence of symptoms), a positive group termination provides a model for future endings in life.

DESIGNING GROUP INTERVENTIONS

In client-centred groups, the importance of thorough and careful planning cannot be overemphasised. The written group plan is called a **group protocol**. It serves as a guide for group sessions and may also be used as a marketing tool. This section will review the steps in designing a group protocol: needs assessment, potential members, therapeutic goals, selecting a frame of reference, logistics (time, place, group size), session outlines, supplies and cost and outcome criteria.

NEEDS ASSESSMENT

An occupational therapy needs assessment explores the problem areas of a potential client population. This information is gathered from documents (such as medical charts), organisational representatives (referral sources), significant others (such as carers) and the clients themselves (written surveys, interviews). In client-centred practice, the clients' collective occupational goals and priorities form the basis for defining needs.

MEMBER SELECTION

Potential members for a group are selected according to commonality of goals, priorities and valued life roles, as well as ability. The purpose of group membership should be discussed with each client prior to the initial session. The protocol outlines the inclusionary (client characteristics, goals or life roles appropriate for the group) and exclusionary (factors making a client inappropriate) criteria for membership in a specific occupational therapy group. Goal refinement is ideally accomplished in an initial meeting with potential members.

GROUP GOALS

Compatible goals of potential members are summarised as the basis for group design. From these **therapeutic goals** a theme emerges, which will guide the selection of appropriate activities. Themes are combined with occupational therapy modalities in creating titles for occupational therapy groups. For example, 'Art for Social Skills', 'Mental Gymnastics for Work Readiness' or 'Movement for Health' each include both goals and methods in a different occupational therapy frame of reference. The group protocol should include a list of at least five therapeutic goals with a rationale for each.

THEORY–BASED GROUPS

Occupational therapy frames of reference guide our clinical reasoning when designing groups. The occupational therapist should **select a frame of reference** that best addresses the therapeutic goals and problem areas of client members. Within the group protocol, the frame of reference should be identified and briefly justified for use with the specific members and goals already described. For example, the **psychodynamic** frame of reference offers guidelines for the application of creative media with goals involving self-awareness, insight or reality orientation, effective expression or control of emotion and developing the skills for maintaining satisfying relationships with others. 'Art for Social Skills' suggests using painting, drawing or sculpture as a way to raise self-awareness as a basis for forming trusting relationships with others.

'Mental Gymnastics for Work Readiness' suggests the use of **cognitive behavioural** exercises to build work skills. The cognitive behavioural frame of reference best suits goals which involve learning or practising skills. In this group example, memory games or problem-solving tasks might be used with individuals who aspire to acquire or return to work. The psychoeducational group uses cognitive behavioural strategies when working with goals like stress management, assertiveness, time management and the modulation of maladaptive occupational patterns such as compulsions or addictions.

'Movement for Health' applies **sensory motor** principles, such as biomechanics or sensory integration, in designing movement activities for groups. Depending on the importance of repetition and practice of skilled movement, the activity portion of the group may be extended to two-thirds and discussion time diminished to one-third, or less if clients have a limited capacity to verbalise. Ross's Five Stage Groups (Ross 1997, Ross & Bachner 2004) use the principles of sensory integration within a structure similar to Cole's seven steps, emphasising non-verbal communication. Ross's groups work on goals such as increasing attention and alertness for clients with minimal cognitive functioning. Bracegirdle (2002) described the advantages of various modes of physical exercise for clients with mental health conditions, such as sports, yoga and relaxation, most of which lend themselves easily to mind–brain–body connection goals in groups. However, the creative use of movement, such as in dance therapy, might better be understood using a psychodynamic frame of reference.

GROUP LOGISTICS: GROUP SIZE, TIMING AND SETTING

The next step in designing a group is to determine **logistics**. Most therapeutic groups should not exceed eight members, with less when the need for more therapist assistance is anticipated. The time and place of group meeting may depend on availability of rooms but contextual factors should also be considered, such as appropriate equipment, privacy or freedom from distractions.

GROUP SESSION OUTLINES

Group session outlines for each session should follow the format in Box 17.1. Activity descriptions should be clear and detailed enough for another occupational therapy leader to follow and lead the group as you intended. At least three open-ended discussion questions should be included for each

Box 17.1 Group session outline using Cole's seven steps

- Title of group (overall theme)
- Title of session (today's activity)
- Number in sequence (e.g. session 3 of 8 total)
- Goals addressed
- Time frame (e.g. warm-up 5 minutes, activity 15 minutes, etc.)
- Supplies (list and include number needed)
- Description:
  Warm-up
  Activity instructions
  Processing questions (at least 3 open questions)
  Generalising questions (at least 3 open questions)
  Application questions (at least 3 open questions)
  Points for summary

of steps 4–6 (see Cole's seven steps described on p 317-320). Points for summary should be anticipated, even though they will change as the session unfolds. Planning at least six sessions is suggested when writing a group protocol.

SUPPLIES AND COST

Supplies and cost can be determined once the session outlines are complete. This information will be needed for marketing the group to hospital or community service administrators. Cost will depend upon the number of members, what might be available free or donated and the average cost of items needed.

OUTCOME CRITERIA

Setting outcome criteria is a way to measure goal achievement. An assessment may be given before the group begins and again at its conclusion to determine what has changed. To assess progress during each session, a check sheet or rating scale may be designed. Occasionally, published assessment tools may fit specific group goals and these may be incorporated into the sessions and discussed with client members. For example, Oakley's Role Checklist (1984) may be incorporated into a retirement planning group as a basis for anticipating changes in role status. In today's cost-conscious health-care environment, occupational therapists need to use outcome criteria to validate the effectiveness of group interventions.

SUMMARY

This chapter has reviewed some ways in which occupational therapy groups may enhance a client-centred mental health practice. Finlay (2002) reminded us that 'group experiences are very powerful and can be destructive as well as beneficial' (p263). A carefully designed group (using Cole's seven steps), application of appropriate theory, prudent selection of members and client participation in goal selection all go a long way toward ensuring positive outcomes.

To handle the challenge presented by clients with mental health issues, occupational therapy leaders need a good understanding of group dynamics as well as good leadership skills. Therapists may wish to write out a group protocol with discussion questions for each step when starting a new group and to practise facilitating member involvement by using some of the techniques described here. Experienced group therapists can then personalise the steps to meet the unique needs of their clients.

Groupwork continues to be a dynamic and cost-effective tool for both evaluation and intervention in occupational therapy.

References

Allen CK, Earhart C, Blue T 1992 Occupational therapy treatment goals for the physically and cognitively disabled. American Occupational Therapy Association, Bethesda, Maryland

Allen CK, Blue T, Earhart CA 1995 Understanding cognitive performance modes. Allen Conferences, Ormond Beach, Florida

Bandura A 1977 Social learning theory. Prentice-Hall, Englewood Cliffs, New Jersey

Barge JK 2003 Leadership as organizing. In: Hirokawa R, Cathcart R, Samovar L, et al L (eds) Small group communication: theory and practice: an anthology, 8th edn. Roxbury Publishing, Los Angeles

Benne K, Sheats P 1948 Functional roles of group members. Journal of Social Issues 2(4): 123-135

Bion W 1961 Experiences in groups and other papers. Basic Books, New York

Bracegirdle H 2002 Developing physical fitness to promote mental health. In: Creek J (ed) Occupational therapy and mental health, 3rd edn. Churchill Livingstone, Edinburgh

Cole MB 2005 Group dynamics in occupational therapy, 3rd edn. Slack, Thorofare, New Jersey

Creek J 2003 Occupational therapy defined as a complex intervention. College of Occupational Therapists, London

Donohue M 1999 Theoretical bases of Mosey's group interaction skills. Occupational Therapy International 6(1): 35-51

Donohue M 2003 Group profile: studies with children: validity measures and item analysis. Occupational Therapy in Mental Health 19: 1-23

Donohue M 2007 Social profile: interrater reliability in psychiatric and community activity groups. Australian Occupational Therapy Journal 54: 49-58.

Eldridge N, Gould SJ 1972 Punctuated equilibria: an alternative to phyletic gradualism. In: Schopf TJM (ed) Models in paleobiology. Freeman, Cooper, San Francisco

Falk-Kessler J, Momich C, Perel S 1991 Therapeutic factors in occupational therapy groups. American Journal of Occupational Therapy 45: 59-66

Finlay L 2002 Groupwork. In: Creek J (ed) Occupational therapy and mental health, 3rd edn. Churchill Livingstone, Edinburgh

Gersick CJ 2003 Time and transition in work teams. In: Hirokawa R, Cathcart R, Samovar L, et al (eds) Small group communication: theory and practice: an anthology, 8th edn. Roxbury Publishing, Los Angeles

Gouran D 2003 Leadership as the art of counteractive influence in decision-making and problem-solving groups. In: Hirokawa R, Cathcart R, Samovar L, et al (eds) Small group communication: theory and practice: an anthology, 8th edn. Roxbury Publishing, Los Angeles

Hersey P, Blanchard K 1969 Life-cycle theory of leadership. Training and Development Journal 23: 26-34

Law M, Baptiste S, Mills J 1995 Client-centred practice: what does it mean and does it make a difference? Canadian Journal of Occupational Therapy 62: 250-257

Levinson D 1978 The seasons of a man's life. Ballantine Books, New York

Mosey AC 1986 Psychosocial components of occupational therapy. Raven Press, New York

Oakley F 1984 The role checklist. National Institutes of Health, Bethesda, Maryland

Poole MS 2003 A multiple sequence model of group decision development. In: Hirokawa R, Cathcart R, Samovar L et al (eds) Small group communication: theory and practice: an anthology, 8th edn. Roxbury Publishing, Los Angeles

Ross M 1997 Integrative group therapy: mobilizing coping abilities with the Five Stage Group. American Occupational Therapy Association, Bethesda, Maryland

Ross M, Bachner S (eds) 2004 Adults with developmental disabilities: current approaches in occupational therapy. American Occupational Therapy Association, Bethesda, Maryland

Schutz W 1958 The interpersonal underworld. Harvard Business Review 36: 123-135

Shaw M 1981 Group dynamics: the psychology of small group behavior, 3rd edn. McGraw Hill, New York

Shiminoff S, Jenkins M 2003 Leadership and gender. In: Hirokawa R, Cathcart R, Samovar L, et al (eds) Small group communication: theory and practice: an anthology, 8th edn. Roxbury Publishing, Los Angeles

Tuckman B 1965 Developmental sequence in small groups. Psychological Bulletin 63: 384-399

World Health Organization 2001 International classification of functioning, disability and health. World Health Organization, Geneva

Yalom I 1995 The theory and practice of group psychotherapy, 4th edn. Basic Books, New York

Chapter 18

Creative activities

Jennifer Creek

INTRODUCTION

Occupational therapists have access to a wide range of activities which can be used with their clients to achieve therapeutic ends. One group of activities, that has gone in and out of fashion over the years but still has an important place in therapy today, is creative activities. Creative activities require the individual to incorporate something of himself into the production of an idea or end product, for example a poem or a piece of embroidery. They therefore have a very personal dimension. Occupational therapists use a full range of creative activities, selecting the most appropriate ones to achieve the goals of particular clients.

This chapter will define creativity, describe the characteristics of creative people and outline the creative process. The therapeutic potential of creative activities will be discussed and some practical pointers given for organising creative therapy sessions. An occupational therapy theory of creativity will be described briefly. The chapter will end with an example of a creative activity used with women with enduring mental health problems.

First, it will be useful to consider what is meant by creativity.

WHAT IS CREATIVITY?

To create is to 'make, form, or constitute for the first time or afresh; produce, give rise to' (*New Shorter Oxford English Dictionary* 1993, p544). To be creative is to have the ability to create, to be inventive or imaginative, to show imagination as well as routine skill (op. cit.). It means being able to think and act independently of the immediate influence of internal and external stimuli (Vygotsky 1994). Stein (1974, p6) defined creativity as 'a process as a result of which novelty is achieved'. This novelty may be in form, appearance or relationship (Beeman 1990). Creative activity is, therefore, activity which involves imagination and has a novel, worthwhile product. The product may be concrete, such as a painting or piece of writing, or it may be an original idea or train of thought.

In order to produce original ideas or solutions to problems, it is necessary to keep an open mind, to let go of stereotypes and to free up the imagination (Flach 1980). This way of approaching the world can be described as playful, in that it 'involves flexibility and spontaneity rather than proficiency in performing specific activities' (Ramugondo 2004, p175).

It is suggested that, although some people have more creative potential than others, everyone has the capacity to be creative. This is called *everyday creativity*: 'an everyday phenomenon found in all people' and 'a facet of personality capable of contributing to the maintenance of mental health' (Cropley 1997, p233).

Everyday creativity represents a departure from a view of creativity as represented only in exceptional and rare accomplishment, such as was found in Mozart or Einstein. In everyday creativity, creativity is considered as a quality or capability that is present to varying degrees in all human beings and that potentially manifests itself in virtually all aspects of daily life (Hasselkus 2002, p116).

Creativity can be differentiated from other types of intellectual ability (Milgram 1990).

1. **General intellectual ability**. This refers to the ability to think in abstractions and to solve problems in a logical and systematic way. This ability can be measured by IQ tests.
2. **Specific intellectual ability**. This is a distinct intellectual ability in a particular area, such as music or mathematics. Such abilities are usually reflected in achievement in particular subjects at school.
3. **General creative thinking**. This is the ability to 'generate ideas that are imaginative, clever, elegant or surprising' (p217) and to produce original solutions to problems.
4. **Specific creative talent**. This refers to the ability to produce socially valued, novel products in areas such as art, writing, science, music, business or politics. Such talents may be evident in children but are not normally fully developed until adulthood.

No correlation has been found between general or specific intellectual ability and general or specific creative ability. This means that a person with a low IQ or someone who has never attained academic qualifications may still be capable of thinking creatively and producing original, creative work. Conversely, a person with high academic achievements or in a very senior administrative job may not perform well in activities that demand creative ability.

Creative activity requires a certain amount of courage and independence (Beeman 1990). Human activities always have a social context and truly original work may appear shocking to others at first. The creative thinker, artist or scientist must be prepared to face disapproval or ridicule before his or her work is accepted. This is not usually the case for most small acts of creation but only for major original works that change the way we see the world. Most people's creativity is shaped by their social environment (Amabile 1990); very few people are able to shape others' perceptions of the world by their work.

Creativity is usually a synthesis or reformulation of existing ideas and experience, therefore a person needs to have experience and knowledge in order to create (Beeman 1990, Cropley 1997).

THE CREATIVE PROCESS

The chapter so far has stressed that although creative activity frequently has an end product, it is a process which takes place over time. Various researchers have described the creative process as consisting of a series of predictable stages (Beeman 1990, Flach 1980, Poincare 1970, Weisberg 1986).

1. **Preparation**. This is a period of time when information is taken in and the individual may be consciously trying to solve a problem or produce a piece of work without success.
2. **Incubation**. The work is put aside and not thought about consciously, but work is continuing unconsciously, sorting and evaluating the information and material that has been absorbed.
3. **Illumination**. If the incubation stage has been successful the individual will experience sudden illumination and a surge of energy to resume work.
4. **Verification**. This is when the solution to the problem is worked out in full, or the painting is completed, or the book written. The insights provided by the illumination stage are put into practice.

The next section looks at how creative ability can be promoted in therapy to assist people to overcome mental health problems.

CREATIVE ACTIVITIES AS THERAPY

When someone is facing difficulties due to illness or disability, a capacity for thinking and acting creatively will influence the way in which problems are approached and will enhance the ability to find solutions. To this extent, creativity is an important aspect of any occupational therapy intervention. There is also a range of interventions which specifically aim to tap into the client's own creative potential. These are often known as creative therapies and include such techniques as art, drama, dance, music, pottery and certain types of writing. Creative activities may be used with people of any age and with any type or level of dysfunction.

Creek (2005) identified four approaches to using creative activities as therapy:

- as a form of psychotherapy, to help people cope with painful or difficult feelings
- for the expression of feelings without the use of spoken language

- as play, for both children and adults, to promote pleasure and spontaneity
- for health promotion, by strengthening emotional resilience.

In this section we will first describe what is meant by creative activities, look at the value of creative activities as therapeutic media and consider how people's creative potential might be supported and expressed. An occupational therapy theory of creative ability is then described.

WHAT ARE CREATIVE ACTIVITIES?

It is possible to approach many of the activities of daily life creatively and use them as vehicles for self-expression (Hasselkus 2002). For example, cooking may be seen as a routine chore or it can be an opportunity for exploration and experimentation. Self-care can be nothing more than a regular habit or it can be a chance to express personality and mood through clothes, make-up, hairstyle, grooming and personal style. Housework, that notoriously dull routine, can be given a creative dimension if the living environment is used as an extension of the personality and as a space for personal expression.

Other activities are valued as carrying a specific potential for creative expression. For example, sewing, knitting, DIY, painting and decorating, pottery, furniture restoration, upholstery, gardening, dancing, writing and cake decorating are all activities which people may engage in for the pleasure of creating as well as, in some cases, because of economic necessity. Adult education classes are often a forum for learning new creative skills or practising existing ones.

The range of creative activities available to the occupational therapist is vast. These may be carried out in hospital occupational therapy departments, on wards, in day centres or in day hospitals. Community facilities may be accessed, for example suggesting an evening class for a client recovering from depression or supporting a person with learning difficulties while he takes a college course in a creative skill. Some of the creative activities that might be used as part of a therapeutic intervention are listed in Box 18.1.

Box 18.1 Creative activities that might be used in therapy

Calligraphy	Making books or journals
Candle making	Marbling
Christmas decorations	Mosaics
Collage	Painting
Conjuring	Papier mâché
Crochet	Patchwork
Dancing	Photography
Decorating Easter eggs	Playing musical
Découpage	instruments
Drama	Pottery
Drawing	Puppetry
Dressmaking	Singing
Embroidery	Stained glass
Enamelling	Tie-dye and batik
Felt making	Weaving
Flower arranging	Woodwork
Gardening	Writing stories or
Juggling	poetry
Knitting	
Macramé	

THE VALUE OF CREATIVE ACTIVITIES

Creativity has an evolutionary value for the human race in that it leads to finding original solutions to problems of survival (Runco & Richards 2002) and, further, contributes significantly to advances in human knowledge and understanding. It also has value for individuals, both for the pragmatic purpose of solving problems in daily life and for enhancing quality of life. Schmid (2005, p27) proposed that people have a biological need to express their creativity and that the expression of creativity 'through everyday activities ... has a major impact on health and well-being'.

Creek (2003, p54) defined health in terms of an ability 'to perform ... daily occupations to a satisfying and effective level and to respond positively to change by adapting activities to meet changing needs'. This definition implies a direct link between creativity and health (Creek 2005, p77): 'If ... creativity is a necessary component of volitional action, then absence of creativity will mean an inability to adapt activities for particular ends and, hence, failure to maintain health'.

When someone has a mental health problem, the ways in which creative activities can be of therapeutic value include the following.

- **Increasing motivation**. People find creative activities pleasurable and will actively seek opportunities to exercise their creative potential. 'Play generates energy because it is a pleasure in itself, an intrinsic end' (Gordon 1961, p119).
- **Enhancing learning**. Reilly (1974) highlighted the importance of a playful approach to learning new skills. She proposed a hierarchy of learning in which playful exploration is the first stage, leading on to practice to a level of competence and finishing with the application of newly learned skills to achieve personal goals.
- **Promoting emotional resilience**. Learning how to think creatively and flexibly in order to solve life's problems or make successful adaptations to circumstances increases the ability to cope with stress and adversity (Flach 1980).
- **Coping with chronic illness**. The psychologist Frances Reynolds (2005) studied how people living with chronic illness and disability use creative activities as part of their coping strategies. She found that the benefits include: renewed sense of agency and control; distraction from symptoms and illness anxieties; provision of meaningful goals; restoring a satisfactory self-image; and providing entry into new social networks.
- **Increasing satisfaction and self-esteem**. It is intrinsically satisfying to produce an original piece of work or an original idea, independent of the personal or social value of the product. Creative activity is therefore an important source of personal satisfaction and self-esteem.
- **Enabling self-expression**. People have a need to express their feelings, whether joyful or painful. Feelings that are not expressed may leak out in inappropriate actions or in overreaction to apparently trivial events. Creative activities are a socially acceptable and controllable medium for expressing strong feelings which may otherwise seem overwhelming.

- **Facilitating projection**. Hagedorn (1995, p120) pointed out that in the field of mental health, creative activities are used projectively, 'to enable the individual to gain insights into his situation'. For example, the client might be invited to paint a picture of how he is feeling. Independently of the conscious use of imagery to express his feelings, he will also project unconscious material into his work which is then available for discussion and analysis.
- **Providing opportunities for sublimation**. The human drive to be creative is so strong that it can be used as an outlet for the feelings arising from frustration of other needs. Hocking (2007, p27) described 'an intensity of emotion' associated with creative self-expression. For example, a client might be encouraged to write a poem about the experience of unrequited love.

ENHANCING CREATIVITY

Although creativity is a natural process and a pleasurable one, there are various factors which might inhibit its expression. Environmental influences, such as an impoverished physical environment during childhood or adults who discourage messy activities, might lead to an unwillingness to risk trying out new ways of thinking or behaving. This can be seen as a form of occupational deprivation (see Chapter 3, p48). Burke (1977) described how the intrinsic urge to act translates into a sense of personal causation – the initiation of action intended to have an effect on the environment. The development of personal causation can be blocked by lack of opportunities to make choices and by repeated experiences of failure. People with a weak sense of personal causation exhibit unwillingness to initiate action and may appear helpless and hopeless.

Du Toit (1991) identified certain personal characteristics which inhibit the expression of creativity, including lack of adaptability, poor self-control, apathy and aloofness. Finally, survival needs take priority over other, higher needs (Maslow 1968); therefore creative expression may be inhibited by physiological need or by feelings of insecurity.

One of the greatest challenges to an occupational therapist is to find activities which tap into the client's creative potential and overcome these barriers. The following list gives some of the conditions which the therapist can provide in the therapeutic environment to facilitate creative expression.

- The environment should be stimulating, containing a variety of attractive objects to look at and handle. Hasselkus (2002, p117) described the importance of the physical environment in stimulating and supporting creativity: 'In some ways, perhaps, one's physical environment acts like a birth mother, providing the host entity and sustenance that enable creativity to be born and to flourish'.
- For an activity which requires a theme or topic, such as creative writing, it may be helpful to brainstorm at the beginning of the session to stimulate the client's own ideas (Hasselkus 2002). For example, the group might be asked to suggest settings for a romantic short story, the more unlikely the better. They may then be asked to think of improbable ways in which the hero and heroine might meet. Introducing an element of absurdity or humour into the exercise demonstrates that it should not be taken too seriously and can help to stimulate creativity.
- Materials and equipment should be of good quality and readily available. For example, if the activity is pottery there should be a plentiful supply of clay ready to use, enough hand tools and turntables or boards for everyone, a water supply, overalls and cleaning cloths. Many materials are attractive and can be displayed advantageously to stimulate clients' interest, such as fabrics, beads, threads and yarns in a sewing room.
- Items that might be copied or might be perceived to set an unachievably high standard should be removed. For example, if clients are having a free painting session, it is not a good idea to have postcards or photographs available to copy. These would focus undue attention on the end product rather than on the process of creativity.

- Participants in any creative activity should be given all the information and instruction they need to complete the activity successfully. For example, when leading a pottery session it is important to emphasise the careful preparation of clay so that air bubbles are removed and the work is not lost in the kiln. The level of ability of the client and his present mental state should always be taken into account in selecting a suitable method for teaching new skills or imparting information.
- The focus of the session should be on the creative process and not on the end product, although every effort should be made to support clients in making products that they can be proud of. The therapist should avoid praising a particular piece of work for its beauty or skilful execution if other clients might compare their own work unfavourably with it and become inhibited.
- Enough time has to be allowed for people to work at their own pace, without pressure. If work cannot be finished during one session, or if the client expresses a wish to continue to practise a new skill, there should be further opportunities to continue.
- The therapist should treat everyone's work with respect, irrespective of the quality of workmanship or stage of completion. This is partly a symbolic valuing of the client himself and partly modelling, so that the client learns to value his own efforts and productions. For example, all pieces of work should be kept unless the client expressly asks for a piece to be destroyed.
  - The environment must be secure and free from casual interruptions. Clients may be inhibited by having other people wandering in and observing them at work. For example, if a small group of clients has been doing creative dancing together for a few weeks, they may have learned to be comfortable with each other but may be extremely embarrassed if an outsider sees them performing.

If people are anxious about trying creative activities it is helpful to provide more structure and a more concrete topic to start with. The amount of structure can be reduced as they become more confident in the activity. The structure may be inherent in the activity used, for example cross-stitch embroidery is a more structured activity than free painting, or it may be in the way the session is organised. For example, a first creative writing session could involve clients in writing a short description of a building they know or writing an imaginary conversation between two people they know. A later session might require them to describe feelings or pretend to be someone else and write in the first person. As the group gains confidence and skill they might progress to writing short stories on topics of their own choice.

AN OCCUPATIONAL THERAPY THEORY OF CREATIVITY

De Witt (1992) demonstrated how the development of creative ability can be used as a framework for therapeutic intervention, drawing on the earlier work of du Toit, a South African occupational therapist. Du Toit (1970) called her model 'Creative ability' and described it as being concerned with the way in which people realise, define and extend themselves by expressing their potential through creative action. Creative ability denotes 'the combination of an inner volition or drive towards action and the externalisation or expression of that volition in action' du Toit 1974, p87).

Creative ability in an individual is manifested in his creation of a tangible or intangible product. The quality of his action (doing) reflects the quality of the volitional component of his 'being'. The level of his 'doing' is characterised by the level of his ability to form relational contacts with materials, people and situations, by the measure of his anxiety control, by his manifestation of originative ability and by the quality of his preparedness to actualise himself through exercising effort in action which makes maximal demands on his potential (du Toit 1970, p39).

Du Toit (1970) described four aspects of creativity.

1. **Creative capacity**: the total creative potential of a particular individual.
2. **Creative response**: the positive reaction which the individual displays towards any opportunity for activity.

3. **Creative participation**: the process of being involved in all activities of life, not just in specific opportunities for creativity.
4. **Creative act**: the endpoint of creative participation, the end product.

Creative action requires a positive attitude towards activity and a willingness to participate, as well as basic creative potential. Creative ability, therefore, affects the degree and quality of the individual's activities in all areas of life: personal care, productivity, social relationships and leisure.

The development of creative ability is a lifelong process, starting at birth and continuing into old age. It is subject to the same influences and constraints as other aspects of human development. Three stages and six substages in the development of creative ability can be identified, as shown in Figure 18.1.

Creative ability is not a static characteristic but varies with the degree to which the individual feels secure and with the demands that are made on him. Mental illness can interfere with creative ability, either temporarily or permanently. Box 18.2 shows the level of function that might be observed in clients operating at the different levels of creative ability.

Creative ability has two components: volition and action. Volition governs action and action is the manifestation of volition, so if either component is deficient then creative ability will be impaired. The therapist assesses the client in terms of these two factors across all areas of daily life activity. Assessment is based on direct observation of the client's performance in a wide variety of situations.

Intervention is planned to stimulate the client's volition or to give a positive direction to actions. The types of activities used will depend on the developmental level of the client's creative ability (de Witt 1992).

Level one

Clients operating at the first level, preparation for constructive action, might include people with profound learning difficulties or those with severe psychosis. At this level, the aims of intervention are to:

- facilitate awareness of the self and of the therapist
- encourage awareness of the environment
- stimulate sensory and motor reflexes to promote biological tone.

Treatment sessions should be short. Alertness and concentration can be maintained through the presentation of stimuli, such as speaking the client's name, presenting objects from the environment to be touched and explored, and changing the client's position and posture. As the client

COMPONENT	Volition	Action
DEFINITION	Inner condition of the organism that initiates or directs its behaviour towards a goal	Exertion of motivation into mental and physical effort resulting in the creation of a tangible or intangible end product
DEVELOPMENTAL STAGES		
I Preparation for constructive action	Tone Self-differentiation	Predestructive Destructive Incidental
II Behaviour and skill development for norm compliancy	Self-presentation Participation: Passive Imitative	Explorative Experimental Imitative
III Behaviour and skill development for self-actualisation	Participation: Active Competitive Contribution Competitive contribution	Original Product-centred Situation-centred Society-centred

Figure 18.1   The development of creative ability (adapted from de Witt 1992).

Box 18.2 Levels of creative ability

Preparation for constructive action
Patients at this level are dependent, unable to provide for or care for themselves in any way. Activity is purposeless and they have little or no control over bodily functions. They lack awareness of the self as a separate being or awareness of others. Language is absent or very basic.

Behaviour and skill development for norm compliance
Patients at this level are exploring and learning about the self and the environment and developing a sense of self. They have many of the skills of independent living and are able to apply them if given support and encouragement. Awareness of others is developing. Conversational skills are improving although conversation may reflect the individual's psychopathology.

Behaviour and skill development for self-actualisation
People at this level are rarely seen as hospital inpatients. They are able to cope independently, to recognise when they have problems and to change their behaviour to meet personal needs. They are able to form consistent and lasting interpersonal relationships although there may be an element of selfishness. They may prefer not to take responsibility or initiate projects with other people. At the lower end of this level, people may have a wide range of interests but organisation of time for adequate relaxation may be a problem.

---

demonstrates increasing receptivity to stimuli, he can be gradually upgraded until he is ready to move on to the next level.

Level two

Clients at the second level, behaviour and skill development for norm compliancy, will include many of the people the occupational therapist works with in a mental health setting. At this level, the aims of intervention are to:

- encourage awareness and exploration of the self and of the physical and social environment
- facilitate the development of personal and social skills to support community living
- encourage awareness of and compliance with social and group norms.

This level covers a wide range of abilities so activities should be graded as the patient's abilities improve. The initial phase of treatment is therapist directed, moving towards patient-directed activities as the patient develops skills and begins to show preferences. It is necessary for the therapist to be encouraging and supportive in the early stages of intervention in order to make the patient feel safe. The patient should be asked for opinions and ideas and given choices about activity. Activities should be varied and will include

personal care, sport and recreational activities, group activities and tasks with a concrete end product, such as art or cooking. Emphasis is placed on the patient's interaction with materials and processes rather than on the end product.

Level three

The third level of creative ability, behaviour and skill development for self-actualisation, is not often seen in people using mental health services since it represents an ability to function in all areas of life. The individual may have a problem but is able to try out new ways of behaving in order to find an acceptable solution. However, occupational therapists working in the fields of primary mental health promotion or community development might find themselves working with people at this level.

ORGANISING CREATIVE ACTIVITIES

Creativity has already been defined as the ability to be inventive or imaginative. Creative activities are therefore those which offer opportunities for the client to produce original work. The skill of the therapist is in adapting or synthesising activities to make it possible for people to access their own creative potential. This section describes how a creative activity session might be organised, using tie-dying as an example.

TIE-DYING AS A CREATIVE GROUP ACTIVITY

This session is planned for a group of women with enduring mental health problems who have never done the activity before. They are attending a day centre on a sessional basis.

Planning and preparation

Half a day is set aside for the activity, allowing for a tea or coffee break while work is in the dye bath or drying. The group know beforehand what activity they will be doing so they can wear suitable clothing. A room is chosen which has good lighting, a sink, tables with washable surfaces, chairs and a washable floor covering. The room is prepared before the group arrive. Buckets, bowls, measuring jugs, kettles, spoons, cold water dyes, dye fixative and salt for preparing the dye are set out on one workbench against the wall. One container of dye may be already mixed for the demonstration. Drying racks, washing powder and an iron are available. Aprons or overalls are available to protect people's clothes. Tables are put together in a square so that everyone can sit together. Fabrics for dying, string, clothes pegs, dye samples, examples of tie-dying, books and any other materials are set out on the main work table.

Running the group

When the group arrive they are invited to sit at the table for a demonstration of the activity. If people arrive early, they may be offered a cup of tea or coffee on arrival and have the opportunity to look at books and samples before the group starts. The therapist tells them what they are going to make and shows examples of finished products. The group are then shown some examples of different tie-dye effects and told how these were obtained. The therapist demonstrates three or four simple methods of tying or clamping cloth to achieve different effects. She points out that there are other methods people can try if they feel confident. She puts her samples into the prepared dye bath and invites people to select their materials and choose a technique to start with. She suggests that they choose different textures and weights of material to see how this affects the finished result.

People are encouraged to work at their own pace on their own pieces of work. The therapist moves around the table, encouraging and offering advice if it is sought. If a piece of work looks as though it is too loosely tied, she will suggest that a better effect may be obtained by tightening the ties. The therapist's manner of approach is important because she wants to ensure that people experience success but wishes to avoid sounding critical of their efforts. If anyone is having difficulty deciding what to do she goes through the alternatives with them again. When someone is ready to put work in the dye bath the therapist asks him to choose a colour and shows him how to mix the dye. Other people are invited to watch the process if they wish to.

When everyone has at least one piece of work in the dye bath, a tea break may be suggested. The session is planned so that everyone can be active throughout, while all working at their own pace. After a break, the first pieces of work should be ready to come out of the dye bath. They are rinsed thoroughly, washed and hung to dry. The drying rack should be near a heater so that the cloth dries as quickly as possible. Once the work is no longer dripping wet, the ties may be cut and the cloth ironed dry. Group members are encouraged to look at each other's work as it is finished.

Ending the session

At the end of the session, some work will still be in the dye bath. The therapist promises to finish the process and leave the work to dry so that people can collect it on another day. Finished work may be taken away.

SUMMARY

This chapter began by considering the nature of creativity as an aspect of human functioning and described the creative process. The therapeutic value of creativity was then discussed, both the value of being able to think of creative solutions to problems and the value of activities which are seen as especially creative, such as art, music and drama. Ways of structuring activity sessions to enhance the expression of creativity were discussed. An occupational therapy theory of creative activity was described briefly. This theory was developed by South African occupational therapists for application with any client group, not just people with mental health problems. The chapter ended with a description of how to set up and run a creative activity group, tie-dying.

References

Amabile TM 1990 Within you, Without you: The social psychology of creativity, and beyond. In: Runco MA, Albert RS (eds) Theories of creativity. Sage, Newbury Park, CA, pp61-91

Beeman CA 1990 Just this side of madness: creativity and the drive to create. UCA Press

Burke JP 1977 A clinical perspective on motivation: pawn versus origin. American Journal of Occupational Therapy 31(4): 254-258

Creek J 2003 Occupational therapy defined as a complex intervention. College of Occupational Therapists, London

Creek J 2005 The therapeutic benefits of creativity. In: Schmid T (ed) Promoting health through creativity: for professionals in health, arts and education. Whurr, London

Cropley AJ 1997 Creativity and mental health in everyday life. In: Runco MA, Richards R (eds) Eminent creativity, everyday creativity and health. Ablex Publishing Corporation, Greenwich, Connecticut, pp231-246

de Witt PA 1992 Creative ability – a model for psychiatric occupational therapy. In: Crouch RB (ed) Occupational therapy in psychiatry and mental health. Lifecare Group, Johannesburg

du Toit V 1970 Creative ability. In: Patient volition and action in occupational therapy. Vona and Marie du Toit Foundation, Hillbrow, South Africa

du Toit V 1974 An investigation into the correlation between volition and its expression in action. In: du Toit V 1991 Patient volition and action in occupational therapy. Vona and Marie du Toit Foundation, Hillbrow, South Africa, 87-97

du Toit V 1991 Initiative in occupational therapy. In: Patient volition and action in occupational therapy. Vona and Marie du Toit Foundation, Hillbrow, South Africa

Flach FF 1980 Psychobiologic resilience, psychotherapy and the creative process. Comprehensive Psychiatry 21(6): 510-518

Gordon WJJ 1961 Synectics. Harper and Row, New York

Hagedorn R 1995 Occupational therapy: perspectives and processes. Churchill Livingstone, Edinburgh

Hasselkus BR 2002 The meaning of everyday occupation. Slack, Thorofare, New Jersey

Hocking C 2007 The romance of occupational therapy. In: Creek J (ed) Contemporary issues in occupational therapy: reasoning and reflection. Wiley, Chichester, pp23-40

Maslow AH 1968 Towards a psychology of being. Van Nostrand, New York

Milgram RM 1990 Creativity: an idea whose time has come and gone? In: Runco MA, Robert RS (eds) Theories of creativity. Sage, Newbury Park

New Shorter Oxford English Dictionary 1993 Clarendon Press, Oxford

Poincare H 1970 Mathematical creation. In: Vernon PE (ed) Creativity. Penguin, Harmondsworth

Ramugondo E l 2004 Play and playfulness: children living with HIV/AIDS. In: Watson R, Swartz L (eds) Transformation through occupation. Whurr, London

Reilly M (ed) 1974 Play as exploratory learning. Sage, Beverly Hills

Reynolds F 2005 The effects of creativity on physical and psychological well-being: current and new directions for research. In: Schmid T (eds) Promoting health through creativity: for professionals in health, arts and education. Whurr, London, CA, pp112-131

Runco MA, Richards R (eds) 2002 Eminent creativity, everyday creativity and health. Ablex Publishing Corporation, Greenwich, Connecticut

Schmid T 2005 A theory of creativity: an innate capacity. In: Schmid T (ed) Promoting health through creativity: for professionals in health, arts and education. Whurr, London

Stein M 1974 Stimulating creativity. Volume 1. Individual procedures. Academic Press, New York

Vygotsky L 1994 Imagination and creativity of the adolescent. In: van der Veer R, Valsiner J (eds) The Vygotsky reader. Blackwell, Oxford

Weisberg R 1986 Creativity, genius and other myths. Freeman, New York

Chapter 19

Play

Deborah Hutton

INTRODUCTION

Within occupational therapy play is commonly believed to be the preferred or primary occupation of young children (Bundy 1993, Knox 2005, Parham & Primeau 1997, Pierce & Marshall 2004, Rigby & Rodger 2006). Play is, however, an enigma, a paradox (Bundy 1993). Whilst play theory asserts that learning through play contributes to the development of social, emotional, cognitive, physical and language skills (Rigby & Rodger 2006), play, unlike work or self-care, is fun, frivolous and has no specific goal. The definition of play therefore has been a problem to theorists who have recognised its significance in child development but who have also viewed it as trivial or irrelevant (Rubin et al 1983).

OCCUPATIONAL THERAPY AND PLAY

Because play is creative rather than technical, joyous rather than serious and allows for a temporary break from reality, those who advocate the value and use of play in therapy run the risk of not being taken seriously (Bundy 1993, Royeen 1997). Perhaps as a consequence, despite the strong association of play with occupational therapy in the founding years of the profession, by the mid-20th century occupational therapists had begun to doubt the importance of play, professional interest instead being eclipsed by more scientifically oriented concerns (Parham & Primeau 1997).

Now particularly in Western culture, the significance of play is widely recognised and play has become greatly valued in the lives of children (Rigby & Rodger 2006). In current occupational therapy literature, play is commonly identified as one of the main occupational performance areas. Kielhofner (2002) considers play along with activities of daily living and work as the three broad 'areas of doing' or occupation. Australian occupational therapists use six classifications of occupation: work, activity, self-care, leisure, *play* and rest (Law et al 2002). Canadian occupational therapists use three different classes of occupation: leisure, productivity and self-care. The Canadian view is that the category of productivity includes, for adults, employment, housework and parenting, and for children, play and school work (Law et al 2002).

Occupational therapists once again are concerned with the occupation of play and with the child developing as a lifelong player (Rigby & Rodger 2006). Wilcock (2006) conceptualised occupation as doing, being and becoming. For children, playing could be viewed as *doing*. During play children could be considered to experience *being* (Ramugondo 2004). As each child is born with the potential to *become*, it is through their life roles, their doing and being (their playing) that this potential emerges (Mandich & Rodger 2006). Wilcock (2006) proposed that occupational therapists are employed to assist people in doing, being and becoming by facilitating their abilities through the performance of meaningful occupations. Consequently, play, viewed as both a childhood occupation and as a therapeutic tool, is of interest to occupational therapists working with children in both mental health and paediatric settings.

Play is not just the preserve of children; play is important at every stage of life (Esdaile 2004). With this view in mind, the first part of this chapter considers play in terms of its definition, purpose and value to the developing individual; the second part examines play in the broader context of the family and in particular the needs of mothers with severe mental illness. Throughout the chapter reference is made to the role of occupational therapists and their use of play as a therapeutic intervention.

THEORIES OF PLAY

The occupations of work and play are often compared and contrasted in order to clarify and define what at first seem to be opposites (for an example, see Primeau 1998). Before we can begin to understand the true nature of play, we need to first consider its relationship with work.

PLAY/LEISURE VERSUS WORK

The practices and activities commonly referred to as play in childhood and youth are typically referred to as leisure in adulthood (Rigby & Rodger 2006), perhaps because leisure is considered to be more respectable than the term *play* in Western culture (Parham 1996).

Whilst the terms *play* and *leisure* are interchangeable in the literature, leisure has been described as offering different kinds of experiences to play, such as involvement in organised activities, clubs and religious worship as well as passive forms of rest and relaxation. The essence of leisure (as opposed to play) for primary school-aged children is the freedom to selectively engage in or discontinue activity participation at any point in time and may include structured or unstructured recreational and cultural activities such as sport, hobbies, and cultural pursuits (Poulson & Ziviani 2006).

Leisure has been defined as an activity that, unlike work, is entered into voluntarily and is intrinsically motivated, whereas work is obligatory or extrinsically motivated (Parham 1996). As such, leisure and play could be seen as being the polar opposite of work yet the two are intricately related. Some play can seem like work and some work has a play-like quality (Anderson 1997). Take, for example, the worker who when asked to do a task as part of his employment becomes so involved that he chooses to go far beyond the requirements of the job (Parham 1996). Or professional sportsmen and women who may view their work as leisure for which they are paid (Anderson 1997, Parham 1996). Equally an occupation could be taken up as a pastime, for reasons of pleasure and relaxation and being productive, but lead to income generation, for example, wood working or textile arts. Clearly play may be enfolded in work and vice versa (Parham 1996).

Reference to the Canadian Model of Occupational Performance helps to distinguish between leisure/play and work by using the different classifications of leisure, productivity and self-care. Leisure is defined simply as any occupation entered into for the purpose of enjoyment, for example, socializing, creative expressions, outdoor activities, games and sports. Productivity, by contrast, involves occupations that make a social or economic contribution or that provide economic sustenance. Examples include play in infancy and childhood, school work, homemaking, parenting and community volunteering (Law et al 2002). Thus play (and parenting) can be viewed as both productive and of social value.

DEFINITIONS OF PLAY

There is no one universal definition of play; each definition devised reflects the theoretical standpoint of its author. Within occupational therapy, Bundy (1991), with a background of sensory integration theory, has proposed a working definition of play as: 'a transaction between the individual and the environment that is intrinsically motivated, internally controlled and free from many of the constraints of objective reality' (p59). This definition includes the key features of intrinsic motivation and suspension of reality (and therefore its consequences) which are common to other definitions. Royeen (1997) adds in the qualities of joy and pleasure as a single criterion of play consistent across all ages.

Characteristics of play

Probably the most common method of defining play is to list traits thought to characterise it or to separate it from other occupations (Bundy 1991). Rubin et al (1983) have identified six widely accepted characteristics of play, borrowed from different theoretical perspectives.

1. Play is *intrinsically motivated*. Play is entered into freely at the will of the player and is not governed by compliance with social demands or inducements external to the behaviour itself.
2. Play involves an *attention to the means rather than the ends*. Play behaviour is spontaneous and its goals can vary according to the salience of the player. For example, a child might choose to build a block tower but the goal may diminish in importance as different ways of stacking the blocks become of greater interest than the production of the standing tower.
3. Play is *organism rather than stimulus dominated*. That is to say that exploratory behaviour is dominated by the stimulus (object) and is orientated towards finding information about it, i.e. what is *it* or what can *it* do? Play in contrast is guided by an organism-dominated quest, the central question being 'what can *I* do with this object?'. Exploratory behaviour occurs when objects are unfamiliar or poorly understood,

play occurs when objects are familiar; it serves to produce stimulation and maintain particular levels of arousal.

4. Play involves *non-literal or simulative behaviour*. Play behaviours are not serious renditions of the activities they resemble; for example, fighting is play fighting and even young children will be able to make this distinction. Instruments too can be used as if they were something else; for example, a chair becomes a car, a horse, a mountain. Play involves pretence.

5. Play is *free from externally imposed rules*. Play is an activity that is controlled by the player. This category differentiates play from games-with-rules, which are less flexible but may be confusing as the developmental relationship between play and games-with-rules suggests the latter may be a later form of play that emerges with the evolving cognitive sophistication of the individual. Therefore, any rules that exist during play are made by the player (and are changeable), rather than those imposed by an adult or even another child.

6. Play requires *active involvement* of the player/s. When a child is truly playing, she is totally absorbed in the activity. This characteristic is used to contrast play from more passive activities such as watching television or lounging around. It does technically exclude the activity of daydreaming but this can be seen by some as active, as it is playing with ideas and may be viewed developmentally as a precursor in young children's active involvement with objects, action or others.

One criticism of this list is that it does not include exploration or sensorimotor play which are seen by many as characteristic of play in infancy and early childhood (Knox & Mailloux 1997).

PURPOSE AND FUNCTION OF PLAY

The value or purpose of play is most often described according to the theoretical bias of the author. Within occupational therapy literature, play is predominantly seen as a skills acquisition process and so a preparation for adulthood. A general summary of the value and purpose of play in childhood from an occupational therapy perspective could therefore be:

Through play children gain mastery about how their body works in relation to the demands of activities and environments and gain knowledge about the world around them. Not only do they learn what they are capable of doing, they learn how to do things and how things work. Play challenges children, stretching their abilities and imagination. (Rigby & Rodger 2006, p180)

The view that play in childhood prepares a child for the role of student and ultimately for the adult worker role is a position that Parham (1996) calls the functionalist view. The functionalist view considers play as important because it is an effective way to develop other functions, such as sensory integrative, motor, social, cognitive or self-care or work skills. From an occupational science perspective, Parham (1996) offers an alternative view, one that states that play is a legitimate end in itself because it is a critical element of the human experience (Parham & Primeau 1997). In viewing play as important for its own sake, Parham (1996) and Parham & Primeau (1997) advocate consideration of play not only as an experience of pleasure in the here and now which can be health promoting but also a view of play as a *vehicle of meaning*. Watching a person at play reveals what is important to him, what provides satisfaction and makes life worth living. From this perspective play becomes a quality of life issue for the present and the future, an active ingredient of a healthy, satisfying lifestyle (Parham 1996).

Three theories of play

Three modern theories of play include play as a socialisation process (Parham & Primeau 1997), an enculturation process (Anderson 1997) and as a type of communication (Royeen 1997).

Play as socialisation

The process of socialisation through play occurs when children play games with their peers and learn social rules and norms. As they take turns and move between roles in a game, they learn to appreciate the perspective of the other players. These changes of roles and perspectives lead to the development of self-identity and the concept of the generalised other – that is, the perspective of the group or wider community (Parham & Primeau 1997).

Play as an enculturation process

Anderson (1997) describes play as an enculturation process, whereby children learn about their culture and how they are supposed to act, cultivating their abilities and habits appropriate in their society. A child learns motor and process skills by participating in cultural practices and equally these skills enable him to participate in the occupations and cultural practices of his family and community (Case Smith 2005). Play can therefore be seen as a way of adults passing on cultural traditions from one generation to the next, ensuring the continuation of a way of life.

Play as a form of communication

Royeen (1997) highlights how play functions as a form of communication, both within the player and among players. This view concurs with those of the theorists in the early 20th century, such as Freud, Piaget and Vygotsky, who proposed that (1) children play in order to express themselves through fantasy or pretence play and that (2) play results, in part, from wish fulfilment, for example wanting to be like... or to have... or to do... (Rubin et al 1983). The notion that play is a form of communication and can be used in therapy, particularly in relation to trauma and conflict, has given rise to the advent of various modes of psychodynamic play therapies, some of which are practised by occupational therapists. Examples of different approaches to play therapy include non-directive or child-centred play therapy, focused therapeutic play or directive play, child psychotherapy, relationship play therapy and family play therapy (Blunden 2001).

CULTURE AND CONTEXT

As play to one person may not be play to another (Royeen 1997), play in one culture may not be considered play in another. From an anthropological perspective Anderson (1997) writes 'All play is cultural. Any student of play must become a student of culture because an understanding of play, its meaning and relevance, must come in the larger context of the culture in which the play is found' (p51).

Culture is a learned phenomenon and occurs as a consequence of an individual's membership of society (Anderson 1997). Cultures vary in many aspects, such as the roles of women and children, values and beliefs about family and religion, family traditions and the importance of health care and education. In contemporary postindustrialist societies, the emphasis is on the individual and individual advancement. In the United States, for example, parents value independence as a primary goal for their children and encourage individual self-expression and independence in their child's thoughts and actions (Case Smith 2005). The indigenous cultures of Australia, by contrast, view the role of family and community as of paramount importance (Darlington & Rodger 2006). The value a people or community places on interdependence among its members versus the importance of the individual thus varies in cultural groups and is a significant determinant of childhood occupations (Case Smith 2005).

The high value placed on play in childhood is essentially a Western one. In situations of poverty, social disadvantage and war, play is often diminished, the struggle for survival robbing children (and families) of the opportunity to be playful (Algado & Burgman 2005, Esdaile 2004, Kronenberg 2005). In Vietnam, for example, young children are required to join their parents in income-generating activities rather than spending their time in education or leisure pursuits (Simmond 2005). Whilst the primacy of the occupation of play in childhood may well be a Western belief, this is not to say that working children do not find ways of integrating play activities and playfulness into their daily occupations (Rigby & Rodger 2006).

PLAY CONTEXT

Simply giving children toys or creating a playful environment does not elicit play (Bundy 1991, Ramugondo 2005). Children need to experience play as a process and this begins during their interactions with their carers when they are infants and develops throughout these interactions during their childhood and youth.

Whilst caregivers have a pivotal role in enhancing or inhibiting a child's play capacity (Ramugondo 2004) there are also environmental factors that can promote play. Such factors have been identified as (1) familiar peers, toys and other materials, (2) freedom of choice, (3) adults who are non-intrusive or directive, (4) safe and comfortable atmosphere, (5) scheduling that avoids times of fatigue, hunger and stress (Rubin et al 1983). Contextual elements that have an inhibiting effect on play include the opposites of those that promote it – for example, too much novelty or challenge, limited choices and overcompetition (Knox 2005). Clearly, any adult wishing to play with a child needs to be mindful of these elements in order for play to occur.

PLAY DEVELOPMENT

Throughout life a person passes through stages of play development. Although there are similarities in how individuals play at various stages in life, social, cultural, and environmental influences along with the individual's own strengths, abilities and interests will result in a unique occupational performance profile for each person. An overview of general play development is given here with these factors and variants held in mind.

INFANCY

From the moment they are born, infants are involved in social interactions with the adults and children in their environment. Some interactions meet their daily care needs. Others are more playful with mutual engagement and synchronised smiles and sounds (Holloway 1997). These social interactions enhance the relationship between the infant and their caregiver but also have developmental benefits; for example, games such as peek-a-boo and tickling promote turn taking and provide a context for language learning (Rubin et al 1983). Through their playful interactions with caregivers, children experience trust, learn to express affection, learn about communication and reciprocal interchange, have the opportunity to explore in a safe environment and learn through caregivers modelling behaviours (Esdaile 2004).

From birth to approximately 2 years of age, a child's play is principally sensorimotor and exploratory (Rubin et al 1983). A baby explores his environment through his senses; as objects become more familiar and his motor skills develop, rudimentary play begins with, for example, banging toys together, stacking blocks, turning pages of books. The toddler's ability to imitate the behaviour and language that surrounds him signals the beginning of pretend or symbolic play, examples being 'feeding' or nurturing dolls, stirring an empty saucepan with a spoon, 'singing' songs and demonstrating actions.

EARLY CHILDHOOD

From the age of 2, symbolic and constructive play continues and develops; stacks of bricks become buildings, trains travel on purposeful journeys along carefully laid-out tracks. Rough and tumble play continues and dramatic play involves the inclusion of superheroes and fictional characters learnt of through watching television and listening to stories. Imaginary or pretence play becomes increasingly more complex and social over time (Case Smith 2005, Rubin et al 1983).

The amount of time spent in pretend play during toddler to elementary school years means pretence is viewed as partially responsible for a plethora of skills, for example abstract thinking, development of self-confidence, self-regulation and self-identity, and knowledge of social rules (Rubin et al 1983).

MIDDLE CHILDHOOD

Play assumes major importance in middle childhood as a processor of social relationships. Peers and peer interaction are very prominent during this time as children learn to influence one another verbally. As a consequence there is an emphasis on games, negotiating the rules of games and an increasing awareness of the need to conform to rules in order to play harmoniously (Florey & Greene 1997).

Play interests also change during middle childhood. Whilst dramatic play with costumes and props is still popular, an interest in sports begins to develop. Craft activities remain of interest to some but assistance is still needed with more complex procedures (Florey & Greene 1997).

ADOLESCENCE

Adolescence is characterised by the development of autonomy and the transition from childhood to adulthood. With that process comes a change of interests, moving away from those centred around family to those in a peer group. For the adolescent the peer group is a source of new information about the world outside and a testing ground for new ideas and behaviours (Kielhofner 2002).

In adolescence the role of friend is increasingly important and may take precedence over the roles of sibling, daughter or grandchild (Rodger & Ziviani 2006). Adolescents spend more time with friends than family and seek out opportunities to be with friends, whether that be at school, after-school clubs or at weekends. Consequently during adolescence there is a transition from the concept of play to that of recreation/leisure (Rodger & Ziviani 2006).

While the single largest leisure activity of adolescence may be socialising, adolescents also spend time watching television, participating in sports, games and hobbies, reading and listening to music (Knox 2005). It is notable that the most popular leisure activities, hanging out with friends and watching television, can be considered passive leisure requiring little energy outlay and demanding few skills or concentration. Solitary, unstructured activities like listening to music or thinking are undemanding, seldom causing the same levels of anxiety that can occur with more active/social events. These easier options may be chosen by the adolescent for their relaxing qualities, in effect as 'time out' from the demands of everyday life (Csikszentmihalyi 1997).

ADULTHOOD

Play is not of course wholly the domain of the child or adolescent and exists in adulthood. Adult play includes a wide range of sports and leisure pursuits that allow for time to be spent in non-work roles. For adults, play provides a break from reality and allows for renewal and reinvigoration (Royeen 1997). Socialising, themed parties, religious festivities all allow adults the chance to dress up, to play and to have fun.

Playfulness

When play in adults is described as a *style* it is referred to as *playfulness* (Bundy 1993). Adults (and adolescents) can be playful in their actions but also through their use of humour and wit, their emotional expressiveness and their levels of curiosity (Rubin et al 1983). A playful approach to activities (and therefore life) is considered by Bundy (1993) as almost more important than the play or leisure activity itself. Whilst Rubin et al (1983) report that there are links to be made with playfulness and creativity, Bundy (1993) argues that playfulness as a style helps people be flexible in their approach to problem solving and as such can be seen as a primary aspect of health and wellness (Royeen 1997).

Play as an occupational role

However, adults are not only players in their own right but are also playmates with children through their familial roles of parent, aunt, grandmother as well as within their occupational roles of, for example, childcare worker, educator or therapist. When play is viewed as a socialisation process, children are not only the recipients of socialisation but can also have an impact upon the adult during the process of play (Anderson 1997). As such, playing can be seen as a two-way process and is of as much importance to the adult as it is the child (Rubin et al 1983).

OCCUPATIONAL THERAPISTS' USE OF PLAY

The way occupational therapists use play in their clinical interventions depends on their chosen frame of reference but generally their use of play can be viewed in two ways: as a treatment modality (play *in* therapy) and as a treatment method (play *as* therapy) (Knox & Mailloux 1997).

PLAY IN THERAPY

Play *in* therapy includes the developmental (Knox 2005) or the human developmental frame of reference (Creek 2002), the goals of therapy being to develop skills in such areas as cognitive, social, emotional and physical development. The therapist uses play materials and activities to engage the child's interest and at the same time facilitate developmental skills, for example, using props in specific role-play scenarios as part of a social skills group (Prior 2001).

PLAY AS THERAPY

Play *as* therapy includes frames of reference that view play as a means as well as an outcome. An example could be the psychodynamic frame of reference (Creek 2002) which utilises exploratory approaches like play to assist with conflict resolution, overcome trauma and assist with the expression of unarticulated emotions. Play sessions will include activities chosen for their symbolic potential and might include projective arts and media such as puppetry, storytelling (Fazio 1997), drawing/painting or, for older children, creative writing. When using an adult-directed approach, the occupational therapist may use activity or task analysis in order to select play activities that a child will most benefit from (Prior 2001, Rigby & Rodger 2006) or may prefer to use a child-directed approach, respecting the child's own choices and working alongside them (Prior 2001). Play as both a treatment modality and as a treatment method may be used in individual work, family work or groupwork.

The chapter so far has considered the free play of normally developing individuals – that is, play which is intrinsically motivated and entered into for its own sake rather than having a specific purpose. When considering the use of play in therapy, a problem arises. While play has been defined as self-initiated, self-directed and flexible, occupational therapists frequently choose to direct a child's play activity to achieve a therapist-driven goal (Holloway 1997). The external constraints placed on therapeutic play by the goals determined by therapists and parents can lead children to perceive the play as more like work (Knox 2005, Knox & Mailloux 1997) and their motivation to engage in it is thus affected.

Child–directed play

For play to be used successfully in any intervention, the child should feel that he is choosing or directing the play (Knox 2005). When a child feels in control of his play and play environment, he is more likely to engage fully in it and thus benefit from its therapeutic value. Intrinsic motivation means engaging in authentic, self-authored and personally endorsed activities, i.e. activities which have personal meaning to the player. When individuals are intrinsically motivated they have high levels of spontaneous interest, excitement, confidence, persistence and creativity (Poulson & Ziviani 2006). Therefore to gain maximum benefit from using play in therapeutic interventions, the occupational therapist needs to pay special attention to how activities are selected or introduced to the child as well as to how the play then proceeds.

Flow

This brings us to the concept of *flow*. Flow occurs when one is immersed and totally absorbed in what one is doing, and is an experience of harmony. Children can experience flow during activities (Mandich & Rodger 2006), for example, when during play they appear completely engrossed in what they are doing and seem oblivious to the external environment, including those around them. In this way flow has close associations with Wilcock's (2006) state of *being*. Whilst many interventions focus on helping children *do* (Wilcock 2006), there is a place for supporting and encouraging children to *be*, so that they can connect with their inner selves, their motivation, their sense of meaning and purpose. *Being* activities are not necessarily passive but rather involve a quieter activity of an inner kind (Mandich & Rodger 2006). Creative pursuits such as art, dance, listening to or playing music can be considered 'being activities' and allow children time to relax, to daydream, simply to *be* themselves (Mandich & Rodger 2006). There are physiological (decreased heart rate, slowing of metabolism) as well as psychological (decreased stress, emotional balance) benefits to such 'down time'. Down time is of particular value when it provides balance to otherwise busy, structured lives (Mandich & Rodger 2006).

In order to experience flow there must be a goodness of fit between the challenges of the activity and the skills of the individual (Csikszentmihalyi 1997). When a challenge is high in relation to low skills, anxiety is experienced. When a challenge is low, in relation to high skills, boredom may be experienced. An important concept of flow is the benefit of achieving arousal, or increased concentration, focus and involvement with what one is doing. This happens when the challenges slightly exceed the skills. This will enable the child to feel a sense of control in the doing. When the level of play skill matches the level of challenge it is called the just right challenge for facilitating play skills (Rigby & Rodger 2006). The occupational therapist is well equipped to grade the level of challenge of activities to ensure goodness of the child–activity fit and enable flow to occur. The experience of flow is important in therapy as it provides motivation, satisfaction and inner rewards (Knox & Mailloux 1997), qualities which may otherwise be lacking in a person's life.

To summarise, to achieve the maximum benefit from using play in therapeutic interventions, the occupational therapist must harness the child's intrinsic motivation by allowing him to feel in control of his play and by the careful selection of play activities which can provide the experience of flow.

The role of an occupational therapist who works with children, however, extends beyond providing individual therapeutic play interventions to include working with the child's family. Therapists can work with families to identify play opportunities within the home setting and thus transfer of the gains of individual therapy into everyday life (Knox & Mailloux 1997, Prior 2001). By actively encouraging and involving parents in play situations with their children, the occupational therapist can help them appreciate their child's strengths and learn the fun of playing with their child, helping to develop habits that will be of benefit throughout their lifetime (Knox & Mailloux 1997, Olson 2001).

PLAY AND FAMILIES

When thinking about play within the family context, it is necessary to view play not just in terms of skill acquisition but in the broader terms of a relationship-enhancing, quality-of-life issue. But first the current social and economic influences that affect modern families need to be considered with regard to children and their opportunities for play.

Across the Western world since the early 1970s, significant changes have occurred in relation to family composition and function (Darlington & Rodger 2006). The average family size is decreasing as women have more control over their fertility, the divorce rate is increasing and family composition is more diverse than in previous generations (Darlington & Rodger 2006). As a consequence, more young children with working parents spend large amounts of time in childcare and experience different play environments and carers/playmates other than their biological parents. The financial pressures on some households coupled with a lack of leisure time or safe outdoor play areas can mean the opportunity for children to play with parents and peers is reduced (Rodger & Ziviani 2006). With working parents commitments being incorporated into the family schedule, rather more out-of-school time is spent in structured activity such as after-school clubs and as such children have less free time to do as they please (Darlington & Rodger 2006). In the case of divorce and separation contact with non-resident parents can bring further complexity to children's lives, disrupting routines and preventing the attendance of social events/activities where play with peers may have been enjoyed (Darlington & Rodger 2006).

Children's leisure time has also been affected by advancements in technology – the use of television, computers and mobile phones means that children have less direct social contact, less physical activity and more exposure to world events (Poulson & Ziviani 2006, Rodger & Ziviani 2006).

In sum, where children play and with whom has changed over the past few years, as has parents' expectations of how their children should spend their leisure time.

FAMILY–CENTRED CARE

In line with these changes over the past two decades much has been written about best practice when working with children and families. One aspect of best practice is the provision of *family-centred care* (Darlington & Rodger 2006). Family-centred care is a philosophy of service provision that emphasises the central role of families in making decisions about the care their children receive (Law et al 2005). In practising family-centred care, the occupational therapist needs to move away from the role of expert to that of collaborator. In this revised role the occupational therapist is better able to view each family as unique and aims to identify the family's individual goals and aspirations for their children as well as the realities of that family's life (Posatory Burke & Schaaf 1997).

FAMILY ASSESSMENT

In order to identify how the referred child, with his abilities, limitations and interests, can be incorporated into activities the family enjoys, the occupational therapist needs to consider the assessment in two parts. First, observation of the child at play within his own home/school will provide valuable information about the child's interests and skills with his peers and family members (Hinojosa & Kramer 1997, Posatory Burke & Schaaf 1997, Prior 2001). The second part of the assessment should include information gathered through discussion with parents about the family's values, needs, resources and routines. Inquiries about play in this way offer opportunities to understand the specific ways a family spends time; how it defines fun, the type of interactions, toys and play materials that are most valued and the use of available play environments (Posatory Burke & Schaaf 1997). Ultimately this combined approach should help the occupational therapist guide families to think of play activities that have meaning to them rather than their feeling compelled to comply with therapist-driven goals (Hinojosa & Kramer 1997).

FAMILY ROUTINES AND TIME TO PLAY

If occupational therapists are to provide family-centred care then they must recognise the family's individual routines and respect its rituals. Family routines are predictable observable behaviours that have an instrumental goal: for example, setting the table before a meal. Routines function to organise and co-ordinate the behaviours and actions of individuals and to bring about order in family life (Segal 2004).

Having identified the kinds of play activities the child and family may wish to undertake,

a second task is to identify when those activities may occur within the family's daily/weekly routine. The different ways in which play can be integrated into the family routines are numerous. The occupational therapist may, for example, advocate one-to-one parent/child play sessions or adult-supervised play times with siblings or family trips out making use of community resources or, as Royeen (1997) recommends, simply finding ways of incorporating play and playfulness into activities of daily living to improve the family's quality of life.

Family strategies

Primeau (1998, 2004) studied parent–child play within the context of family routines in the home. She described two main strategies used by parents to incorporate play into daily routines at home: strategies of *segregation* and strategies of *inclusion*. In strategies of segregation, the child's play takes place as an entirely separate activity from parental household work and the parent either takes a break from work to play with the child or they work whilst the child plays independently – for example, the adult cleans up whilst the child plays with toys nearby. In strategies of inclusion, the child's play is embedded in the parent's work – for example, the parent does housework and plays with the child at the same time, allowing the child to participate playfully in the work task such as in helping to prepare a meal.

Primeau (1998, 2004) found that when a child participated in adult chores, the parents would often structure and support (or scaffold) the activity so that the child could perform as much of it as possible; the situation therefore becomes one in which the child develops skills under the parent's guidance. Parents thus use play embedded in housework as a strategy to play with their children whilst managing to complete household work and maintain family routine.

Family rituals

Family rituals differ from routines in that they are a symbolic communication of who we are and give a sense of belonging to a family and continuity across generations (Segal 2004). Rituals may include mealtime routines, weekend leisure activities, bedtime stories, birthday celebrations. Segal (2004) reported that routines give life order while rituals give it meaning.

Darlington & Rodger (2006) suggest that occupational therapists need to consider both family *doing* and *being* goals as the key aspects of occupation-based family-centred interventions. Occupational therapists have a role in assisting families to *be* through promoting and facilitating engagement in rituals to enable them to create meaning. The introduction of play into family rituals and routines is one way of bringing meaningful occupation into the family unit and so supporting individual family members in *being* a family. This in turn promotes family occupations, health and well-being (Darlington & Rodger 2006).

MOTHERING AND MENTAL ILLNESS

The skills required in mothering change over time according to the age and developmental needs of the children. Early on with preschoolers, the emphasis is on caretaking activities and meeting basic needs whereas with young adults, emotional and supportive activities are more in demand. A mother who experiences recurring bouts of mental illness will require different help depending on the age and developmental demands of her family.

The presence of severe mental illness may affect a mother's capacity to care for her child in a range of ways, including parenting skills, her perception of the role of parent and her control over her emotions (McKay 2004). Parents with mental illness may be emotionally unavailable and withdrawn from their child and therefore less sensitive to their child's behaviour and needs (Bassett et al 2001). The consequent effects of maternal mental illness on children may include a lack of stimulation, neglect and isolation which can result in developmental delay (McKay 2004). Depending on their age, children with mentally ill parents may adopt the role of carer and have little time or capacity for play; they may withdraw from social situations, develop difficulties in social skills or engage in inappropriate behaviours in an effort to gain a desired parental response (Bassett et al 2001). In addition, children from families with these difficulties may also experience times of separation and loss during their parent's admissions to hospital, incurring different carers/living situations and thus loss of access to familiar toys and peers.

ROLE OF OCCUPATIONAL THERAPY

Occupational therapists have a part to play in supporting women with severe mental illness in their roles as mothers (Bassett et al 2001, McKay 2004). This may include practical support or developing effective coping strategies to deal with the pressures of mothering. From a community perspective, occupational therapists may be involved with mothers in structuring their day, maximising their abilities to encourage appropriate play and create environments that facilitate their child's development (Knox & Mailloux 1997, McKay 2004). Occupational therapists may also help mothers engage in local mother/toddler groups at churches and community centres, thus reducing their isolation and providing more play opportunities for their children.

Depending on the kind of service offered, the occupational therapist may also provide parenting programmes that include an opportunity for mentally ill parents to interact with their children in both structured and unstructured playtime (Bassett et al 2001). Within sessions therapists can model play behaviour for parents to observe, identify and discuss a child's play skills as they occur and encourage parents to enter into play episodes with the necessary support and supervision (Knox & Mailloux 1997). Occupational therapists can also help parents think of ways of stimulating children and expand their resources through creative activities.

The use of play within the mother/child dyad has been utilised by many occupational therapists with various client groups. Esdaille (2004) has developed a community-based family-focused programme with disadvantaged mothers in the UK using toy making to facilitate mother–child interactions. Ramugondo (2004, 2005) has used play to enrich the lives of children living with HIV/AIDS in South Africa, providing their mothers with both support and the opportunity to be playful with their children. In the United States Olson (2001) has also used parent–child activity groups to encourage parents of children with emotional disorders to play together and therefore experience pleasurable interactions within a family context. Clearly the scope for occupational therapists in using play with families, mothers and children is wide ranging and full of potential.

SUMMARY

If the development of a healthy capacity to play is a life task (Esdaile 2004) then occupational therapists need to be aware of the need for play and leisure activities throughout the life cycle. The role of player begins in infancy and continues into old age, shaped by cultural and social expectations along with personal interests and skills. What a person *does*, that is, which activities and occupations they engage in during their life, defines their identity and impacts on who they *become*

(Mandich & Rodger 2006). When people lose their ability to play in the ways they choose, they lose important pieces of who they are (Bundy 1993). Mental health problems, poverty, social disadvantage, physical disability and cognitive impairment all reduce a person's ability to play and thus benefit from the renewal and reinvigoration the experience of play can provide.

Bundy (1991) argues that occupational therapists should actively and systematically promote play and leisure in their clients' lives. Furthermore, play used as a therapeutic medium needs to be taken seriously (Bundy 1993). It is proposed here that play ought not to be seen just as a skills acquisition process but rather viewed in its broadest terms, as a quality-of-life issue. This chapter has attempted to outline some of the ways in which play can and is being used as a medium for therapeutic interventions with children and families. The descriptions here serve only as an introduction for clinicians wishing to explore the topic of play further.

References

Algado SS, Burgman I 2005 Occupational therapy intervention with children survivors of war. In: Kronenberg F, Algada SS, Pollard N (eds) Occupational therapy without borders: learning from the spirit of survivors. Churchill Livingstone, Edinburgh, pp245-260

Anderson R 1997 The anthropological study of play. In: Chandler BE (ed) The essence of play: a child's occupation. American Occupational Therapy Association, Maryland, Bethesda, pp51-63

Bassett H, Lampe J, Lloyd C 2001 Living with under fives: a programme for parents with a mental illness. British Journal of Occupational Therapy 64(1): 23-28

Blunden P 2001 The therapeutic use of play. In: Lougher L (ed) Occupational therapy for child and adolescent mental health, Churchill Livingstone, Edinburgh, pp67-86

Bundy A 1991 Play theory and sensory integration. In: Fisher AG, Murray EA, Bundy AC (eds) Sensory integration: theory and practice. FA Davis, Philadelphia, pp46-67

Bundy A 1993 Assessment of play and leisure: delineation of the problem. American Journal of Occupational Therapy 47(3): 217-222

Case Smith J 2005 Development of childhood occupations. In: Case Smith J (ed) Occupational therapy for children, 5th edn. Mosby, St Louis, pp88-116

Creek J 2002 Approaches to practice. In: Creek J (ed) Occupational therapy and mental health, 3rd edn. Churchill Livingstone, Edinburgh

Csikszentmihalyi M 1997 Finding flow: the psychology of engagement with everyday life. Basic Books, New York

Darlington Y, Rodger S 2006 Families and children's occupational performance. In: Rodger S, Ziviani J (eds) Occupational therapy with children: understanding children's occupations and enabling participation. Blackwell, Oxford, pp22-40

Esdaile SA 2004 Toys for shade and the mother–child co-occupation of play. Esdaile SA, Olson JA (eds) Mothering occupations: challenge, agency and particpation. FA Davis, Philadelphia, pp95-114

Fazio LS 1997 Storytelling, storymaking and fantasy play. In: Parham LD, Fazio LS (eds) Play in occupational therapy. Mosby, St Louis, pp233-247

Florey LL, Greene S 1997 Play in middle childhood: a focus on children with behavioural and emotional disorders. In: Parham LD, Fazio LS (eds) Play in occupational therapy. Mosby, St Louis, pp126-143

Hinojosa J, Kramer P 1997 Integrating children with disabilities into family play. Parham LD, Fazio LS (eds) Play in occupational therapy. Mosby, St Louis, pp159-170

Holloway E 1997 Fostering parent–infant playfulness in the neonatal intensive care unit. In: Parham LD, Fazio LS (eds) Play in occupational therapy. Mosby, St Louis

Kielhofner G 2002 Introduction to the model of human occupation. In: Model of Human Occupation, 3rd edn, Lippincott Williams and Wilkinson, Baltimore

Knox SH 2005 Play. Case Smith J (ed) Occupational therapy for children, 5th edn. Play Mosby, St Louis, pp571-586

Knox SH, Mailloux Z 1997 Play as treatment and treatment through play. In: Chandler BE (ed) The essence of play: a child's occupation. American Occupational Therapy Association, Bethesda, Maryland, pp175-204

Kronenberg F 2005 Occupational therapy with street children. In: Kronenberg F, Algada SS, Pollard N (eds) Occupational therapy without borders: learning from the spirit of survivors. Churchill Livingstone, Edinburgh, pp261-276

Law M, Polatajko H, Baptiste S, et al 2002 Core concepts of occupational therapy. In: Townsend E (ed) Enabling occupation: an occupational therapy perspective. Canadian Association of Occupational Therapists, Ottawa, pp29-56

Law M, Missiuna C, Pollock N, et al 2005 Foundations for occupational therapy practice with children. In: Case Smith J (ed) Occupational therapy for children, 5th edn. Mosby, St Louis, pp53-87

Mandich A, Rodger S 2006 Doing, being and becoming: their importance for children. In: Rodger S, Ziviani J (eds) Occupational therapy with children: understanding children's occupations and enabling participation. Blackwell, Oxford, pp115-135

McKay EA 2004 Mothers with mental illness: an occupation interrupted. In: Esdaile SA, Olson JA (eds) Mothering occupations: challenge, agency and participation. FA Davis, Philadelphia, pp238-258

Olson LJ 2001 Child psychiatry in the USA. In: Lougher L (ed) Occupational therapy for child and adolescent mental health. Churchill Livingstone, Edinburgh, pp173-191

Parham D 1996 Perspectives on play. In: Zemke R, Clarke F (eds) Occupational science: the evolving discipline. FA Davis, Philadelphia, pp71-80

Parham LD, Primeau LA 1997 Play and occupational therapy. In: Parham LD, Fazio LS (eds) Play in occupational therapy. Mosby, St Louis, pp2-21

Pierce D, Marshall A 2004 Maternal management of home space and time to facilitate infant/toddler play and development. In: Esdaile SA, Olson JA (eds) Mothering occupations: challenge, agency and participation. FA Davis, Philadelphia, pp73-94

Posatory Burke J, Schaaf RC 1997 Family narratives and play assessment. In: Parham LD, Fazio LS (eds) Play in occupational therapy. Mosby, St Louis, pp67-84

Poulson A, Ziviani J 2006 Children's participation beyond the school grounds. In: Rodger S, Ziviani J (eds) Occupational therapy with children: understanding children's occupations and enabling participation. Blackwell, Oxford, pp280-298

Primeau LA 1998 Orchestration of work and play within families. American Journal of Occupational Therapy 52(30): 88-195

Primeau LA 2004 Mothering in the context of unpaid work and play in families. In: Esdaile SA, Olson JA (eds) Mothering occupations: challenge, agency and participation. FA Davis, Philadelphia, pp115-133

Prior K 2001 Occupational therapy with school aged children. In: Lougher L (ed) Occupational therapy for child and adolescent mental health. Churchill Livingstone, Edinburgh, pp132-150

Ramugondo EL 2004 Play and playfulness: children living with HIV/AIDS. In: Watson R, Swartz L (eds) Transformation through occupation. Whurr, London, pp171-185

Ramugondo EL 2005 Unlocking spirituality: play as a health-promoting occupation in the context of HIV/AIDS. In: Kronenberg F, Algado SS, Pollard N (eds) Occupational therapy without borders: learning from the spirit of survivors. Churchill Livingstone, Edinburgh, pp313-325

Rigby P, Rodger S 2006 Developing as a player. In: Rodger S, Ziviani J (eds) Occupational therapy with children: understanding children's occupations and enabling participation, Blackwell, Oxford, pp177-195

Rodger S, Ziviani J 2006 Children, their environments, roles and occupations in contemporary society. In: Rodger S, Ziviani J (eds) Occupational therapy with children: understanding children's occupations and enabling participation. Blackwell, Oxford, pp3-21

Royeen CB 1997 Play as occupation and as an indicator of health. In: Chandler BE (ed) The essence of play a child's occupation. American Occupational Therapy Association, Bethesda, Maryland, pp1-14

Rubin KH, Fein GG, Vandenberg B 1983 Play. In: Mussen PH (ed) Handbook of child psychology. John Wiley, New York, pp693-774

Segal R 2004 Family routines and rituals: a context for occupational therapy interventions. American Journal of Occupational Therapy 58: 499-508

Simmond M 2005 Practicing to learn: occupational therapy with children of Viet Nam. In: Kronenberg F, Algado SS, Pollard N (eds) Occupational therapy without borders: learning from the spirit of survivors. Churchill Livingstone, Edinburgh, pp277-286

Wilcock A 2006 An occupational perspective of health, 2nd edn. Slack, New Jersey

Chapter 20

Life skills

Mary Roberts

INTRODUCTION

Onlookers watch with fascination as a lump of clay is transformed into a beautifully shaped pot by an experienced potter at the wheel. People cheer and extol the virtues of the winning competitor in a sport. In each case exceptional skills have been displayed, usually resulting from a combination of talent, practice and hard work. Everyday activities also require a vast repertoire of skills which are gained with effort as a person develops. Whether exciting or mundane, skills are an essential part of a human being's interaction with his environment.

Mental illness can cause disruption and deficit in an individual's skills. The processes which enable the growth of potential talents or skills may be inhibited. Abilities which are used daily and which are taken for granted can become impaired and deteriorate.

An occupational therapist aims to enable the client to function at his optimum level when mental health problems arise. This invariably means that the client will be assisted either to learn new skills or to re-establish old ones. The ability to apply skills training in the context of therapy is a skill in itself, and one that an occupational therapist has to acquire. This chapter will examine the occupational therapist's role and perspective in skills training.

WHAT ARE LIFE SKILLS?

DEFINITION OF SKILLS

Skills enable people to operate as individuals and contribute to their functioning as part of the society in which they belong. Some skills are needed to help a person survive, for example being able to obtain and/or prepare food. There are also skills which help individuals to follow and develop a sense of self-identity, such as being a wage-earner or artist.

Skill, according to the *Shorter Oxford Dictionary* (1993), is an ability to do something well. Skills are involved in achieving tasks and are dependent on abilities. Hence a skill is something we know how to do and feel comfortable with when putting it into action. Once learned, it often becomes automatic, for example applying the brakes when driving a car. Initially the driver will learn where the brake is in relation to the foot, how hard to press it and on what occasions to do this. With practice, the driver will learn to differentiate between, for example, slowing down in traffic and doing an emergency stop, until he can stop without hesitation in a way that is appropriate to the situation. Skills have physical and mental components which link closely together – an ability to tie shoelaces is hindered not only if a person does not have the motor skill to manipulate the laces but also if he feels too anxious to learn how to do so.

In occupational therapy, a skill is defined as a performance component which evolves with practice. Skills are grouped according to the emphasis of the occupational therapy approach used, for example psychosocial function or cognitive ability. They form the basis of performance, behaviour, cognition and social interaction. A description of these concepts will provide further clarification.

Performance

The concept of *performance* is one used frequently in occupational therapy. In relation to skills, it is the process or manner of functioning, which incorporates what a person does and how it is done. Performance is the outward expression of skills.

It also includes the degree to which an individual is competent; that is, whether there is achievement or failure in doing an activity. A person's perception of competence can vary according to the demands of the situation and his view of himself.

Behaviour

Studies in psychology have provided insights into behaviour which have enabled interventions such as systematic desensitisation. Behaviour is defined as acting or reacting in a specific way. This can be particular to the individual but there are also behaviours which are common to human beings in general.

Complex interactions within the human being produce behaviour, often in patterns. For example, walking into a room full of people in a meeting and being able to show the right amount of formality and confidence requires previous knowledge, an ability to judge a situation, appropriate body language and so on.

Behaviour includes the response of an individual based on attitudes and values, verbal and non-verbal communication. Sometimes it is innate, developing under the influence of heredity, and sometimes it is produced by environmental factors or a combination of both (Argyle 1978). Behaviour can be changed by re-education, illness or trauma.

Cognition

Cognition involves the mechanisms of knowing and perceiving. It includes the skills of reasoning, mental processing, thinking, remembering, planning and problem solving. Aspects of cognition are essential to the development of performance. Associated skills are restricted if there are problems in cognition. In psychology and occupational therapy literature, cognition is well documented (Chapter 16).

The development of cognitive skills as a therapeutic goal can be effective in dealing with some mental health problems.

Social interaction

Social interaction is the process by which individuals communicate, react and behave with one another in society. Doble & Magill Evans (1992) described it as the ability to receive and selectively attend to social information in the environment, by which a person is able to interpret situations and adapt his responses accordingly. The processes required for this are: receiving and interpreting social messages, planning social output, interactional style and social enactment.

A person will use various combinations of verbal and non-verbal communication, assertiveness, negotiation and co-operation in his interactions (Mosey 1986). His responses will partly depend on personal goals – that is, what he is trying to accomplish in the interaction. They are also guided by cultural expectations – the rules of behaviour outlined by group norms (Franklin 1990). For example, in one culture it may be acceptable to greet someone by shaking hands but in another it may be considered offensive to touch another person in public.

These skills contribute to competent social behaviour, enabling the person to be comfortable in society. They also facilitate the making and sustaining of interpersonal relationships. Difficulties in social interaction are often an aspect of mental health problems and, as such, are commonly dealt with by occupational therapists.

ACQUISITION OF SKILLS

Theorists in social psychology, language and sociology identified stages of growth and development in the areas described above as they explored human development from birth to maturity. For example, physical motor, social language, activities of daily living and sociocultural skills were identified by Gesell, areas of psychosocial development were described by Erikson, while Grant and Freud developed psychodynamic theories. Needs were linked to motivation by Maslow, and Piaget explained cognition (Llorens 1991). Such theories form a basis of knowledge and understanding of how skills are acquired.

Early work in skills training emphasised social behaviour. The work was mainly done by social psychologists and included research into behaviour, verbal and non-verbal communication, behaviour modification and the ability to change. Jones (1967, in Argyle 1978) analysed social behaviour. Rogers (1967, in Gadza & Brooks 1985) researched social and life skills training which formed the basis of the first training model in social skills developed by Carkhuff (1969, in Gadza & Brooks 1985). Trower et al 1978 began to categorise what was described as social inadequacy and formulated social skills training programmes to deal with it.

Social skills training is well documented and described elsewhere (Argyle 1978, Franklin 1990). A plethora of social skills exercises are used by a number of different professions, including those working in prisons and the probation service, personnel and business management and education, as well as those working within mental health. The occupational therapist is advised to search psychology literature for specific topics and ideas relating to particular interventions.

Evolution of skills concepts in occupational therapy

When we consider the contribution of occupational therapy to life and skills training, it is interesting to explore how the profession's theories have come to complement and progress the concepts discussed above. The early work in both psychology and occupational therapy has been built on by others, such as Mosey and Kielhofner, to formulate models and approaches for practice. Ayres' work (Llorens 1991), which later became sensory integration theory, described the function and dysfunction of the central nervous system relating to purposeful activity. Llorens (1976), also with an emphasis on activities, synthesised developmental theories. Her work added to our understanding of the nature of the acquisition of skill for mastery, the role of trauma in disrupting the developmental cycle and the idea of using activities, tasks and interpersonal interactions to reinstate skills.

The use of purposeful activity

Activities are characteristic of, and necessary to, human existence (Cynkin & Robinson 1990). Knowledge about skills has developed within the context of the way occupational therapists use activities to achieve multiple and complex treatment aims (Creek 1996). The foundational knowledge of occupational therapy is in the meaning of occupation and purposeful activity (Gillette & Kielhofner 1979).

Purposeful activity is an integrated part of therapy and is meaningful in its relation to the treatment goal (Golledge 1998). If an activity has no meaning for the client it does not have a therapeutic value (Creek 1996). Purposeful activity provides the incentive and opportunity for the individual to achieve mastery, thus gaining a sense of inner assurance and competence (Fidler 1981). The occupational therapist and client co-operate to produce change and development (Breines 1984, Dickerson 1995).

Learning skills is seen as integral to an individual's relationship with *doing*. Fidler described doing as purposeful activity (in contrast to random activity), which is a process of investigating, trying out and gaining evidence of one's capacities for experiencing, responding, managing, creating and controlling, in order to become a competent and contributing member of society (Fidler & Fidler 1978). Doing provides the means to develop and integrate sensory, motor, cognitive and psychological systems. It allows an individual to experience reality, to achieve, to fail, to explore and to grow (Stewart 1994). Mind, body and social self are developed through what we do (Creek 1996).

Skills are, therefore, attained through development, learning and practice. There are inherent characteristics in these processes which affect the direction of skill acquisition. For instance, in order to ride a bicycle a child will need to develop the appropriate level of musculoskeletal size and strength, co-ordination and balance and, later, the ability to appreciate safety measures. Incapacity in any of these areas will influence the acquisition of the skill.

A skill has to be internalised and this is done either through learning by copying someone else or by gaining knowledge and understanding of the process required for the skill. Either way, the process has to be experienced and practised regularly, repeating each stage until competence is achieved. For example, when making a cake, repeatedly following the same recipe, rectifying mistakes and acquiring knowledge on the way usually achieves a good result in the end.

Good results at each stage are important, both to increase understanding and to build up confidence. Poor results and a sense of failure can mean that attempts at learning the skill are abandoned. Success and achievement are important factors in supplying the incentives to learn a skill. These are closely followed by self-esteem and approval. All these contribute to motivation (see Chapter 6), which is the driving force behind occupational behaviour and therefore an essential element in acquiring skills. It prompts the individual to seek out and master new skills. It contributes to the 'urge to explore and master the environment, i.e. fitness and responsiveness to external demands and to personal drives for competence' (Kielhofner 1985, p14).

The ability to learn is, therefore, an important element of skill acquisition and is facilitated by appropriate instruction and training. An understanding of the learning process and the difficulties experienced in this area by clients with mental health problems are essential for occupational therapists involved in any form of skills training.

LEARNING THEORY

Learning may be defined as a change in behaviour that occurs as the result of experience.

Learning theory offers an explanation of how individuals reach a particular level of competence in cognitive performance, rather than looking at patterns common to all. The overall level of competence achieved is seen as important, rather than the age at which skills are developed.

A major difference between cognitive developmental theory and learning theory is that, in the latter, skills are thought to be acquired through the individual's interaction with the environment and are not dependent on prior learning of more basic skills.

Learning theory presents a model of how skills are learned and also suggests ways in which learning can be facilitated. Learning is seen to take place through a variety of experiences, including:

- habituation
- conditioning
- transfer of learning.

Habituation

Habituation is learning not to react to stimuli that are constant or irrelevant, for example, not to listen to the background hum of traffic noise. New sights and sounds attract immediate attention but, once the judgement is made that they are irrelevant, the individual learns to ignore them.

This has implications for the design of a therapeutic environment. Small changes, such as turning off the radio, can be used to reactivate a client's attention.

Conditioning

Conditioning is the acquisition of conditioned responses or the making of new associations between elements in the environment. There are two types of conditioning: classical conditioning and operant conditioning. Both these techniques are used to change people's behaviour; that is, to teach new skills. In classical conditioning, a behaviour normally produced in response to one stimulus is transferred to another stimulus. For example, a client with severe learning difficulty feels pleasure when he drinks coffee. By always giving him a cup of coffee at the end of a treatment session, the therapist teaches him to associate therapy with coffee and he learns to feel pleasure when attending a treatment session.

Operant conditioning increases or decreases the likelihood of a behaviour being repeated by applying a positive or negative stimulus immediately after the behaviour. For example, if the therapist praises a client every time he performs a task, he is more likely to repeat it. If she ignores him when he shouts inappropriately, he is less likely to shout. Behaviour can be shaped towards a desired pattern by rewarding any operant behaviour that approximates to the desired behaviour.

Transfer of learning

Learning one skill often affects the learning of other skills, either by facilitating or by interfering with their acquisition. When earlier learning has a positive effect on later learning it is called transfer of learning; for example, learning to use a gas stove in the occupational therapy department will help a person to learn to use the gas cooker in his new flat. When the effect is negative, it is called negative transfer; for example, learning how to use one type of computer in occupational therapy can make it difficult to get used to a different one at home. Negative transfer effects can slow down the learning process when new skills are being learned but they do not usually persist.

Transfer occurs because of similarity of content, the way in which the skill is learned and the principle behind solving the problems, or a combination of these.

Simulated tasks give preliminary practice when dangerous skills are being learned or when the real situation is inaccessible. However, simulation is only useful if there is positive transfer from the simulated task to the real one and no negative transfer (Munn 1966). For example, an occupational therapist designed an activities of daily living (ADL) assessment unit for stroke victims in which all the fitments were adjustable so that the essential features of the home environment could be simulated. It was found that even confused clients responded automatically to familiarly positioned features, demonstrating that learning was transferred from the home environment to the unit. It could therefore be assumed that further learning would transfer from the unit to the home environment and this was found to be the case (Smith 1979).

SKILL DEFICITS CAUSED BY MENTAL ILLNESS

The process of mental illness can itself undermine the individual's performance, behaviour, cognition and social interaction. Secondary factors of illness may mean that skills in these areas have not been developed; for example, a dysfunctional family background may have affected the learning process early in the person's life. Institutionalised methods of providing care instead of an enabling approach (whether in a hospital or community setting) can inhibit the individual's development of skills in all these areas.

The occupational therapy approach is important because it helps to maintain an adequate level of skills and prevent deterioration. Certain skill deficits apparent in the major categories of mental illness are the focus of intervention. The following descriptions of such skill deficits are not definitive, as the problems in reality are complex, but some of the main areas of difficulty are indicated.

Psychotic disorders

During an acute onset of psychosis, when the symptoms such as hallucinations are florid, functional ability can be grossly impaired because of the effect of thought disorder. Perceptual difficulties will mean that the person is unable to interpret some aspects of reality. Action, learning and performance are therefore disrupted, sometimes in unexpected ways. For example, a patient may be unable to peel potatoes because they transform into snakes before his eyes. There may also be difficulty in filtering out irrelevant stimuli or information when doing a task. These problems result in poor acquisition of skills. There is some evidence to suggest that elements of sensory integration may be affected, such as co-ordination, balance and manual dexterity, which will also influence physical performance (King 1974).

A deterioration in skills may also be experienced if the illness emerges over a long period of time. This can be particularly true during the slow onset of negativism, when symptoms take on a chronic form. The sufferer may have developed problems early in life and therefore school work and learning would be affected. Often, further education and career pursuits are interrupted and a work history will show a downward trend towards less skilful and demanding jobs. Behaviour may be bizarre and social and life skills may be lacking. Interests and hobbies are not pursued so that social and emotional withdrawal is increased. Alternatively, a person may have become excessively involved with an interest which has become part of his delusional system so that skills required for anything other than this interest, for example looking after himself, may not have been acquired. The general disorganisation caused by the symptoms affects the maintenance and growth of skills in cognition, performance, behaviour and social interaction.

Affective and neurotic disorders

Illnesses in this category are characterised in the acute phase by strong emotional responses such as anxiety, guilt, self-reproach, despair and, as a result, can also cause temporary deterioration in some existing abilities. Skills may be lacking initially for a number of reasons associated with the factors contributory to the illness. As a consequence, the individual may habitually respond to situations in a maladapted way, for example, by overreacting or with learned helplessness.

Mood swings can interfere with a person's judgement. Abilities may be viewed in an unrealistic way, either under- or overestimating them. Similarly, the person may have no notion of his own potential to develop skills. Behaviour may be inconsistent as a result of mood swings. These difficulties affect the person's motivation to learn or cope with problems for which he needs new skills. The feeling of being controlled by emotional responses or irrational thought undermines confidence to increase skills. Physical discomfort, such as tiredness and lethargy, hinders the development and maintenance of some skills and therefore they deteriorate. Conversely, activity may be speeded up through agitation so that mistakes and failures occur or things are left incomplete. These also lead to a loss of confidence and a sense of failure, often out of proportion to the event. This will mean that more courage is required to respond to the challenge of learning a new or different way of doing something. Apathy may consequently occur, resulting in a vicious cycle of few skills leading to less effort to attain skills and therefore further reduction in skills.

Preoccupation with worries can undermine learning, causing a lack of attention which prevents the absorption of information, thus interfering with memory (retention and recall). The application of skills is also hampered through lack of attention and concentration.

In chronic form these illnesses often have associated social and family problems, making the person's situation unstable. Energy is used up coping with social and environmental problems and stressful situations, with few resources left to accommodate change. This affects skill development and consolidation. Sometimes, there is a store of skills in the premorbid personality but, due to secondary gain, energy is devoted to maintaining the sick role.

There are other problems indirectly caused by the after-effects of illness which can interfere with skill training and acquisition. Often, clients may be unable to apply themselves: they may have days when they are feeling particularly unwell or troubled, the side-effects of medication may produce difficulties such as tiredness or discomfort, or time-keeping can be erratic. Consequently, occupational therapy sessions are not attended regularly and this interferes with the learning process.

THE OCCUPATIONAL THERAPIST'S ROLE IN SKILLS TRAINING

The occupational therapist has several contributions to make in enabling people to acquire and reacquire skills after mental illness. The focus of occupational therapy in this context is the skills that the client needs to promote mental health and wellness. The emphasis is either on how to improve quality of life, if there are permanent difficulties, or on how to draw out potential abilities. The therapist has a role as mediator, enabler, guide and teacher.

As a mediator, an occupational therapist will structure and organise the learning experience and provide feedback to the learner on his performance (Christiansen & Baum 1991). This has to be done in a way which will draw on the person's strengths, bearing in mind their vulnerability and insecurity. By facilitating the learning process, the therapist acts as an enabler, empowering the client to gain and use skills. It is, therefore, important to understand any barriers to learning, such as the effect of the person's illness or previous learning problems. She can then help the learner to work through them and overcome them. The therapist directs the learning process, thus acting as a guide, providing and encouraging appropriate activities and creating an environment in which the individual, with his unique abilities and deficits, can learn. The ability to teach at an appropriate level, including providing relevant instruction and materials, is also essential.

It is necessary to apply a 'just right challenge' (Robinson 1977) in order to build a sense of achievement and restore confidence in skills. Individual or group sessions are used to do this, depending on the needs of the client or the resources available. For some, individual sessions with the therapist will remove the threat of comparison with others and provide the appropriate situation to build concentration and confidence. In other cases, using group interactions and process will enhance learning by providing stimulation and social contact. Careful planning is required, not only to enable the person to learn or relearn a skill in a supportive environment, but also to take into account the needs of an individual affected by illness and, sometimes, a variety of difficult social circumstances. Some of these points are highlighted in the history of Mrs X, in Box 20.1.

FACILITATING CHANGE

Learning causes changes in behaviour (see p363) and occupational therapy can contribute to change by teaching new and adaptive skills. Building confidence enables a person to respond to a situation

---

Box 20.1 Case example 1

Mrs X was an outpatient, aged 45, recovering from depression which recurred periodically. One of the contributory factors to her illness was chronic social problems. She also suffered from anxiety, especially when required to do something new, and became very negative about her own abilities. Her self-confidence and self-esteem were low.

Aims of intervention
- To build confidence and increase self-esteem.
- To provide opportunities and support for doing something new.
- To improve her concentration and memory by following written instructions.

Activity chosen: patchwork
Mrs X had previously attended anxiety management and enhancing self-esteem courses and had shown herself to be well motivated, but she needed to apply her knowledge in practical situations. She wanted to try patchwork because she had seen her friend make a quilt. Mrs X used sewing as a means of relaxing and managing stress. By attempting patchwork, she was using skills already familiar to her in a challenging new way. Mrs X also wanted to improve her concentration and memory in order to resume her hobby of reading.

Approach of therapist
Care was taken to make the task manageable, ensuring successful stages, to reduce anxiety and anticipation of failure. Although Mrs X wanted to make a quilt, after discussion with the therapist it was agreed that a patchwork pattern on her nephew's cot cover would be easier to begin with. Support and encouragement were given initially to help her through hindrances to learning such as her negative overreaction to difficulties. The activity was also used to remind her of relevant issues she needed to practise from the previous courses.

Environment
This was arranged to minimise any possibility of failure because Mrs X was so nervous that she could easily have been put off. There was sufficient space to cut out and sew. The environment had to be clean and dust free. The scissors were sharp; the needles and thimble were of a size which was comfortable and the same sewing cotton was available for each session. Seating was arranged to accommodate Mrs X's back problem and she was situated where there was good lighting. She was placed slightly apart from others, initially, because she was too shy to let them see her work. As her confidence grew she became more sociable and was able to allow others to see and comment on her work.

Teaching methods
Mrs X was shown each stage as she was ready for it, by demonstration and verbal instructions. To reinforce these and to help her work independently, she also had written instructions and pictures. The process was adapted when she took fright at the prospect of making her own template. In order to avoid this becoming an obstruction to the whole learning process, she was provided with one made by the therapist.

Progress
Gradually Mrs X became confident enough to work on her own, succeeded in making the patchwork and designed and completed the cot cover on her own at home. She was very pleased with the finished article and subsequently made some draught excluders out of patchwork, on her own, solving the problem of templates by buying plastic ones!

in new ways. This produces different feedback and can stop the vicious cycle of failure, thus increasing self-esteem. An increasing awareness of abilities gives the individual new expectations of himself (Kanfer & Goldstein 1981) and this can affect the attitude to learning. By providing opportunities to develop skills and observe the results, the therapist enables the client to become competent through doing, thus changing attitudes which affect behaviour.

There is also a need to be able to cope with an inability to change. Change may not occur for a number of reasons, for example the prognosis of the illness, failure of medical treatments, the client's fear of change or social circumstances. Consequently, it is important to enable the client to have a quality of life within the limits of his difficulties, to make adjustments and to be able to gain skills which provide a sense of satisfaction.

PROFESSIONAL EVOLUTION AFFECTING HOW OCCUPATIONAL THERAPISTS FACILITATE SKILL ACQUISITION

It will be useful at this point to take into account some areas of the profession that have been affected by the closure of the large psychiatric hospitals at the end of the 20th century. Occupational therapists have had to re-evaluate the way they work and make many adjustments.

Since around 1998, an increasing number of changes and areas of concern have been debated and discussed in the British and international occupational therapy journals. This discussion centres around defining the role of occupational therapists in community mental health teams, whether they should work generically or maintain a specialist emphasis on occupational performance. Professional identity was felt to be under threat, the occupational therapy process was being affected and the core skills of the profession had to be identified (Box 20.2.). Occupational therapists may be managed and supervised by someone of a different profession (see Chapter 39) and there are calls for strong occupational therapy leadership, consultation and networking to support staff as they seek to clarify their roles.

Funding services can be a problem, such as having to seek joint funding with voluntary agencies, having only a very small petty cash budget or even needing to ask for materials from day centres. These problems can be overcome to a certain extent by working with agencies, such as Restore (see Other resources, p379) or adult education departments, but overall the profession's autonomy can be undermined by these difficulties. Skill acquisition needs a starting point. For the occupational therapist to provide opportunities for people to begin a process, it is often easier if it is by doing, making, experiencing. As stated earlier, these need appropriate materials and equipment in order to provide just the right challenge.

It is disappointing that the occupational therapist's role in day resource units has diminished due to funding difficulties. Resource centres often have equipment and facilities readily available for practical activities and can offer an easily accessible route to vocational training and work opportunities.

However, despite these challenges and the need to adapt working practices, it remains the case that occupational therapists enable people to acquire or maintain skills. It can be argued that

Box 20.2 Some essential core skills of occupational therapists in mental health (adapted from points made at a Berkshire occupational therapists' liaison group study day, February 1991)

- Assessments and interventions for performance dysfunction
- Approaches to facilitating group processes
- Use of activity and task analysis
- Adaptable teaching techniques
- Use of creative and practical activities as means to improving occupational performance
- Empowerment through problem solving

occupational therapy models are reality based and therefore fit better within a community setting. Occupational therapists are coming into their own by doing community work, and the activities focus is even more important.

The service user is no longer expected to be passive in the intervention process so that part of the occupational therapist's work is to empower the service user in their progress towards improved function or adaptation. Occupational therapists see themselves as agents of change, providing opportunities for clients to try things out, building a sense of achievement and competence. For example, after discussions about goal setting in relation to improving physical health, a depressed person may choose to incorporate swimming into their weekly structure, thus having control over what activity to use and when.

The development of the profession is ongoing, with more research being needed into its contribution to mental health needs and skill acquisition. Occupational therapists must continue working to prevent their own skills being diminished and diluted, thus preserving their unique contribution to health.

SKILLS FROM THE PERSPECTIVE OF FOUR PRACTICE MODELS AND APPROACHES

As has been stated earlier, a goal of occupational therapy is to enable people to function at their optimum level, and there are a number of practice models which highlight ways to bring this about. Each model has its own perspective on how to develop and harness certain skills. More detailed information about the models is dealt with elsewhere but certain aspects are relevant here. Generally, problems are explained in terms of dysfunction and maladaption. It is suggested that each model has its contribution to make in facilitating the acquisition or re-establishment of skills, depending on the individual's circumstances. A pragmatic and holistic approach in their use is therefore advised.

The Model of Human Occupation

In this model (Kielhofner 1985), the outward manifestations of skills are evident in performance. These in turn are driven by volition and habituation.

Volition

Volition has three components which are personal causation, values and interests.

1. **Personal causation** is a person's self-perception of his effectiveness in the environment, including his belief in his skills, his ability to exert control and his anticipation of results.
2. **Values** are those principles or standards by which the person judges things or actions to be good, right and important.
3. **Interest** is the disposition to find occupations pleasurable. It is generated by action and the individual's personal experience of an activity.

Some interests are preferred to others, and this is related to the degree of enjoyment and complexity in the activity and its appeal to the senses. If the experience of an activity is a good one, interest grows and the inclination for future action is increased. Interest, therefore, acts as an important factor in motivation. The development of an individual's interests has been informed by the values of family, peer groups, culture and educational background. Interests are affected by a person's openness to new experiences, his developmental level and the available opportunities in the environment. Matsutsuyu (1969) stated that interests are influenced by early experience, stimulate positive and negative emotional responses, sustain action and are part of a person's self-image. Roberts (1994) noted that interest seems to be associated with the inherent processes of an activity and how that activity is valued. Achievement is also a significant factor, since interest is increased when a successful end product or goal becomes a likely outcome of doing an activity. Roberts also found that clients were strongly motivated to overcome difficulties by interest in an activity.

Habituation

Behaviours become habituated into roles (expectations of behaviours which accompany particular functions), habits and routines. These work in conjunction to produce skilled behaviour expressed outwardly as performance.

Performance

The components of performance are skills and skill constituents.

1. **Skills**, in this context, are defined as abilities that a person has which lead to accomplishment of a goal under variable environmental conditions. These include: perceptual motor skills, which are those of manipulating the self and objects; process skills, which are problem-solving and planning abilities, and communication/interaction skills for co-operating and interacting with people.
2. **Skills constituents** are subcomponents of skills, which are symbolic (images which guide performance), neurological (actions produced by the central nervous system) and musculoskeletal (the production of movement).

It can be seen, therefore, that when volition and habituation are affected by mental illness, performance in certain areas will also break down. This model gives some guidance as to which skills need to be repaired or developed and what motivates the client in particular areas. A person's sense of effectiveness, belief in skills and routines can be affected by mental illness. It is often the case that the person's roles and interests are also disrupted and the model can contribute towards making a profile of what the client is normally like and potential areas for development.

Functional Information–Processing Model

This model is also known as the Allen theory of cognitive disability. Allen (1982) described cognitive limitations caused by chronic illness and identified the remaining functional ability. She advocated certain crafts to assess cognitive function because of the type of memory and problem-solving skills required. The person's cognitive progress is seen as a continuum of motor and verbal performance linked by attention.

There are six cognitive levels (ACLs), which range from 0.0 (coma) to 6.0 (normal). Within each ACL are a number of modes characterised by variations in:

- attention
- apparent purpose
- experience
- behaviour
- duration and process of action.

The ACLs identify the highest level at which a person can function so that the expectations of the client are realistic. Screening tools are designed to provide an initial estimate of cognitive function. They are confirmed by observation of the client's performance in tasks associated with his usual or intended environment. There is a particular emphasis on task analysis so that the cognitive dimension of performance is known. This provides the means for a task to be adapted to match the maximum ability of the individual. Since an individual can then gain a sense of achievement, the distress caused by failure is reduced. For instance, a client functioning at the model's Level 4 may be able to learn the process of chopping vegetables by copying and repetition. He can then make an acceptable contribution (with guidance) towards group cooking in a hostel but would not be expected to cook meals on his own.

Theories about cognitive disability continue to evolve. Recent modifications include further clarification of the performance modes. Several studies have also been done with elderly people and those with brain damage, in addition to those with functional mental health problems. A biological element has been recognised in the cognitive dysfunction of some people who are affected, and permanent impairment is assumed. A deeper appreciation of two roles in the information-processing capacity of the brain has enhanced the effectiveness of the model. These are working memory and procedural memory.

Working memory enables a person to process new information and therefore to adapt within a changing environment, such as at home or in the workplace. Working memory has to be assessed to gain a clear picture of the client's cognitive ability.

Procedural memory enables habitual tasks to be performed, such as activities of daily living, and a routine inventory assessment tool has been produced to assess this (Allen 2002).

This model differs from other approaches in psychiatry in its acceptance of residual disability.

The management of permanent residual limitations is the focus of the model, rather than improvement or alteration. It therefore provides guidance for enabling clients to function at their optimum level without putting them under undue stress. The expected skills are laid out clearly in the model handbook (Allen 2002, Allen et al 1992) and task-orientated activities are used for gaining achievement. It can be argued that if an individual is able to build and apply skills within his cognitive limitations, this will also have a positive effect on his behaviour.

Adaptive skills approach

Mosey's (1970) work is specific to mental health. It identifies, in depth, psychosocial functioning and the problems associated with lack of skills and learned maladaptive responses in this area. These are described as affecting task planning, performance, interactions and ability to identify and satisfy needs. The skills required are called performance components, of which there are four.

1. **Sensory integration**. This is the process of receiving and utilising sensory stimuli, including tactile subsystems, postural and bilateral interaction and praxia.
2. **Cognitive function**. This refers to the cortical processes which use information for thinking and problem solving. These include: attention, thought processes, levels of conceptualisation, intelligence, dealing with factual information and ability to identify and follow through a plan to deal with problems.
3. **Psychological function**. This deals with the processing of information from past events plus that currently available in the environment in order to view self and others realistically. This is seen as a dynamic state which includes needs, emotions, values, interest and motivation.
4. **Social interaction**. This is the ability to engage with others in casual and sustained relationships, to interpret situations socially and to structure social interplay. Social skills are defined as the capacity to relate to others in ways that are satisfying to the self and others. They include communication and dyadic and group interaction skills.

An individual uses performance components in occupational performances that are described as 'organised patterns of behaviour through which an individual engages in and meets the demands of the environment' (Mosey 1986, p64). They are categorised as family interactions, activities of daily living, school/work, play/leisure/recreation and temporal adaptation. Role behaviour in relation to these performances is seen as dynamic because it is changeable and capable of being redefined.

From these concepts, Mosey developed three models for practice, of which **recapitulation of ontogenesis** is the one particularly relevant to the acquisition of skills. The term itself means returning to an earlier stage of development to rectify maladaption. It is linked to cognitive and social learning theory and uses aspects of the developmental and humanistic frames of reference. Mosey identified six adaptive skills:

- perceptual motor
- cognitive
- dyadic interaction
- group interaction
- self-identity
- sexual identity.

These skills are acquired sequentially, linked chronologically and evolve in complexity and adaptive potential. They are subdivided into skill components which are the stages in which they are learned. Mosey advocated the use of experiential learning through activity (individually and in groups) to adapt responses and improve skills.

This approach provides a means of checking on which stages of skill acquisition have been missed or where the individual is stuck. It is then possible to place the person into a learning situation where skills can be extended by starting at a natural stage of development.

Adaptation through occupation

This model, developed by Reed & Sanderson (1984), centres on skills assessment, development and retraining, and this is seen as the main concern of occupational therapists. It is based on problem solving and emphasises autonomy, actualisation and accomplishment. Occupations are identified as natural vehicles for normal human development and adaptation for the primary learning of skills. Participation in occupation enables adaptive responses. Occupational performance results from developmental motivation and the learning of many skills. Component skills are integrated into patterns and are configured appropriately to the requirements of the situation, for example, particular roles. Skills in this context are:

- motor activities
- sensory and cognitive functioning
- psychological and emotional behaviour
- social awareness
- work adjustment
- avocational interests and leisure activities.

Occupational performance is influenced by environmental factors, which are physical, biopsychological and sociocultural. The context and content of these may enhance or impede learning or performance. When a person has the occupational skills, and is able to use them to fulfil needs and meet demands, he has achieved a state of adaptation and health.

A person may lack motor, sensory, cognitive, intrapersonal or interpersonal skills and, in this model, the occupational therapist aims to develop, improve, re-establish or maintain skills in order to prevent, remediate or minimise dysfunctional performance.

The general focus on skills development makes this model suitable for use with both psychiatric and physical conditions.

METHODS OF SKILLS TRAINING

ADAPTABLE TEACHING TECHNIQUES

There is little documentation about the planning, organisation, knowledge of teaching methods and care for detail which an occupational therapist needs in order to provide opportunities for clients to acquire appropriate skills. It is nevertheless a major function of the occupational therapist to do this. She has to be adaptable and flexible in the methods used, bearing in mind the specific needs of the client. One of the core skills of an occupational therapist is to design a unique therapeutic programme of activities for the client (Hagedorn 1992), often including a means to enable the client to achieve

or adapt specific skills. To do this, an occupational therapist has to attend to the approach used, the learning environment and the teaching methods.

The attitude and approach of the therapist

The therapist aims to build a sense of achievement and confidence in the client so that motivation is enhanced, learning takes place and skills are increased. The therapist's own attitude and approach are a crucial part of this process. There is collaboration between client and therapist so that information is not imposed on the client but a means is found to begin at a stage appropriate to the client's learning needs.

Many aspects of being a therapist will also come into play in the skills training role. In particular, the therapist will draw from the conscious use of self as described by Mosey (1986), which means that interactions with the client are planned. Acknowledging the individuality of the learner, the therapist reflects carefully on her approach and that approach will depend on the situation. It may not be possible to take the same approach with the client in every session. The client's moods and condition are unpredictable and so the therapist has to be accommodating and well prepared, having reviewed a number of options of how to teach particular aspects of a skill.

Consideration has to be given to how facts and concepts are communicated. It is important to instruct the learner at a level which will make understanding easy, using words and concepts which are familiar to him and working at his pace. This is done in a way that is non-patronising, protecting the client's dignity, acknowledging his inherent capacity but bearing in mind the possible cognitive difficulties brought about by illness.

It is necessary to allow the learner freedom to learn by avoiding criticism and embarrassment. The therapist offers the learner respect, acceptance and a sense of security by being patient and non-judgemental. The aim is to alleviate fear and to provide reassurance and encouragement. The client needs support as he tries out new skills, experimenting with abilities which do not yet feel comfortable. Support is withdrawn at an appropriate time when he becomes competent. In fact, it is appropriate in the latter stages of intervention to provide or seek out opportunities which challenge the learner to increase the new skill.

The therapist's manner should be relaxed so that the learner feels free to make mistakes without feeling as though it is a disaster. Equally, it is important to give sufficient guidance so that the learner avoids making so many mistakes that he becomes disheartened and learning does not take place. To avoid pressurising the learner, the therapist remains objective about his progress, keeping expectations balanced and realistic. The therapist also has to have knowledge of the skills to be acquired or provide an appropriate instructor. If support workers or instructors are involved in the situation, mutual co-operation is important to ensure consistency of approach.

The learning environment

The occupational therapist not only has to design a unique programme, that incorporates suitable intervention procedures in a therapeutic sense for each individual, but also has to create a specific learning environment to facilitate the person's optimum ability to learn while handicapped by illness or residual dysfunction. The intention is to eliminate as many external barriers to learning as possible. The following should, therefore, be arranged with care.

- Attention to the details of basic comfort – such as appropriate heating, lighting, ventilation, room layout and seating arrangements – is essential for all learning. This will help to alleviate some of the general problems already discussed (pp364, 365) such as lack of concentration, preoccupations, anxiety and fatigue.
- Particular consideration is also given to the atmosphere. Is the atmosphere conducive to thinking and reflection? Is the encouragement of conversation and discussion desirable? What things will distract the learner? Certain distractions will negate the learning process, for example, observers, people wandering in and out, excessive extraneous stimuli. How much noise is acceptable? For some, a hub of conversation, music or background noise may be comforting. For others, silence and a sense of calm will be necessary. Willson (1987) advised selective

stimulation with clients who cannot filter out stimuli. This means that the environment is organised so that it only contains those things which will enhance the learning process.

- Space is also a relevant issue. The close proximity of others, including the therapist, may make the client feel tense. Therefore, in order to learn, he may need to be provided with sufficient body space as well as work space around him. There are occasions when a place for time out is important so that the learner can take a break when fatigued or experiencing difficulty.
- Consideration has to be given to the best setting in which to achieve learning goals. To enhance motivation, reduce frustration and ensure achievement in acquiring practical skills, there needs to be availability of adequate areas, suitable and functioning equipment, relevant materials and choice.

Ultimately, the client needs to feel secure in order to be motivated and engaged in intervention (Cook & Howe 2003). Therefore, tailoring the environment for the client's benefit is an accepted part of the occupational therapy process. This remains the same wherever the venue.

The traditional occupational therapy department had a role in providing the client with a safe environment and a routine in which to initiate some skills. It gave a structure and place for occupational therapy intervention. Funding was available to provide equipment and materials. Any amount of opportunity was provided for creativity and doing, with support. It can be argued that these departments were havens from reality and contributed to the institutionalisation of patients. Activities were used from the perspective of providing therapy (Roberts 1994) to deal with the specific symptoms of mental illness, such as poor concentration, chaotic thought processes, social withdrawal, low self-image and sense of failure. Currently, the use of real activities in daily life provides the learner with opportunities to develop and practise skills in real situations in the community. This can lead to a changed lifestyle, involvement in society and a return to paid employment or voluntary work.

Since the closure of traditional occupational therapy departments, occupational therapists are to be commended for the creative ways in which they are using their local communities as part of the intervention. A variety of places are now used: the client's home, GP surgeries, group rooms of mental health units, public amenities such as libraries and leisure centres, adult education facilities, community halls, portacabins, cafés, parks, day activity centres or resources centres.

A number of the points in the above sections are summed up in the requirement for careful preparation, both in the therapist's approach and in the organising of the environment. Careful preparation is also necessary in the application of teaching techniques.

Teaching methods

The methods employed to convey information are of paramount importance because, if chosen appropriately, they will increase the client's chances to learn and acquire skills. Each person learns in his own individual way. Since this process can be impeded by mental health problems, the occupational therapist will use teaching techniques that take into account the presenting problems of the client. She will need to know what the client's premorbid personality was like, and aspects of his educational background and previous learning capacity. This will be evident in part from his school achievements, work history and interests, but also in his ongoing response to activities and the learning process. This information is used to devise teaching techniques individualised for the client's learning needs. The method will allow for the client's fluctuating condition and be readily adapted when required, as illustrated in the case example in Box 20.3.

In order to provide personalised learning situations for the client, it is advantageous to be aware of various teaching techniques. Techniques which enhance the learner's own learning strategies, increasing the sense of achievement and confidence, are summarised in Box 20.4.

There are also teaching strategies which are particularly useful when dealing with the implications of mental ill health and its effect on learning. Some of these are described below.

Box 20.3 Case example 2

Mr Y is in hospital having his medication adjusted. He suffers from hallucinations, which are causing him intense distress at present. At times, when he concentrates hard, he is able to do an activity despite them. He and the occupational therapist agree that an interesting activity would help alleviate some of his distress. He begins to learn how to do marquetry (which he could continue at home and develop as a hobby). There are times when he is able to follow verbal instructions and can be left to work alone. On other occasions he finds this difficult and, until his condition is more settled, the therapist sits next to him and works with him, helping him to do one small section at a time.

Box 20.4 Helpful teaching techniques (paraphrased from Christiansen & Baum 1991)

Learning strategies can influence successful acquisition of performance skills by teaching techniques that help learners to:
- use self-motivation and reinforcement to sustain interest in what is being learned
- focus attention and concentration on relevant and important information (and ignore irrelevant and distracting information)
- acquire, organise and interpret new information
- enhance memory
- use rational principles and problem solving to make their own decisions (for helping themselves).

- **Clear verbal instructions and repetition.** These techniques allow the learner time to absorb what is being said. Make short comments which describe the procedure or concept succinctly, avoiding lengthy explanations. Check if the learner has understood what has been said. Repeat the points when necessary.
- **One concept at a time.** Break a process down into stages so that the learner is shown one concept and masters that before going on to the next stage. In this way learning is split into achievable tasks. The challenge for the learner,

Table 20.1 Breaking down a process to teach a task (Example: using a wood plane correctly, when the user is right-handed)

Method	Key points
• Take a firm stance, facing the bench with your feet slightly apart. This enables you to swing the weight of your body from one side to the other. • Hold the handle of the plane in the right hand and the knob in the left hand. • Start the stroke with your weight on the right foot, then, keeping an even pressure on the knob, follow the body through, finishing with the weight on the left foot. • When planing the ends of a piece of wood, work inwards to the centre from one end and repeat the process for the other end. If you plane straight across from one end, the edges will splinter. • Give the movement smoothness and rhythm and do not force the plane.	• Always keep the cutting edge of the plane sharp. • Always plane with the grain, not against it, or the wood will split. • Avoid letting the plane slip from the horizontal, either at the beginning or the end of the stroke, or the ends of the work will become rounded.

therefore, is not so great that he gives up and he is able to feel in control (see Table 20.1).

- **Key points.** It may sometimes be necessary to state the obvious and draw attention to main points because this will reinforce learning. This will also help to clarify a process and enable the learner to progress.

- **Instant feedback.** Feedback should be positive, constructive and as immediate as possible to indicate to the learner where he is succeeding and what errors he is making. It is preferable to deal with errors by first pointing out what has been done well and then suggesting improvements. This is especially necessary when a practical task is being attempted, for example the use of tools.

- **Reinforcement.** It is essential to provide or find a means of making opportunities to practise newly learned skills. This is important not only to reinforce what has been learned until the learner is competent but also to overcome the inhibiting factors of illness. Low levels of motivation and lack of confidence make practising techniques difficult. Tasks which are set to reinforce learning are sometimes best negotiated with the client so that they become achievable. Again, feedback and discussion on the results should be a part of the process to encourage a continuous progression.

- **Demonstration.** Showing the learner how to do something is often an advantage because it enables the learner to understand a process more clearly than if it is just explained. If a demonstration takes place it may bypass some of the cognitive difficulties inherent in illness, such as a short attention span. By using this technique the therapist can also spend time with the learner, providing encouragement and support.

- **Experiential learning.** This will provide the learner with an experience that enhances the learning process. Examples of this are the therapist going with the client to practise using a library or doing a role play. A client with a mental health problem may not have the motivation or courage to initiate an experience on his own, such as going to an adult literacy course. It is important for the therapist to facilitate secure situations where the learner can gain the experiences that he needs.

- **Duration of session.** Timing is an essential element in the learning process. It is important to arrange sessions so that they are not so long as to overwhelm the learner in terms of length of time, fatigue and attention span. The time allocated for a session also has to allow learners to reach a point of clarity in learning so that they do not leave feeling confused, which would inhibit the process of acquiring a skill.

- **The individual within a group context.** Teaching techniques will be required which suit the individual as he learns a skill, either alone or in a group. When the occupational therapist runs a group, whether it is practical or not, she takes into account the learning needs of each group member. The group is planned so that the participants are compatible and the size is comfortable. The group process and the activity are used to meet clients' emotional and learning needs in order to facilitate the development of skills (Mosey 1973). Consequently, there will be learning goals for each individual as well as for the group as a whole.

Some of these points are highlighted in Box 20.5. where the teaching techniques for two people are compared. One person has no mental health problems and the other is suffering from a psychosis.

Emotional skills

Strategies which make it easier to teach emotional skills, such as anxiety or anger management or building self-esteem, are also worth contemplating.

Much of the material available for the average person – such as handbooks, leaflets and tapes about acquiring skills – usually has plenty of information relating to a subject, often more than is required in order to add interest. Methods of teaching which convey very detailed information pose difficulties for some people with mental health problems. In the same way that clients cannot cope with too much sensory stimulation in the environment, they can also find that too much information clouds an issue for them, so that they cannot select what they need. Simpler information, if it is available, is often childish and can undermine the client's self-respect. It is better, therefore, to design information which will suit the occasion. In this way a balance between easily understood information and a respect for the client's adulthood can be attained.

For those clients who require it, the following points may be helpful.

- In some cases, when the client may have one main issue to deal with more than any other, it is advisable to use the previously mentioned technique of one concept at a time and break down ideas into individual elements. For example, a

---

Box 20.5 Teaching techniques for making a coil pot, adapted to clients with different needs

A client of average ability and not affected by illness
- Ensure that the environment has adequate light and is comfortable, and have enough appropriate tools to hand.
- Give clear, concise instructions.
- First, demonstrate hand wedging.
- Second, show how to roll out coils of clay, prepare base and pinch coils into place.
- Third, advise on care of clay by covering with a damp cloth to prevent cracking.
- The client may finish these processes in one or two sessions, depending on size of pot and time available.

A client of similar ability recovering from a psychotic episode
- Add to these points the need to organise the environment to be quiet and not overstimulating. Seat the client on his own to reduce distractions.
- In addition to this, be calm, supportive and encouraging but do not fuss. Give the client his required space.
- Demonstrate hand wedging and show pictures of this (and the next stages), thus reinforcing the information.
- Expect to work through one stage at a time, depending on the degree of tolerance, attention and preoccupation observed in the client.
- Repeat the relevant movements of each process if necessary and give as much guidance as required to ensure success.
- Allow for a lower standard than may be assumed for the age and expected ability of the client. If the client is able to tolerate it, move on to the next stage, but end with a complete stage to ensure achievement.

client may need to learn how to breathe slowly, so that he can deal with panic, but be unable to cope with exploring all the facts relating to the fight and flight mechanism, which must be held back until a later date. Simple written information and handouts which summarise the main points will serve as an easy reminder when required.

- Some clients have reached a stage when they are ready to assimilate information regarding their emotional needs. They are able to utilise cognitive techniques to enhance their insight and motivate themselves to use coping strategies. Other clients, especially those with enduring mental health problems, may experience strong symptoms that make them feel helpless. In this case, particular help is needed to raise awareness of how to isolate the problem and deal with it. This process can be facilitated by use of symbolism (Reilly 1974) conveyed by visual aids, games and aspects of creative therapies, such as paints and clay.
- Alternatively, the situation may need to be depersonalised in order to gain a perspective on it that will enable the client to progress. Story telling is a good way of accomplishing this, for example a story about how a fictional person achieved his aim by setting goals. Another means is to provide opportunities to discuss real-life events by, for example, showing a video. Sometimes discussion is inappropriate because the person needs the experience of success before being able to move forward. The best teaching technique, therefore, is to provide opportunities for active participation.

USE OF ACTIVITIES TO TEACH SKILLS

As indicated above and in the section on models and approaches, activities and the process of doing are a natural part of daily life and therefore a dynamic means by which skills can be taught. Activities are used to provide structure, develop routines and roles, learn organisational skills, build self-esteem and improve concentration. Reilly (1974) viewed activity as an intrinsic part of the learning process and Fidler (Fidler 1981, Fidler & Fidler 1978) advocated *doing* for the development of performance skills.

Doing is an integral part of self-expression and becoming 'I'. The human being's interaction with objects in the environment provides him with the opportunities to experiment and gain feedback. Doing is defined as 'enabling the development and integration of the sensory, motor, cognitive and psychological systems; serving as a socialising agent, and verifying one's efficacy as a competent, contributing member of one's society' (Fidler & Fidler 1978). Understanding the nature and relevance of *doing* to human adaptation can enhance the teaching strategies of an occupational therapist.

Chugg & Craik (2002), in their study of the factors that influence occupational engagement for people with schizophrenia, concluded that occupational therapists need to research more deeply into why people do things so they can further enable their clients to engage in doing. There are many ways in which an occupational therapist will apply the process of doing in order to develop a client's skills. Task-orientated activities and parallel groups are two useful examples.

Task–orientated activities

Traditionally, in occupational therapy, task-orientated activities are associated with the concept of doing, be it a practical, functional or creative activity. A task is a constituent part of an activity. Young & Quinn (1991) stated that a sequence of tasks combine to form an activity. It is through the precise analysis of activities broken down into tasks that the learning process in occupational therapy is often facilitated. The therapist will therefore encourage the client to do a task as part of the skill acquisition process, whether it is participation in a craft group or role playing a job interview. The activity is graded, sequenced and adapted to enable the learner to succeed (Cook & Howe 2003; see also Chapter 6). Thus, the learner is more motivated and becomes engaged in doing.

Providing the learner with just the right challenge enables him to set goals and achieve small tasks first (see Chapter 6). For example, it is better to have the initial meeting between the client and occupational therapist in the person's home, doing something simple like having a cup of tea and agreeing on some goals, before attending a venue for an activity.

Mosey (1973) identified task skills which serve as a guide to what is normally expected and how the therapist can enable their development. They are:

- a comparable rate of performance
- appropriate use of tools
- willingness to engage in tasks
- sustained interest
- following instructions (verbal, written or demonstration)
- acceptable tidiness
- appropriate attention to detail
- problem solving and organisational abilities related to the task.

Parallel groups

The process of doing tasks can also serve as a stepping stone towards the development of group interaction skills. A way of achieving this is to use the parallel group concept.

The participant in a parallel group works at a task in the presence of other group members (Mosey 1986). There is a small amount of interaction with other members of the group, in that tools are shared. The therapist provides support to the group and is a strong leader. The activities are well within the clients' abilities and assistance is given when required. Two or more participants doing the same activity is encouraged because this increases interaction.

Parallel groups are a useful means of skills training because they provide a secure forum for doing tasks, giving opportunities for guidance and support while the client is doing the task and learning to interact. Also, the environment and therefore the degree of stimulation can be controlled. For clients with enduring mental health problems, parallel groups can be a starting point for developing both the task and interaction skills that they need.

SUMMARY

Skills are an essential part of the human being's interaction with the environment and form the basis of performance, behaviour, cognition, social interaction and participation. Skills are acquired by development, learning and practice. Mental illness affects a person's skills in varying degrees, causing deficits or difficulties in relation to them. Occupational therapy has a role in enabling the person to recover, adapt or acquire new skills. The occupational therapist facilitates the learning process by a combination of enabling, guiding, teaching and mediating.

Practice models argue for the necessity to develop skills in order to be able to function, and highlight different perspectives on how to achieve this.

Occupational therapists use particular methods of teaching to facilitate skills training. They are adaptable and flexible, taking into account the individual needs of the client while affected by illness and providing a suitable level of challenge. The approach of the therapist, the learning environment and the use of activities are important factors in this process.

References

Allen CK 1982 Independence through activity: the practice of occupational therapy (psychiatry). American Journal of Occupational Therapy 36(11): 731-739

Allen CK 2002 Structures of the cognitive performance modes. Allen Conferences, Florida. Available online at: www.allen-cognitive-levels.com 25 May 2002

Allen CK, Earhart CA, Blue T 1992 Occupational therapy treatment goals for the physically and cognitively disabled. American Occupational Therapy Association, Rockville, Maryland

Argyle M 1978 The psychology of interpersonal behaviour. Cox and Wyman, London

Breines E 1984 The issue is: an attempt to define purposeful activity. American Journal of Occupational Therapy 38(8): 543-544

Christiansen C, Baum C (eds) 1991 Occupational therapy: overcoming human deficits. Slack, Thorofare, New Jersey

Chugg A, Craik C 2002 Some factors influencing occupational engagement for people with schizophrenia living in the community. British Journal of Occupational Therapy 65(2): 67-74

Cook S, Howe A 2003 Engaging people with enduring psychotic conditions in primary mental health care and occupational therapy. British Journal of Occupational Therapy 66(6): 236-246

Creek J 1996 Making a cup of tea as an honours degree subject. British Journal of Occupational Therapy 59(3): 128-130

Cynkin S, Robinson AM 1990 Occupational therapy and activities health: towards health through activities. Little Brown, London

Dickerson AE 1995 Action identification may explain why the doing of activities in occupational therapy effects positive changes in clients. British Journal of Occupational Therapy 58(11): 461-464

Doble SE, Magill Evans J 1992 A model of social interaction to guide occupational therapy practice. Canadian Journal of Occupational Therapy 59(3): 141-150

Fidler GS 1981 From crafts to competence. American Journal of Occupational Therapy 35(9): 567-573

Fidler G, Fidler J 1978 Doing and becoming: purposeful action and self-actualisation. American Journal of Occupational Therapy 32(5): 305-310

Franklin L 1990 Social skills training. In: Creek J (ed) Occupational therapy in mental health: principles, skills and practice. Churchill Livingstone, Edinburgh

Gadza GM, Brooks DK 1985 The development of the social/life skills training movement. Journal of Group Psychotherapy, Psychodrama and Sociometry 38(Spring): 1-10

Gillette N, Kielhofner G 1979 The impact of specialization on the professionalization and survival of occupational therapy. American Journal of Occupational Therapy 33: 30

Golledge J 1998 Distinguishing between occupation, purposeful activity and activity. Part 1. Review and explanation. British Journal of Occupational Therapy 61(3): 100-105

Hagedorn R 1992 Occupational therapy: foundations for practice, models, frames of reference and core skills. Croom Helm, London

Kanfer FH, Goldstein AP 1981 Helping people change. Pergamon Press, Oxford

Kielhofner G (ed) 1985 A model of human occupation, theory and application. Williams and Wilkins, Baltimore

King LJ 1974 Sensory integrative approach to schizophrenia. American Journal of Occupational Therapy 28: 529-536

Llorens LA 1976 Application of developmental theory for health and rehabilitation. American Occupational Therapy Association, Rockville, Maryland

Llorens LA 1991 Performance tasks and roles throughout the lifespan. In: Christiansen C, Baum C (eds) Occupational therapy: overcoming human deficits. Slack, Thorofare, New Jersey

Matsutsuyu JS 1969 The interest checklist. American Journal of Occupational Therapy 23(4): 323-328

Mosey AC 1970 Three frames of reference for mental health. Slack, Thorofare, New Jersey

Mosey AC 1973 Activities therapy. Raven Press, New York

Mosey AC 1986 Psychosocial components of occupational therapy. Raven Press, New York

Munn NL 1966 Psychology: the fundamentals of human adjustment, 5th edn. Houghton Mifflin, Boston

Reed KL, Sanderson SN 1984 Concepts of occupational therapy. Williams and Wilkins, Baltimore

Reilly M (ed) 1974 Play as exploratory learning. Sage Publications, London

Roberts ME 1994 Doing a task orientated therapeutic activity – the client's response. Unpublished MSc dissertation, University of Exeter

Robinson A 1977 Play: the arena for acquisition of rules for competent behavior. American Journal of Occupational Therapy 31: 248-253

Shorter Oxford Dictionary 1993 Clarendon Press, Oxford

Smith ME 1979 Familiar daily living activities as a measure of neurological deficit after stroke. Unpublished fellowship thesis. College of Occupational Therapists, London

Stewart A 1994 Empowerment and enablement: occupational therapy 2001. British Journal of Occupational Therapy 57(7): 248-254

Trower P, Argyle M, Bryant B 1978 Social skills and mental health. Methuen, London

Willson M 1987 Occupational therapy in long term psychiatry, 2nd edn. Churchill Livingstone, London

Young M, Quinn E 1991 Theories and practice of occupational therapy. Churchill Livingstone, Edinburgh

Other resources

Restore working for mental health. Available: Restore, Fleetmeadow, Sandringham Road, Didcof, Oxfordshire, OX11 8TP

SECTION **6**

Client Groups

Chapter 21

Loss and grief

Clephane A. Hume

INTRODUCTION

Loss encroaches on all aspects of life and is a topic which is highly relevant in the field of mental health. Indeed, all clients will have experienced a sense of loss because of their inability to cope with the demands of life and consequent referral for help.

Bereavement is a specific response, usually regarded as the feelings experienced as the consequence of the loss of a significant individual, but many of these feelings are typically features of other types of loss. This chapter therefore aims to take account of coping with any type of loss.

Paradoxically, the prevalence of AIDS and recent incidences of wars and natural disasters have increased public awareness about some of the issues related to loss. Despite this universality of experience, and the increasing amount of literature about bereavement, it is still an area about which many people are reticent. Social taboos and discomfiture persist, adding to the painful feelings of the individual concerned.

In the context of illness, losses might include alteration in roles and reduction in cognitive or physical abilities, choices, self-esteem and hope. Some people will be additionally distressed by loss of faith.

Unacknowledged loss, or feelings which are ignored, may lead to future mental health problems and the occupational therapist therefore requires an understanding of some of the issues facing clients.

Much documented work about the impact of loss on health relates to terminal illness, bereavement and unemployment.

The aim of this chapter is not simply to repeat material which already exists about the theory of loss but rather to consider the nature of loss, people's reactions and factors which may influence mental health and well-being. The impact of loss on occupation – alteration of roles or occupational deprivation – will be considered. Case examples of loss consequent on ill health and bereavement are included and attention is given to how such losses may add to existing feelings of loss for patients and relatives. It has to be recognised that the intensity of the grief reaction may sometimes necessitate specialist intervention, therefore some sources of help are included.

TYPES OF LOSS

In considering the nature of loss, it is helpful to identify some of the most common contexts in which loss may be experienced. Bereavement and redundancy are obvious examples, illness less so. However, the recurrence of schizophrenia or depression after a symptom-free period can be a real blow.

Social pressures and expectations may also contribute to feelings of loss. For example, in a success-oriented society, those who do not come first may lose everything. Being second does not secure the job.

Sometimes the loss may be felt retrospectively or may reflect a gap in the person's life: a living loss, as illustrated in Box 21.1. Marris (1974) wrote of the 'crisis of discontinuity' and Morley (1996) wrote movingly about her feelings of loss in relation to not being a parent.

BOX 21.1 Living Loss

Sarah was an elderly lady with a long history of mild arthritis which would not have been a problem to most people. Her considerable gifts as a pianist were much enjoyed by those round about her. She, however, experienced lifelong grief because her physical illness had deprived her of her career as a professional pianist. This led to bouts of depression and withdrawal and repeated hospital admissions for psychiatric intervention.

In practical day-to-day terms, loss may occur as the result of various situations which cause changes in relationships. Table 21.1, contexts of loss, is not a hierarchy of the gravity or severity of any loss, since each individual's experience is entirely personal. Clients will have their own examples.

Mitchell & Anderson (1983) divided loss into six types.

1. **Material**: loss of possessions, for example, theft, breakage; loss of income and consequent further loss.
2. **Relationship**: an unavoidable aspect of human life; change in social status.
3. **Intrapsychic**: loss of self-image because of a change in circumstances such as bereavement, completion of a task, failure.
4. **Functional loss**: loss of autonomy; occupational deprivation.

Table 21.1 Contexts of loss

Cause of loss	Examples of loss
Bereavement	Spouse, parents, siblings, friends, child
Miscarriage, stillbirth	Expectations of parenthood
Death of a pet	
Unemployment/ redund-ancy	Major role, financial security, daily routine
Divorce	Also affects children and grandparents
Breakdown of a relation-ship/friendship	
Remarriage	From the child's perspective, loss of previous relation-ship with a parent
Ill health	Enduring or recurrent illness, sudden accident
Loss of familiar environment	Move to another town, to long-term care
Failure	Not getting a job or passing exams
Empty nest syndrome/ retirement	
Loss of relationships through neglect	The busy parent/spouse who has little time for the family
Loss of opportunities	Childlessness
Loss of valued objects	Loss of precious mementos, due to breakage or theft

5. **Role loss**: retirement; acquiring new roles or responsibilities; becoming a patient.
6. **Systemic loss**: loss of function within an existing system, for example, a child leaves home, a family member dies, retirement or illness impacts on the function of the entire family.

Of these, types 3, 4 and 5 have particular significance in relation to loss of health. The other categories may also be sources of stress and are therefore of relevance in occupational therapy.

The particular situation of refugees – loss of familiar environment, loss of status, deskilling because of difficulty in communication, memories of terrifying experiences – merits specific consideration. This includes situations where there is uncertainty about the status of family members who have gone missing.

CHARACTERISTICS OF LOSS

Features of the presenting situation affect the characteristics of the loss experience. Using as an example a teenage girl who sustains a spinal cord injury, the loss may be:

- **avoidable or unavoidable?** This is debatable. Her mother says: 'If only I had prepared a meal for her before I went out she wouldn't have had to go the chip shop and that car wouldn't have knocked her down...'.
- **temporary or permanent?** She will never be able to walk again.
- **actual or imagined?** This example is a fact. It has happened.
- **anticipated or unanticipated?** This injury was not expected. Insidious conditions or terminal illness may have given the individual time to anticipate further loss.
- **static or deteriorating condition?** Unlike a degenerative illness, once rehabilitation is complete and occupational adjustment has occurred, this girl should be able to lead an active, albeit altered, life.

TIMESCALE

As reactions to loss vary according to the individual situation, so too does the timescale during which the intensity of feelings may be experienced. It may reasonably be expected that sad and painful feelings will diminish with time, as usually happens in bereavement, but it would be wrong to assume that they will completely disappear. Grief may persist for a long time, as shown by the personal anecdote in Box 21.2

Loss may be experienced in terms of the following timescales.

- **Immediate.** Instant feelings of loss in response to trauma or diagnosis which, in the case of an accident, may be mingled with relief that the person is still alive.
- **Anticipatory.** Response to an expected loss, when the person begins the grieving process in advance of the actual loss, for example following diagnosis of terminal illness or dementia in a loved one.
- **Episodic.** Feelings experienced from time to time, particularly in relation to lack of achievement of normal milestones, for example, by the parents of the young man who, but for his head injury, would have been graduating with his peer group.
- **Future.** The parents of this young man are now unlikely to be grandparents.
- **Anniversaries.** 'It was on this date, 5 years ago, that X was diagnosed/Y died/Z had his birthday.'

It is documented by hospital chaplains in the field of general medicine that within the bereavement process there is generally a 2-year average period of adjustment, and it could be speculated that this would be comparable in the context of illness (Ainsworth Smith & Speck 1982). However, opinions vary. My own experience has indicated that, for some people, loss is an enduring feature of disability, such as the artist who is unable to paint. This view was described by Monteith (1987,

Box 21.2 Persistent grief

My collar hides a scar. The surgeon did an impressively neat job and the line is not nearly as visible as it used to be, so that a lot of people do not notice it. However, I know that it is there and I shall always be aware of it. Sometimes it twinges.

p10) in respect of inability to participate in normal childhood activities.

In contrast, Whalley Hammell (1997), writing in the field of spinal cord injury, found reduction in expression of loss after a period of time similar to that described in relation to bereavement. She suggested that, for some people, the experience of physical disability enhances quality of life and unexpected opportunities may result. This latter point is supported by Darke (2005), who became a wheelchair user following an infection and then a member of the British Adaptive Ski Team.

It should be noted that feelings of loss will fluctuate and apparently small losses may add to the cumulative experience which leads to seeking help. Breaking a mug given by a deceased person may trigger a grief reaction which far outweighs that which might have been expected, due to the symbolic meaning of the object.

The implications of multiple bereavements are obvious, but any experience of loss may contribute to mental health problems or act as a precipitating factor in the onset of illness. Illness may give rise to further, secondary experiences of loss and these merit attention as consequent changes in occupational roles may in themselves be significant.

REACTIONS TO EXPERIENCES OF LOSS: THE GRIEF PROCESS

Theories of loss have been documented by authors working in different contexts and are continually evolving. Some authors describe similar patterns of functional and psychological reactions (Bowlby 1985, Livneh & Antonak 1997). Theories in relation to bereavement have been developed by doctors and counsellors, including Kubler Ross (1970), Parkes (1986) and Worden (2003). Briefly, these theories describe common features and pathways towards the resolution of grief.

- **Denial**: disbelief and numbness
- **Anger**: usually directed towards God or towards the person for going away
- **Depression**: the pain of reality and realisation of the permanence of the situation
- **Acceptance**: gradual accommodation to the situation

Bereaved people will often express feelings of guilt: 'If only I had...'. These stages have been described in relation to terminal illness by Kubler Ross (1975) and can be translated into experience of loss consequent on disability.

- **Denial**: 'When I get home everything will be all right.'
- **Anger**: 'What have I done to deserve this? Am I being punished?'
- **Bargaining**: 'If I become a better sort of person ... maybe things will work out.'
- **Depression**: 'I'm no good to anyone like this.'
- **Acceptance**: 'Being able to get out again makes me feel I can still be of some use.'

People will not follow these stages neatly; they may swing between them or follow a circular course. Mitchell & Anderson (1983) described the pattern of grief as spiral, not linear, with distortion of time.

Work by Stroebe & Schut (1999) introduced the Dual Process Model of bereavment which demonstrates that, during the grief process, people oscillate between emotional (loss-oriented grief work) and practical aspects of readjustment (restoration-oriented changes in tasks and roles).

Machin & Spall (2004) described the development of a measurement tool for mapping grief. The Adult Attitude to Grief scale (AAG), used with older adults, provides the basis for a six-stage process that focuses on responses on a continuum ranging from overwhelmed, through balanced to controlled.

The realisation of loss and grief may occur suddenly. The woman who returned home having purchased bananas, which she did not eat but which were a favourite food of her mother who had recently died, stated that this was when it really hit her that her mother had gone for ever. Isolated events may trigger feelings of loss at any time, possibly producing unexpected flashback reactions which demonstrate the fickle and enduring nature of the experience

The cumulative effect of multiple losses should be recognised, and grief may also be regarded as a crisis of coping. Talking of his wife's final admission after years of treatment for cancer, Ian said, 'The dog died just 2 days before she went back into the hospice'. This left him completely alone. Caplan (1969), who pioneered the development of crisis theory in community psychiatry, noted that subsequent crises rekindle the feelings associated with earlier losses.

The usual experience and process of grieving as a reaction to loss may be summarised as: disbelief; acknowledgement of the reality of the situation; experience of pain and grief; and rebuilding over a period of time unique to the individual. There can be no predicted time by which the process will be complete.

RISK FACTORS AND PROBLEM REACTIONS

Grief is a *normal* reaction to loss; however, there are certain factors which can be recognised as putting the person at greater risk of developing problem reactions. Karaban (2000) presented concepts of complicated grief, including examples of difficult social contexts and disenfranchised loss, in which the person experiences a stigmatised or unacknowledged loss. Inadmissible grief, such as may occur where the mourner is the unacknowledged widow(er) of a gay partnership, may be particularly hard to bear.

Mitchell & Anderson (1983) described some impediments to grieving, including intolerance to pain, in the sense that the individual does not allow himself to feel it. This may be linked to a need to maintain control, and therefore acceptability, according to cultural and family influences, or to external factors such as lack of privacy or of supportive listeners. The expression of distress may also be hindered by intellectualising or masked by the use of sedatives, which medicalises a normal response.

Some people may employ coping tactics, such as the use of humour or keeping busy as a distraction/avoidance technique. A few may fling themselves into a new lifestyle with no apparent regrets: the merry widow syndrome. Such behaviour may create more difficulties for the observer than for the bereaved individual, who may be cocooned in a state of denial or preoccupied with maintaining a fragile front.

Further risk factors include traumatic death, other recent losses and problems arising due to the nature of the relationship, for example, the parent/child relationship in which there are tensions or a marriage in which the couple are totally enmeshed with each other. Those relieved of a burden of care may feel guilty for feeling thankful, whereas post-traumatic grief may give rise to feelings of guilt in those who have survived the accident. Shared grief may lead to bonding experiences in which onlookers find themselves excluded.

While these reactions have their origins in the context of bereavement, they are also valid for the person struggling to come to terms with loss of health. Bright (1996), a music therapist and grief counsellor, stressed the need for the person to grieve over disability and not to be overwhelmed by an approach coloured by therapeutic optimism.

COPING WITH DISABILITY AND ILLNESS

Previous work in relation to psychiatric rehabilitation (Hume & Pullen 1994) identified that how someone copes with a physical disability depends on a variety of factors, which can also apply to mental illness:

- the nature of the onset of the disability/illness
- the nature of the disability/illness
- what the disability/illness means for the person
- the reaction of others to the disability/illness.

A similar perspective was taken by Livneh & Antonak (1997), who proposed four classes of variables which must be considered in relation to outcomes of psychosocial adaptation:

1. the disability itself
2. sociodemographic characteristics of the individual
3. personality attributes of the individual
4. characteristics of the physical and social (external) environment.

From this classification, they devised a model of psychosocial adaptation to chronic illness and disability (CID). This incorporates functional performance, quality of life and medical status as indicators of level of adaptation.

In addition to the indicators included in the CID, other factors might influence individual responses and outcome. Those with curious and intellectual minds (expert patients) may search the Internet looking for answers to questions about the nature of their experience of loss, and then ask for definitive solutions when none are in fact possible. This is an experience unique to the individual. In addition, responses will depend upon age of onset, stage of life the person has reached and general social circumstances: 'If this had happened when I was younger, I don't know what I would have done ...'.

The physical and social environment may or may not be readily adaptable. Friends and family may be in/flexible in their outlook and each individual will have personal resources with which to cope with what has happened (Hume & Pullen 1994). Many people will be living on their own and, when it comes to public transport and other resources, there is a world of difference between being alone in a rural area and in the city.

Previous experience and particular circumstances necessarily have an impact on reactions; for example, the families of siblings diagnosed with the same life-threatening illness face the prospect of multiple bereavements. A family where the prospect of redundancy threatens will be susceptible to extra strain imposed by the worry of having a sick family member.

GUIDELINES FOR WORKING WITH PEOPLE WHO GRIEVE

The pain of grief, whether individual or shared and however it is expressed, cannot be avoided and needs to find expression within a supportive environment (see Box 21.3). However, grieving is a lonely experience and the world can be very critical of people who have not recovered after a period of time. People must be allowed to grieve at their own pace, according to the nature of their loss and their changed role.

Worden (2003) suggested four tasks to be undertaken in bereavement:

1. accept the reality of the loss
2. work through the pain of grief
3. adjust to an environment in which the deceased person is missing
4. emotionally relocate the deceased and move on with life.

Box 21.3 Grieving with support

Joan's husband died unexpectedly following minor surgery. Surrounded by a supportive family and friends, she was able to express her feelings and to pick up the threads of life again, without any medical intervention.

For the therapist working with a bereaved person, this means providing a supportive environment for the expression of painful feelings. People may feel a lack of support from others (real or perceived), so listening is of paramount importance. Perceptions of support are crucial to the progress of the grieving individual. Careful attention to the person's use of language can identify those at risk of self-harm or suicide: 'I wish I could see *the* light at the end of the tunnel' does not mean the same as 'I wish I could see *a* light at the end of the tunnel'. When someone says, 'I would like to get away from it all', does this mean for a holiday or for ever?

Gomez (1987) outlined a problem-solving process very similar to that of a treatment-planning cycle, in which the person is encouraged to identify areas of difficulty. Possible alternatives are then considered and a course of action planned. Re-evaluation of the outcome leads to any other problems being identified.

The Dual Process Model of bereavement (Stroebe & Schut 1999) is highly relevant for occupational therapists. Restructuring of life, including occupational readjustment, might include the acquisition of practical skills and building social networks. Support and encouragement in undertaking new roles or in doing things alone should lead to increasing confidence and self-esteem for the individual adjusting to altered status.

PRACTICAL CONSIDERATIONS

A client-centred approach is essential. What the bereaved person seeks, above all, is someone who has time to listen in a non-judgemental way, who will accept the painful feelings and anger which need to be expressed. Worries about upsetting the person or saying the wrong thing are natural, but tears need to be shed and it is preferable for this to happen in a supportive environment. Giving helpful advice should be resisted. The suggestion, albeit from another widower, to get broadband and a dog was of questionable benefit to Peter whose wife had recently died and who had his own, different ways of restructuring his life.

Most people will want to talk about the person who has died, in a realistic rather than idealised way, and to avoid this can be hurtful. Some will want a hand to hold or a touch on the shoulder and this must be sensitively gauged. Non-tactile people can usually make their feelings obvious!

Start where the person is and let him take the lead. Give him time to talk and be gentle in encouraging self-disclosure. Use the deceased person's name and ask questions which demonstrate an interest in knowing what s/he was like. The reality of the loss has to be acknowledged, both in the present and in what the future will now mean.

Asking what the grieving person does not miss may help to promote expression of anger or negative thoughts, which may be concealed as being unacceptable when other people are focusing on the positive attributes of the deceased.

It may be necessary to cover the same ground more than once and it is important to realise that, once the initial period of numbness and shock is passed, when society thinks the person is back to normal again, feelings of grief may actually be more painful.

Never be tempted to compare your own experience of grief with the person and say, 'I know how you feel'. You do not. Although your experiences may help you to understand, the person's sense of loss is unique to him.

In summary, be there for the person and stay there. People may choose not to accept help; it is their right to refuse offers of assistance but they suffer more when others avoid them than they do from supportive attempts to help. Do not take an initial refusal of an offer of support as an indicator of total rejection. The person may welcome help at a later date.

LOSSES DUE TO DISABILITY AND ILLNESS

It is necessary to consider the consequences of loss in practical terms. What effect has the loss had on the individual's life? For example, news of a serious or fatal diagnosis is usually delivered in a supportive context and counselling for the newly diagnosed eliminates the referrals for psychiatric help which were previously not uncommon. Reality, which might mean a confirmed diagnosis, however bleak that may be, can be easier to cope with than uncertainty, for it gives a clear starting point for action. However, realisation that the diagnosis means long-term dependence upon medication may provoke a grief reaction or a form of Russian roulette in which erratic compliance becomes problematic.

The following examples of the consequences of having a disability or chronic illness are by no means comprehensive but are a starting point for understanding and, therefore, for intervention.

Psychological and emotional consequences

The emotional suffering caused by loss in all its forms always merits consideration, but especially loss of control over one's life, isolation, abandonment or inability to carry out normal roles. Difficulties related to sexual expression may not readily be talked about and loss of friends, just when most needed, is painful: 'It's interesting who has helped. Some unexpected people have helped while others, whom I thought would do so, have stayed away'.

Occupational deprivation may be interpreted as 'I'm not doing anything'. Inability to work or to maintain previous levels of activity may create feelings of worthlessness and alter social status. It can feel as though nothing will ever be the same again.

Cognitive consequences

Processing information, organising thoughts and making decisions may all take extra time and energy and detract from other activities. Perplexity and anxiety may result. For example, a man with schizophrenia said, 'I can listen to the content of the conversation or determine whether or not the other person is friendly, but not do both at the same time'.

The problems of deteriorating memory are more easily understood but are painful for those who experience them, both sufferers and carers. Depression may be a reaction to failing memory.

> **Box 21.4 Living loss**
>
> Paul contracted encephalitis at the age of 17. This left him with a limited field of vision in his right eye, some arm movement and the ability to move three fingers in his dominant hand. His parents and siblings cared for him devotedly but his girlfriend's visits diminished and eventually she stopped coming to see him. Likewise, his hopes for going to university faded.

> **Box 21.5 Loss of important relationship**
>
> Freda threatened to pour boiling oil over her young daughters in order to purify them. In later years they expressed their feelings of terror and sense of loss of their mother as a real mother rather than being someone strange and frightening.

Physical and perceptual consequences

Problems may be visible or invisible. They can affect movement, mobility and function and, therefore, will impact on activities, levels of independence, social relationships and career prospects (see Box 21.4). Fatigue may also seriously restrict activity.

Loss of sensory function, for example sight or hearing, may also lead to profound feelings of grief, as in, 'I'll never be able to see what my grandchildren look like'.

Spiritual consequences

Formerly a neglected area, the spiritual dimension of treatment is receiving more attention from health professionals (Hume 1999). In the context of psychotic illness, people may become confused by religious ideology or make statements such as 'I've lost God'.

In the secular world, spirituality is acknowledged as having a wider meaning than organised religion, so that the individual's beliefs about health care, thoughts about the meaning of life and personal values will be recognised as having an influence on his spiritual needs. The Mayers' Lifestyle Questionnaire (Mayers 1998) and the framework of the Canadian Model of Occupational Performance (Townsend et al 1999) provide ways of giving attention to this dimension of care.

Social consequences

Alteration in interpersonal relationships and social activities must be considered, both on account of the individual's feelings and because these experiences will be shared by relatives and friends. Withdrawn,

unpredictable or antisocial behaviour can seriously curtail social contacts, while role reversal can give rise to difficulties in relationships. Leisure activities or holidays may be impossible due to various factors such as difficulties in access, financial constraints or ongoing medical problems.

Consequences for carers and family

Those closest to the individual have their own experience of loss. Karaban (2000) referred to 'ambiguous loss' where the person becomes lost to family and friends through a disease process such as dementia. Carers say, 'He's not the person he used to be', 'I've become his carer, not his wife' or 'My mother doesn't recognise me – it's like she has already died'. Box 21.5 gives an example of how psychosis can affect other family members.

Such feelings may be particularly difficult where the problems are not immediately obvious to others, for example in early dementia or a relationship confused by delusional ideation. Occupational therapists can provide practical assistance and opportunities for people to share their complex feelings, either individually or in a supportive group context.

It is also necessary to remember the future which may not now happen and the hopes and ambitions for the family that cannot be realised due to the limitations imposed by disability or financial constraints (Bright 1996, Hume 1994).

The importance of support and respite for carers, who may also be elderly people, is well recognised.

Loss and the elderly

Footballing grannies and jet-setting pensioners notwithstanding, old age can be a time of loss through alteration in roles and occupational deprivation. This is multifactorial, including memory,

> **Box 21.6 Retirement as bereavement**
>
> Jim had a very responsible job in banking. On his retirement, he became seriously depressed, believing that he was no longer of any use. Reassurance from his friends that they would welcome his company on the golf course had little effect. Fortunately, a course of antidepressant medication was effective and his wife was able to persuade him to go to America to visit his grandchildren. On his return, he took up voluntary work and began to enjoy life again.

physical health, stamina, cognitive ability. Friends may die or become lost through illness. For those unable to live at home, loss of symbols, objects, possessions and, perhaps, a pet exacerbate feelings of incompetence at relinquishing independence.

The special needs of those growing old in an alien culture, who may never return to their roots, should be acknowledged.

Loss in old age comes in many guises but can be summarised as leading to loss of control over one's life, roles and choices, any of which may give rise to feelings of isolation and abandonment and to reduced self-esteem (see Box 21.6).

SOURCES OF HELP

There will be occasions when someone needs to be referred for more specialised help. This is not an admission of failure on the part of the therapist but rather a mature professional judgement. There are specialist organisations to which people may be referred for bereavement counselling in relation to specific circumstances. The best known in the UK is Cruse, the bereavement care organisation, which has branches throughout the country. There are also groups such as WAY (Widowed and Young), SOBS (Survivors of Bereavement by Suicide), SANDS (Stillbirth and Neonatal Death Society), Compassionate Friends (death of a child) and the Miscarriage Association.

Self-help groups may provide support for those experiencing loss in relation to a specific diagnosis and fellow sufferers can also offer practical advice on coping strategies. These groups are too numerous to list but may be contacted through local libraries, voluntary organisations, information officers or resource workers.

CARE FOR THE THERAPIST

Working with people expressing loss can be distressing and may awaken memories of grief experienced by the therapist. Identification with clients may, to some extent, be helpful in creating empathy but it may also tempt thoughts of self-disclosure. While this is useful in some instances, too much equates to stealing the person's problem and may be embarrassing to the client. It may create loss of confidence as the person has doubts about the ability of the therapist, who has apparently not dealt successfully with her own problems, to help.

If the therapist finds herself personally distressed and unable to respond to loss situations in others, it would be wise to discuss things with a supervisor. It is only the stony-hearted who remain unmoved by the pain of others but overwhelming reactions are counterproductive to therapy.

A FINAL CAVEAT

The reaction of the individual may not be consistent with what the loss implies to others. For example, the treatment team congratulated themselves on curing Jimmy's hallucinations. But Jimmy, after 30 years of hearing companionable voices, reported feeling lonely and did not perceive the change as totally beneficial.

SUMMARY

Loss encompasses many aspects of everyday life. It is important that all therapists are aware of the implications of reactions to loss, both for clients and their families, as well as for the individual therapist. An understanding of ways in which such reactions may encroach upon the treatment process is also valuable. This chapter has reviewed the context and characteristics of a variety of situations and outlined common grief reactions. Examples of reactions to bereavement and loss of health have been described.

References

Ainsworth Smith I, Speck P 1982 Letting go: caring for the dying and bereaved. SPCK, London

Bowlby J 1985 Attachment and loss, vol 3. Loss: sadness and depression. Penguin, London

Bright R 1996 Grief and powerlessness. Jessica Kingsley, London

Caplan G 1969 An approach to community mental health. Tavistock, London

Darke C 2005 'What's for you won't go by you'. Able Magazine, January/February, p33

Gomez J 1987 Liaison psychiatry. Croom Helm, London

Hume C 1994 Working with terminally ill people and their relatives. Therapy 20(50): 6

Hume C 1999 Spirituality: a part of total care? British Journal of Occupational Therapy 62(8): 367-370

Hume C, Pullen I (eds) 1994 Rehabilitation for mental health problems. Churchill Livingstone, Edinburgh

Karaban R 2000 Complicated losses, difficult deaths. Resource Publications, San Jose, California

Kubler Ross E 1970 On death and dying. Tavistock, London

Kubler Ross E 1975 Death, the final stage of growth. Prentice-Hall, New Jersey

Livneh H, Antonak R 1997 Psychosocial adaptation to chronic illness and disability. Aspen, Maryland

Machin L, Spall B 2004 Mapping grief: a study in practice using a quantitative and qualitative approach to exploring and addressing the range of responses to loss. Counselling and Psychotherapy Research 4(1): 9-17

Marris P 1974 Loss and change. Routledge and Kegan Paul, London

Mayers C 1998 An evaluation of the Mayers' Lifestyle Questionnaire. British Journal of Occupational Therapy 61(9): 393-398

Mitchell K, Anderson H 1983 All our losses, all our griefs. Westminster Press, London

Monteith G 1987 Disability, faith and acceptance. St Andrew Press, Edinburgh

Morley B 1996 Grieving for what has never been. Contact, the Interdisciplinary Journal of Pastoral Studies 120(2): 22-25

Parkes CM 1986 Bereavement: studies of grief in adult life, 2nd edn. Penguin, London

Stroebe M, Schut H 1999 The Dual Process Model of coping with bereavement: rationale and description. Death Studies 23: 197-224

Townsend E, de Laat D, Egan M et al 1999 Spirituality in enabling occupation: a learner centred workbook. Canadian Association of Occupational Therapists Publications, Canada

Whalley Hammell K 1997 Spinal cord injury: quality of life; occupational therapy: is there a connection? British Journal of Occupational Therapy 58(4): 151-157

Worden J 2003 Grief counselling and grief therapy: a handbook for the mental health practitioner, 3rd edn. Routledge, London

Chapter 22

Acute psychiatry

Robert Hawkes, Valerie Johnstone, Lynn Yarwood

INTRODUCTION

Acute mental health problems are typically characterised by sudden onset and marked symptoms, and they may affect an individual's cognitive process, beliefs, perceptions and outward behaviour. The acute episode may be a first presentation or occur as a relapse of a pre-existing or ongoing mental health problem. One in six people will experience mental health problems during their life, ranging from distress to severe illness. These problems include depression, anxiety, eating disorders, psychosis, schizophrenia, bipolar disorder and dementia (NIMHE 2005).

In the past, options for treatment available to people with acute mental health problems were limited and often meant an admission to an inpatient unit. In 1990, mental health services in the UK began a major shift towards care in the community (DoH 1990). More recently, publications such as the *National Service Framework for Mental Health* (DoH 1999) and the *NHS Plan* (DoH 2000) have outlined priorities, strategies and the vision for working-age adults. Additional policies and guidance to support the development and improvement of specific services for people with acute mental health problems have been produced by the Department of Health (2002).

The *Mental Health Policy Implementation Guides* (DoH 2002) are intended to ensure the delivery of a local, flexible, focused mental health system. Specific implementation guides describe new models of service provision such as crisis resolution, assertive outreach and early intervention in psychosis, as well as providing guidance for improving existing services such as adult acute inpatient care. The development of new community-based mental health services and a reduction in the traditional reliance on inpatient services are central to the process of modernising mental health care.

This chapter gives an overview of the main types of services for people with acute mental health problems, both community provision and inpatient care. It discusses the nature of occupational therapy in acute inpatient settings and describes the occupational therapy process with this client group.

COMMUNITY PROVISION IN ACUTE PSYCHIATRY

A client with acute mental health problems may access or have ongoing contact with mental health services in a variety of ways. Local policies and resources, along with client need, determine the nature of the intervention and the treatment setting. The acute inpatient setting will be the main focus of this chapter but outlined below is a brief introduction to some of the community services that address the needs of people experiencing an acute episode of mental illness. Community mental health services are described in more detail in Chapter 27.

COMMUNITY MENTAL HEALTH TEAMS AND PRIMARY CARE

Community mental health teams care for the majority of people with mental illness in the community. These teams are multiprofessional and, typically, give priority to those clients with severe and enduring mental health problems whose needs are often complex and who require specialist psychiatric care. Practice is guided by care co-ordination and Care Programme Approach (CPA) principles, as social and health-care services are integrated. Alongside primary health care, these teams are the key source of referrals to the specialist teams described below, and they provide the core around which other services are developed.

Providing services for adults with the less complex and disabling mental health problems, such as depression and anxiety disorders, may be part of the function of community mental health teams. An alternative model is a separate primary mental health-care service operating within a local health centre and working closely with GPs and other professionals.

ASSERTIVE OUTREACH

Assertive outreach teams, known also as assertive community treatment teams, provide intensive support, normally 7 days a week, for an identified client group of adults with severe and persistent mental illness who do not effectively engage with other mental health services. There is usually a history of repeated use of inpatient care so the aim is to reduce the frequency and duration of hospitalisation and to improve engagement in therapeutic interventions. Using a team approach, workers aim to establish a trusting relationship with each client in a flexible, creative and needs-focused way. This enables the delivery of a care package which fits each client's specific needs. A low ratio of workers to service users allows intensive frequency of client contact compared to standard community mental health services.

CRISIS RESOLUTION AND HOME TREATMENT TEAMS

These teams provide services for adults with severe mental health problems who are experiencing an acute psychiatric crisis. They offer rapid assessment and, if required, provide intensive treatment in the least restrictive environment, 24 hours a day, 7 days a week. The aim is to avoid hospital admission and to act as gatekeepers to other mental health services. Interventions are time limited and the turnover of clients is often high.

EARLY INTERVENTION IN PSYCHOSIS

Early intervention services are in the main for people aged 14–35 either at a first presentation of psychotic symptoms or during the first 3 years of psychotic illness. Intervening early in the course of psychosis is crucial for all aspects of the individual's life as it can prevent initial problems and improve long-term outcomes. Early intervention services are best provided by a specialist team, with the emphasis on recovery. Use is made of local resources such as mainstream educational, recreational and vocational agencies.

ACUTE INPATIENT SETTINGS

Improvements in community care mean that many clients receive treatment in their home environment. However, hospital admission may be necessary if there is risk of harm to self or to others, self-neglect or medication issues. Clients who are admitted to an acute psychiatric inpatient unit are usually severely ill and have experienced deterioration in their ability to fulfil their normal daily roles.

The purpose of an adult psychiatric inpatient service is to provide a high standard of humane treatment and care, in a safe and therapeutic environment, for service users in the most acute and vulnerable stage of their illness. It should be for the benefit of those service users whose circumstances or acute care needs are such that they cannot, at that time, be treated or supported at home or in an alternative less restrictive residential setting (DoH 2002). Adult acute inpatient units are commonly placed within either psychiatric or general hospitals. Some only admit patients with a particular illness while others take patients with a wide variety of diagnoses.

The main purposes of admission are to:

- provide a thorough assessment
- initiate treatment
- reduce symptoms
- provide a place of safety
- plan discharge and reintegration into the community.

The main features of the inpatient environment are the ward, the multidisciplinary team and the legal and policy framework of care.

THE WARD

A mental health ward is run by registered mental health nurses (RMNs) with support from healthcare assistants (HCAs). The main purpose of admission is to provide a period of assessment so the length of stay may vary; those patients detained under the Mental Health Act 1983 may be in hospital from 28 days to 6 months (and longer in certain situations). Most people require only a brief period of hospitalisation, on average around 6 weeks. During this time, patients are encouraged to maintain their independence: making their own beds, attending to their own laundry, making tea and coffee and, in some cases, making meals and snacks. The HCA plays a vital role in ensuring that patients do not become dependent on staff, a skill that requires a great deal of expertise, as it is often easier just to get on and do things for people.

Each patient has a named nurse who is responsible for ensuring that the treatment outlined in the nursing care plan is provided. Each nurse will be the named nurse for several patients. The nursing staff on an acute ward need to be skilled at challenging difficult behaviour, as some patients may be angry at being detained in hospital, although others like the security of being in hospital and are anxious about leaving.

Treatments available on acute wards include medication, electroconvulsive therapy (ECT) and one-to-one work, such as cognitive behavioural therapy and psychosocial interventions. The occupational therapist works closely with nursing staff, balancing the need to contribute to generic team tasks with maintaining a specific professional role.

Ensuring safety, privacy and dignity

Service users report that many inpatient units feel neither safe nor therapeutic. In order to provide a safe, relaxed and comfortable environment of care, the following factors need to be considered.

- Ward size
- Good bed management systems
- Risk management, with detailed risk assessments
- Cultural needs
- Gender needs, e.g. single-sex accommodation
- Meaningful activity

The importance of upholding the individual's right to privacy can create problems when patients need close observation for their own safety. Careful consideration has to be given to the design of the accommodation to minimise potential risks and allow discreet observation of the occupants by staff.

THE MULTIDISCIPLINARY TEAM

A typical multidisciplinary team on an acute inpatient unit may include nursing and medical staff working closely with psychologists, social workers, physiotherapists, art therapists and occupational therapists. In order to plan for effective services for the after-care of clients, community staff, such as community psychiatric nurses, social workers and community-based occupational therapists, should also be recognised as vital team members.

Generic working has become a fact of professional life for many community occupational therapists but the situation is very different for those working in acute mental health. Here, the luxury of profession-specific working allows therapeutic activities to be embraced as the tools for assessment, treatment and evaluation of those with mental health needs.

THE MENTAL HEALTH ACT 1983

The majority of clients are admitted to hospital on an informal basis, which means that they come into hospital voluntarily. However, some clients who have a mental illness may be detained formally under a section of either the Mental Health Act 1983 or the Mental Health (Scotland) Act 1984 for assessment or treatment. These Acts are utilised where there are concerns regarding the health and safety of the client and/or there is a need to protect others. The Mental Health Act Commission monitors the working of the Act by visiting people who are detained under one of its sections. This is to ensure that the correct procedures have taken place and that the rights of individuals under the Act are upheld.

All areas of occupational therapy practice in acute inpatient psychiatry are influenced by operation of the Mental Health Act 1983 or the Mental Health (Scotland) Act 1984. It is essential for the occupational therapist to be familiar with those sections of the Act relating to professional and ethical practice, which may include issues of consent to treatment and therapeutic relationships. The occupational therapist may be expected to contribute to legal procedures, including:

- inpatient assessment
- hospital managers' hearings
- Mental Health Act review tribunals
- treatment requiring consent or a second opinion
- leave arrangements
- statutory after-care planning.

NICE GUIDELINES

The National Institute for Health and Clinical Excellence (NICE) produces clinical guidelines outlining good practice for different mental health conditions and covering diagnosis, care and treatment and referral pathways. To date, guidelines have been produced for the following diagnostic categories in adult mental health: anxiety, bipolar disorder, depression, eating disorders, obsessive-compulsive disorder, post-traumatic stress disorder, schizophrenia and self-harm. There is also a guideline on the short-term management of disturbed or violent behaviour. Health-care professionals are expected to be aware of and to follow these guidelines.

CURRENT ISSUES WITHIN ACUTE INPATIENT PSYCHIATRY

There are a number of current issues in acute inpatient psychiatry that require attention from all professions, including occupational therapy. These issues will have an impact on every aspect of service delivery. The key issues are explained below and the implications for occupational therapy will be discussed in the next section.

Integrated inpatient care within a whole–systems approach

The inpatient stay must form part of a planned and integrated whole system with effective co-ordination and communication, particularly with community teams. Plans for after-care should be included in the initial care plan in order to avoid delayed discharge. Planned and co-ordinated multidisciplinary and multiagency input to treatment programmes during an inpatient stay can facilitate home leave and early discharge.

Social inclusion

Inpatient units have the delicate task of providing both a shelter from the burden of responsibilities and relationships and, at the same time, holding on to fragile connections with family, employers and friends. Staff members have a crucial role to play in supporting patients to maintain and maximise these connections with their local community. Those staff providing therapy groups for inpatients should be mindful of this, as people with mental health problems are often at greatest risk of social exclusion (Huxley & Thornicroft 2003).

Clinical effectiveness

Research is urgently needed on the effectiveness of interventions in the area of inpatient psychiatry. However, there is a range of evidence-based interventions and skills that are particularly relevant to inpatient work, for example, family and carer

support interventions, medication management strategies, coping strategy development, risk management and safety interventions. Inpatients should have access to these interventions as a matter of priority.

Informed and involved service users and carers

Service users report that admission can be a distressing and demeaning experience, with both the patient and the family not knowing what support is available or what is expected of them. Information should be provided in an appropriate and accessible format and there should be a commitment to service user and staff collaboration. This should include clear arrangements and support to facilitate feedback about any concerns that patients or their relatives may have and about ways of making improvements.

The planning and philosophy of care need to be service user focused, with patients involved in all aspects of the planning and review of their care. For occupational therapists, service user choice of occupation must be considered paramount (Frances 2006).

Structured activity and engagement focus

The service user experience of acute inpatient admission can be strongly influenced by the amount and type of therapy available on the ward. 'Because of the numerous pressures that staff and patients are under, inpatient stays tend to be characterised by an absence of therapeutic, or even recreational, engagement' (Janner 2006, p5).

Inpatient environments where there is a programme of activities that meet the needs of individuals and a culture of staff engaging with service users diminish disturbance, violence and boredom (DoH 2002, Garcia et al 2004, Mental Health Act Commission 2006, MIND 2004, National Institute for Health and Clinical Excellence 2005).

Inpatient units that provide appropriate stimulation and structure as part of individual care plans have a more therapeutic and safe environment. Yet a recurring theme in most reports on inpatient care is 'lack of something to do' (as one report put it, 'a sort of suspended animation'). Each inpatient service needs to have a clear focus on the timetabled accommodation of therapeutic activity and engagement of service users, both on and off the ward. Meaningful activity should be determined within an individual care plan negotiated with the service user. (DoH 2004, p15)

There is also recognition of the role of the occupational therapist in establishing such a culture.

Occupational therapists have a specific expertise in assisting this care planning and in the determination and facilitation of a range of appropriate activity inputs onto the ward. Some of these interventions need to be adapted and specifically modified to practise within the constraints of working in an inpatient setting where an increasing number of service users are detained and many compulsory inpatient stays are of a relatively short duration.

With clarity of whole-system working and clear care pathways many of those interventions can be continued post discharge. (DoH 2004, p14)

OCCUPATIONAL THERAPY SERVICES IN ACUTE INPATIENT PSYCHIATRY

Occupational therapists are not primarily concerned with diagnosis or the application of a medical model but they do work within medical settings where their role is to analyse the relationship between health, illness and occupational functioning. It is essential that the profession retains a sound understanding of illness, disability and concepts of health. Mental illness usually develops as a result of a combination of biological, psychological and social influences. The occupational therapist, therefore, has to examine the relationship between clinical presentation and function from a biopsychosocial perspective.

The range of disorders encountered in an acute psychiatric setting is diverse. Although similarities exist between diagnostic groups, each client will differ in presentation. For example, no two clients who have schizophrenia are the same or have the same needs. For example, during the acute phase,

two clients may both hear voices but, for one, this symptom results in high levels of distress and agitation whilst the other withdraws from daily life and spends most of his time in bed.

The art of occupational therapy is to collaborate with the client to examine the impact of illness on function and to define associated needs. It is inappropriate for an occupational therapist to treat each patient according to diagnosis. Instead, every client should be approached as an individual, with emphasis placed on how their symptoms affect their ability to function in daily occupations.

Therapists working in the acute mental health sector need to adapt to constant change in the presentation of the people they work with, and this must be taken into account when setting up and developing inpatient services. Therapy must reflect the needs of the client in a care package that can adjust to change and yet still be stable enough to inspire confidence in the service user.

THEORIES USED TO INFORM PRACTICE

Occupational therapists are experts in matching meaningful occupations and wellness to a person's performance level of daily activities (Helbig 2005). The profession believes that people can live a meaningful and satisfying life despite serious mental illness (Mahler 2001).

The literature review for a strategy for occupational therapy in mental health services in the UK, *Recovering Ordinary Lives*, identified two approaches to mental health and illness (College of Occupational Therapists 2006). Both are encountered within acute psychiatric services and both have their place. However, they offer different ways of working for the occupational therapist.

- **Crisis and compulsion**: in this approach, mental health problems are treated as illnesses that have to be controlled or managed. Occupational therapists may extend their roles to include such activities as prescribing medication, providing cognitive behavioural therapy and acting as case managers.
- **Recovery and hope**: in this approach, resources are directed towards promoting positive mental health and improving well-being. Occupational therapists work

with individuals, carers, organisations and communities to develop their skills and resources. The focus is on health promotion, community development, social inclusion, rehabilitation and employment.

When an individual experiences an acute psychiatric illness, it is likely that his ability to engage in the meaningful daily activities that support his usual range of occupations is diminished. If the individual is admitted to hospital, he will also experience a significant and relatively sudden environmental change which lessens his chances of maintaining any degree of normal daily life and routine. In this situation, the medical model can dominate treatment: a reductionist approach is used and there is pressure to identify symptoms and alleviate illness. The occupational therapist has an essential role to play in the promotion of independent and meaningful occupations and activities.

A sound understanding of illness allows the occupational therapist to appreciate the client's situation and work in parallel with the multidisciplinary team. However, the occupational therapist must also understand occupational therapy concepts of health to be able to offer a unique contribution to intervention that is grounded in the philosophical basis of the profession.

Occupational science

Occupational science is the discipline that aims to study systematically all aspects of the relationship between humans and occupation (Wilcock 1991, Yerxa 1993). It searches for evidence of the influence of occupation and activity on health that can be used to justify the historical assumptions and beliefs of the occupational therapy profession and to inform practice. Furthermore, there seems to be increasing emphasis on the idea that health is not just the absence of illness but is a state which reflects quality of life and experiences of well-being (Wilcock 2006, Yerxa 1998).

When an individual begins to show signs of mental ill health, attention is commonly focused on symptom reduction, medical treatment and protection of the client within a safe, caring and supportive environment. This practice is essential and can be extremely effective; however, the occupational needs of individuals are also paramount at this time and occupational scientists suggest that occupational deprivation can be detrimental to health (Wilcock 2006). Some inpatient wards may produce a situation of occupational deprivation simply by not taking into consideration the boredom produced by a lack of daily structure and meaningful occupations. Alleviation of symptomatology and illness, without paying attention to occupational needs, is insufficient for a healthy recovery.

Flow is a subjective psychological state that exists when an individual is totally involved in an activity (Emerson 1998). To achieve flow, individuals must be engaged in the 'just right' challenge; therefore the essential skill of the occupational therapist is to find activities which can engage people in the acute stage of illness.

During an acute illness, clients can become immersed in symptoms and distress. It can be argued, however, that to reach some level of flow state can not only reduce symptoms but can promote a healthier state of mind. Although the symptoms and worries of the client do not disappear, some quality time out can ease their distress and allow them to feel more able to cope with their situation.

Motivation and change

Motivation theory has been widely researched, particularly in the field of psychology (Bernstein et al 1988). The word motivation comes from *movere*, the Latin word meaning 'to move'. It can be defined as the influences that account for the initiation, direction, intensity and persistence of behaviour (Geen et al 1984). The study of motivation focuses on the internal and external influences that might drive a person to act.

Motivation is a key focus in acute psychiatry, as an understanding of what it is that motivates each individual is essential for treatment to be effective. Sociologists have explored ideas that include the sick role and the patient career. In practice, this is often referred to when it is thought that an individual has a preference for living in a hospital setting, seemingly enjoying the benefits of illness. This is a crucial time to revisit concepts of motivation and, with the client, explore patterns and stages of change.

DiClemente & Prochaska (1998) developed a model of change that is particularly useful to consider when the client is thought to have some degree of control over his behaviour. Stages of change identified in this model include precontemplation, contemplation, action and maintenance (see Chapter 29). Intervention will vary depending on the stage the client is at – for example, motivational interviewing during precontemplation or support to develop coping strategies during maintenance.

Solution-orientated therapies promote change by inviting the client to use his own strengths and resources to move towards a better future, remembering that behaviour change, or lack of it, is not just the patient's problem (Rollnick et al 1999). The occupational therapist has a role to play in behaviour change by providing treatment that is stimulating, client centred, challenging and person specific, and that takes into account the individual's current needs. The therapist must also be approachable, friendly and fun to be around, whilst allowing the patient to see the serious nature of therapy.

The main treatment tool used by occupational therapists is meaningful activity which meets clients' goals. However, the context and the nature of the activity must be carefully considered, agreed and planned in collaboration with the client. Failure to work collaboratively could result in resistance, since the goals could be wrong or the stage of change could be misjudged.

OCCUPATIONAL THERAPY PROCESS

The occupational therapist working in an acute inpatient unit needs to develop specific skills in:

- rapid assessment of needs
- goal setting
- prioritising key problems
- exploring and highlighting relevant strengths and resources
- providing effective short-term interventions
- discharge planning that takes into consideration the long-term functional needs of the client.

Referral

Some units operate a system of blanket referral whereby all patients admitted are assessed by the occupational therapist. More commonly, patients are referred according to individual need, following discussion with the multidisciplinary team. The preferred system will depend on a number of factors, including staffing, resources, unit capacity and service philosophy. On receipt of the referral, the occupational therapist must first consider the level of priority of the client's needs. This is essential when, as is often the case, the demand for occupational therapy outweighs the resources available.

Consent to treatment

Central to occupational therapy philosophy is the importance of working closely with clients to determine treatment goals and desired outcomes. This collaborative relationship can be influenced in an acute psychiatric setting by:

- an individual refusing treatment or not being able to participate in the process
- the medical model
- client need as perceived by the team versus the client's personal wishes
- the constraints of the Mental Health Act 1983.

These are areas that must be addressed by the multidisciplinary team and therefore any decisions the occupational therapist takes regarding treatment must be well justified and ethical.

Assessment

Once the referral has been discussed and agreed, the process of assessment is initiated. Information about a client's needs must be gathered and analysed within a short time by the occupational therapist working in the acute inpatient setting. Occupational therapists use a variety of assessment tools, the choice of which will be influenced by:

- the reason for admission
- the client's mental state
- areas of need identified by the team
- areas of need identified by the client

- the preferred theoretical framework of the occupational therapy service and the team
- service constraints
- the therapist's professional strengths.

Assessment tools

Assessment tools and methods may include:

- brief, regular contact with the client
- observation
- interview
- activity
- standardised assessment tools
- specific assessments, for example, assessment of domestic skills
- observing the individual in his normal everyday environment.

Further information about methods of assessment can be found in Chapter 5.

Throughout the assessment the occupational therapist gathers information about the client's:

- productivity, self-care and leisure roles
- normal daily routine
- occupations of productivity, self-care and leisure
- perceptions of the factors which influence their function and occupations
- hopes, aspirations and goals
- strengths, abilities and achievements.

The occupational therapist works with the client to determine what can reasonably be accomplished in a short time, ensuring that goals are specific and realistic and using initial and ongoing assessment findings to formulate a plan of intervention.

Assessment of safety and risk

Whether the occupational therapist is working with a client on a ward, in the community or in the client's home, she must constantly be aware of the client's and her own safety and ensure that measures are in place to minimise risk. The following factors must be carefully considered and all decisions discussed and documented prior to contact with any client who has an acute mental health problem.

- policies and procedures regarding safety and risk, e.g. observation policy
- outcomes of risk assessment
- views of the multidisciplinary team
- location of meeting place
- action plan in case of emergency
- leaving information about whereabouts and expected time of return
- alarm systems
- access to equipment or tools
- client history of violence
- content of hallucinations or delusional beliefs
- history of substance misuse
- risk of suicide and history of self-harm.

Planning therapeutic programmes

Many wards now have activity workers whose role is to provide structured programmes of activity for inpatients. The activity worker and the occupational therapist must work closely together to avoid duplication of treatment and to ensure that activities are therapeutic and client led.

Recreational activities are a major component in mental health care yet many therapists now seem to avoid them, feeling that they must undertake activities or therapeutic techniques that appear more complex if they are to be taken seriously as professionals. However, occupational therapists have a unique understanding of the power of activities, and activity analysis is perhaps the tool that most differentiates the approach of the occupational therapist from the activity worker. When selecting activities for their therapeutic value, consideration is given to the client's aims and objectives for the intervention (see Chapter 6) and, in group activities, to ensuring that every session is therapeutic and meaningful to all group members. Molineux (2004) suggested that confident, skilled and articulate occupational therapists are proactive in promoting health and quality of life through creative occupations.

The range and level of the client's occupational performance indicate the type of intervention required. For example, an individual with depression may have reduced occupational performance in the area of self-care, lacking the motivation to take care of his personal appearance and take an adequate diet. Job satisfaction and performance may fall, or the low mood could mean that the person no longer wishes to go out to work and be with others. The daily routines for taking care of the home often become less of a concern for someone with depression, as there seems no point to life. Leisure activities may decline as the person may take less pleasure from life and mixing with others, and may withdraw from society, spending more time at home.

Interventions should allow the inpatient to return to independence as quickly and effectively as possible so every effort is made to ensure that the therapeutic plan reflects individual need. For example, the patient with depression may just need time to talk at first, so intervention may be slow to begin with. Mood is often linked with motivation so the client could be asked to monitor and record his mood level to help him regain control. Working with a client at the time of day when his mood is higher will make therapy more effective.

Most clients prefer to have opportunities to explore the reasons behind their low mood or other problems on an individual basis, even if group work is the preferred intervention. Individual sessions lasting around 30 minutes are more productive than longer interviews for people in the acute stage

of illness. They should begin with the client taking control by listing in order his main concerns since becoming ill and the things he wishes to work on. Those difficulties outside the therapist's remit may require referral to other areas.

Box 22.1 describes the process of problem identification and treatment planning with an inpatient, Darren.

Intervention

The range of interventions used in an inpatient setting is wide and varied, so it is impossible to describe and justify every possibility. Instead, some general guidelines are given for how to approach the provision of occupational therapy in an acute inpatient setting, then an anger management group is described.

General guidelines

The type of occupational therapy programme provided on an inpatient ward is influenced by a variety of factors, including the resources available, the skills of staff, the therapist's caseload and national treatment guidelines. For example, the NICE guidelines on schizophrenia (National Institute for Health and Clinical Excellence 2002) state that:

Box 22.1 Darren

Darren was a 28-year-old man who had been on the ward for a week when he first came to the activity sessions held in the occupational therapy department. He expressed an interest in finding out what else was available, so the occupational therapist offered an assessment of his current needs. Darren agreed to this and they began to explore those areas he found most problematic.

These were his low self-esteem, anxiety, low mood and lack of confidence, which were recorded on a problem sheet and developed into a treatment plan. For Darren to feel fully involved, as part of this treatment, he was asked to rate his problem areas, starting with those causing him the greatest concern. He identified two main problems. First, he began to lose confidence after his girlfriend of 3 years finished their relationship and he had to find new accommodation. Second, he no longer attended football practice with his Sunday league team and was reluctant to go to join a group of friends at the local pub on Friday nights.

Darren was offered therapy groups with other patients experiencing similar problems. These sessions occurred three times per week and were run by an occupational therapist and a co-worker from the nursing staff. In order to ensure that these sessions were of maximum benefit, Darren was also given weekly one-to-one sessions where he could discuss the more private aspects of his life. This enabled the therapist to help Darren challenge his previous methods of problem solving.

As Darren had worked well during his time in occupational therapy, the therapist decided to refer him to the community team for a short period of follow-up after he was discharged.

> Social, group and physical activities are an important aspect of comprehensive service provision for people with schizophrenia as the acute phase recedes, and afterwards. All care plans should record the arrangements for social, group and physical activities. (p10)

> Supported employment programmes should be provided for those people with schizophrenia who wish to return to work or gain employment. However, it should not be the only work-related activity offered when individuals are unable to work or are unsuccessful in their attempts to find employment. (p21)

Most patients need to learn or to develop skills to help them deal with the difficulties of modern life. People with mental health problems commonly face problems with life skills such as assertiveness, anxiety awareness, goal setting, problem solving, confidence, anger management, raising self-esteem and tackling distorted thinking. Provision of skills training is an important part of the occupational therapy programme (see Chapter 20).

Following the assessment of individual needs, looking at problem areas and completion of the treatment plan, group work may be the most effective method with which to reach the greatest number of people in a short space of time. These could be groups that allow people to discuss their thoughts and feelings and to realise that other people are facing similar problems. Art sessions may also allow for expression and self-discovery. Life skills workshops can challenge and help participants to make effective behaviour changes. Further information on facilitating groups can be found in Chapter 17.

Groups work best when a light-hearted approach is used alongside a more serious one. People need to feel comfortable talking about their innermost thoughts as many patients are new to discussing private and personal matters. Therefore light-hearted introductory activities such as coffee mornings, crafts, art, games and cooking allow staff and patients to become comfortable with each other. This, in turn, allows the therapist to assess and monitor those patients who might benefit from individually planned therapeutic programmes.

An anger management group

In order to determine the need for an anger management group, the therapist reviews the individual treatment plans for patients, looking for common themes. If such a group would be relevant for a number of patients, the next task is to set aims and objectives for the group. These aims and objectives will meet as many individual patient goals as possible. An aim could be as simple as: 'After people leave the session, they will have a greater understanding of the effect that anger has upon them'. Objectives are the steps taken to reach the overall aim, such as: 'learning to recognise how we display anger' or 'learning to recognise what makes us angry'.

Group rules are given out in writing prior to the first session so that group members have the chance to read and digest the information. At the beginning of the first session, people are encouraged to add their own rules and discuss them with the group.

Each session should begin on time and start with the therapist explaining the focus of the session; for example, 'For the next hour we will explore anger and the effects it has upon our lives'. The group are then warmed up before starting to work on the main objective for the session. This requires skill, as the therapist has to ensure that group members feel safe enough to disclose personal information. An example of a warm-up might be asking people to pull their most angry face, scream or shout. This can lighten the mood of the session prior to focusing on the main task of the group.

Following the warm-up, group members are given a quiet time to think about their anger and an opportunity to write their thoughts. The therapist monitors the group to see if anyone is losing concentration. It is a matter of professional judgement to decide on the right moment to invite group members to share their thoughts with the group. People need a balance between getting their thoughts down on paper and taking turns to talk, in order to maintain their focus. The therapist ensures that everyone is given the same amount of time to talk and asks at least one question to show that she is listening actively.

As the group comes towards the end, participants need to be aware of time. The therapist does not stop the session suddenly but guides members through the last few minutes.

During the last 10 minutes, it is helpful to ask participants what has been most useful and what could have been left out of the session. Members' suggestions are then used to develop the content of future sessions. Another method of asking for feedback is to give out evaluation forms, either at the end of each session or after a series.

Evaluation

The occupational therapist must examine both the processes and outcomes of interventions in order to provide clients with a high-quality service that is up to date and effective. Finlay (1997) suggested that evaluation of what we do is fundamental to our integrity and confidence as therapists.

Occupational therapists working in an acute psychiatric setting have the responsibility to ensure that interventions are effective in meeting the needs of their client in a short period of time. Any occupational therapy programme should be regularly reviewed and evaluated to ensure that the needs of the client group at any time are being met.

Evaluation should include:

- evaluation of the self, for example, through reflection and supervision
- regular evaluation with clients through the use of, for example, outcome measures and questionnaires
- evaluation of the service, for example, by clinical audit, consumer surveys, outcome measures and soliciting the views of the multi-disciplinary team.

Discharge planning

Discharge planning begins at the point when the patient is admitted to hospital. In order to contribute effectively to this process, the occupational therapist needs to have a good knowledge of community resources. She would also hope to ensure that clients are safe to return home and adequately prepared to cope with their normal environment. However, one of the frustrations often encountered by occupational therapists working in acute inpatient settings is that patients are discharged before successful completion of occupational therapy interventions.

To alleviate this problem, short-term care must be viewed as part of the total spectrum of services. Managers should plan services that allow for cross-boundary working and flexibility in service provision, with the inpatient occupational therapist being able to offer short-term follow-up or to refer the client on to community-based occupational therapists for longer term intervention.

Box 22.2 describes some of the issues around discharge for Sally, a young woman admitted to hospital following an overdose.

Box 22.2 Sally

Sally awoke in the accident and emergency department of her local hospital and was transferred to a medical assessment ward. The nursing staff felt that she needed to be seen by the self-harm team, who arranged for her transfer to the mental health unit as an inpatient for a period of assessment.

After losing her job, Sally had begun to spend less time with her friends and stopped going to the gym. She began spending longer periods alone in her small flat, staying in bed for long periods during the day and being unable to sleep at night. Eating became unimportant to her so that her energy levels reduced even further. Sally could see no alternative but to end her life. After taking an overdose of her antidepressant medication, with a large amount of alcohol, she was found by her father when he came to visit.

While on the ward, Sally was encouraged to attend the occupational therapy department. After a number of sessions, the therapist felt that the priority should be for Sally to look for employment. With the help of the therapist, Sally began to explore what jobs might be appropriate for her. She did not wish to look at the issues relating to her depression after discharge from hospital, but agreed to close monitoring by her community nurse.

SUMMARY

This chapter has described the importance of meaningful activity in acute adult psychiatric wards and the role of the occupational therapist in this area. The multidisciplinary team and current influences in this field have been introduced, whilst inviting the reader to consider the attitudes, principles and core beliefs that define practice. The occupational therapy process within this setting has been described, with some practical examples.

Within the ever-changing climate of health care, the future of occupational therapy in acute inpatient psychiatry is dependent on efficient service delivery which is evidence based and responds to current trends. The challenge is paramount.

References

Bernstein DA, Roy A, Srull TK et al 1988 Psychology. Houghton Mifflin, Boston

College of Occupational Therapists 2006 Recovering ordinary lives. College of Occupational Therapists, London

Department of Health 1990 National Health Service and Community Care Act 1991. HMSO, London

Department of Health 1999 National service framework for mental health. HMSO, London

Department of Health 2000 NHS national plan. HMSO, London

Department of Health 2002 Mental health policy implementation guides: adult acute inpatient care provision. Department of Health, London

Department of Health 2004 Mental health policy implementation guide – developing positive practice to support the safe and therapeutic management of aggression and violence in mental health in-patient settings. Department of Health, London

DiClemente CC, Prochaska JO 1998 Toward a comprehensive, transtheoretical model of change: stages of change in addictive behaviours. In: Miller WR, Heather N (eds) Treating addictive behaviors, 2nd edn. Plenum, New York

Emerson H 1998 Flow and occupation: a review of the literature. Canadian Journal of Occupational Therapy 65(1): 37-44

Finlay L 1997 The practice of psychosocial occupational therapy. Stanley Thornes, Cheltenham

Frances K 2006 Outdoor recreation to improve quality of life for people with enduring mental health problems. British Journal of Occupational Therapy 69(4): 182-187

Garcia I, Kennett C, Quraishi M et al 2004 Acute Care 2004: a national survey of adult psychiatric wards in England. Sainsbury Centre for Mental Health, London

Geen RG, Beatty WW, Arkin RM 1984 Human motivation: physiological, behavioural and social approaches. Allyn and Bacon, Boston

Helbig K 2005 The graded skills development programme. Mental Health Occupational Therapy 10(2): 51-53

Huxley P, Thornicroft G 2003 Social inclusion, social quality and mental illness. British Journal of Psychiatry 182: 289-290

Janner M 2006 Editorial In: Star wards: another Bright idea. Bright, London

Mahler J 2001 The recovery model. Psychosocial Journal of Rehabilitation 16(4): 11-24

Mental Health Act 1983 HMSO, London

Mental Health Act Commission 2006 In place of fear? Eleventh Biennial Report 2003–2005. Stationery Office, London

Mental Health (Scotland) Act 1984 HMSO, London

MIND 2004 Ward Watch – MIND's campaign to improve hospital conditions for mental health patients. MIND, London

Molineux M 2004 Occupation for occupational therapists. Blackwell, Oxford

National Institute for Health and Clinical Excellence 2002 Schizophrenia: core interventions in the treatment and management of schizophrenia in primary and secondary care. National Institute for Health and Clinical Excellence, London

National Institute for Health and Clinical Excellence 2005 Violence: the short-term management of disturbed/violent behaviour in in-patient psychiatric settings and emergency departments. National Institute for Health and Clinical Excellence, London

National Institute for Mental Health in England 2005 Outcome measures implementation best practice guidance. National Institute for Mental Health in England, Leeds

Rollnick S, Mason P, Butler C 1999 Health behaviour change. A guide for practitioners. Churchill Livingstone, Edinburgh

Wilcock AA 1991 Occupational science. British Journal of Occupational Therapy 54(8): 297-300

Wilcock A A 2006 An occupational perspective of health, 2nd edn. Slack, New Jersey

Yerxa E 1993 Occupational science: a new source of power for participants in occupational therapy. Occupational Science Australia 1(1): 3-10

Yerxa E 1998 Health and the spirit of human occupation. American Journal of Occupational Therapy 52(6): 412-418

USEFUL WEBSITES

National Institute for Health and Clinical Excellence: www.nice.org.uk

Sainsbury Centre for Mental Health: www.scmh.org.uk

Chapter 23

Approaches to severe and enduring mental illness

Simon Hughes

CHAPTER CONTENTS

INTRODUCTION

This chapter gives an overview of the context for working with people with severe and enduring mental health problems and gives guiding principles to shape and inform practice. Terminology will be briefly reviewed and the context will be drawn predominantly from policy drivers in England and Wales. There will be an overview of psychosis which focuses on people with a diagnosis of schizophrenia. The role of the occupational therapist in working with positive and negative symptoms will be highlighted.

The contribution of generic and profession-specific working will be explored as well as models that help to inform practice. The models will include stress vulnerability, rehabilitation, recovery and the social model of disability. Working with individuals will look at engagement, self-maintenance, leisure and productivity. There will be an extended look at employment as a key area where there is robust evidence for an effective intervention, in terms of positive outcomes for mental health status as well as an area that is central to the concerns of service users.

The chapter will emphasise that positive attitudes and values are key to working with people with severe and enduring mental health problems to counter stigma, promote social inclusion and work within a spirit of hope and optimism to foster recovery. It will conclude with a description of the experience of one young man.

CONTEXT

The importance of delivering high-calibre health care by the use of evidence-based practice has been gathering momentum for over 20 years. In the UK it is espoused in the policy documents and in addition, values-based practice is an emerging aspect of policy documents with a move towards socially inclusive practice where, through a collaborative approach, the service user is central to the process.

TERMINOLOGY

A wide range of terms is used to describe people with mental health problems, each with a different emphasis and perspective. Clients, consumers, ex-patients, experts by or through experience, patients, people with mental health problems, people with experience of mental and emotional distress, people with a mental illness, psychiatric survivors, service users, sufferers, survivors and users are all commonly used terms. People may well have negative connotations about terms used about them or apply a particular term themselves. The use of language can portray underlying values and attitudes, so respecting the person and understanding their perspective can help to work towards client-centred practice where the individual's preferences, concerns and expectations are understood.

POLITICAL CONTEXT

Key documents that highlight the priority for mental health services in the UK are the *NHS Plan* (DoH 2000a), the *National Service Framework (NSF) for Mental Health* (DoH 1999), *The Ten Essential Shared Capabilities* (DoH 2004a) and *Modernising Mental Health Services* (DoH 1998). These set out an agenda of user involvement and user-focused services, a promise of government investment in the process with a timetable of targets to be achieved. The vision is for comprehensive, effective and co-ordinated services that are able to offer appropriate interventions around the clock.

Modernising Mental Health Services

Modernising Mental Health Services (DoH 1998) proposed local services that were safe, sound and supportive. To do this it had 10 guiding principles. Services should:

- involve users and their carers in the planning and delivery of care
- deliver high-quality treatment and care, which is known to be effective and acceptable
- be well suited to those who use them and non-discriminatory
- be accessible, so that help can be obtained when and where it is needed
- promote the safety of service users and that of their carers, staff and the wider public
- offer choices which promote independence
- be well co-ordinated between all staff and agencies
- deliver continuity of care for as long as it is needed
- empower and support staff
- be properly accountable to the public, users and carers
- reduce suicides.

National Service Framework and NHS Plan

The NSF expanded on the policy ideas in *Modernising Mental Health Services* with models of care and treatment defined, with timescales to measure progress. The standards in the NSF targeted at people with severe mental illness were: to ensure that each person with severe mental illness receives the range of mental health services they need; that crises are anticipated or prevented where possible; to ensure prompt and effective help if a crisis does occur, and timely access to an appropriate and safe mental health place or hospital bed, as close to home as possible. The *NHS Plan* (DoH 2000a) set out a number of pledges for mental health services including the provision of assertive outreach, early intervention and crisis resolution home treatment teams. These documents viewed together give a comprehensive plan for mental health services.

The Ten Essential Shared Capabilities

The Ten Essential Shared Capabilities (DoH 2004a) describes the capabilities necessary to achieve best practice for all staff who work in mental health services (see Chapter 12). The capabilities are geared towards the cultural changes in services, providing choice, being person centred and mental health promotion. The 10 key capabilities are listed below.

- **Working in partnership**. Developing and maintaining constructive working relationships with service users, carers, families, colleagues, lay people and wider community networks. Working positively with any tensions created by conflicts of interest or aspiration that may arise between the partners in care.
- **Respecting diversity**. Working in partnership with service users, carers, families and colleagues to provide care and interventions that not only make a positive difference but also do so in ways that respect and value diversity including age, race, culture, disability, gender, spirituality and sexuality.
- **Practising ethically**. Recognising the rights and aspirations of service users and their families, acknowledging power differentials and minimising them whenever possible. Providing treatment and care that is accountable to service users and carers within the boundaries prescribed by national (professional), legal and local codes of ethical practice.
- **Challenging inequality**. Addressing the causes and consequences of stigma, discrimination, social inequality and exclusion on service users, carers and mental health services. Creating, developing or maintaining valued social roles for people in the communities they come from.
- **Promoting recovery**. Working in partnership to provide care and treatment that enable service users and carers to tackle mental health problems with hope and optimism and to work towards a valued lifestyle within and beyond the limits of any mental health problem.
- **Identifying people's needs and strengths**. Working in partnership to gather information to agree health and social care needs in the context of the preferred lifestyle and aspirations of service users, their families, carers and friends.
- **Providing service user-centred care**. Negotiating achievable and meaningful goals, primarily from the perspective of service users and their families. Influencing and seeking the means to achieve these goals and clarifying the responsibilities of the people who will provide any help that is needed, including systematically evaluating outcomes and achievements.
- **Making a difference**. Facilitating access to, and delivering, the best-quality, evidence-based, values-based, health and social care interventions to meet the needs and aspirations of service users and their families and carers.
- **Promoting safety and positive risk taking**. Empowering the person to decide the level of risk they are prepared to take with their health and safety. This includes working with the tension between promoting safety and positive risk taking, including assessing and dealing with possible risks for service users, carers, family members and the wider public.
- **Personal development and learning**. Keeping up to date with changes in practice and participating in life-long learning, personal and professional development for one's self and colleagues through supervision, appraisal and reflective practice.

Mental Health and Social Exclusion

The Social Exclusion Unit report into mental health and social exclusion (Office of the Deputy Prime Minister 2004) identified five main reasons why mental health problems too often lead to and reinforce social exclusion:

- Stigma and discrimination
- Low expectations
- Lack of clear responsibility
- Lack of ongoing support to enable people to work
- Barriers to engaging in the community

People from ethnic minorities, young men, parents and adults with complex needs were found to face particular barriers to having their needs addressed.

Stigma and discrimination are present everywhere with little positive change in attitudes despite numerous mental health promotion campaigns. Health-care professionals continue to have low expectations of what individuals may achieve and inadequate awareness that returning to work and overcoming social isolation are associated with better outcomes. There is a lack of clear responsibility for promoting vocational and social outcomes and subsequently services do not always work effectively together. The lack of ongoing support to enable people to work means people may miss out on services that are beneficial or end up using services that do not best meet their needs. Barriers to engaging in the community can limit people's access to housing, transport, arts, sport, education and leisure providers. In an address to the European Conference on Promotion of Mental Health and Social Inclusion in Tampere in 1999, David Byrne, Commissioner for Health and Consumer Protection, stated 'We have to move to escape from the tendency to deal with mental health in the narrow confines of our healthcare systems. Of course, our healthcare systems have a critical role to play, especially in addressing mental illness. But, as you know, the real gains are often to be made in our education systems, in housing provision, in employment policies and perhaps most of all in how society perceives mental health' (Mental Health Europe 2001).

The values and beliefs of occupational therapy along with the knowledge and skills of individuals provide opportunities for occupational therapists to be at the centre of developments with service users, in tackling issues of social exclusion. With a policy arena that raises the importance of occupation and involvement in social and leisure activities, there is a clear role and direction available if occupational therapists are prepared to take the lead.

UNDERSTANDING MENTAL ILLNESS

Mental health is quite clearly no longer a matter of simple biology and therefore treatment which endeavours to rectify a chemical imbalance in the brain. The emerging evidence base for psychological and social approaches means that understanding complexity and being open to a range of possible explanations are essential. The recognition that bad things happen to people and that this can cause difficulties in living which can appear like madness is simplifying the complexity; however, a human response is essential. Occupational therapists believe that health and well-being can be achieved through occupation, through everyday living, through recovering ordinary lives (College of Occupational Therapists 2006).

PSYCHOSIS

Psychotic experiences can be present in a range of diagnoses but people with a diagnosis of schizophrenia are likely to be the predominant group among those with severe and enduring mental health problems. Around one in every 100 people will be diagnosed with schizophrenia at some time in his life. It is commonly diagnosed during a person's 20s, although it may be diagnosed earlier or later. After first being diagnosed, around one in five people will not experience psychosis again. About seven out of 10 people will experience a further period of psychosis, usually within 5–7 years of the first occasion. Some people will continue to experience some symptoms that come under the diagnosis of schizophrenia, whilst others may be free of symptoms. A few people will experience long-lasting periods of psychosis.

The previous dominance of the medical model as the primary explanation for psychosis is changing to a broader multifaceted view. The contribution of brain chemistry, genetics, neurodevelopment, cognitions, behaviours, the environment and life experiences, and the person's world view can all be factors in helping the individual to understand his situation using his own frames of reference to help explain unusual experiences, heightened sensations, suffering, confusion and disorganisation.

There are still tensions between individual practitioners and groups with a bias towards a particular view. However, as robust evidence is produced across the different domains and with the influence of evidence-based policy, the emergence of a bio-psychosocial explanatory model is becoming central to mainstream mental health services. The National Institute for Clinical Excellence (2002) guidelines for schizophrenia illustrate this, encompassing medication, occupation and family and individual cognitive behavioural therapy-based approaches. The biological, psychological and social causes of psychotic experiences are all important and interact with many potential factors in a complex way.

As a way of understanding schizophrenia, symptoms have been categorised into positive and negative symptoms. The positive symptoms are those which would be described as psychosis.

Positive symptoms

Symptoms of psychosis include hallucinations, delusions and thought disorder.

- Hallucinations occur when someone can hear, see, feel, smell or taste something that isn't there. The experience is totally real to the individual.
- Delusions are seen as fixed false beliefs that are not open to persuasion.
- Thought disorder is where an individual has problems with thinking. Thoughts may feel pressured or blocked or people may have beliefs about their thoughts, for example, that they are being inserted or removed by others or broadcast for others to hear.

There are a number of effective interventions for helping people cope with psychotic experiences, including medication and specific psychological approaches. The relationship between engagement in meaningful occupation and health status is also recognised, giving occupational therapists a role in working positively with people with psychosis (British Psychological Society 2000).

Negative symptoms

Research into negative symptoms continues to develop. There is a view that a distinction can be made between primary and secondary negative symptoms, the belief being that primary negative symptoms may be intrinsic to the disturbance of schizophrenia and that secondary negative symptoms may be related to psychological, social and spiritual causes which are potentially treatable (Watkins 1996). However, the exact definition of primary negative symptoms and the ability to clearly distinguish them from secondary symptoms has not been clearly proven.

Negative symptoms include:

- decreased range and intensity of emotional responsiveness which is described as blunting or flattening
- poverty of thought which is reflected in the limited amount of spontaneous speech, brief and concrete replies
- loss of motivation or drive which is shown in a lack of interest in and ability to initiate goal-directed activities
- diminished capacity to experience pleasure, including recreational interests, relationships or sex
- social isolation and withdrawal whereby a person may be uncommunicative and prefer to be alone.

Negative symptoms are not unique to schizophrenia; they may have many causes and, more importantly, can often be prevented or alleviated. Watkins (1996) identifies a number of strategies including several that occupational therapists will readily identify with, such as gradually to increase activity and responsibility, maintain a structured routine of activity, find a balanced level of stimulation, adopt a healthy lifestyle and learn effective coping skills.

RISK

The need for comprehensive risk assessment and risk management through the Care Programme Approach (CPA) process, with effective strategies for collaboration across agencies, is established practice (NHSE/SSI 1999). Although the

CPA process is partly about risk, it is also about person-centred care, in which an individual's needs are assessed and progress is reviewed regularly and the negotiated plan of care is communicated to all relevant parties. Media focus on tragic incidences, creating fear in the general public, takes attention away from actuarial risk. Severe self-neglect receives little attention as does the vulnerability of service users who may be the victim rather than the perpetrator of risky behaviour.

Risk assessment broadly looks at suicide and self-harm, aggression and violence, neglect and other areas including exploitation, abuse, harassment and specific identified behaviours. Assessment should include an attempt to contextualise the risk using historical and contemporary information. Risk management recognises that risk may well be minimised rather than eliminated; it can include strategies to manage current risk and plans of action for predicted risk. It is recognised that when working in a model of recovery, there is a need to consider positive risk taking, with the rationale for decisions being clearly documented.

HOMELESSNESS

Occupational therapy with people who are homeless and have mental health problems is an area that has developed over the last decade. People may well have complex and diverse needs without necessarily being able to or wanting to access support services. Homeless populations have an increased incidence of people with physical health needs and increased problems with alcohol and drug use. People who are homeless may be roofless or residing in hostels, shelters or other temporary housing environments.

The occupational therapist may be working with people who have a chaotic lifestyle, with habilitation and rehabilitation needs. The focus of intervention is obviously individualised. Areas may include activities of daily living, meeting employment needs, developing adaptation skills, financial management, skills and opportunities to develop and sustain relationships, structuring time and developing routines. Primary needs may well be centred on securing permanent accommodation and maximising finances.

LIFESTYLE ISSUES

Dealing with lifestyle issues is an area where, without awareness of one's own values and prejudices, it is possible that subjective views and opinions may be imposed on the individual as well as the imposition of standards and values. Working with individuals in a respectful manner whilst working towards a society that tolerates difference and welcomes diversity can be difficult when there are a number of complex factors involved. Factors may include stigma, prejudice, socially acceptable behaviour, culture, illness, illicit behaviour, expressing sexuality and self-harm.

When working in a collaborative way and negotiating with people, a common approach may initially be around damage limitation and harm reduction, particularly when dealing with issues such as drug and alcohol use and self-harm. Using motivational interviewing (Miller & Rollnick 2002), discovering dissonance and moving from precontemplation to contemplation of change are commonly used methods within this area.

The *NHS Improvement Plan* (DoH 2004b) places health promotion and the management of long-term conditions as a priority for the health service in England; it put an emphasis on tackling obesity, smoking and sexually transmitted infections because of the preventable health consequences. The role of the occupational therapist in exploring the individual's valued occupations, roles, routines and activities in the context of the environment can be invaluable in enabling individuals to work towards positive change.

SERVICE SETTINGS AND CONFIGURATIONS

People with severe and enduring mental health problems will be seen in a range of service settings including inpatient, day services and community settings. Roles and settings are covered comprehensively elsewhere in this book (Chapters 12, 22, 27). The trend for occupational therapists working with people with severe and enduring mental health problems is, as across the whole of mental health care, a move to more community-orientated interventions. Posts are often for sole practitioners rather than as part of an occupational therapy team. New posts may well be in developing service areas and non-traditional settings where there may be limited evidence or previous expectation to guide the role of the occupational therapist. There is a need for the occupational therapist to be aware of the myriad influences and from this, agree roles within the team or service.

GENERIC AND PROFESSION-SPECIFIC WORKING

There has been much debate over recent years around generic mental health work and specialist occupational therapy (Cook 2003, Harries & Gilhooly 2003, Harrison 2003, Lloyd et al 2004, Parker 2001). This is a multifaceted debate with many areas of discussion, including the retention of the framework of occupation and utilising best evidence. In services where the occupational therapist may be the sole practitioner, there is an argument that if much of their time is given to generic mental health work, those individuals who need the specialist interventions of an occupational therapist may lose out. The point here is not about professional protectionism but about how occupational therapists, as part of a team, can best meet the needs of individuals.

Policy has been driving practice towards a greater blurring of roles with the focus on streamlined workforce planning and development stemming from the needs of the individual, not professionals (DoH 2000b). However, the need for profession-specific skills and expertise is seen as integral to the implementation of the *National Service Framework for Mental Health* (Sainsbury Centre for Mental Health 2000). The *Code of Ethics and Professional Conduct for Occupational Therapists* (College of Occupational Therapists 2005) has an expectation that shared team roles will be balanced with a priority towards people with occupational performance difficulties. Specifically, under section 5.3 Collaborative Practice 5.3.4 states that 'occupational therapists shall identify their core skills and roles and ensure that they are not undertaking work that is deemed to be outside the scope of occupational therapy practice or their

competence' (College of Occupational Therapists 2005, p15).

The difficulty in defining which interventions are part of generic work and which are part of specialist occupational therapy was raised by Cook (2003). Harrison (2003) argues in favour of occupational therapists being more flexible and responsive to best meet the needs of service users and that this approach can be consistent with maintaining an occupational focus whilst also contributing to the development of the profession. Common shared roles include care co-ordination under the CPA, interventions such as psycho-education, cognitive behavioural therapy, family therapy and brief solution focused therapies, duty work that may involve routine or crisis assessments, being on call or dealing with telephone calls during office hours, taking the lead in chairing meetings or taking minutes.

MULTIAGENCY WORKING AND CROSS-BOUNDARY PARTNERSHIPS

Partnership working in mental health is expected across a variety of organisations including health, social services, criminal justice system, housing, voluntary and independent sector enterprises, local government departments, user and carer groups, housing, training and support agencies (DoH 1999).

Partnership working has become accepted practice when working with people with long-term mental health problems. It is recognised that the diverse needs of individuals cannot be met, and indeed should not be met, by a single provider or totally within mainstream provision. The background is one of a focus on service user-centred delivery of service with individual choice a key driver. This approach provides occupational therapists with the opportunity to work creatively and innovatively in finding solutions in partnership with local communities in their widest sense.

MODELS, APPROACHES AND FRAMES OF REFERENCES

Occupational therapy models, approaches and frames of reference will be briefly mentioned but a detailed exploration is outside the scope of this chapter and is covered in depth elsewhere in this book (Chapter 4).

Within occupational therapy there are numerous approaches to practice, including neurodevelopmental, adaptive, compensatory, behavioural, habilitative and rehabilitative. Common frames of reference utilised in mental health settings include human developmental, psychodynamic, sensory-motor and psychosocial. Models of practice used in mental health settings include the Canadian Model of Occupational Performance, the Model of Human Occupation and the Reed & Sanderson Occupational Performance Model. Models are seen as useful tools if used considerately (Creek 2003), but 'adhering to one model without critical thought and evaluation can lead to routine practice rather than reasoned and reflective practice' (Creek 2003, p35).

STRESS VULNERABILITY

The stress vulnerability model of schizophrenia described by Zubin & Spring (1977) sees individuals as having a predisposition or vulnerability to developing psychosis and that the individual's exposure to stress may precipitate a psychotic experience. This simple model shows that individuals who are more vulnerable may need fewer stressors to develop a psychotic reaction. Individuals who are less vulnerable may need more stressors to develop psychosis. This model allows a normalisation approach to be used and can help to break down 'us and them' barriers by suggesting that any individual could develop schizophrenia given enough stressors in relation to their own vulnerability.

From an occupational therapy perspective, interventions may be targeted at the level of stress or vulnerability. Personal stress may be reduced by working collaboratively with the person on activities that they find relaxing. Environmental stress may be addressed directly through changes to that environment or indirectly by removal to other less stressful environments. Vulnerability can be tackled by working on issues such as problem-solving skills, coping skills, social skills and developing support networks.

The stress vulnerability model is able to incorporate biological, psychological and social elements. This biopsychosocial approach enables the model to bring together different health-care workers using a shared understanding of schizophrenia. A major criticism of the model is that if the focus of interventions revolves around minimising or avoiding stress it may lead to risk-aversive practice, contributing to having low expectations of what individuals can achieve. This may reinforce a maintenance model approach rather than a focus on recovery.

RECOVERY

Traditionally services for people who are seen as having severe and enduring mental health problems have focused on medication and the maintenance of a settled mental state. Opportunities offered have tended to be restricted to those provided within mental health services, with few routes away from and out of the mental health system. The concept of recovery is now becoming key to working with this client group; it is seen as an active process, often described as a personal journey. The journey is travelled with a spirit of hope and optimism. Recovery is about reclaiming and rediscovering what may have been lost at one stage: occupations, roles, expectations, self-determination. It is about attaining a valued lifestyle, not about cure or the absence of symptoms.

Recovery is a concept unique to each individual; it is not static (Birchwood et al 2000). As the person grows and achieves his goals and dreams, he may feel that even greater levels of recovery and understanding of himself can be reached. Recovery has an outlook of growth through adverse experience.

Issues which influence recovery include:

- a sense of security, financial security and good housing
- social networks, friends and family, the ability to sustain relationships and resolve conflicts
- employment or having meaningful vocational opportunities
- the desire to progress in life and make changes where necessary to achieve goals and dreams

- a sense of belonging to a group or community and having a valid role to play in that group
- spiritual growth and finding an individual philosophy to live by.

REHABILITATION

Rehabilitation has been defined in various ways, often being described as a process, with important elements being maximising function, maximising quality of life, adaptation to and prevention of disability. An emphasis is placed on developing and maintaining respectful relationships with the person. Rehabilitation is increasingly seen as a community-based rather than a hospital-based process. Petterson (2004) recorded the following point:

> Rehabilitation psychiatry is a philosophy, not necessarily a set of services – it is a way to 'do' community psychiatry. It applies to *all* people experiencing mental health problems and is about working with people in their social context, over long periods of time if necessary, helping them to get the most from life and to manage their illness as well as they can. (p3)

A definition from Barton (1999) of psychosocial rehabilitation described it as a range of social, educational, occupational, behavioural, and cognitive interventions to increase the role performance of persons with serious and persistent mental illness and enhancing their recovery. Empowerment, competency and recovery are seen as key concepts with recovery of vocational goals as an essential element.

The Royal College of Psychiatrists (2004) commissioned a report on rehabilitation and recovery. The report looked at the transition of services from being focused on traditional hospital-based rehabilitation to modernised services where concepts of recovery drive the rehabilitation process. They identified six principles to guide and inform service development.

- Enhancing the strengths and resilience of long-term service users and their families.
- Maintaining optimism for individual growth and recovery.

- Treating disability with respect and acceptance.
- Improving the holistic quality of life for those with the most severe disabilities.
- Reducing stigma and promoting social inclusion.
- Therapeutic risk taking to promote personal responsibility.

These principles fit well with the values of occupational therapy and can be incorporated into many areas of practice.

In general, when asked what they would like from services, users report that they would like somewhere decent to live, enough money to get by, something meaningful to do, including work, and the opportunities to form relationships (Rogers et al 1993). When asked what getting better means to them, rehabilitation service users identified many factors including improved physical and material well-being, empowerment, confidence and self-worth, more involvement in activities and work, coping with everyday life, having help and support available, improved mental state and improved relationships (Meddings & Perkins 2002). This complex, holistic view of what getting better means is something that occupational therapists should be readily able to identify with and should work collaboratively towards it with service users.

THE SOCIAL MODEL OF DISABILITY

The World Health Organization (WHO 2001) *International Classification of Functioning* defines disability as the outcome of the interaction between a person with impairment and the environmental and attitudinal barriers he may face. This places disability in the context of the environment rather than the individual. This fits with the social model of disability which recognises that society, through government, agencies and individual citizens, has a duty to remove barriers and that disabled people have the same rights to full equality as all other citizens. The European Congress on People with Disabilities (ECPD 2002) produced the Madrid Declaration that 'non-discrimination plus positive action results in social inclusion'. The vision is of an inclusive society for all: 'A society that shuts out a number of its members is an impoverished society. Actions to improve conditions for disabled people will lead to the design of a flexible world for all' (ECPD 2002).

The promotion of the use of the *International Classification of Functioning* within occupational therapy is relatively recent, generally underdeveloped and mainly focused in physical health settings, but research into its use in mental health settings may prove fruitful.

PSYCHOSOCIAL INTERVENTIONS

Psychosocial interventions can have a number of definitions, broad and narrow. Aspects of occupational therapy can be seen as a psychosocial intervention within a broad definition. For the purposes of evidence-based health care, a narrow definition is generally seen as therapeutic approaches that improve outcomes for people with psychosis and their carers. Interventions include assertive case management, family interventions and psychological approaches to deal with psychotic symptoms.

Evidence from systematic reviews (Bustillo et al 2001, Razali et al 2000) shows that family therapy and assertive community treatment have a clear effect on the prevention of relapse and on rates of rehospitalisation, but there is no reliable effect on positive or negative symptoms, social functioning or employment status. Social skills training improves social skills but has no clear effect on relapse, symptoms or employment. Supportive employment using a 'place and train' model improves employment outcomes. Cognitive behavioural therapy used to address delusions and hallucinations has been shown to lead to symptom reduction. The role of information processing and the arousal system is also felt to be an important mechanism in the process for people experiencing psychosis, which may be due to the inability to filter out extraneous background stimuli.

Developing skills in narrowly defined psychosocial interventions enables occupational therapists to enhance their generic mental health skills in an area of robust evidence-based practice. These interventions may then be used alongside occupational therapy skills to provide an effective individualised approach.

WORKING WITH PEOPLE WITH A DIAGNOSIS OF SEVERE AND ENDURING MENTAL ILLNESS

The values and person-centred approach of occupational therapy, where practice is socially inclusive and demonstrates an understanding of the person's lived experiences and influences, is crucial to effective collaboration in working towards recovery. Engagement is a key element of the recovery process and engagement with the person's carers is also important. The occupational therapist utilises activities in the domains of self-maintenance, leisure and productivity to achieve the goals of the individual. In the sphere of productivity, work is an area where there is robust evidence; people in general want to work and work is protective to people's mental health.

ENGAGEMENT

Engagement is an important process in working with people with severe and enduring mental health problems, whether this be the first contact or continuing engagement. Working at the individual's pace in a respectful and collaborative way enables an effective therapeutic relationship to develop. Taking time to listen to people, to discover their narratives and to see their world view can help the therapist to understand where people are coming from and the changes they want to make on the journey ahead.

Chugg & Craik (2002) found that there are many factors that influence occupational engagement and that these are often poorly understood. They call for greater creativity and more consideration of the timing and the chosen environment for activities, to enable individuals to engage in a range of occupations. The use of activity as a way of engaging with an individual may be enhanced if some thought, planning and preparation have gone into the process. The more experienced therapist may well be going through these stages intuitively.

When working with people in an assertive outreach setting, engagement is seen as fundamentally important to developing a collaborative relationship. Suggested characteristics of a first meeting are described by Morgan (1993) and include:

- positive atmosphere, focus on strengths, abilities and interests not deficits
- equal power, attempting to establish similar agendas
- comfortable atmosphere, active listening, attention to non-verbal signals
- breaking down of barriers through appropriate self-disclosure
- fun, discussion of lighter subjects or humorous circumstances.

The need for caution and discretion is highlighted in particular for the last two points with a reminder that the purpose is the benefit of the client. (See Chapter 13)

USER AND CARER INVOLVEMENT

One of the guiding values and principles of the *National Service Framework for Mental Health* (DoH 1999) is that service users and their carers, where acceptable to the service user, may be involved in the planning and delivery of care. The NSF also calls for user involvement in research that develops and evaluates a range of occupational activities to maximise social participation, enhance self-esteem and improve clinical outcomes.

The involvement of users and carers is consistently advocated in recent policy documents from a range of agencies. Involvement is encouraged at all levels from individualised care planning to representation as a key stakeholder on the national Mental Health Taskforce Board and involvement in research and development projects. The emphasis is on making the best use of the knowledge and experience of users and carers and keeping a focus on the issues and concerns that are important to them. To enable this to happen effectively, a range of information and support may need to be in place as well as attitudes that demonstrate commitment to user and carer participation and are not tokenistic.

SELF-MAINTENANCE, LEISURE AND PRODUCTIVITY

The self-maintenance, leisure and productivity activities that are chosen when working with people with severe and enduring mental health problems will be based on negotiation and collaboration with the individual. Basic principles apply in the use of purposeful activities to promote health and well-being, to achieve a balance of roles within a meaningful lifestyle.

When working in partnership with people with enduring mental health problems, a range of issues may be relevant to establishing self-maintenance, leisure and productivity goals. The occupational therapist thinks about the individual's motivation and how that can be harnessed to start the process of recovery and that exposure to a variety of activities may be necessary for individuals to start to exercise free choice and identify their own purpose and meaning. The occupational therapist needs to be sensitive to the possibility that long-term users of services may have been exposed to environments of low expectations and that the process of recovery, in raising their hope and expectations, may initially be alien and counter to underlying beliefs and values.

EMPLOYMENT

Occupational therapy has an established role in work rehabilitation. Seebohm et al (2002) felt that occupational therapists can act as key figures within the vocational system, by being a resource for community teams, day services, wards and even GP practices, bringing vocational expertise to every corner of the mental health service.

Employment is an important issue from a number of perspectives including the evidence base, current policy and service user wishes (Mental Health Foundation 1998). Unemployment in general is linked to mental ill health. It can therefore be argued that those with mental health problems have more need for work than others (Seebohm et al 2002) and that people with mental health problems experience high unemployment rates, less than 15% being economically active. People with mental health problems want to work and with the right level of support, they are able to do so. A range of services is required to meet the needs of individuals (Grove et al 2005).

Barriers to work and employment include low expectations from staff, negative employer attitudes, difficulties moving from benefits to a wage and lack of support for job retention.

The development of user employment in the NHS is supported by the Department of Health itself (DoH 2000b). By employing suitably qualified people who have mental health problems, the contribution of expertise through experience can enhance the acceptability and accessibility of services, thereby improving the quality of services.

Reynolds & Higgins (1997) give a concise description of a range of employment service models.

- **Social firm**: a business created for the employment of people who are disadvantaged in the labour market. At least 30% of employees fit this description. Work opportunities should be equal between disadvantaged and non-disadvantaged employees.
- **Community business**: a business with a legal structure whereby profits are invested in its employees, overseen by a group of directors.
- **Co-operative**: a legal structure for a company which is owned and managed democratically by its employees.
- **Supported employment** involves clients working in open employment with support from a job coach or other support staff. Clients are paid the going rate for the job which can be full or part time.
- **Work placement**: as above, but clients are not paid the standard hourly rate. Some projects will engage in this practice while an individual's benefits are being assessed or while clients are having work experience.
- **Supported Placement Scheme (SPS)**: SPS is a national scheme provided by the Employment Service. The scheme offers long-term support in the workplace to people with disabilities who are otherwise unable to obtain or retain jobs in the open market.
- **Sheltered employment**: people with disabilities/disadvantages are engaged in work with other people with disabilities/disadvantages.
- **Sheltered workshop**: where clients are engaged in work activities in a sheltered setting but due to a variety of factors do not receive a wage at the going rate for the job, but might receive therapeutic earnings, for example.
- **Vocational training**: clients are taught vocational skills and qualifications. Projects are often located in colleges or training centres or involve workplace training.

- **Vocational guidance** refers to projects whose main activity is vocational guidance and counselling.
- **Rehabilitation centre**: usually for people recovering from mental illness, offering specialist assistance, assessment and training.

The range of options available locally should allow individuals to construct their own path towards employment, permitting them to progress at their own pace. Services should be user focused and aim to balance commercial concerns with the needs of the individual who may have to cope with periods of fluctuating productivity, performance and attendance.

The National Institute for Clinical Excellence (2002), in its clinical guidelines for schizophrenia, recommends that an individual's ability and access to work is assessed. Section 1.4.6, Employment, states that the overall aim of mental health services is to help service users get back to living an ordinary life as far as possible. The *National Service Framework for Mental Health* (DoH 1999) requires an individual's enhanced CPA care plan to include action needed for employment, education or training or another occupation.

Occupational therapists' involvement in work and employment-based activities is clearly established historically and also a clear role remains as services modernise and new ways of working are established.

TONY'S EXPERIENCE OF MENTAL HEALTH SERVICES

The following story illustrates the journey through the mental health services of a young man experiencing a severe and enduring mental illness.

Tony is a 23 year old who has been in contact with mental health services for the last 5 years. He describes an uneventful childhood but feels his father pushed him to succeed whilst his mother was more easy-going. He has a younger brother with whom he used to get on well, however, over recent years Tony feels more like the younger sibling as his bother has achieved more in his life – he has been to university, owns a car and has a career. They still get on but don't spend much time with each other any more.

Tony's difficulties began in his late teens when he started to struggle at school and was not attaining the predicted grades he required to achieve his father's ambitions. Tony had discovered music and sex; he learnt to play the guitar competently and played in local rock bands and had numerous short-lived relationships. He started drinking alcohol regularly and experimenting with drugs, taking whatever drugs were available but particularly using cannabis excessively.

His parents describe a period of about 18 months where Tony became moody, irritable, isolated and latterly suspicious. At times he displayed bizarre behaviour and was unable to express himself. Initially his parents thought this was typical adolescent behaviour and believed it to be a phase that he would come through.

Tony came into contact with mental health services following his detention by the police when he was wandering in the town centre late at night. He was obviously intoxicated and believed that he was on a special mission, appearing to be responding to voices or visions. He firmly believed that the magic mushrooms and cannabis that he had been taking were natural and pure and that no one could object to that.

Tony spent the next 2 years in and out of hospital. He would be admitted to hospital, generally under section 2 of the Mental Health Act 1983, where he would be medicated, his mental state would then stabilise and he would be discharged. Following discharge, Tony would stop taking his medication, withdraw from services and resume taking illicit drugs. His alcohol consumption would gradually increase from social drinking with friends and band members to needing a drink to start the day.

Eventually, on one of his admissions Tony did not respond rapidly to the reintroduction of the medication and his section 2 was converted to a section 3 and he was then referred to the local rehabilitation and recovery services. Prior to this admission Tony had been kicked out of the band, his parents were struggling to know what to do to support him and his latest relationship had ended acrimoniously after he had been unfaithful.

Whilst in hospital Tony would frequently go absent from the ward without permission, usually returning some hours or occasionally days later, often intoxicated and becoming more aroused, suspicious and verbally hostile. This behaviour would usually settle down after a week or so. On his return to the ward Tony would be asked to submit to a blood or urine screen and each time he did so he was found to have taken cannabis and occasionally other substances.

Tony was keen to get out of hospital; he wanted to get on with his life like his brother, get a job, a car and settle down. He felt that there was nothing wrong with him, that he should be left alone to get on with his life, he did not need any help and if people just let him be, he would be fine.

When he was in the rehabilitation and recovery services he would often be bored and frustrated on the unit. This frustration was used as a way to engage with Tony and explore his likes and dislikes and how he would utilise his time whilst he waited to get out of hospital. His love of music was a key area; he could identify songs and lyrics that were meaningful for him, he kept in touch with the local music scene and went to gigs with staff members. This engagement enabled some more in-depth work to be initiated. Tony started to identify through motivational interviewing that perhaps there was a link between his drug use and his mental health. He came to the conclusion that he was sensitive to cannabis and that it may be better if he avoided it, but he reserved the right to party and suffer the consequences if he so wished.

Work was an area that Tony was adamant he would be able to sort out for himself, believing that if he put enough time and effort into his music, he would make it as a rock star. On other occasions he saw his music as a hobby and he wanted a job to be able to fund his hobby. Over time Tony was willing to test out his work readiness by attending a local workshop and through this he discovered a new interest and skill. After attendance at the workshop for an agreed 3-month period, the local disability employment advisor was approached for advice and support. Tony was placed on a course to develop his computer skills and offered a job through a supported employment scheme working in a large supermarket warehouse. This computer course was more acceptable to Tony as he preferred to go on a course offered through work. He had felt stigmatised considering a similar course through mental health services. He also accepted the job as this would allow him the flexibility to negotiate shifts to fit in with his musical ambitions.

The computer course was a success and Tony enrolled on a further course at a higher level. The job started off well but after 4 months he stopped going after he had 'an absolute bender'. The computer course was due to start at this time and was also abandoned. Tony had been about to move to his own flat around this time and was able to acknowledge that he was feeling stressed about this and had coped with it by doing what he knew best!

Tony was again suspicious and aroused and irritable but he recognised that he was responsible for his actions and his theory about being sensitive to cannabis may well be true. He reattended the workshop whilst arranging with the DEA to explore work options again. He felt that the computers could wait for a while as he believed he needed to work on some areas he had been worrying about but not talking about, to do with moving on. He sought out the occupational therapist to practise his shopping, cooking and budgeting skills as a way to boost his confidence in order to move into his own place.

This was done in collaboration with the community-based occupational therapist working with the assertive outreach team who were going to support him after his discharge from the rehabilitation and recovery services. His contact with the assertive outreach services led him to meet other service users who attended a hearing voices group. Tony started to attend the group, but did not want to discuss it as 'it's my stuff for me'; however, he said that it helped and that he understood things even more now.

Tony continues in his job at the supermarket warehouse and follows music more often than playing music. He is developing pride in his domestic skills and feels he is sorting his head out through the voices group. He describes feeling 'on the edge' a lot of the time but knows how to stay there and not fall off. His relationship with his parents has improved as he feels under less pressure and that it is OK to be who he is.

SUMMARY

Policy places the role of the occupational therapist centrally within modern health care where the value of social and functional recovery is highlighted. The occupational therapist can utilise a variety of models and interventions in order to support service users in working towards recovery. Positive attitudes and values are central to working with people with severe and enduring mental health problems to move towards respectful practice which embraces diversity and the unique contribution of the individual's personal experience.

Key themes outlined in this chapter are as follows.

- User involvement, client-centred practice, choice and mental health promotion within a context of social inclusion are key to recent policy.
- Understanding psychosis and the implications for the individual in terms of cognition, arousal and the impact of positive and negative symptoms will enable occupational therapists to work more effectively. Occupational therapists work actively with positive and negative symptoms.
- The complexity of needs gives rise to complex solutions where partnership working across agencies may be necessary.
- The stress vulnerability model, concepts of rehabilitation, recovery and the social model of disability can be used to inform practice across a range of disciplines and gain the involvement of service users.
- There is a current emphasis on the concept of recovery. Understanding the principles of recovery and where they converge with the principles of occupational therapy will enable practitioners to work effectively in this area.
- The balance between generic working and profession-specific working is one that is highly debated. Generic mental health skills can be enhanced by developing psychosocial intervention skills.
- Engagement is an important process when working with people with severe and enduring mental health problems and is also central to occupational therapy practice.
- Self-maintenance, leisure and productivity goals are highly individualised and may be subject to the influences of others' values and attitudes as well as the environment.
- Developing motivation and exposure to activity to promote meaningful choice may be important factors in working towards recovery.
- Individual employment needs is an area that occupational therapists should be addressing to work towards evidence-based practice and reflecting the concerns of service users.

References

Barton R 1999 Psychosocial rehabilitation services in community support systems: review of outcomes and policy recommendations. Psychiatric Services 50: 525-534

Birchwood M, Fowler D, Jackson C 2000 Early intervention in psychosis: a guide to concepts, evidence and interventions. Wiley, Chichester

British Psychological Society 2000 Recent advances in understanding mental illness and psychotic experiences. A report by the British Psychological Society Division of Clinical Psychology. British Psychological Society, Leicester

Bustillo J, Lauriello J, Horan W et al 2001 The psychosocial treatment of schizophrenia: an update. American Journal of Psychiatry 158(2): 163-175

Chugg A, Craik C 2002 Some factors influencing occupational engagement for people with schizophrenia living in the community. British Journal of Occupational Therapy 65(2): 67-74

College of Occupational Therapists 2005 Code of ethics and professional conduct for occupational therapists. College of Occupational Therapists, London

College of Occupational Therapists 2006 Recovering ordinary lives, the strategy for occupational therapy in mental health services 2007–2017, a vision for the next ten years. College of Occupational Therapists, London

Cook S 2003 Generic and specialist interventions for people with severe mental health problems: can interventions be categorised? British Journal of Occupational Therapy 66(1): 17-24

Creek J 2003 Occupational therapy defined as a complex intervention. College of Occupational Therapists, London

Department of Health 1998 Modernising mental health services: safe, sound and supportive. Department of Health, London

Department of Health 1999 National service framework for mental health: modern standards and service models. Department of Health, London

Department of Health 2000a The NHS plan. Department of Health, London

Department of Health 2000b Looking beyond the labels: widening the employment opportunities for disabled people in the new NHS. Department of Health, London

Department of Health 2004a The ten essential shared capabilities – a framework for the whole of the mental health workforce. Department of Health, London

Department of Health 2004b The NHS improvement plan: putting people at the heart of public services. Department of Health, London

European Congress on People with Disabilities 2002 Available online at: www.madriddeclaration. org/en/dec/dec.htm

Grove B, Secker J, Seebohm P 2005 New thinking about mental health and employment. Radcliffe Publishing, Oxford

Harries P, Gilhooly K 2003 Generic and specialist occupational therapy casework in community mental health. British Journal of Occupational Therapy 66(3): 101-109

Harrison D 2003 The case for generic working in mental health occupational therapy. British Journal of Occupational Therapy 66(3): 110-112

Lloyd C, Bassett H, King R 2004 Occupational therapy and evidence-based practice in mental health. British Journal of Occupational Therapy 67(2): 83-88

Meddings S, Perkins R 2002 What 'getting better' means to staff and users of a rehabilitation service: an exploratory study. Journal of Mental Health 11(3): 319

Mental Health Act 1983 Department of Health, London

Mental Health Europe 2001 Available online at: www.mhe-sme.org/en/european-projects/promoting-social-inclusion-of-people-with-mental-health-problems.html

Mental Health Foundation 1998 Mental Health Foundation Briefing No.19. Welfare to work: what works for people with mental health problems. Mental Health Foundation, London

Miller W, Rollnick S 2002 Motivational interviewing: preparing people for change. Guilford Press, New York

Morgan S 1993 Community mental health: practical approaches to long term problems. Chapman and Hall, London

National Institute for Clinical Excellence 2002 Schizophrenia. Core interventions in the treatment and management of schizophrenia in primary and secondary care. National Institute for Clinical Excellence, London

NHSE/SSI 1999 Effective care co-ordination in mental health services – modernising the care programme approach. Department of Health, London

Office of the Deputy Prime Minister 2004 Mental health and social inclusion, Social Exclusion Unit report. Office of the Deputy Prime Minister, London

Parker H 2001 The role of occupational therapists in community mental health services: generic or specialist? British Journal of Occupational Therapy 64(12): 609-611

Petterson L 2004 An interview with Geoff Shepherd, Royal College of Psychiatrists. Social and Rehabilitation Psychiatry Faculty Newsletter 5: 3-4

Razali S, Hasana C, Khan U et al 2000 Psychosocial interventions for schizophrenia. Journal of Mental Health 9(3): 283-289

Reynolds S, Higgins G 1997 ERMIS European Economic Interest Grouping – Database, 2nd edn. InformaTECH, Glasgow

Rogers A, Pilgrim D, Lacey R 1993 Experiencing psychiatry – users' views of services. MIND/Macmillan Press, Basingstoke

Royal College of Psychiatrists 2004 Rehabilitation and recovery now. Council report CR121. Royal College of Psychiatrists, London

Sainsbury Centre for Mental Health 2000 The capable practitioner: a framework and list of the practitioner capabilities required to implement the National Service Framework for Mental Health. Sainsbury Centre for Mental Health, London

Seebohm P, Grove B, Secker J 2002 Working towards recovery: putting employment at the heart of refocused mental health services. King's College Institute for Applied Health and Social Policy, London

Watkins J 1996 Living with schizophrenia. An holistic approach to understanding, preventing and recovering from negative symptoms. Hill of Content, Melbourne

World Health Organization 2001 International classification of functioning, disability and health. World Health Organization, Geneva

Zubin J, Spring B 1977 Vulnerability: a new view of schizophrenia. Journal of Abnormal Psychology 86(2): 103-126

Chapter 24

Older people

Jackie Pool

CHAPTER CONTENTS

INTRODUCTION

Ageing is a continuing part of lifespan development. Life expectancy, that is, the length of time a person can expect to live as predicted at the moment of birth, alters according to factors such as health, social circumstances and social trends. These must be favourable if life expectancy is to be achieved. The study of demographic trends shows that people are living longer as the barriers to achieving life expectancy are removed.

The 2001 census of Great Britain showed that the UK has an ageing population. The population grew by 6.5% in the last 30 years or so, from 55.9 million in 1971 to 59.6 million in mid-2003. The percentage of people aged 65 and over increased from 13% in mid-1971 to 16% in mid-2003. This ageing is primarily the result of past patterns in the number of births, although decline in mortality rates also contributes.

Continued population ageing is inevitable during the first half of this century, since the number of elderly people will rise as the relatively large numbers of people born after the Second World War, and during the 1960s baby boom, become older. It is predicted that this trend will continue and that by 2026 the number of people aged 65 years and over will have increased by 30%. The greatest increase will be in the number of very old people, that is, those aged 85 years and over (see Table 24.1). The 2001 population census revealed that, at that time, there were about 336,000 people aged 90 and over and, of these, nearly 4000 were providing 50 or more hours of unpaid care per week to another family member or friend. Although only 26.2% of people aged 90 and over living in households were men, they made up just over half of the carers in this age bracket.

In addition to the increase in an ageing population, the working-age population will also fall in size as the baby boomers move into retirement, since relatively smaller numbers of people have been born since the mid-1970s. The implication for occupational therapists when considering these facts and figures must be that older people need to be assisted to live independently for as long as possible.

Well-being depends on a balance of physical and mental health and social support. A breakdown of any one of these factors can lead to a breakdown of all three, therefore a holistic approach to working with older people is essential. Occupational therapists, with their wide range of knowledge and skills, are well equipped to work in this field.

There is a commonly held belief that old age is a time of mental decline but, as Twining observed in

Table 24.1   Projected change in population 1989–2026, England and Wales (source: Office for National Statistics 1991)

Age group	1989	2026	Absolute change millions	Percentage change
0–4	3.3	3.4	0.1	3
5–14	6.1	6.7	0.6	10
15–24	7.7	6.7	-1.0	-13
25–44	14.6	13.9	-0.7	-5
45–64	10.9	13.6	2.7	25
65–74	4.5	5.5	1.0	23
75–84	2.8	3.7	0.9	33
85+	0.8	1.3	0.5	66
All ages	50.6	54.8	4.2	8

1988, 80% of those who live to be 80 years or more show no sign of dementia. Indeed, only a small percentage of older people consult general practitioners about mental health problems in comparison with other conditions such as circulatory or respiratory diseases (Fig. 24.1).

Occupational therapists working in the mental health field can offer a range of services to older people. This may be within the National Health Service, in specialist inpatient units for assessment and treatment purposes, or in day hospitals. There may be a respite care service offered and this is often coupled with the use of counselling skills to support the relatives and carers of this client group.

The implementation of the Care in the Community Act (DoH 1990) in 1993 expanded the role of occupational therapists working with their clients living in the community. In addition, the *National Service Framework (NSF) for Older People*, published on 27 March 2001, set new national standards and service models of care across health and social services for all older people, whether they live at home or in residential care or are being looked after in hospital. The standards within the NSF highlight the need to promote an active and healthy life for all older people (standard 8) and that older people with mental health problems need access to integrated specialist services (standard 7).

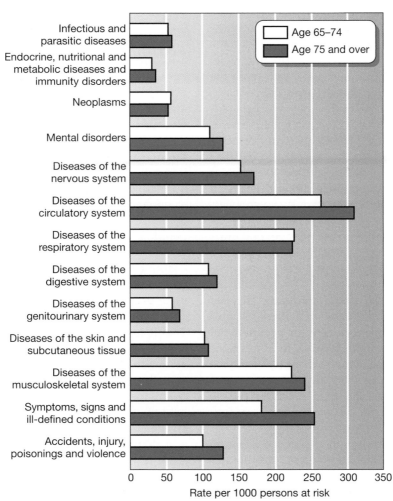

Figure 24.1   Causes of general practitioner consultations among people 65 years and over (Office of Population, Census and Surveys 1983).

In the Department of Health resource document, *A New Ambition for Old Age* (Philp 2006), it is stated that there are still deep-rooted negative attitudes and behaviours towards older people and that there have been high-profile cases of poor treatment of older people in care homes. The aim of the government is to take the next steps in implementing the NSF and to renew the commitment to ensure that older people and their families will have confidence that, in all care settings, older people will be treated with respect for their dignity and their human rights.

Intermediate care is seen as an essential way of meeting these needs by providing a range of integrated services to promote faster recovery from illness, prevent unnecessary acute hospital admission, support timely discharge and maximise independent living (DoH 2002). Equally, the White Paper *Our Health, Our Care, Our Say* (DoH 2006) sets a new direction for the whole health and social care system. It confirms the vision set out in the Department of Health Green Paper *Independence, Well-being and Choice* (2005), that there will be a radical and sustained shift in the way in which services are delivered, ensuring that they are more personalised and that they fit into people's busy lives.

Older people who do not present themselves for treatment from the NHS may receive an occupational therapy service from social services-employed therapists. This may be achieved by direct referral and, in some cases, the general practitioner may be involved initially. This is often the case when relatives and carers seek professional help directly from their social services department. As the Care in the Community Act has become more widely implemented, there has also been an increasing opportunity for occupational therapists to tender their services in a freelance capacity. Whatever the employment status of the occupational therapist, this diversity of career opportunities enables the needs of older people with mental disorders to be met in a variety of ways.

This chapter is set out in three sections. The first section looks at the ageing process. It promotes the concept of ageing as a positive experience and discusses theories of normal ageing, including biological theories, disengagement theory and activity theory. The social-psychological effects of ageing, cultural patterns and the multipathology of old age are also explored. The next section looks at mental disorders of old age, setting out the epidemiology, aetiology, pathology and clinical features of each. The final section explores ways of working with older people with mental disorders. Values and principles of practice are discussed, then the occupational therapy process of assessment, treatment and care planning, implementation and evaluation is applied to this client group. In summary, the chapter looks at the challenge of working with older people with mental disorders in terms of changing attitudes, ensuring quality care and the need for ongoing research in this field.

THE AGEING PROCESS

ATTITUDES TOWARDS AGEING

An understanding of normal ageing is essential if we are to understand mental disorders in old age. The mental capacity of older people is often underestimated. Provided they escape dementia and other brain diseases, healthy old people retain the ability to make their own decisions and to run their own lives. Old age can and should be a positive experience, with more time available to engage in enjoyable activities, to spend with the family and to reflect. Unfortunately, some old people accept the belief that old age is a time of decline and this then becomes self-fulfilling. For example, there is a belief that all old people are incontinent, therefore an old person may accept incontinence as inevitable when there is probably a physiological cause that can be treated. This is just one example of how attitudes to old age affect old people's self-attitudes so that they accept the avoidable as the inevitable and thus contribute to the negative stereotype of old age.

This negative attitude to old age is not only held by older people but reflects the view of society generally. We have inherited ageist attitudes and dogmas from our history and are applying them to today's society. However, Professor Eric Midwinter (1993), former director of the Centre for Policy on Ageing, suggested we should be adopting a completely revised concept of old age. Midwinter suggested that the construct of stages rather than ages is more useful and proposed three: childhood and socialisation, child-rearing and paid work, and the third stage in which people retire from one or both of these tasks.

WHAT IS AGEING?

Physiological ageing

An ageing process is any process in the individual which increases the likelihood of death in a given time interval. Ageing starts when physiological maturation stops. The ageing of individual organs depends on their type and cellular structure. For example, the heart wall becomes more rigid and the elasticity of large arteries is reduced. Lung capacity remains unchanged but vital capacity falls and there is a reduction in the elasticity of tissue. Muscle bulk and innervation are also reduced, causing myopathy and reduced muscle power. Muscle bulk can be increased by exercise but not the muscular cell count. There is, on average, a 1% reduction in physical function per year from the age of 30 years.

Reliable information about the structure of the normal brain in old age is difficult to find; many brains examined at post-mortem are likely to show the abnormalities of disease as well as normal ageing changes. These age-related changes may include reduced weight and volume of the brain, enlarged sulci and ventricles, thickening and hardening of blood vessels and the meninges, fewer neurones in some areas, and reduced amounts of neurotransmitters (Roberts 1989).

Psychological effects of ageing

Observations of healthy older people reveal evidence that there are only slight changes in memory function. Short-term memory is affected more than long-term but these effects are more apparent for recall than for recognition. If older people are given choices or cues their performance improves.

Learning tends to be slower but this is sometimes due to a tendency to persist with poor strategies. Slower learning does not necessarily mean that the final level of skill will be less, just that the older person may take a little longer to get there.

Some thought processes are more affected by old age than others. The most noticeable change is in the speed of reacting to something unfamiliar. Crystallised intellect (wisdom) changes less than fluid thinking (lateral thinking/problem solving).

These changes are not enough to affect everyday functioning but may be influential if the older person is under any type of stress, including physiological. Continuity characterises the personality in old age, with patterns emerging from maturity onwards. Therefore, marked personality changes are a sign of illness and not of ageing.

Old people are not all the same but there are differences between young and old people due to differences in background and upbringing. These are known as cohort differences.

Cultural patterns of ageing

Social conditions have had the greatest effect on the transition from a young to an ageing population in the UK. This country was the first to make the transition because it was the first to have an industrial revolution, which led to improved living conditions. Whereas in developed countries the demographic transition has evolved, in developing countries the ageing population has been achieved artificially, by reducing the birth rate and improving the mortality rate, even among adverse social and environmental conditions. In some developing countries, even though poor social conditions still exist, the mortality rate from disease has fallen because of an increase in the availability of vaccinations and treatment. In some countries women have chosen to reduce their birth rates by being sterilised. This practice is encouraged by medical practitioners who receive fees for carrying out this service.

Attitudes to old age in the West can be seen as discriminatory, with older people being viewed as a financial drain on society: unproductive, dependent and in need of costly health care. In the East there is a tradition of viewing older people with respect and valuing their wisdom and experience. Unfortunately, this is now changing as the ageing population increases. In Japan, for example, it has been estimated that by the year 2020 one in four citizens will be over 65 years of age. The Japanese have become so worried about the cost of supporting their ageing population that they are considering exporting it. Retirement cities in low-cost countries have been built as a way of moving large groups of old people out of Japan.

In the West, there is a noticeable absence of positive images of old age in the media and an increasing obsession with methods of avoiding old age through diet, exercise, use of chemicals and surgery. When older people are used in advertising they usually support the negative stereotype rather than reflect the reality.

THEORIES OF AGEING

Theories that explain the processes involved in ageing have been produced by psychologists, biologists and sociologists. Aspects of these theories should be incorporated into the knowledge base of occupational therapy to increase therapists' understanding of the functioning of their older clients and to enhance clinical judgement, effective treatment and informed prognosis.

Developmental theories

Human development has fascinated men of literature and science throughout the centuries. The various developmental theories are dealt with in more depth in other books, such as Lewis's *The Mature Years* (Lewis 1979). Human development follows a sequence, which may be viewed as occurring in stages. Arrival at each stage depends on many factors, including the maturity of the individual, gender, culture, class and the experiences they have encountered. Although the sequence of development is orderly, some individuals will reach these stages ahead of others.

There are several theories of stages of development. Two that are particularly helpful when working with people with dementia are cognitive development and social development. Developmental theory is widely used in occupational therapy practice (Pollock & McColl 2003) and forms the basis of such therapeutic techniques as reminiscence and validation. These can be used, for example, to help resolve the final developmental crisis of old age: the search for meaning in one's life in order to achieve integrity (Erikson 1959).

Biological theories

While a deep understanding of genetic and cellular structure is not essential for an occupational therapist, an awareness of biological changes and associated psychological factors is important for individual assessment. Equally important is a recognition of the sociopsychological impact that biological ageing can have. Relationships and status can alter as people begin to interact differently with the visibly ageing individual, sometimes to the extent that the psychological well-being of the older person is affected. This phenomenon is even more evident when the ageing individual is also displaying signs of a dementing illness. This will be discussed further in the section on working with older people with mental disorders.

Genetic theories

There are three hypotheses about the genetic factors which may cause ageing.

1. **Error accumulation** describes the formation of abnormal proteins which cause abnormal enzymes to rise to critical levels, leading eventually to death.
2. **Mutation** describes more spontaneous changes which, again, cause abnormalities to reach a critical level and lead to death.
3. **Programmed ageing** suggests that all individuals have a biological clock which is set at the moment of conception to run for a given length of time.

Cross-linkage

This theory suggests that abnormal bonds formed in collagen fibres lose their elasticity and eventually cause the organ to cease functioning.

Free radical

Oxygen molecules have pairs of orbiting electrons. Sometimes abnormal molecules are produced which have one electron missing. The remaining free electron acts like a magnet, attracting an electron from a neighbouring molecule. This sets off a sequence of cells changing their molecular structure and, as a result, body tissue becomes altered. The effect may be of ageing or of disease, such as cancer. The theory proposes that certain substances, including some linked to smoking, may increase the production of abnormal oxygen molecules and that others, such as vitamin E, may reduce them.

Social disengagement theory

This theory proposes that there is a mutual withdrawal of society from the individual (due to compulsory retirement, children growing up and leaving home, and so on) and of the individual from society (reduced social activities and a more solitary life). It is mainly based on a 5-year study of 275 people aged 50–90 in Kansas City (Cumming & Henry 1961). However, the theory attracted criticism because it assumes that withdrawal from society is an inherent part of ageing. A follow-up study, including 55% of the original 275, showed that although increasing age is accompanied by increasing disengagement, the most socially engaged people were the most happy (Havighurst et al 1968).

Disengagement may be cohort specific, that is, it may have been adaptive to withdraw from an ageist society in the 1950s when the original study was carried out but withdrawal may not be necessary now. Many of the social conditions which forced older people into restricted environments in the past have changed so that more active and socially engaged lifestyles are now possible (Turner & Helms 1989).

However, some older people do prefer to disengage and activity can decline without adversely affecting morale. A more leisurely lifestyle with fewer responsibilities can be seen as one of the rewarding aspects of old age.

Activity theory

This is the major alternative to social disengagement theory and is sometimes called re-engagement theory. It asserts that the natural tendency of most older people is to associate with others, particularly in group and community affairs (Lemon et al 1972, Maddox 1963). By becoming more socially active, older people engage more in leisure activities. The achievement of leisure goals serves to sustain the older person's self-esteem and morale.

Social exchange theory

This theory criticises both disengagement and activity theories for not taking into account the physical and economic factors which may limit an individual's choice of how he ages. On retirement, an older person enters into an unwritten contract with society, exchanging the role of an economically active member of society for increased leisure and less responsibility (Hayslip & Panek 1989).

The hypothesis underpinning this theory is that the contract is achieved through mutual consent. In reality, retirement from paid work is artificially set by legislation which does not account for the disparate abilities and aspirations of older people. At the same time, although this exchange of leisure and work enables a society to utilise the work potential of younger people, unfortunately it does not encourage younger people to value their elders.

An evaluation of all of these theories suggests that each may refer to a legitimate process by which some individuals come to terms with the changes which accompany ageing. Therefore, each theory may be seen as an option and it will very much depend on the personality of the individual as to which option is chosen.

MENTAL DISORDERS IN OLD AGE

Altered patterns of disease in old age

As a person ages, physiology alters, which often only becomes apparent when an individual organ becomes stressed and has a diminished reserve of function with which to cope. Homeostatic mechanisms also become defective with ageing so that, although they may function adequately under normal conditions, they lose their reserve under stress. For example, temperature regulation is impaired and the facility for shivering is diminished; the thirst sensation is reduced, which may cause an older person to be liable to dehydrate. Together, reduced physiological reserves and impaired homeostatic mechanisms, when confronted with a stress factor, can contribute to tipping the balance into failure of the system.

In an older person this can cause the presentation and pattern of disease, and the reaction to it, to be different from the experiences of a younger person. In many cases the disease will present less dramatically, with vague, non-specific symptoms such as falling or collapse. Thus, information which conflicts with conventional medical ideology may lead to an inaccurate diagnosis.

The symptoms which most often lead to hospital admission are instability, incontinence and cognitive failure. These can be caused by a range of conditions, both physical and mental, and are often a combination of several. The occurrence of several different pathological processes together is common in old age and is called multiple pathology. The diseases may be related or can be totally separate.

Older people are susceptible to the same range of mental disorders as younger people, although they may present in a different way. These include: personality disorders, neuroses, psychoses and organic conditions. For many old people there may not be a clear disorder, but a breakdown of their physical health and/or social network can cause them to be vulnerable to mental ill health. For example, deafness combined with arthritis leads to social withdrawal, which causes loneliness and a state of ill-being.

With all mental disorders in old age, the important point to consider is the wide range of potential differential diagnoses and the altered patterns of presentation. It is essential to work with each person as an individual and to carry out a comprehensive assessment. The specialist needs of this client group require the special skills of experienced multidisciplinary team members who embrace supervision and continued learning to keep abreast of current trends and research opportunities.

The most common organic and functional disorders affecting older people are described below.

ORGANIC DISORDERS

Organic disorders are disorders resulting from damage to, or changes in, the brain. Dementia, or mental deterioration, is caused by disease of the brain, usually of a chronic or progressive nature, leading to multiple disturbances of higher cortical function, including impairment of memory, thinking, orientation, comprehension, learning ability, language and judgement. These changes occur in clear consciousness, which assists in differentiating between dementia and acute confusional states.

The term 'dementia syndrome' is used to describe the clearly evident progressive decline of these cortical functions over at least a 6-month period. There is a group of organic disorders with similar signs and symptoms but with many different causes, and pathology and prognosis will vary according to the cause. However, the concept of a single cause is no longer viable and mixed pathologies are common, especially in late-onset dementia syndrome. In 2006, the Alzheimer's Society estimated that there were over 750,000 people in the UK affected by dementia. Approximately 18,000 people with dementia are under the age of 65 but the incidence of dementia increases with age, affecting one person in 20 over the age of 65 and one person in five over the age of 80. The number of people with dementia is steadily increasing.

ALZHEIMER'S DISEASE

- **Epidemiology.** The most common cause of dementia is Alzheimer's disease (AD), which probably accounts for around 55% of all dementia cases.
- **Aetiology.** Despite major advances in the study of Alzheimer's disease, the cause is not known. Epidemiological studies have confirmed that old age, a family history of AD, and the presence of Down's syndrome are all risk factors (Henderson 1988). As with many diseases, it seems that the aetiology of AD is multifactorial. Genetic influences, in combination with environmental factors, lead to the development of the disease.
- **Pathology.** A concrete diagnosis of Alzheimer's disease can only be achieved at post-mortem, when generalised cerebral atrophy is evident along with shrunken gyri and widened sulci. Under microscopic examination, neuronal cell loss, plaques and tangles can be seen. The plaques are extracellular and consist of swollen, degenerating nerve structures with

a central core of protein called amyloid. This protein is bound to aluminium silicate, hence the research into aluminium as a possible causal factor. The tangles are intracellular and consist of bundles of abnormal fibres. Plaques and tangles occur throughout the cortex but are particularly abundant in the temporal and parietal lobes, thus affecting memory and cognitive function.

- **Clinical features.** A particular feature of Alzheimer's disease is a steady decline of intellect and function as the disease progresses.

The onset of the disease is marked by loss of recent memory, affecting the individual's ability to carry out intellectual tasks of daily living, such as planning, financing and shopping. As with other types of dementia, the disease can manifest in a variety of ways depending on the area of the brain which has been affected (Table 24.2). The final outcome for people with Alzheimer's disease is death within 2–20 years from the onset of the illness. This large variation in prognosis may be due to the effect of psychosocial factors.

Table 24.2 Lesion sites and neuropsychological deficits

Lobe	Dominant hemisphere	Non-dominant hemisphere
Frontal	Expressive aphasia Agraphia Verbal apraxia Motor apraxia	Motor amusia Motor apraxia
Temporal	Sensory amusia Receptive aphasia Auditory agnosia Alexia Agraphia	Sensory amusia Metamorphosia Constructional apraxia
Occipital	Right hemianopia Alexia Colour agnosia Receptive dysphasia Constructional apraxia Dyscalculia Visual object agnosia Simultanognosia	Prosopagnosia Alexia Colour agnosia Dysgraphia Topographical disorientation Dressing apraxia Visual object agnosia Left hemianopia
Parietal	Tactile agnosia Constructional apraxia Visual object agnosia Visual spatial agnosia Agraphia Acalculia Right/left discrimination Finger agnosia Gerstmann's syndrome Somatognosia Asymbolia Ideomotor apraxia Ideational apraxia Simultanognosia	Tactile agnosia Constructional apraxia Visual object agnosia Visual spatial agnosia Agraphia (possibly) Acalculia (possibly) Right/left discrimination (possibly) Apractognosia Amorphosynthesis Unilateral neglect Dressing apraxia Prosopagnosia Topographical disorientation Anosognosia Alexia (possibly) Spatial relations syndrome

DEMENTIA WITH LEWY BODIES

- **Epidemiology.** This type of dementia, which occurs in association with Parkinsonian features, was thought to be very rare until recent studies of the pathology of people with dementia at post-mortem revealed that it is the second most common type of dementia, being roughly twice as common as vascular dementia (Perry et al 1989).
- **Pathology.** There is a degeneration of the substantia nigra in the midbrain region. Normally, the substantia nigra is populated by nerve cells which contain a dark brown pigment. In Lewy body dementia these cells die and so the substantia nigra appears abnormally pale. Remaining nerve cells contain abnormal eosinophilic (pink-staining) structures called Lewy bodies. These spread in the brainstem and in the cortical areas. As with Alzheimer's disease, there is some loss of neurones and plaques are present. However, neurofibrillary tangles are relatively sparse.
- **Clinical features.** With this condition there is a development of dementia with features overlapping with those of Alzheimer's disease. The person with dementia with Lewy bodies will have a mild form of Parkinsonism with rigid limbs, tremor, bradykinesia and shuffling gait. Memory function may be less impaired than in Alzheimer's disease, but psychiatric symptoms, including visual and auditory hallucinations, are common. There is a sensitivity to antipsychotic medication. The main feature differentiating dementia with Lewy bodies from Alzheimer's disease and from vascular dementia is the variability of the symptoms, both at onset and as the disease continues.

VASCULAR DEMENTIA

- **Epidemiology.** This type of dementia, which may be a result of either multi-infarcts or of vascular failure, accounts for about 15% of dementia cases.
- **Aetiology and pathology.** Multi-infarct dementia is caused by cerebral arteriosclerosis disrupting the blood supply to the brain, causing the death of brain cells in the affected areas. Vascular disease may also be a result of the ageing process which leads to cerebrovascular failure and, subsequently, a decay of white brain matter. Both these causes of vascular dementia are most common in people who have general vascular problems, and may be preventable. Unfortunately, as with other dementias, once the symptoms of this dementia have occurred they are not reversible.
- **Clinical features.** Multi-infarct dementia caused by cerebral arteriosclerosis often has a rapid onset and a stepwise progression as further vascular accidents occur. Cerebrovascular failure is likely to have a more insidious onset and a smoother progression. The features of vascular dementia will vary according to the site of brain damage.

A comprehensive comparison of the further features of vascular dementia with Alzheimer's disease can be found in a good psychiatric textbook, for example *An Introduction to the Psychiatry Of Old Age* (Pitt 1982).

NEW-VARIANT CREUTZFELDT–JAKOB DISEASE (CJD)

- **Epidemiology.** The total number of suspect cases referred to the National CJD Surveillance Unit at 2 April 2001 was 1330. At this date the number of deaths of definite and probable cases of new-variant CJD was 97.
- **Aetiology and pathology.** This dementia is caused by prions, which are small infective agents made of proteins. Infection can occur between humans, for example following an injection of growth hormone from human pituitary glands which are contaminated with prions, or during neurosurgery. Infection can also occur through ingestion of infected food. In sheep, prions cause scrapie and, in cows, bovine spongiform encephalitis (BSE), commonly known as mad cow disease. The disease is known to pass to cows when they graze on pasture infected by sheep. There is understandable concern that BSE is being contracted by humans, in the form of new-variant CJD, if they eat infected neural matter from cows.

There is evidence to support this but other theories are also being investigated. Once a person has been infected with prions it may be decades before the onset of dementia but, when the symptoms of dementia and ataxia develop, the process of the disease is usually very rapid (Livingston 1994).

- Neuropathologically there is spongiform change, neuronal loss and astrocytic gliosis, which is most evident in the basal ganglia and thalamus. The most striking pathological feature is amyloid plaque formation extensively distributed throughout the cerebrum and cerebellum.
- **Clinical features.** There is an early age of onset or death, the average being 27.6 years with a range of 18–41 years. The average duration of the illness is 13.1 months, with a range of 7.5–24 months. There is a predominantly psychiatric presentation, including anxiety, depression, social withdrawal and behaviour changes. Nearly all patients are referred to a psychiatrist early in the clinical course. After a period of weeks or months there is a development of cerebellar syndrome with gait and limb ataxia. Forgetfulness and memory disturbance develop later in the clinical course, progressing to severe cognitive impairment and a state of akinetic mutism. Myoclonus develops in the majority of patients and, in some, this is preceded by choreiform movements.

HIV-ASSOCIATED DEMENTIA

The ability of the retrovirus known as HIV to attack the brain directly was first reported in 1987 by Price and Navia of Cornell University. The virus infects the central nervous system and causes a brain disorder which slows the individual's thought processes and affects the ability to remember and to concentrate. This is one of the major complications of HIV infection, affecting most AIDS patients.

There are also motor features with leg weakness, loss of balance and unsteady gait. The individual becomes apathetic and socially withdrawn. If untreated, the infection progresses quickly and the patient will survive for only 6 months or less. However, there has been a dramatic decline of at least 50% in the incidence of HIV-associated dementia, as there has been in the incidence of all AIDS-related illnesses, since the introduction in 1996 of highly active antiretroviral therapy (HAART).

HIV-associated dementia tends, by its nature, to affect a younger age group than the other dementias.

OTHER ORGANIC DISORDERS

A variety of pathologies accounts for the remaining 5% of dementia cases, including space-occupying lesions, hydrocephalus, neurosyphilis, systemic disorders, such as hypothyroidism and drug toxicity, and Korsakoff's syndrome. The last is not strictly a dementia as it does not have a global cortical effect. It is caused by alcohol abuse resulting in a lack of thiamine and leading to memory impairment.

FUNCTIONAL DISORDERS

In functional disorders there is no evidence of damage or disturbance to the brain. As research adds to our knowledge and understanding of the process of these disorders, it may be found that what was once termed a functional disorder is actually an organic one. For example, damage due to chemical changes may be discovered.

Older people may experience the same functional disorders as younger people but they may manifest in different ways or, as with certain physical problems, may be dismissed as a natural part of the ageing process. The functional disorders which particularly affect older people are set out here.

REACTIVE DEPRESSION

Reactive depression, sometimes termed neurotic or exogenous depression, is associated with major life events, especially those involving loss. Older people may experience many losses, including the loss of spouse, friends, financial security, physical health, sensory acuity, cognitive powers, social independence or work status. Surgery, acute illness or being institutionalised may also be significant, as studies have shown that older people are less able to tolerate acute stress than they are chronic stress (Fogel 1991).

Estimates of the prevalence of reactive depression in people over 65 vary widely, but depression may be more common in older people as it is this age group that experiences the most negative life events. Interestingly, as old people age further their coping strategies improve and they have lower rates of depression than younger old people.

PSYCHOTIC DEPRESSION

The most significant difference between psychotic depression – also termed endogenous or unipolar depression – and reactive depression is the presence of delusions which may, for example, be of persecution, disease, sin, death or poverty.

Older people with a psychotic depression are likely to have had previous experience of it at a younger age. They often show a history of psychiatric illness and, possibly because of this, may also show signs of institutionalisation.

Diagnosing depression in an old person can be difficult because it often presents an atypical picture. It may be necessary to establish that there has been a change from the individual's usual mood and behaviour, which may perhaps have occurred years ago if the depression is of long standing. The fact that functional illnesses are treatable makes this thorough assessment worthwhile, particularly if there are signs of depression or if the old person displays insight, for example, reporting that they cannot remember rather than simply giving a wrong answer. If care is not taken, depression may be wrongly diagnosed as dementia because there are similarities between the two conditions (Table 24.3).

PARAPHRENIA

This condition, which is usually treatable, is characterised by delusions of persecution that are often accompanied by auditory hallucinations. The older person with paraphrenia will present as preoccupied, suspicious and sometimes aggressive. Unfortunately, the stereotype of old age as having these very characteristics may cause this condition to be accepted as normal and go untreated. Alternatively, the older person may be labelled as having this condition when the problem is due to hearing loss.

WORKING WITH OLDER PEOPLE WITH MENTAL DISORDERS

The multidisciplinary team

Working with older people requires a holistic approach in a multidisciplinary team, in order to make a complete assessment and meet the possibly complex needs of this client group. The membership of the multidisciplinary team will vary according to the needs of the individual and the service setting. Commonly, a health service team would include a consultant in the psychiatry of old age, nurses, occupational therapists and social workers. A social services team may consist of social workers, home carers and occupational therapists. There is often an overlap between the two services, therefore good communication channels are essential. Increasingly, multidisciplinary teams are also including service providers from the voluntary and independent sectors, if they are involved in an individual's care. The older person is the central figure in the team and, as such, he, or an advocate, should be consulted and informed about the care package.

When working with older people, team members should agree on common principles which meet their clients' basic needs and uphold their fundamental rights.

Values and principles of practice

Older people have the same basic rights to dignity, privacy, choice, independence and fulfilment as people of any other age group. When an older person experiences a mental health disorder these fundamental rights may easily be undermined by those giving care. Until the early 1990s there were few theories of care giving and most work with older people was based on clinical experience. However, a theory of personhood and well-being has now been developed, in response to the

Table 24.3 Similarities between depression and dementia (Macdonald 1980)

	Depression	Dementia
Decline in mental functioning	Can't make effort to think or remember. Only remembers bad things: preoccupied with past misdeeds or regrets; ruminates about failure or death. Does not attend to surroundings. May have mental slowing	Unable to connect similar ideas or to absorb new ones
Withdrawal	Feels isolated and sometimes deservedly rejected. Can't make effort to join in social activities. May have retardation, physical and mental. Apathetic, hopeless or despising themselves	Thought processes too disordered for communication. Shallow, transient feelings, or feelings reduced generally
Inappropriate social actions	May have persecutory ideas, may hear accusing voices. May have impulses to abase themselves. Early morning wakening with maximum depression of mood leads to wandering and suicide attempts	Stereotyped (purposeless, repetitive) movements and behaviour. Disorientation in time leading to nocturnal activity
Wandering	Searching (grief). Restlessness, agitation, anxiety, compelling thoughts. Early morning wakening or general poor sleep	Disorientation as to place. Misrecognition of unfamiliar places and people
Poor memory	Mental slowing, or too agitated and preoccupied with gloomy thoughts. Can't make effort, gives up easily	Direct effect of underlying physical brain deterioration. Wrong replies given readily
Others	Crying, incontinence, weight loss, angry outbursts	

particular needs of older people with dementia (Kitwood & Bredin 1992). This theory emphasises the primary importance of a sociopsychological approach to care giving. It explains how the prevailing social psychology, which depersonalises the person with dementia, results in care which is well intentioned but lacking in insight and understanding and which contributes to the dementing process. Personhood is essentially social and refers to the human being in relation to others, having status and being worthy of respect. When the individual is not accorded appropriate social interaction, well-being will suffer.

The theory proposes that a dementing illness is not necessarily a process of inevitable deterioration. Some people with dementia will score low on cognitive tests but will still function well as people, whereas others whose cognitive impairment is less severe will fare less well. A dementing condition tends to be compounded by depression, anxiety, apathy or discouragement. Therefore, a person with dementia may be in a state of well- or ill-being regardless of the degree of cognitive impairment. Kitwood proposed that there are four states of well-being: self-esteem, or a global feeling of personal worth; agency, that is, the ability to control personal life in a meaningful way and to produce and achieve; social confidence, or being at ease with others, and a fourth state of hope, or the retention of confidence that security will remain, and of optimism. There are 12 indicators that the person with dementia is experiencing one of these states:

1. the assertion of desire or will
2. the ability to experience and express a range of emotions
3. initiation of social contact
4. affectional warmth
5. social sensitivity
6. self-respect
7. acceptance of other dementia sufferers
8. humour
9. creativity and self-expression
10. showing evident pleasure
11. helpfulness
12. relaxation.

If social psychology, which views the person with dementia as a problem and not as a person to be related to, can contribute to the dementing process, it follows that human interaction can bring about some return of mental function. The indicators of well-being enable caregivers to evaluate the quality and effectiveness of their interventions within a theoretical framework.

People with dementia are missing out on the increasing resources for rehabilitation and intermediate care. It has long been the view of many that rehabilitation and dementia are not compatible, although there is now growing evidence that a variety of rehabilitation approaches can be effective in improving the cognitive, physical, social and emotional function of people with dementia (Marshall 2005). The aim of these approaches is to facilitate the person with dementia to achieve a state of well-being in one or all of these functions. Occupational therapists are well placed to use rehabilitation approaches, including life story work, cognitive rehabilitation, the use of environmental aids and adaptations, and the use of assistive technology to facilitate an occupational approach to well-being in dementia (Perrin & May 2000).

The occupational therapy process

The fundamental principles, philosophy and process of occupational therapy are the same when working with older people as with other age groups. However, practice draws on a broad range of theories, including physiological, behavioural, psychodynamic and cognitive concepts, and reflects the complexity of the physical, intellectual, emotional and social needs of older people. With this broad theoretical base, a variety of approaches may be used when working with older people with mental disorders. The key to successful intervention is to apply the occupational therapy process of assessment, treatment planning, implementation and evaluation in order to select the most appropriate approach and ensure a high-quality service.

ASSESSMENT

In order to assist the older person to become as independent as possible, it is first necessary to assess the individual's abilities, problems, wishes and interests. A problem-orientated assessment alone is too narrow, focusing on difficulties, whereas the treatment plan should also incorporate the person's abilities in order to use and maintain them. It is possible to motivate clients to be involved in therapy by building the programme of intervention on their wishes and interests.

A range of assessment methods may be used, including interviews, observation techniques and standardised tests.

INTERVIEWS

Interviewing an older person can be a lengthy process if a full history is to be obtained. When communication skills have been affected by mental disorder, it may be tempting to interview the client's relatives or carers but, if the therapist utilises all her communication skills, it is possible to achieve an informative interview with even the most dysphasic person.

The therapist should pay attention to the older person's non-verbal responses, including reactions, expressions, posture and tone of voice. The therapist also needs to use simple language and to ask closed questions when interviewing a person with dementia. The client must always be given time to respond. Possible sensory deficits should always be considered; it should be standard practice to allow for hearing or visual impairment. Making sure that a client is wearing his hearing aid, and that it is switched on and working, could prevent or correct a misdiagnosis of depression or dementia.

OBSERVATION

Observing the older person carrying out everyday functional tasks can reveal not only the person's level of ability in achieving an end result but also the presence of specific deficits for which treatment can then be planned. A functional assessment may be carried out in an occupational therapy department or in the familiarity of the person's own home. The therapist needs to be aware of the different demands on the client in each location.

In unfamiliar environments a person will be relying on higher cognitive level skills to solve problems and to carry out executive functions, whereas in a familiar environment the person may be performing actions by relying on procedural memory and familiar patterns of movement. Each assessment will reveal a very different set of information: in the unfamiliar environment the true level of cognitive ability and disability will be observed and in the familiar environment the therapist will be able to note how the person can function despite any cognitive disability. Both sets of information are important for planning therapeutic interventions.

The activity that the therapist and client select as an appropriate assessment task will use the therapist's skills in task analysis and activity analysis. For example, making a cup of tea is an activity which tests the person's orientation, sequencing, memory, safety, perception and visuospatial skills. Many occupational therapy departments have developed their own assessments of activities of daily living and, although these are not standardised, they do have a valid place in the department's battery of assessments.

STANDARDISED TESTS

These are tools used to detect impairment and should be used in addition to interview and observation in order to gain a full picture of the client. As the name indicates, the tests are designed to measure the client against set standards. They can be useful for determining the older person's baseline function and can then be reapplied after intervention to measure any changes. Not all standardised tests have been validated, but four which are well documented as valuable and reliable are the Allen Cognitive Level Screen (Allen et al 1992), the Pool Activity Level (PAL) Instrument (Pool 2008), the Dementia Rating Scale (Mattis 1988) and the Middlesex Elderly Assessment of Mental State (MEAMS; Golding 1989).

The Allen Cognitive Level Screen

The Allen Cognitive Level Screen (ACLS) uses a simple functional task as a screening assessment to analyse the level of cognitive ability. The assessment supports the theoretical model of functional information processing. This is an occupational therapy model used when working with people with cognitive impairments, including those caused by dementia, developmental delay, mental health problems, such as depression or schizophrenia, and acquired brain injury.

The model proposes that there are six cognitive levels, each of which can be described in terms of limitations associated with the medical condition and remaining abilities, as seen in patterns of behaviour in everyday tasks (Allen et al 1992). The levels range from level 6, where functioning is normal and no intervention is required, to level 1, where the person is profoundly impaired. An analysis of the results aids understanding of the client's behaviour when carrying out everyday tasks. Optimum environmental stimulation and support can then be planned and implemented to decrease confusion, maximise functional capacities and help the person retain a sense of competence despite impairment.

For more information on the Functional Information-Processing Model, see Chapter 20.

The Pool Activity Level (PAL) Instrument

The Pool Activity Level (PAL) Instrument (Pool 2008) has become the framework for activity-based care systems in a variety of settings for people with dementia and other cognitive impairments. The instrument is now standardised following a research study to assess the validity and reliability of the PAL Checklist for use with older people with dementia (Wenborn et al 2008). The Checklist was designed for use by care staff to assess performance in nine everyday activities. It indicates an individual's cognitive ability to engage in activity, using four activity levels: planned, exploratory, sensory and reflex.

In the *National Clinical Practice Guideline for Dementia* (National Institute for Health and Clinical Excellence 2006), the PAL Instrument is recommended for activity of daily living skill training and for activity planning.

The PAL Checklist and action plan are based on the underpinning hypothesis that people with cognitive impairments have a potential for development and that occupation is the key to unlocking this potential. The theory of developmental process for cognition, sensorimotor and interaction skills is applied in practice to working with people with cognitive impairments, by presenting care workers with tools to identify the developmental level and the activity level of the person.

Completing the PAL Checklist enables caregivers to recognise the ability of a person with cognitive impairment to engage in activity. Any individual who knows the person well, by considering how he generally functions when carrying out activities, particularly those involving other people, can complete it. These observations should have been made in several situations over a period of 1 week. If the person lives in a group setting, such as a home, the observations may need to be a compilation from all involved caregivers. In this way, the variation of abilities and disabilities, which can occur in an individual over a period of time, is taken into account and an occupational profile can be made. The occupational profile gives an overview of the way in which a person best engages in activities and how to create a facilitating environment.

Because there are many factors affecting an individual's ability to engage in an activity (cognitive integrity, the meaningfulness of the task, the familiarity of the environment, the support of others), it is likely that an individual will reveal a variation in his level of ability in different activities. The PAL Instrument acknowledges the importance of this and provides the opportunity to create an individual action plan that allows for a varying degree of support in some of the personal activities of daily living.

Dementia Rating Scale

The Dementia Rating Scale (DRS) is a rapid but comprehensive measure of cognitive status for adults between the ages of 65 and 81 who have cortical impairment (Mattis 1988). It provides an accurate assessment of the progression and level of the person's behavioural, neuropathological and cognitive competence and can be used to plan programmes to maximise quality of life and to enhance intact abilities.

Middlesex Elderly Assessment of Mental State

The Middlesex Elderly Assessment of Mental State (MEAMS) is a screening test used to detect impairment of specific cognitive skills in older people and is designed to assist professionals working with older people to differentiate between functional and organic conditions (Golding 1989). The MEAMS requires the subject to perform a number of simple tasks, each sensitive to the functioning of a different area of the brain. It is therefore useful in treatment planning and as an indicator for further investigations.

OCCUPATIONAL THERAPY ASSESSMENT IN THE MULTIDISCIPLINARY TEAM

Assessment is a complex process requiring contributions from different members of the multidisciplinary team in order to obtain as accurate a picture as possible. The occupational therapist may be the first person to note a particular deficit which indicates that a specific area of the brain has been affected. Alternatively, the therapist may already have received a pathology report from colleagues, detailing the areas affected. She can then assess the implications of these findings for the person's functional ability.

The occupational therapist is often asked to provide information about a person's basic living skills, for example stating whether or not a person is safe to live at home alone or whether he requires the assistance of a home carer, but can make a much wider contribution to the overall assessment of the client's abilities and needs. For example, the therapist may offer guidance to carers on how to help the older person to carry out tasks to his maximum potential. The occupational therapist will be able to advise not only whether the help of a home carer is required but also how that help should be given (Box 24.1).

The *National Service Framework for Older People* (DoH 2001) has raised awareness of the role of occupational therapists in providing rehabilitation services to older people. This applies equally for people with mental health problems as well as for people with physical needs. Standard 3 of the NSF states that individuals will have access to a range of intermediate care services, at home or in designated care settings, to promote their independence by providing enhanced services from the NHS and local authorities. The aim of intermediate care is prevent unnecessary hospital admission and to provide effective rehabilitation services to enable early discharge from hospital and prevent premature or unnecessary admission to long-term residential care.

TREATMENT AND CARE PLANNING

When information about the older person's abilities, needs, wishes and interests has been gathered through the assessment process, it can be used to formulate a plan of treatment. This is called a treatment or care plan. Where possible, the client should be involved in the treatment planning process, since understanding the aims of the programme will increase motivation to participate.

The treatment plan should follow the same format as for any other client group, with goals and objectives clearly defined so that all members of the team, including the client and his family or carers, are fully informed (see Chapter 6).

Traditionally, leisure activities have been the main treatment medium for older people. However, the key point when planning treatment is that the activity should be purposeful, both in achieving the goals of therapy and in the meaning it has for the individual. A basic living task can be just as effective in achieving therapeutic goals

---

Box 24.1 Case example 1

Mr Scott lived in a long-stay hospital unit for people with dementia. He had been diagnosed as having Alzheimer's disease, and CT scans showed lesions in the temporal and parietal lobes of the left hemisphere. Nurses were having difficulty helping Mr Scott to carry out many everyday tasks, although physically he was able to function well. Staff described him as lazy and deaf, since he did not respond to repeated instructions from his carers and he was becoming increasingly withdrawn.

The occupational therapist carried out an assessment with Mr Scott by observing him getting dressed and watering the unit's plants. She found that Mr Scott was not deaf and responded to a calm, reassuring tone of voice by making eye contact and smiling. It was evident that Mr Scott had a receptive aphasia and was therefore unable to follow the verbal instructions of his carers. In addition, the therapist observed that Mr Scott would start to get dressed but would abruptly stop and remain holding a sock as if unsure of his next move. Given the site of his brain damage, this indicated the possibility of an ideational apraxia. She advised the carers to remain with Mr Scott while he dressed and to give him physical, rather than verbal, prompts when he was seen to falter, but to allow him to physically carry out the task himself. She also suggested that appropriate praise should be used to reinforce his achievements. In this way, Mr Scott was able to get dressed as independently as he was able, his self-confidence improved and he became less withdrawn.

as a leisure activity, and it may be more appropriate for the older person who has never had time to participate in leisure activities and may feel uncomfortable being involved in them. A light domestic task, such as dusting, watering plants or cleaning shoes, can be as effective as a leisure activity and the older person may feel more in control by engaging in a familiar activity.

Activity media should motivate the older person to participate in the treatment programme. For some people, this may require that it is age specific whereas, for others, it may be more important that it is therapeutically specific. For example, when games are used, such as bowls or skittles, for those who would be undermined by childish activities they should be played with adult equipment and not children's versions bought from toy shops. However, for a person whose cognitive impairment is such that they are most able when they are engaging with media that capture their attention because of bold colour or design, media from children's departments may be most appropriate. The approach used by the therapist when introducing the activity will enable the older person to feel comfortable with the chosen medium.

TAKING RISKS

Older people may be so protected by their carers that they are prevented from achieving fulfilment in their lives. There can be a temptation to stop someone attempting anything which may result in harm, particularly when they have a

mental illness such as dementia. The relatives of the older person often wish for this protection, mistakenly believing that their father or mother is at risk of injury through carrying out certain activities. The Mental Capacity Act 2005 sets out the requirement to determine the capacity of an individual to make decisions and to act in the best interests of people without capacity, using the least restrictive option. This Act clearly guides all professionals, including occupational therapists, to consider these issues for people with cognitive impairments. If relatives are involved in the treatment planning process then they should have the opportunity to discuss the use of any activities which involve an element of risk. Through discussion, agreement or compromise may be reached.

Appropriate risk taking is a normal part of everyday life and adds quality to the subjective experience. When we take a risk we usually consider the advantages and disadvantages and only act if, on balance, the reason for taking the action is worth the element of risk. The older person's right to take appropriate risks should be considered and appropriate opportunities built into the treatment plan. An older person with a mental disorder has the same legal and civil rights as anyone else. Restraining someone from carrying out an activity may constitute abuse. Protecting an older person from taking appropriate risks may do them more harm than enabling them to do so; this is the balance which needs to be considered (Box 24.2).

Box 24.2 Case example 2

Mrs Jones lived in a residential home for older people. She was diagnosed as having a dementia and was ataxic. Mrs Jones had a walking frame but constantly forgot to use it and was having frequent falls. The manager of the home applied to the occupational therapist for a chair from which Mrs Jones would find it difficult to rise, thus preventing her from walking about and protecting her from falling.

The occupational therapist worked with the staff and manager of the home, helping them to recognise Mrs Jones's right to get up and move around and the importance of mobility to her physical health. The therapist then assisted the staff to plan Mrs Jones's care so that they reduced her risk of injury from falling by assisting her to walk at planned times and prompting her to use her frame at others. To compensate for times when staff were not available, another resident, who was a friend of Mrs Jones, was encouraged to prompt her to use the frame.

In this way, Mrs Jones's care was planned so that appropriate risk taking was built in but the element of risk was reduced to a minimum.

TREATMENT IMPLEMENTATION

A variety of media and methods is covered comprehensively in Section 5 of this book. In addition, there are many relevant publications, some of which are recommended for further reading at the end of this chapter.

SOME TECHNIQUES

This section will consider some of the techniques which are frequently used with older people with mental disorders. Each of these approaches employs effective communication as its vehicle. Without good communication, treating the older person with respect for his dignity and individuality, all these approaches fail. It may be the process of these therapies, rather than the outcome, that is important because if the basic values underpinning good practice with older people are carried out then their personhood and well-being will be assured.

Anxiety management

Older people may experience anxiety, which affects their ability to function, in the same way as people of other age groups. The cause of this disorder in an older person may be a reaction to loss or to the onset of disease, or it may be a disorder which has carried on from a younger age. Anxiety management and relaxation techniques can be used to assist older people, even those with dementia, to take control of their own feelings in the same way as they are used to assist younger people.

Reminiscence

Reminiscing was once thought to be an indication of mental deterioration but it is now viewed as a positive experience which should be encouraged. Reminiscence has value as a way of preserving one's identity, searching for meaning and relevance in one's life, or reviewing past experiences of solving problems in order to solve current ones. Reminiscence can therefore be therapeutic and can be utilised by occupational therapists to assist clients to resolve conflicts or maintain self-esteem, as well as being a social or recreational activity.

A vast selection of media can be used to trigger reminiscence, including material published for this purpose in the form of videos, audio tapes, photographs and pictures. Libraries, museums and community groups are also useful sources of archive material.

The use of a life story book can help an older person to piece together his past in order to preserve a sense of identity. The information can also be shared with others, for example as a living history project with schoolchildren or simply with carers. Appreciating the history of the older person promotes his self-esteem and enables others to be empathetic.

Reality orientation

Reality orientation (RO) is a treatment method which aims to stimulate people to relearn basic facts about themselves and their environment by systematically presenting and reinforcing relevant information. It is therefore only appropriate to use this method with people who are able to learn and it is not suitable for a person with dementia who has lost this cognitive skill. Rimmer (1988) offered a useful assessment tool which uses interview to assess the older person's level of orientation and to determine if RO is appropriate. Reality orientation is traditionally used with people with a dementia but it is also helpful for others who are disorientated, perhaps because of living in a long-stay unit and becoming institutionalised.

Reality orientation can be practised in two ways. The 24-hour approach involves all members of the treatment team consistently reinforcing information which helps the older person to orientate himself. The person is always addressed by his preferred name and cues, such as clocks, calendars and notice boards, are also used. Individuals who are severely cognitively impaired, and who may have become so disorientated that they are not self-aware, may respond to direct sensory stimulation which aims to increase awareness of self.

Group RO is a selective approach used with a small group of people of a similar level of ability. The group meets regularly and each meeting lasts for about half an hour. The aim of group RO is to stimulate each of the participants' senses selectively in order to assist them to become more aware of their surroundings and themselves. The occupational therapist should identify the people most likely to benefit from this approach. An individual who can no longer store new memories, for example someone in the later stages of dementia, may be put under undue pressure by this approach while a person who does still have the ability to learn may benefit.

Cognitive rehabilitation

Cognitive rehabilitation uses the therapist's understanding of cognitive functioning to support people so that they can deal with the problems that arise because of cognitive changes and to facilitate them to participate in interactions and engage in activity within their own personal and social context (Clare 2005). This approach therefore fits well within the *International Classification of Functioning, Disability and Health* (ICF) (WHO 2001), which describes how people live with their health condition.

Cognitive rehabilitation interventions include a range of methods and techniques, such as spaced retrieval and errorless learning. These methods can be used independently or combined to enable a solution-focused approach that can make a considerable difference to individuals with dementia, promoting a sense of hope, agency, self-confidence and self-esteem that all contribute to a state of well-being.

Spaced retrieval

Spaced retrieval (SR) is a memory intervention technique that gives individuals with memory deficits practice at successfully recalling important information over progressively longer intervals of time. Clinical research using SR has demonstrated that individuals with Alzheimer's disease can be taught to remember compensatory strategies that help facilitate safety and greater levels of independence.

The use of this technique has helped individuals with memory impairments learn how to use a daily calendar, to effectively and safely use adaptive equipment, to remember the names of objects and items related to basic and medical needs, to perform activities of daily living at higher levels of independence and to learn safer swallowing behaviours (Brush & Cameron 1998).

Errorless learning

This is a method of acquiring implicit knowledge of the performance of a specific task or activity through repetition of a pattern of movement and actions. In this way, the learning bypasses the cognitive system and is stored as procedural memory in the joints and muscles. If the action to be learned is identified as important to the older person, he may feel that the effort involved is worthwhile for the desired outcome. This approach is useful for an individual who has lost the ability to store and access explicit memories. It can also be utilised by therapists when advising on environmental layout to optimise the performance of familiar activities such as personal care and other activities of daily living. A person can develop a pattern of movement that relies on the consistent layout of the media required by practising the same movements each time. For example, when getting washed, the facecloth, soap and towel are always located in the same places and the person is led through the same order of the stages of the task, until the task becomes familiar.

Validation therapy

This approach was developed to give validity and dignity to the feelings expressed by disorientated older people who can no longer benefit from reality orientation. The concept of validation may be used with a wide group of people and may also be seen as an issue of good practice. However, validation therapy can assist the client to begin to resolve past conflicts by expressing his feelings to someone who empathises. It is thus possible to reduce problem behaviours which are symptomatic of internal conflicts.

Sensory stimulation

It is commonly accepted that sensory stimulation is necessary for physical and mental health. The concept of sensory deprivation relies on the theory that environmental stimulation leads to an appropriate response. Without this stimulation, no response will be forthcoming. This theory has been explored in relation to people with dementia and taken further to propose that sensory deprivation may add to, or even cause, dementia, and that it is possible to use sensory stimulation to reverse, or at least slow down, the disease process. Sensory stimulation can be achieved in many ways. At a simple level, the opportunity for sensory engagement with the environment can be enhanced by presenting everyday features to individuals. These environmental features may include objects, such as ornaments, fabrics, plants, flowers or animals. Food is particularly valuable because it can be multisensory, incorporating opportunities for visual, olfactory, tactile, auditory and gustatory stimulation. Occupational therapists who recognise this can bring the environment to the person and ensure that the full value of the experience is derived by encouraging exploration.

In addition to using everyday environmental features, it is possible to use special environments and objects which aim to elicit specific responses. Originally developed as a leisure experience for people with severe learning difficulties and sensory disabilities, Snoezelen is a facility which is now used on a much wider scale. It is a non-directive approach which presents items of sensory equipment for exploration and development. Whole rooms can be dedicated to the arrangement of Snoezelen equipment, but small portable items can be presented to individuals in their own homes.

The use of Snoezelen with people with dementia is relatively new, but positive therapeutic outcomes have been described (Pinkney & Barker 1994). In addition to stimulating and maintaining the body's ability to receive information through all the sensory modalities, and thus stimulating neurological responses, Snoezelen promotes the development of a therapeutic relationship between the person with dementia and his caregiver. In fact, the relationship becomes a partnership in which the caring role is exchanged for one of equality as both participants are engaged in exploring and enjoying the environment.

Music is a medium which has therapeutic benefits going far beyond the immediate one of auditory stimulation. While language deterioration is a feature of cognitive disability, musical abilities can still be preserved. This may be because the fundamentals of music are not based in the lexical and semantic functions of naming and reference but in tone and rhythm (Aldridge & Brandt 1991). Music has a history as a means of communication, and varying tones and rhythms elicit primitive responses in mood and basic physiological functions such as heart and respiration rates. These are subcortical responses which can be stimulated even in people who have severe cortical damage but whose subcortex remains intact.

Behavioural therapy

This systematic approach may be used to reduce problem behaviours associated with dementia, such as aggression, inappropriate urinating, undressing or shouting. An assessment is carried out to determine the nature, frequency, triggers and consequences of the problem behaviour. This information is then used to plan a staged intervention until the desired new behaviour is elicited and the undesirable behaviour removed.

GROUP VERSUS INDIVIDUAL TREATMENT

The decision to use an individual or a group approach should depend on the needs of the older person. Groups may be appropriate for some activities, particularly those which aim to promote social skills and verbal interaction, but the group must be carefully selected for size and composition. If the group is too large or has members of varying levels of ability, it can be frustrating for participants. Large group outings can also be counterproductive as they may not promote a positive image of older people but rather contribute to negative stereotypes of old age. Often, an individual approach for a short length of time will be more beneficial, and will enhance the client's personhood and well-being more, than a longer period in a group.

USING VOLUNTEERS

Group, rather than individual, treatment or care is sometimes selected in an attempt to provide a service for a larger number of old people. Lack of staff may mean that the needs of the individual cannot always be met. If this is the case, it is worth considering the use of volunteers. When a treatment or care plan has been formulated with clear objectives, the volunteer can be guided to help the older person to achieve these. The volunteer will also find it beneficial to work to a plan and will appreciate being given direction. Most volunteers tend to give up because of having too little, rather than too much, to do.

ENVIRONMENTAL ADAPTATION

In addition to using the treatment techniques described, occupational therapists have a role to play in adapting the older person's environment to promote function at the optimum level. This may require the provision of equipment to enable the person to overcome a physical problem. For example, large-handle cutlery may be provided for someone with arthritis, or a raised garden constructed for someone in a wheelchair.

Alternatively, the adaptation may meet the psychological needs of the person. The design of residential or day units for people with dementia can affect their orientation, mood or thought processes. The occupational therapist can advise on the use of colour, plants or ornaments to act as environmental clues. She may also apply her knowledge of perceptual deficits when advising about décor. For example, functional problems arising from an inability to discriminate between a figure and its background can be overcome by the careful use of colour and lighting. The provision of quiet areas and areas which are stimulating to the senses will affect the user's mood and, in the case of people with dementia, their levels of expressed emotion.

ASSISTIVE TECHNOLOGY

Assistive technology ranges from very simple tools, such as memory aids and simple-to-use telephones, to high-tech solutions such as satellite-based navigation systems to help find someone who has got lost. Unobtrusive wireless sensors can be placed around the home to raise the alarm if there is a potential problem inside the home of the person with dementia. If the sensors detect possible smoke, gas, flood or fire, they sound an audible alarm as well as alerting a carer, keyholder or 24-hour monitoring service.

Assistive technology can make a huge difference to the lives of people with dementia and their carers, enabling them to stay put in their own home and to live safely. However, some people might find the presence of the equipment distressing, either because it reminds them that they have a problem or because they cannot learn how to use it. Some technological solutions may be unnecessarily complex or expensive and small changes in daily activities may be enough to overcome a problem. Importantly, the use of assistive technology should never replace the opportunity for social interactions and will only be effective when combined with good care.

EVALUATION

The occupational therapist must continuously monitor the outcomes of her intervention with clients to determine the effectiveness of the treatment or care plan. The evaluation should include a reassessment using the standardised tests which were used to establish the client's baseline of function. It will then be possible to make a comparison between the client's level of function before and after therapeutic intervention.

In this way the therapist can evaluate the effectiveness of her treatment. If the evaluation shows that occupational therapy is not effective, then the programme may need to be modified. This may involve the deletion of unattainable goals or the modification of goals partly achieved. It is also important to modify the programme of intervention when evaluation shows that therapy is being effective, as new goals will need to be added as progress is made.

Consultation with the client is important to determine his level of satisfaction with his treatment or care. Although in cases of chronic dementia a cure will not be possible, it is possible to promote a positive outlook in the client by involving him in the evaluation process and reinforcing when goals have been achieved.

SUMMARY

This chapter has focused on the positive aspects of old age and on the rights of older people to be treated in the same way as other client groups. Part of the challenge of working with older people is to change the attitudes of others, and of old people themselves, by disproving the myths and negative stereotypes of old age.

The impact that mental disorders in old age can have on physiological and social well-being should not be overlooked. Multipathology calls for skilled care and treatment by experienced occupational therapists, and requires application of the occupational therapy process within a framework of appropriate theories.

The field of work with older people with mental disorders is becoming increasingly stimulating as levels of knowledge about conditions and methods of intervention improve. Occupational therapists have a role to play in clinical practice and have much to contribute to research in this area. Demographic trends have led to older people constituting an increasingly large number of occupational therapists' clients. An opportunity therefore exists to test out hypotheses about intervention, to evaluate new techniques and to document and publish findings.

Finally, the role of occupational therapists in educating others working with older people is clear. Apart from providing education about the wider role of occupational therapy, there is also scope for educating others, including colleagues, relatives and carers, about the potential of older people for functioning independently and the techniques which can be used to achieve this.

References

Aldridge D, Brandt G 1991 Music therapy and Alzheimer's disease. British Journal of Music Therapy 5: 28-36

Allen CK, Earhart CA, Blue T 1992 Occupational therapy treatment goals for the physically and cognitively disabled. American Occupational Therapy Association, Rockville, Maryland

Brush J, Cameron J 1998 Spaced retrieval: a therapy technique for improving memory. Menorah Park Center for Senior Living, Beachwood, Ohio

Clare L 2005 Cognitive rehabilitation for people with dementia. In: Marshall M (ed) Perspectives on rehabilitation and dementia. Jessica Kingsley Publishers, London, pp180-186

Cumming E, Henry WE 1961 Growing old: the process of disengagement. Basic Books, New York

Department of Health 1990 NHS and Care in the Community Act. HMSO, London

Department of Health 2001 National service framework for older people. HMSO, London

Department of Health 2002 NSF for older people: intermediate care – moving forward. HMSO, London

Department of Health 2005 Independence, well-being and choice: our vision for the future of social care for adults in England. Department of Health, London

Department of Health 2006 Our health, our care, our say: a new direction for community services. Stationery Office, London

Erikson EH 1959 Identity and the life cycle: selected papers. Psychological issues (monograph). International Universities Press, New York

Fogel BS 1991 Depression and ageing. Neuropsychiatry, Neuropsychology and Behavioural Neurology 4(1): 24-35

Golding E 1989 The Middlesex Elderly Assessment of Mental State. Thames Valley Test Company, Bury St Edmunds, pp 7–9

Havighurst RJ, Neugarten BL, Tobin SS 1968 Disengagement and patterns of ageing. Middle age and ageing. University of Chicago Press, Chicago

Hayslip B, Panek PE 1989 Adult development and ageing. Harper and Row, New York

Henderson AS 1988 The risk factors for Alzheimer's disease: a review and a hypothesis. Acta Psychiatrica Scandinavica 78: 257-275

Kitwood T, Bredin K 1992 Towards a theory of dementia care: personhood and well-being. Ageing and Society 12: 269-287

Lemon B, Bengtson VL, Peterson JA 1972 An exploration of the activity theory of ageing: activity types and life satisfaction among in-movers to a retirement community. Journal of Gerontology 27

Lewis SC 1979 The mature years: a geriatric occupational therapy text. Slack, New Jersey

Livingston G 1994 Understanding dementia: the rarer dementias. Journal of Dementia Care 2(3): 27-29

Macdonald A 1980 Depression and elderly people. Mind, London

Maddox GL 1963 Activity and morale: a longitudinal study of selected elderly subjects. Social Forces 43: 195-204

Marshall M 2005 Perspectives on rehabilitation and dementia. Jessica Kingsley, London

Mattis S 1988 Dementia rating scale. NFER-NELSON, Windsor

Midwinter E 1993 A voyage of rediscovery. Third Age, London

National Institute for Health and Clinical Excellence 2006 Supporting people with dementia and their carers. National Institute for Health and Clinical Excellence, London

Office for National Statistics 1991 Census of population and housing – Great Britain – 1991. Office for National Statistics, London

Office of Population, Census and Surveys 1983 Morbidity statistics from general practice, 1981–1982. Office of Population, Census and Surveys, London

Perrin T, May H 2000 Wellbeing in dementia: an occupational approach for therapists and carers. Churchill Livingstone, Edinburgh

Perry RH, Irving D, Blessed G et al 1989 Clinically and neuropathologically distinct form of dementia in the elderly. Lancet 335: 166

Philp I 2006 A new ambition for old age: next steps in implementing the National Service Framework for Older People. Department of Health, London

Pinkney L, Barker P 1994 Snoezelen – an evaluation of a sensory environment used by people who are elderly and confused. In: Hutchinson R, Kewin J (eds) Sensations and disability. Rompa, Chesterfield.

Pitt B 1982 An introduction to the psychiatry of old age. Churchill Livingstone, Edinburgh

Pollock N, McColl MA 2003 How occupation changes. In: McColl MA, Law M, Stewart D et al (eds) Theoretical basis of occupational therapy. Slack, Thorofare, New Jersey, pp63-88

Pool J 2008 The Pool Activity Level (PAL) Instrument for Occupational Profiling. Jessica Kingsley, London

Rimmer L 1988 Reality orientation: principles and practice, 2nd edn. Winslow Press, Bicester, Oxfordshire

Roberts A 1989 Systems of life. Nursing Times 85(49): 57-60

Turner JS, Helms DB 1989 Contemporary adulthood, 4th edn. Holt, Rinehart and Winston, Fort Worth, Florida

Twining TC 1988 Helping older people: a psychological approach. Wiley, Chichester

Wenborn J, Challis D, Orrell M 2008 Reliability and Validity of the PAL Checklist. In Pool J. The Pool Activity Level (PAL) Instrument for Occupational Profiling. Jessica kingsley, London, pp 21-34

World Health Organization 2001 International classification of functioning, disability and health. World Health Organization, Geneva

USEFUL WEBSITES

Information about Alzheimer's disease, the Alzheimer's Society and related websites: www.alzheimers.org.uk

Information about dementia with Lewy bodies: www.ccc.nottingham.ac.uk and link to lewyhom

Information about new-variant CJD: www.cjd.ac.uk

Information about the Functional Information-Processing Model and Allen's cognitive levels and assessment battery: www.allen-cognitive-levels.com

Chapter **25**

Child and Adolescent Mental Health Services

Lesley Lougher, Deborah Hutton, Donna Guest, Alan Evans

INTRODUCTION

To work with children is to be there at the beginning. Children do not arrive fully formed but develop in the context of their relationships, roles, activities and routines. Some occupational therapists work with mothers and young babies, helping to develop the vital early relationship, others with parents struggling to create patterns in their family lives. Equally, some will be touched by a child struggling to make sense of abuse and neglect through the process of play, whilst others engage with adolescents trying to find their own identity. In Child and Adolescent Mental Health Services (CAMHS), occupational therapists have the opportunity to use their knowledge of the importance of occupation in the creation of a secure family environment and the development of a child's identity. As the context of a child's life is always important in any intervention, so must CAMHS be seen as one of the network of agencies working with the child.

This chapter looks at the history of occupational therapy with children and child psychiatry and the legislative changes and national priorities for CAMHS in the United Kingdom. This is followed by an overview of the types of problems experienced by children and their families. The final section addresses the role of occupational therapy in the tiered system of CAMHS delivery: from community work to specialist services.

HISTORY OF OCCUPATIONAL THERAPY IN CAMHS

Child psychiatry emerged as a specialty in the 1930s, when child guidance clinics were established to provide a community-based inter-disciplinary service, staffed by psychiatrists, psychiatric social workers and educational psychologists. Occupational therapy specifically for children with mental health difficulties is first mentioned in the literature in the 1950s (Rockey 1987), with therapists working mainly in inpatient units. However, Wilcock (2001, 382), writing about the social reformer Octavia Hill, suggested that 'it is in the way she helped the children to develop and grow through the occupations they pursued that she can be regarded as a pioneer occupational therapist working in community health'. Many of the current trends in occupational therapy concerned with child mental health, in non-statutory agencies and in community development, are similar to the work of Octavia Hill over 150 years ago.

Within the last few years the occupational science literature has examined the activities and tasks involved in the occupation of parenting (Pierce 2000, Primeau 1998), the development of children's occupations (Humphrey 2002, Lawlor 2003) and leisure occupations (Csikszentmihalyi 1993, Passmore 2003). Occupational therapists now have the theory base to underpin their interventions (see Chapter 19).

NATIONAL AGENDA FOR CHILDREN IN ENGLAND AND WALES

In recent years, there has been an increased national interest and understanding of the role of CAMHS in the UK. The following publications are used in planning priorities in England and Wales but it is important for all occupational therapists to be aware of the political influences on their services, wherever they work.

Together We Stand

For many years, children's mental health was a little known and underfunded specialty but it was brought to greater prominence by the publication of a service review, *Together We Stand* (Health Advisory Service 1995), which analysed some of the difficulties inherent in the many small, poorly resourced services. This document introduced the concept that child and adolescent mental health is everyone's business and recognised that all children's agencies are working to promote children's mental health. Occupational therapists were mentioned as members of the core teams.

The National Service Framework for Children, Young People and Maternity Services

The *National Service Framework (NSF) for Children, Young People and Maternity Services* (DoH 2004) includes a standard (9) for the mental health and psychological well-being of children and young people. This describes a four-tier strategic framework (Table 25.1) which indicates the functions of the agencies delivering services to children and families. Occupational therapists are only mentioned in specialist CAMHS (tiers 3 and 4), which represents a conservative view of the profession, as will be explained later.

The vision of the NSF is to see:

- an improvement in the mental health of all children and young people
- multiagency services, working in partnership, promote the mental health of all children and young people, provide early intervention and also meet the needs of children and young people with established or complex problems
- that all children, young people and their families have access to mental health care based upon the best available evidence and provided by staff with an appropriate range of skills and competencies.

Table 25.1 The four-tier strategic framework

Tier	Professionals providing the Service Include	Function/Service
Tier 1 A primary level of care	• GPs • Health visitors • School nurses • Social workers • Teachers • Juvenile justice workers • Voluntary agencies • Social services	CAMHS at this level are provided by professionals working in universal services who are in a position to: • Identify mental health problems early in their development • Offer general advice • Pursue opportunities for mental health promotion and prevention
Tier 2 A service provided by professionals relating to workers in primary care	• Child and Adolescent Mental Health workers • Clinical child psychologists • Paediatricians (especially community) • Educational psychologists • Child & Adolescent psychiatrists • Child and adolescent psychotherapists • Community nurses/nurse specialists • Family therapists	CAMHS professionals should be able to offer. • Training and consultation to other professionals (who might be within T1) • Consultation to professionals and families • Outreach • Assessment
Tier 3 A specialised service for more severe, complex or persistent disorders	• Child & adolescent psychiatrists • Clinical child psychologists • Nurses (community or in-patient) • Child psychotherapists • Occupational therapists • Speech and Language therapists • Art, music and drama therapists • Family therapists	Service offer: • Assessment and treatment • Assessment of referrals to T4 • Contributions to the services, consultation and training at T1 and 2.
Tier 4 Essential tertiary level services such as day units, highly specialised out-patient teams and in-patient units		• Child and adolescent in-patient units • Secure forensic units • Eating disorders units • Specialist teams (eg. for sexual abuse) • Specialist teams for neuro-psychiatric problems

Every Child Matters: Change for Children

This document (Department for Education and Skills 2004), underpinned by the legislation of The Children Act 2004, specified five outcomes which are to be targets for all services working with children.

• Be healthy
• Stay safe
• Enjoy and achieve
• Make a positive contribution
• Achieve economic well-being

(See Box 25.1. What the outcomes mean.)

In the UK, services for children have belonged to different organisations, such as health, education and social welfare. *Every Child Matters: Change for Children* (ECM) lays out principles for the integration of universal services. Targeted and specialist services are to be made available nearer to home and effective case management is to be established, led by professionals working in multidisciplinary/multiagency teams.

The Common Assessment Framework

A multiagency assessment, the Common Assessment Framework (CAF) (Department for Education and Skills 2006a), has been developed to ensure that children are referred to the appropriate specialist services. It is used by all agencies, in partnership with the family, and covers the context of a child's problems.

Box 25.1 What the outcomes mean

Be healthy	Physically healthy
	Mentally and emotionally healthy
	Sexually healthy
	Healthy lifestyles
	Choose not to take illegal drugs
	Parents, carers and families promote healthy choices
Stay safe	Safe from maltreatment, neglect, violence and sexual exploitation
	Safe from accidental injury and death
	Safe from bullying and discrimination
	Safe from crime and antisocial behaviour in and out of school
	Have security, stability and are cared for
	Parents, carers and families provide safe homes and stability
Enjoy and achieve	Ready for school
	Attend and enjoy school
	Achieve stretching national educational standards at primary school
	Achieve personal and social development and enjoy recreation
	Achieve stretching national educational standards at secondary school
	Parents, carers and families support learning
Make a positive contribution	Engage in decision making and support the community and environment
	Engage in law-abiding and positive behaviour in and out of school
	Develop positive relationships and choose not to bully and discriminate
	Develop self-confidence and successfully deal with significant life changes and challenges
	Develop enterprising behaviour
	Parents, carers and families promote positive behaviour
Achieve economic well-being	Engage in further education, employment or training on leaving school
	Ready for employment
	Live in decent homes and sustainable communities
	Access to transport and material goods
	Live in households free from low income
	Parents, carers and families are supported to be economically active

Many children continue to be referred to specialist CAMH services with problems arising from their familial and social environments, which may be more appropriately helped in the social care or voluntary sector, whereas there are other children with developmental disorders who go unnoticed.

A comprehensive assessment which actively involves the family should ensure referral to the appropriate agency from the start but will not take the place of specialist assessments of occupational or psychological performance or for psychiatric diagnosis.

MENTAL HEALTH PROBLEMS AND DISORDERS OF CHILDREN AND YOUNG PEOPLE

In England and Wales, 10% of 5–15 year olds have a diagnosable mental disorder, which indicates that around 1.1 million children and young people under 18 would benefit from specialist services. It is estimated that only about 60% of children with a disorder receive the appropriate service. Another 10% of children and young people have less serious mental health problems and will be helped by services in primary health care, social care, education and the voluntary sector. Some children are at greater risk of developing mental health problems or disorders, for example, looked-after children. That is, children in care of local authorities are five times more likely to have a mental disorder and children with significant learning disabilities are 3–4 times more likely. Forty percent of young offenders have been found to have a diagnosable mental disorder (DoH 2004).

PRESENTING PROBLEMS

Children and young people experience similar mental disorders to adults but changes in behaviour may be the first sign of difficulties. A young child struggles to concentrate in class and distracts other children or an adolescent has uncharacteristic outbursts of anger. Another child may complain of aches and pains and refuse to go to school. There could be many reasons for a child's distress so it is important that a general assessment is made initially, which will cover the family circumstances and stresses as well as the child's individual needs.

Case example

A 6-year-old boy is restless in class and cannot concentrate on his work. His mother says that she is at the end of her tether and that something must be done to sort out his difficult behaviour. There could be many factors explaining this child's problems.

- He has a new teacher and struggles with her different approach, then takes out his frustrations at home.
- He is being bullied in the playground but does not tell anyone.

- His family has moved to a hostel and are sharing one room.
- His father has left the family and is not seeing his son.
- His favourite grandparent has died recently.
- His mother has postnatal depression following the birth of the new baby.
- He has unidentified developmental problems which affect his social or intellectual abilities.
- His parents disagree on how to manage their child's behaviour.

A full assessment will show which agency would be best placed to help this family: education, housing, mediation service, adult mental health, community paediatrician or a parenting programme run by the voluntary sector. Primary mental health workers and professionals from specialist CAMHS offer advice, training and consultation to primary care agencies so that they are aware of mental health issues and the services available. Children and young people referred to specialist CAMHS will receive additional assessment for diagnostic and treatment purposes.

TYPES OF MENTAL DISORDER IN CHILDREN AND YOUNG PEOPLE

Evans (2001) suggested that occupational therapists in CAMHS need a working knowledge of diagnostic categories but warned that a developmental framework and a family assessment are also needed. Children and young people experience the same range of emotional disorders as adults, such as depression, anxiety and obsessional disorders. Emotional disorders account for 25–33% of CAMHS clinic attendees, whilst eating disorders represent 2–5% (Evans 2001). Anorexia nervosa is identified in 0.5–1% of 12–19 year olds and is 8–12 times more common in girls than boys.

Conduct disorders in young children consist of oppositional behaviour at home and/or school and can lead to antisocial behaviours in adolescence, such as violent and aggressive behaviour, theft or fire setting. However, they can also be a reaction to bullying, frustration or abuse, as some young people cope with sadness or fear by showing aggression. There is debate within CAMH services as to where children and young people exhibiting difficult behaviour are best helped, since other agencies may have more useful skills in this area. Youth services may provide local projects aimed at groups of young people to encourage multicultural activities. Sports programmes could help young people expend their energies in a healthier direction. Positive Activities for Young People (PAYP) programmes were established to reduce criminal activity (Department for Education and Skills 2006b).

Neurodevelopmental disorders are conditions where the child's brain functioning is affected. These include learning disabilities, autistic spectrum disorder (ASD) and attention deficit hyperactivity disorder (ADHD), which all affect cognitive processing and social functioning.

Children who have had a poor or non-existent relationship with a carer in the first few months and years of life may develop an attachment disorder; however, this is a description of a relationship problem rather than a difficulty within the child. This is not uncommon in looked-after children who may have had several carers from a young age. This can affect future relationships and the associated behaviour difficulties are sometimes confused with other diagnoses, such as ADHD.

CHILDREN IN FAMILIES

The most important factor in the mental health of all children is the nature of their care. A sensitive parent/carer who is responsive to the child's needs and reciprocates communications will aid the development of the child's psychological well-being. The family is the first source of personal and social identity and provides a structure of habits and routines from which the child develops a sense of self, learns essential skills and builds relationships.

In a healthy family, the structure and routines are sufficiently flexible to respond to the differing needs of growing children. Preschool children require clear and consistent boundaries to protect and nurture them, whereas adolescents need more freedom to experiment and take risks in order to learn by experience. There are many styles of families according to culture and circumstances.

Families headed by one parent are increasingly common. The risk factors attributed to this type of family are more likely to be associated with the effects of poverty, poor housing and isolation than

with the quality of relationships. In some cultures the extended family plays a major role in child rearing, whereby grandmothers or aunts will care for children of working mothers, but there can also be differences of opinions on appropriate methods of bringing up the children. Step-families, where one or both parents have established a new partnership, may give the children a broader experience of family styles and access to a larger extended family or may be a source of conflicting views and loss of contact with a parent.

OCCUPATIONAL THERAPY IN CAMHS

Occupational therapists work in all areas of CAMHS and may be employed by a variety of agencies. Both the Health Advisory Service review (1995) and the NSF (DoH 2004) recommended that occupational therapists should be represented in core CAMHS teams. CAMHS occupational therapists in the UK may be employed by mental health trusts, primary care trusts, education services or the voluntary sector, which consists of charities established to provide services for children and their families independently from statutory organisations. CAMHS mapping exercises, carried out between 2003 and 2005, found around 120 occupational therapists working in CAMHS, although this does not include those working as primary mental health workers (www.camhsmapping.org.uk). These surveys were also unlikely to have counted occupational therapists working in the voluntary sector, education or children's centres.

The first British conference for occupational therapists in CAMHS, held in 2004, attracted over 100 delegates working in all aspects of CAMHS: primary mental health, specialist outpatients and residential services. Although they make up a small proportion of the profession, occupational therapists in CAMHS use a wide range of approaches and therapeutic interventions. Polichroniadis (2004) surveyed occupational therapy practice in CAMHS and found that respondents were enthusiastic and committed to their work, and were continuing to develop their professional role.

Many theories are used to inform practice so that three occupational therapists working in a service could use different frames of reference and approaches, influenced by the type of setting, service aims and their own area of interest. For example, one may use a psychosocial approach in working with adolescents or play therapy with younger children, another may use a sensory integrative approach for children with ADHD, and a third may use a community development approach in neighbourhood settings. All, however, will have assessed the child/young person's present range and balance of occupations and occupational performance, and each therapist will be using a theory of occupation, shifting their perspective from occupation, to activity, to task, to skill and back again (Creek 2003).

The approach used is influenced by the underpinning theories, so that the occupational therapist working with adolescents will be focusing on activities and tasks in order to achieve the goal of improving social skills, whereas her colleague treating children with ADHD has a greater focus on skills development. The occupational therapy process may appear very different when the underlying shifts of perspective are not visible to a colleague from another discipline or to parents of children attending CAMHS. Such a variety of approaches may confuse other staff, and even possibly other occupational therapists, as to the role of occupational therapy in CAMHS.

In the UK, as mentioned above, there has been guidance from the government to differentiate between the universal and more specialised services available for children and young people with mental health problems (DoH 2004, Health Advisory Service 1995). The emphasis is on agencies working together to provide a more co-ordinated service, but with greater clarity as to the contribution of each agency. Occupational therapy has a role at each level of intervention.

TIERS 1 AND 2: HEALTH PROMOTION AND EARLY INTERVENTION

In 1995, the Health Advisory Service acknowledged the contribution made by universal services/primary care and community projects to children's emotional well-being. Health visitors have always advised new mothers on how to care for their babies and meet their needs, both practically and emotionally, school nurses advise on bedwetting

and behaviour problems and teachers encourage children to learn social skills as well as teaching more curriculum-based activities. Agencies in the voluntary sector, such as Homestart, NSPCC, NCH and the Family Welfare Association, to name only a few, have been running children's projects for many years and provide practical support for families and children. Now, a new role of primary mental health worker (PMHW) has been created in order to provide consultation, training, joint assessments and mental health promotion programmes for these services. Occupational therapists have taken up this new role of PMHW and have been able to expand the contribution of occupational therapy in CAMHS.

> I think I am MORE of an occupational therapist since becoming a Primary Mental Health Worker! Practically everything I do with families or professionals involves a functional assessment of occupation, be it play, parenting or paid employment. (Anderson 2004, personal communication)

Wilcock (1998a) proposed a wider role for occupational therapy in public health by suggesting that health and well-being result from individuals being in tune with their occupational nature.

Scaletti (1999) described a community development model for child, adolescent and family mental health services designed to be practised along a continuum from developmental casework to the client's involvement in community and social movements. 'The link between mental health, occupation and community is reinforced through a community development approach that empowers clients to develop their occupational roles of choice' (Scaletti 1999, p46).

Watson (2004, p6), writing about community-based rehabilitation in South Africa, suggested that:

> Making positive choices about occupations that have personal meaning for the individual, that are health promoting and that are also valued by others, can change a way of life. How this becomes part of occupational therapy practice, and what to change so that the needs of individuals, groups and populations can be addressed, has not yet been fully established.

Scriven & Atwal (2004) described three levels of health promotion.

- **Primary health promotion**: targets whole populations, aiming to prevent ill health by health education campaigns or legislation, for example, anti-smoking campaigns.
- **Secondary health promotion**: targeted at individuals or groups who may be at risk due to their health-damaging habits, for example, healthy eating programmes for overweight people.
- **Tertiary health promotion**: client-centred approaches for those who already have a specific condition or disability, for example, a rehabilitation programme.

Scriven & Atwal suggested that occupational therapists make a considerable contribution to health promotion action at a secondary and a tertiary level but that it would necessitate a paradigm shift in perception of roles and professional practice to become involved in primary health promotion. It is this shift in paradigm that Wilcock proposed:

> ... practitioners focusing on promoting the health-giving relationship of occupation have to consider or explore all levels by focusing on what and how it can improve physical, mental, social, spiritual and environmental wellbeing. (Wilcock 2006, p312)

In working with children, there is already a movement away from an illness treatment model to a mediating, enabling and advocating role, whether working within or outside the health service. Occupational therapists are in a strong position to apply the principles of occupational choice in health promotion and community development by taking on the new posts being established, such as primary mental health workers, or positions in children's centres and community projects run by the voluntary sector. This echoes the call in *Together We Stand* (Health Advisory Service 1995) for the mental health of children and adolescents to become everyone's business rather than the preserve of specialist CAMHS teams, and recognises the need for early intervention before patterns of illness are established. Occupational therapists may use their knowledge and skills directly with children and families or in training or consultation with other workers to promote the mental health needs of children.

Occupational therapy in tiers 1 and 2

Occupational therapists working in the field of early intervention, health promotion and community development to address the mental health needs of children and adolescents may focus on an individual child and family, on the local community or on the wider population.

The individual child and family

Interventions include the development of personal skills to facilitate occupational potential and are similar to tertiary health promotion. Wilcock (2006) suggested two aspects: the promotion of health and well-being and the prevention of illness and disability. Interventions may involve working with an individual within the family or with groups of peers. For example, an occupational therapist in the role of PMHW may suggest activities for parents and children which will help the child's sensory processing, where this seems to be contributing to the child's behaviour problems (Saunders 2004, personal communication). An occupational therapist/PMHW based in a school devised an anti-bullying programme that involved role play and activities on developing skills in anger management, assertiveness and self-awareness (Harrison 2004, personal communication, Killett 2004, personal communication).

Such programmes also enable young people to learn how to establish mutual support networks.

Community development approach

Community development involves 'Community consultation, deliberation and action to promote individual, family and community-wide responsibility for self sustaining development, health and wellbeing' (Wilcock 1998b, p238). This includes the facilitation of occupational change and the growth of community contacts, according to the child or family's perceived needs. For example, occupational therapists working in children's centres might respond to the requests from parents on how to promote the emotional and behavioural development of their preschool children by running groups on the use of play. Within children's centres parents have the opportunity to access accredited learning programmes should they wish to develop a career in child care (Bovan & O'Rafferty 2004, Larcombe 2004, personal communication). Children may join a school group and learn about traffic rules and safety issues, later becoming part of the school crossing patrol team (Scaletti 1999).

Wilcock (2006) suggested that community development needs to be combined with concern for eco-sustainability. For example, groups of young people may be involved in cleaning out a pond or designing an eco shelter out of straw bales as a meeting place (Benjamin 2006).

Social justice

A wider population approach involves 'Promotion of social and economic change to increase individual, community and political awareness, resources and equitable opportunities for health (Wilcock 1998b, p235). This has led to occupational therapists coining the term *occupational justice* (see Chapter 3), which includes the concept of occupational deprivation.

Children may lack occupations due to understimulation from caregivers or due to their status as asylum seekers with restricted freedom of movement. In order to promote occupational justice, occupational therapists may need to become involved in social and political lobbying for change of policies toward occupational equity. For example, in New Zealand, occupational therapists in CAMHS suggested enabling adolescents to become involved in youth councils and their parents to act as school governors so that they are able to influence the policies that affect their communities (Scaletti 1999).

These are examples of occupational therapy concerned with the mental health needs of children and adolescents being directed towards community-oriented programmes and, as such, they represent small steps towards a major redevelopment of professional focus.

TIER 3: SPECIALIST CAMHS OUTPATIENT TEAMS

Working in CAMHS requires occupational therapists to make significant adjustments in their attitude towards the concept of mental health and

to extend further their clinical knowledge base. Some of the challenges faced by an occupational therapist wishing to specialise in child mental health are:

- learning to view clients, that is, children and adolescents, within the context of their families rather than as autonomous individuals
- gaining a greater knowledge and understanding of childhood difficulties, disorders and child-specific therapies
- developing the ability to work, often in professional isolation, within a multidisciplinary team.

Each of these challenges could apply to the occupational therapist working in any CAMH service but here they are considered with respect to working in a specialist or outpatient CAMH service.

Children within the family context

Because of their immaturity, children and, to a lesser extent, adolescents depend on others to meet their emotional, social and physical needs. In recognition of a child's level of dependence most CAMHS interventions include meetings with family members and/or carers in order to get a full history of the presenting problems and current concerns. Attending a clinic for an initial assessment may be a stressful experience for both the child and family. However, having all family members attend the assessment appointment can provide some emotional security for the referred child, as well as starting to involve parents/carers in the planning of their child's therapy.

It is essential to engage the parents/carers at an early stage of treatment as they may be vital to the successful outcome. Parents may need to be involved in the child's therapy in a number of differing ways, ranging from providing transport for the child/adolescent so that they can attend appointments to becoming involved themselves in meetings of a therapeutic nature. Whilst some clinicians prefer to see parents/carers alone for the first meeting, others invite the whole family and then spend time separately with the older child/adolescent as part of the joint appointment.

Regardless of the preferred assessment format, a child or adolescent will be viewed as part of a family system in order for the clinician to best understand how problems may have arisen and how they have been addressed previously. Sometimes during an initial assessment the family will recognise how relationships or past experiences have directly or indirectly affected their child; these kinds of insights may lead to parents also becoming clients and undertaking therapy with their child. This may be in family therapy or separately, for example, by attending a parenting group.

This way of working requires the occupational therapist to be able to consider the emotional needs of several members of a family simultaneously in order to develop a trusting working relationship with each family member. Such working relationships may include parents who are not directly involved in the child's day-to-day care, such as may be found in divorced/separated families or with children in foster care. In order for the occupational therapist to work collaboratively with both children and their families in this way, she will need to be proficient in her use of self (Hagedorn 1995, 2001) and have well-developed interpersonal communication skills.

The occupational therapist working in CAMHS will also require a thorough knowledge of the emotional development of children with respect to their familial and social relationships, in order to identify appropriate goals of treatment. This knowledge will help to inform the occupational therapist's assessment of the child's progress in therapy, the probable duration of the intervention and the likely outcome.

Working with a child on an individual basis, whilst taking account of the family context, requires the therapist to provide parents/carers with regular feedback about their child's welfare and ongoing needs. Any feedback given regarding the child's progress in therapy should be informative whilst ensuring an appropriate level of confidentiality for the child. In all instances, occupational therapists are advised to make use of both clinical and managerial supervision within their particular CAMH service, in order to ensure their clients' privacy whilst at the same time sharing appropriate information with the wider systems/services that provide care for them.

Childhood difficulties, disorders and child–specific therapies

Working in child mental health can present the occupational therapist with an opportunity to work with problems she would not encounter in any other service. Some presenting problems are unique to childhood, for example:

- child abuse, i.e. emotional, sexual and physical abuse and neglect
- conduct or behavioural problems
- elimination disorders, i.e. enuresis and encopresis
- attention deficit hyperactive disorder (ADHD).

Some of the problems referred to a tier 3 CAMH service begin in childhood or adolescence but either take a long time to address, and therefore lead into adulthood, or are resolved in the short term but then re-emerge later in life, for example eating disorders, including both anorexia nervosa and bulimia nervosa, anxiety states and phobias, deliberate self-harm and depression. It is here that occupational therapists need to use their knowledge of the characteristic emotional and cognitive development of adolescence in order to understand the difficulties faced by their clients at this transitional stage of their lives. Careful liaison with adult mental health services may be required in order for the occupational therapist to ensure continuity in the care of older adolescents when they are transferring to adult services, which may not routinely cater for the needs of young people.

Given the speed of the development which occurs in childhood and adolescence, it is not surprising that there is a considerable variety of needs within this client group. While some clinicians have a range of ages in their caseload, many prefer to specialise in an age group, frequently choosing either primary school-aged children or adolescents in order to focus on the psychodynamic issues that pertain to each.

Many occupational therapists who attend to the needs of primary school-aged children develop skills in play therapy, in recognition of play being a process inherent in normal child development (Lougher 2001). There are several forms of play therapy, the most commonly practised being structured or focused play therapy (Carroll 1998, Wilson et al 1992) and non-directive play therapy

(Wilson et al 1992). Since occupational therapists use activities to meet developmental goals in therapy (Hagedorn 1995), many are comfortable with the use of structured/focused play therapy methods. In structured/focused play therapy the clinician chooses an activity that she believes will have some therapeutic value for the client. Examples of such activities vary from those intended to develop self-esteem through the acquisition of specific skills to activities selected for their value as projective tools, for example those used to facilitate the expression of thoughts and feelings.

It is a matter of debate where occupational therapy that utilises play activities ends and play therapy begins but some clarity can be found when the therapist adopts a specific play therapy approach such as non-directive play therapy. Non-directive play therapy is based on Rogerian principles and, as such, fits well with the philosophy of humanism that is evident in occupational therapy (Bruce & Borg 1993). Unlike the structured/focused play therapy commonly used in CAMH services, in non-directive play therapy it is the child who selects what to play with, sets the agenda for each session and determines the pace of the therapy. In this truly client-centred approach, the therapist follows the child's lead and does not ask any questions nor offer encouragement or praise.

Although appearing simple in principle, non-directive play therapy in practice requires a great deal of self-discipline, insight and self-awareness on the part of the clinician (Lewis & Miller 1990). Postgraduate training is highly recommended for the occupational therapist who wishes to specialise in play therapy; only courses accredited by the British Association of Play Therapy (BAPT) provide a licence to practise as and use the (as yet unprotected) title of play therapist.

According to Erikson's theory of psychosocial development (Pownall 2001), adolescence is a time of individuation, of identity formation, a time of transition from childhood to adulthood. In CAMHS, the occupational therapist may adopt the developmental view of adolescence, seeing it as characterised by the need for an individual to acquire both practical and emotional independent living skills, for example the

organisation of leisure or work activities and the development of social and sexual relationships. Within the developmental approach, occupational therapists recognise the importance of interpersonal relationships during adolescence and may provide group work in order to facilitate peer group experiences (Flanigan 2001) alongside individual cognitive behavioural therapy and family work.

The occupational therapist may work in the community to help an adolescent develop the independent living skills he requires, alongside school support staff, social workers and youth workers. As a matter of course, the occupational therapist will liaise with all those involved in the adolescent's care (including the family) while perhaps affording a greater level of confidentiality than they would to younger children, in recognition of the different level of maturity of the adolescent.

Matters concerning child protection still pertain to adolescents and, once again, supervision can assist the occupational therapist in the management of cases when such situations arise. All occupational therapists working in CAMH services must be able to recognise signs of abuse in children/adolescents and familiarise themselves with the child protection procedures that exist within their local authority.

Multidisciplinary team working

Multidisciplinary team working is commonplace in mental health services and is typical of both inpatient and outpatient services. Multidisciplinary teams vary in size but due to the degree of co-working required, most will have a shared case review system in which care/treatment plans are discussed with the whole team. Multidisciplinary teams usually consist of the professionals found in most other areas of mental health, for example psychologists, psychiatrists and mental health nurses.

Often, professionals in tier 3 CAMH services find that they need to advance their knowledge base and clinical skills by undertaking postgraduate training in child-related therapies such as play therapy or family therapy. As a consequence, multidisciplinary teams can consist of team members with a number of different professional backgrounds and titles, in addition to various trainees, assistants and those with generic titles, such as child therapist.

In some CAMH services, multidisciplinary teams have been created to address specific disorders and conditions, for example ADHD. Tier 3 services are typified by therapy being provided by more than one clinician – that is, a multidisciplinary approach. Often, families using CAMH services undertake programmes of therapeutic interventions offered in parallel, for example family work running alongside individual sessions, or in tandem, for example a parenting group occurring after family sessions. As a multidisciplinary team member, the occupational therapist may act as a case manager, overseeing a multidisciplinary treatment/care plan agreed for her clients on her own caseload.

The culture of the multidisciplinary team and its approach will affect the professional development of the occupational therapist and the services she offers. Many CAMH services are behavioural or psychodynamic in orientation, which fits well with occupational therapy practice that uses an object relations frame of reference (Bruce & Borg 1993). However, the occupational therapist who aims to provide a truly client-directed approach may find it difficult to reconcile these values with those of the medical model usually found in consultant-lead teams (Hagedorn 2001). The need to compromise professional ideals in order to form an eclectic team approach has led to multidisciplinary team working being criticised for bringing about role confusion (Lougher 2001).

The challenges for an occupational therapist working in a tier 3 CAMH service are no more or less than those of any other professional but are perhaps emphasised by her professional isolation, as she will often be the only occupational therapist in the team. Equally, the variety of models used by different occupational therapists in one CAMH service can cause confusion for colleagues and referrers alike, as the overarching occupational therapy philosophy which underlies their practice is obscured by their differing treatment modalities and approaches. The need for professional cohesion and networking, particularly with other CAMHS occupational therapists, is of continuing importance.

TIER 3: ATTENTION DEFICIT HYPERACTIVITY DISORDER

Attention deficit hyperactivity disorder (ADHD) is a complex neurodevelopmental disorder characterised by excessive inattentiveness, hyperactivity and impulsiveness, which has significant impact on a child's everyday life at home and at school. There is no single aetiology. Various studies have highlighted differences in brain anatomy, genetic links and chemical imbalances in the attention centre of the brain. It is a hidden disability that only becomes recognisable through behavioural manifestations (Dowdy et al 1998).

The main symptoms of ADHD are as follows.

- **Inattention**. Inability to sustain concentration on any activity requiring focused thought. Cognitive tasks that have frequent rewards, for example computer games, are attended to much better.
- **Hyperactivity.** An excess of motor activity compared to what is demanded of the situation.
- **Impulsivity.** A tendency to act on sudden urges or desires.

Many research studies have looked at the prevalence of ADHD and results vary from 2% to 7% of the school-age population (Barkley 1998). A prevalence of 5% would indicate that there are 345,000 children in England and 21,000 children in Wales who have the disorder. These figures make ADHD one of the most common disorders of childhood and adolescence. It is also considered to be one of the most significant causes of educational and social failure.

Studies also demonstrate a wide range of boy: girl ratios ranging from 3:1 to 9:1. Certainly, in most clinics there is a higher number of boys on clinicians' caseloads. Girls with ADHD tend to present with less hyperactivity and as a result are less disruptive than hyperactive boys. It has been suggested that many girls with ADHD are not being identified and treated.

Historically, children with ADHD have been seen within the general CAMH services and within community children's health services. This has often resulted in isolated interventions. Due to the complex nature of the condition, services for children with ADHD have adopted a more multidisciplinary team approach. Many services have developed specialist teams to offer a more seamless service to the children and their families. Occupational therapy for children with ADHD is a developing field in the UK (Chu 2002).

Assessment

Specialist teams dedicate considerable time to the detailed assessment of children who attend clinics. It is good practice to gather information from home and school in the initial stages and the teams offer school observations, school liaison, home assessments, evaluation of rating scales and developmental assessments to gather a detailed history of symptoms. The disorder is most prominent in day-to-day adaptive functioning in the classroom and social domains, so information from school provides more reliable information for making a diagnosis (Barkley 1994). Occupational therapists contribute important information which may help with the diagnosis of ADHD or suggest other reasons for the presentation of symptoms.

Assessment of motor skills, perceptual skills, sensory integration, visual-motor integration skills, executive control processes and communication skills helps to establish the child's general development level. The use of standardised assessment tools can assist in the identification of difficulties, for example the Winnie Dunn Sensory Profile (Dunn 1999) or ABC Movement Assessment Battery for Children (Henderson & Sugden 1992), as can clinical observations in school, at play and at home. This assessment will also help with identification of co-morbidities such as developmental co-ordination disorder (DCD), autistic spectrum disorders and specific learning difficulties.

Diagnosis is often lengthy and painstaking and is made following careful analysis of information provided by all team members. It is important that other medical conditions, developmental disorders or family/social circumstances are excluded before a diagnosis of ADHD is made, as many other reasons may contribute to a similar pattern of behaviour. These include social pressures, which could include drug use, domestic violence and crime, along with parenting styles, family arrangements and mother–child attachment.

In order for ADHD to be diagnosed, the criteria in the *Diagnostic and Statistical Manual of Mental Disorders* (DSM IV; American Psychiatric Association 1994) or the *International Classification of Diseases* (ICD-10) need to be considered. These include:

- onset before the age of 7 years
- persistent symptoms for at least 6 months
- symptoms present in at least two environments
- symptoms causing significant functional impairment.

Multiagency meetings are essential in making sense of the information gathered from assessments. It is important that all significant parties involved with the child (parents/carers, school, health) meet to review the information, identify a suitable diagnosis and agree on a management plan.

Intervention

Attention deficit hyperactivity disorder is a complex neurobiological disorder which can manifest itself in varying degrees of difficulty. It can have a huge impact on the day-to-day functioning of individuals and their families, peers and teachers. None of the treatments and interventions currently available provide any cure for the disorder, they only provide symptomatic relief. Multidisciplinary and multiagency teams have been recognised to be essential in the delivery of an effective service, and the treatment of ADHD requires the partnership of the health team, the family and school.

Medical management

The National Institute of Clinical Excellence published guidelines (National Institute of Clinical Excellence 2000) which recommended that the first-line treatment for children with ADHD is the use of stimulant medication, for example, methylphenidate (Ritalin). This medication works by stimulating the brain to improve concentration and reduce hyperactivity and impulsiveness. Studies have shown a 70–75% probability of improvement in a child who has been diagnosed with ADHD.

Methylphenidate is a licensed drug and needs careful monitoring. Hospital clinics monitor a child's growth, weight and blood pressure regularly.

Parent support

Parent support is vital through the diagnosis and intervention stages. Psychoeducation and behaviour management skills are necessary to support medical intervention. A study carried out by the Attention Deficit Disorder Information and Support Services (ADDISS 2006) of 500 parents of children with ADHD highlighted that two-thirds of the parents had divorced, separated or experienced marital distress due to their child's disorder. Fifteen percent of parents had lost their job as a direct result of caring for their ADHD child, and almost half had been treated for depression (ADDISS 2006).

School support

Regular liaison with teachers, teaching assistants and the special educational needs co-ordinator (SENCo) is essential to ensure that appropriate strategies are used to manage the symptoms of ADHD. The ADDISS study (2006) highlighted that 39% of children with ADHD had had a fixed-term exclusion from school, with 11% being excluded permanently.

Occupational therapy for ADHD

Occupational therapy is still a developing field in this area (Chu 2002) but the results of a national survey indicated that 8.5% of occupational therapists were involved in a designated service for children with ADHD in the UK (Chu 2003). The only clear evidence base is for using sensory integrative approaches, which have proved to be extremely effective. Occupational therapy interventions using this approach to treat the symptoms of ADHD are practical and usually enjoyed by children. Further research is essential so that occupational therapists continue to build their skills to provide effective interventions to the children with this condition, and their families.

Occupational therapy is concerned with improving a person's occupational performance (self-care, work, play). In a paediatric setting, the occupational therapist deals with children whose occupations are usually as players, preschoolers or students. Attention deficit hyperactivity disorder can significantly affect all these areas and there is a range of approaches that can be used to improve daily function.

Typically, children with ADHD have a sensory-seeking profile. This means that the child has an underaroused central nervous system and they are observed engaging with their environment in order for their brains to have the necessary input to work. Interventions to manage this condition may include:

- a series of sensory integration sessions with an occupational therapist in a sensory integration unit
- school/home-based interventions such as the ALERT self-regulation programme (Williams & Shellenbeger 1994)
- the use of sensory circuits – a selection of activities in a circuit to provide alerting, organising and calming sensory input. These are used at the beginning of the school day and sometimes after lunch
- sensory diet – individual activities chosen for a specific child to manage arousal levels. These can be done throughout the day to help regulate attention. For example, using fidget toys, threading (rubber ribbon which can be used around chair legs to provide sensory input whilst seated), heavy work activities to provide proprioceptive input and regular movement breaks incorporated into daily activities
- participation in sports.

Teachers often appreciate suggestions to help modify behaviour because they fit well into classroom routines (Chu 2004). These include (Chu 2002):

- room arrangements – for example, position in class, distractions, personal space, buddy systems
- classroom organisation – for example, alternating activities which require high levels of concentration with tasks that require less effort, such as a seated literacy activity followed by a practical task involving more movement
- curriculum modification – volume of work, different recording methods, modification of task
- performance-promoting strategies – for example, clear step-by-step instructions, using other methods of recording, encouraging repetition

- behavioural management strategies – for example, rewards, punishments and feedback, specific praise.

Many children with ADHD do not engage in activities such as after-school clubs because their behaviour has led to them being banned from participating. Recent studies have highlighted the use of sport to manage ADHD symptoms and increase self esteem in an individual (Lopez-Williams 2005). This is an area which needs to be investigated more by occupational therapists, as there is little research available at present.

During assessment, co-morbid conditions may have been highlighted that may also need input. For example, impaired visual-motor integration resulting in untidy, slow, laborious handwriting may benefit from a handwriting programme.

TIER 4: SPECIALIST CAMH TREATMENT SETTINGS

Tier 4 services are described as essential tertiary services (Health Advisory Service 1995) and include day units, highly specialised outpatient teams and inpatient units for older children and adolescents who are severely mentally ill or at risk of suicide. Specialist services include: eating disorder services, specialist treatment teams based in community settings, youth offending teams and looked-after children's services. These services are infrequently used and may need to be provided on a supra-district level, as not all districts could expect to offer this level of expertise.

Since the publication, in 1995, of the Health Advisory Service review, debate has raged about how essential tertiary services should be constituted, especially in relation to the role and function of inpatient adolescent units, which have in many areas predated the development of outpatient teams. More recently, the change agenda has transformed services and challenged traditional patterns of service delivery. Investment and service planning have been targeted towards providing equitable access to services nationally and towards providing greater access to short-term therapies, such as cognitive behavioural and solution-focused therapy.

There has always been a belief that inpatient care for young people should be avoided wherever possible, alongside recognition of the importance of maintaining a degree of developmental normality in the young person's life and the danger of institutionalisation. It is also argued that inpatient care is less effective than outpatient care; for example, research in the field of adolescent eating disorders casts doubts on the benefits of inpatient care versus outpatient treatment (Gowers et al 1994).

Inpatient services have responded to such criticisms and are now demonstrating a willingness to change and develop. For example, newly developed inpatient eating disorder services are planned nationally, as specialist units offer an intensity of treatment that is uneconomic to deliver locally. Many such units offer a wider variety of treatment options than just inpatient beds, with link workers from outpatient teams following the child or young person into the unit and providing continuity of care (Jacobs & Green 1999). They are now seen as areas of specialism that can offer group work, day care and a useful link to early-onset services.

Occupational therapy in tier four

In the 1960s, Philip Barker, a child psychiatrist, outlined a role for occupational therapists in inpatient care (Barker & Muir 1969). As a historical document, this paper is interesting for highlighting changes that have impacted on services and on the profession itself. It is also interesting to note that treatment media have changed while many of the early objectives of treatment have stayed the same. Dr Barker warned the profession against seeing ourselves as psychotherapists and reminded us of the need to use our core skills, a message as relevant now as then.

In the 1990s, Flewker-Barker & Stephenson (1996) explored the role of the occupational therapist in child mental health within their own service in Aberdeen, where the overlapping of roles across paediatrics and child mental health helped them to define a practice that is truly holistic and integrated. They made special mention of the role that the occupational therapist has in assessing motor skills, apart from the more traditional responsibility to offer group therapy.

More recently, Flanigan (2001) discussed the task of being a therapist within a child and adolescent unit and defined the skills she believed occupational therapists need to work in such settings: retaining an activity focus and coming to terms with their own adolescent issues.

The latter two accounts describe different theoretical approaches, sensory motor skills in Aberdeen and family and psychodynamic work in Flanigan's accounts, but both describe a large area of overlapping common practice and both mention the importance of group work skills.

Occupational therapists in inpatient units embrace tasks that sit comfortably with the focus of the profession. Inpatient units have an important assessment function: young people are available for assessment and a detailed report of functional ability can be undertaken, prior to beginning treatments that are supported by the whole treatment team. Clients referred to the specialist tier 4 services often have complex pathologies and require a range of assessments. The occupational therapist's knowledge of motor skills assessment and of sensory and cognitive functioning can be vital in gaining an understanding of why a child is struggling with a range of difficulties.

A comprehensive range of treatments has been identified as essential in inpatient units, including drug therapy, cognitive and behaviour therapies, group therapy and family therapy (Hartwell et al 2005). Parent training, psychodynamic psychotherapy, social skills training, play therapy, art, music and drama therapy are all desirable options. Occupational therapists use many of these interventions but will work from an occupational performance perspective; it is unlikely that cognitive behavioural therapy offered by an occupational therapist will incorporate the same content or media as that offered by another member of the treatment team. (See Chapter 16)

Adolescents struggle to negotiate the transition from child to adult, reviewing their roles and redefining themselves as responsible young adults. This takes place against the background of mental ill health and the skills of the occupational therapist to negotiate, process and liaise with the environment of the young person are very important. Wider networks need to be involved in the young person's rehabilitation, including youth workers community workers, teachers, Connexions advisors and parents.

SUMMARY

This chapter has examined the contribution made by occupational therapy to children's mental health. Occupational therapists have opportunities to use their skills in mental health promotion as well as in specialist interventions. They contribute their understanding of the value of occupation in order to support children accessing the range of activities required for their health and development, as well as using activities in therapy.

All work with children entails working closely with parents or carers. The emphasis on cross-agency working and opportunities to work in non-statutory settings fit well with the profession's philosophy of engaging with a person within his own context.

Future advancements in the use of sensory integration in the neurodevelopmental field and health promotion in community settings suggest that occupational therapists interested in children's mental health will be able to contribute to development of occupational therapy practice.

References

ADDISS 2006 ADDISS families survey. Available online at: www.addiss.co.uk

American Psychiatric Association 1994 Diagnostic and statistical manual of mental disorder, 4th edn. American Psychiatric Press, Washington

Barker P, Muir A 1969 The role of occupational therapy in a children's inpatient psychiatric unit. American Journal of Occupational Therapy XX: iii

Barkley RA 1994 Programme manual for Video 'ADHD – what can we do? Guilford Press, New York

Barkley RA 1998 ADHD – a handbook for diagnosis and treatment, 2nd edn. Guilford Press, New York

Benjamin A 2006 Eco shelter gives teens a place to go. Guardian, London

Bovan T, O'Rafferty J 2004 The role of the occupational therapist in Sure Start. NAPOT Journal 8(3): 30-31

Bruce MA, Borg B 1993 Psychosocial occupational therapy: frames of reference for intervention, 2nd edn. Slack, New Jersey

Carroll J 1998 Introduction to therapeutic play. Blackwell Science, Oxford

Chu S 2002 Occupational therapy for children with ADHD – a neuropsychobehavioural model. Lecture notes, NAPOT Conference

Chu S 2003 Occupational therapy for children with ADHD: a survey on the level of involvement and training needs of therapists. British Journal of Occupational Therapy 66(5): 209-218

Chu S 2004 Occupational therapy for children with ADHD: research protocol training course manual.

Creek J 2003 Occupational therapy defined as a complex intervention. College of Occupational Therapists, London

Csikszentmihalyi M 1993 Activity and happiness – towards a science of occupation. Occupational Science 1(1): 38-42

Department for Education and Skills 2004 Every child matters: change for children. DfES Publications, London

Department for Education and Skills 2006a The common assessment framework for children and young people: practitioner's guide. DfES Publications, London

Department for Education and Skills 2006b Positive activities for young people – national evaluation. DfES Publications, London

Department of Health 2004 National service framework for children, young people and maternity services. Department of Health, London

Dowdy CA, Patton JR, Smith TEC et al 1998 ADHD in the classroom – a practical guide for teachers. Pro-ed, Austin, Texas

Dunn W 1999 Sensory profile – user's manual. Harcourt Assessment, San Antonio, Texas

Evans A 2001 Problems and disorders found in child and adolescent mental health. In: Lougher L (ed) Occupational therapy for child and adolescent mental health. Churchill Livingstone, Edinburgh

Flanigan A 2001 Occupational therapy with adolescents. In: Lougher L (ed) Occupational therapy for child and adolescent mental health. Churchill Livingstone, Edinburgh, pp151-170

Flewker-Barker J, Stephenson E 1996 The role of occupational therapy in child psychiatric units. In: Chesson R, Chisholm D (eds) Child psychiatric units at the crossroad. Jessica Kingsley, London, pp124-144

Gowers S, Norton K, Halek C et al 1994 Outcomes of outpatient psychotherapy in a random allocation treatment study of anorexia nervosa. International Journal of Eating Disorders 15: 165–177

Hagedorn R 1995 Occupational therapy: perspectives and processes. Churchill Livingstone, Edinburgh

Hagedorn R 2001 Foundations for practice in occupational therapy, 3rd edn. Churchill Livingstone, Edinburgh

Hartwell E, Dugmore O, Palmer L et al (eds) 2005 Quality network for inpatient CAMHS (QNIC) service standards 2005/2006. Royal College of Psychiatrists/Royal College of Nursing, London

Health Advisory Service 1995 Together we stand – the commissioning, role and management of child and adolescent mental health services. HMSO, London

Henderson S, Sugden D 1992 The movement assessment battery for children (movement ABC) – user's manual. Harcourt Assessment, San Antonio, Texas

Humphrey R 2002 Young children's occupations: explicating the dynamics of the developmental process. American Journal of Occupational Therapy 56: 171-179

Jacobs B, Green J 1999 In-patient child psychiatry – adapting for the future. Young Minds Journal 36: 14

Lawlor MC 2003 The significance of being occupied: the social construction of childhood occupations. American Journal of Occupational Therapy 57: 424-434

Lewis M, Miller SM (eds) 1990 Handbook of developmental psychopathology. Plenum, New York,

Lopez-Williams A, Chacko A, Wymbs BT 2005 Athletic performance and social behaviour as predictors of peer acceptance in children with ADHD. Journal of Emotional and Behaviour Disorders 13(3): 173

Lougher L (ed) 2001 Occupational therapy for child and adolescent mental health. Churchill Livingstone, Edinburgh

National Institute for Clinical Excellence 2000 Technology appraisal guidance no.13. Guidance on the use of methylphenidate (Ritalin, Equasym) for attention deficit hyperactivity disorder (ADHD) in childhood. National Institute for Clinical Excellence, London

Passmore A 2003 The occupation of leisure: three typologies and their influence on mental health in adolescence. OTJR: Occupation, Participation and Health 23(2): 64-71

Pierce D 2000 Maternal management of the home as a developmental playspace for infants and toddlers. American Journal of Occupational Therapy 54(3): 290-299

Polichroniadis S 2004 A survey of occupational therapy practice in child and adolescent mental health services in the United Kingdom. Unpublished

Pownall S 2001 Aspects of child development. In: Lougher L (ed) Occupational therapy for child and adolescent mental health. Churchill Livingstone, Edinburgh, pp33-47

Primeau LA 1998 Orchestration of work and play within families. American Journal of Occupational Therapy 52(3): 188-195

Rockey J 1987 Occupational therapy with children. British Journal of Occupational Therapy 50(10): 341-342

Scaletti R 1999 A community development role for occupational therapists working with children, adolescents and their families: a mental health perspective. Australian Occupational Therapy Journal 46: 43-51

Scriven A, Atwal A 2004 Occupational therapists as primary health promoters: opportunities and barriers. British Journal of Occupational Therapy 67(10): 424-429

Watson R 2004 New horizons in occupational therapy. In: Watson R, Swartz L (eds) Transformation through occupation. Whurr, London

Wilcock A 1998a Occupation for health. British Journal of Occupational Therapy 61(8): 340-345

Wilcock A 1998b An occupational perspective of health. Slack, Thorofare, New Jersey

Wilcock A 2001 Occupation for health, volume 1: a journey from self health to prescription. College of Occupational Therapists, London

Wilcock A 2006 An occupational perspective of health, 2nd edn. Slack, Thorofare, New Jersey

Williams MS, Shellenberger S 1994 How does your engine run? A leader's guide to the Alert programme for self regulation. Therapy-Works, Albuquerque, New Mexico

Wilson K, Kendrick P, Ryan V 1992 Play therapy – a non-directive approach for children and adolescents. Baillière Tindall, London

FURTHER READING

Colby Trott M, Laurel M, Windeck S 1993 Sense-abilities: understanding sensory integration. Communication Skills Builders, Arizona

Green C, Chee K 1999 Understanding ADHD – the definite guide to attention deficit hyperactivity disorder. Random House Ballantine Publishing Group, New York

Lougher L (ed) 2001 Occupational therapy for child and adolescent mental health. Churchill Livingstone, Edinburgh

Wilcock A 2006 An occupational perspective of health, 2nd edn. Slack, Thorofare, New Jersey

USEFUL WEBSITES

ADDISS (Attention Deficit Disorder Information and Support Services): www.addiss.co.uk
British Association of Play Therapists: www.bapt.uk.com
CHADD (Children and Adults with Attention Deficit/Hyperactivity Disorder): www.chadd.org
COT Specialist Section – Children, Young People and Families: www.cot.co.uk
Sensory Integration Resources Centre: www.sinetwork.org
The Out Of Sync Child: www.out-of-sync-child.com
Young Minds: www.youngminds.org.uk

Chapter 26

Learning disabilities

Anne Fleming

INTRODUCTION

This chapter is intended as a practical guide to those entering this specialty. It is not intended to be either definitive or prescriptive in content. The text aims to serve as a reference and to direct the reader to other information that has been adequately provided and discussed elsewhere.

The Department of Health (2001) defined learning disability as including the presence of:

- a significantly reduced ability to understand new or complex information, to learn new skills (impaired intelligence), with
- a reduced ability to cope independently (impaired social functioning)
- which started before adulthood, with a lasting effect on development.

This definition applies to people with a wide range of abilities, and it can be argued that it is this range of ability which both challenges and satisfies occupational therapists in the application of their knowledge, skills and experience (Fleming & Mackintosh 2004).

The author has chosen to adopt a case study approach in order to illustrate the clinical reasoning involved in any period of intervention. The hope is that this approach will be both useful and stimulating, and that readers will find the chapter relevant regardless of the setting in which this population is encountered. The intention is to bring the reader up to date with the current philosophy of care and service provision, as determined by legislation and social policy, and to demonstrate some of the factors that make working in this specialty so interesting.

LEARNING DISABILITY SERVICES IN CONTEXT

The way in which services are provided to meet the needs of people with a learning disability is governed by the wider policy and legislative framework of the time. Hence, we have seen provision of services that utilise custodial, medical and social models of care.

Since 2000, both policy and legislation have been reviewed with significant impact on both service provision and the lives of people with a learning disability. The overarching principles of these reviews have been to:

- ensure that health and social services and other agencies work in partnership
- deliver robust and flexible community-based services for people with a learning disability
- develop an inclusive society, which respects the rights and values of all its members.

Some specific policies and pieces of legislation currently directing services in Scotland are detailed in Table 26.1. Comparable documents exist in England, Wales and Northern Ireland in most instances – for example, *The Same as You?* (Scottish Executive 2000a) equates to *Valuing People* (DoH 2001) in England and *Fulfilling the Promise* (National Assembly for Wales 2001) in Wales.

TERMINOLOGY

The definition of learning disability quoted earlier demonstrates an increasing move away from a medical model of care and the associated intelligence quotient (IQ)-related terms. While measuring IQ alone has never been sufficient to diagnose a learning disability, and the terms mild, moderate, severe and profound are still used, it is now more common to find specific descriptors of levels of need(s) in addition to specific syndromes and genetic disorders. The Scottish Executive (2000a) defined these levels as: everyday need, extra needs because of the presence of learning disability; and complex needs arising from both the learning disability and other difficulties such as physical and sensory impairment, mental health problems or behaviours which challenge services. There is also recognition that to meet any of these needs, the level of support required will vary. This level of support may range from occasional and short term to that of a constant and highly intensive nature.

There are many drivers continuing to bring about changes in legislation, service delivery and terminology, including:

- the *International Classification of Functioning, Disability and Health* (ICF) (World Health Organization 2001), which moves classification away from a consequence of disease to a component of the health system. This classification facilitates the standardised description of body functions and structures, ability to perform activities, participation in life situations and the environmental factors that can support or hinder performance
- the increasing involvement of people who use services, and their carers, in service planning, delivery and monitoring (Scottish Executive 2001)
- an increasing awareness that, in order to be able to offer people appropriate support, more must be known about their health needs (Cooper et al 2004).

The biopsychosocial model presented in the ICF recognises the importance both of activity in supporting participation and of the context in which it is carried out. This is, in turn, more consistent with the civil rights legislation listed in Table 26.1,

Table 26.1 Legislative framework in Scotland

Year	Title and purpose	Outcome(s)
2000	*Community Care: A Joint Future (Scottish Executive 2000b)* Recommends that agencies work in partnerships in localities through operational and strategic planning, joint budgets, services and systems	Integrated community learning disability teams Single shared assessment
2000	*The Same as You? A Review of Services for People with Learning Disabilities (Scottish Executive 2000a)* Recommends the closure of long-stay hospitals and the development of effective community-based services. Emphasis on the need for robust health needs assessment to underpin these services, and the need to involve people who use services and their carers in service planning, monitoring and development	Joint learning disabilities strategies Health needs assessments Person-centred services Development of independent advocacy services
2002	*Promoting Health, Supporting Inclusion (Scottish Executive 2002a)* Specific focus on the nursing contribution to services for people with learning disabilities. Sets out a five-tier model of care and support that is applicable to all service providers from primary care to highly specialised area services	Learning disability liaison nursing Improved awareness of learning disability issues in primary care and mainstream services
1995	*Disability Discrimination Act 1995* Details the requirements to make goods and services accessible to all members of society regardless of their ability. Includes access to buildings, transport, education, employment and information	Public awareness of disability issues raised Improved building design Increased opportunity to access desired services, amenities and facilities
2000	*Adults with Incapacity (Scotland) Act (Scottish Executive 2000c)* Makes provision for decisions to be made on behalf of adults who lack the capacity to act for themselves with regard to finances, property or personal welfare. Includes capacity to consent to treatment. The principles require that any decision must be of benefit to the adult, require minimum intervention, take account of the wishes of the adult and encourage the adult to exercise residual capacity	Multidisciplinary assessment of capacity The adult's condition and capacity to consent are kept under regular review Very specific powers of attorney can be granted
2002	*Community Care and Health (Scotland) Act (Scottish Executive 2002b)* Progresses the joint working arrangements between social and health care, and includes recommendations for charging/not charging for services, provision of accommodation and direct payments. Places a duty of care on staff to assess carers with regard to their needs and ability to provide care	Increases individual choice Recognises the demands on unpaid carers
2003	*Mental Health (Care and Treatment) (Scotland) Act (Scottish Executive 2003)* Affords new rights to people with mental health disorders, including those with a learning disability. Right of access to independent advocacy is particularly relevant, as is the right to appeal against excessive security	Robust procedures in place Duties and responsibilities of staff clearly defined

which demands that barriers in the environment to participation for people with disabilities are removed through inclusive design and changes to management procedures.

All terminology will eventually become dated and be seen as inappropriate. We need to be aware that we are dealing with individuals whom it is difficult to categorise using a non-specific term, and that people referred to occupational therapy have individual needs and should not be seen in terms of a rigid diagnostic label. The ICF comes closer than earlier classifications to reflecting the potential variations of individual complexities and needs that develop in respect of life experiences, and is more consistent with the philosophy of occupational therapy.

PREVALENCE OF PEOPLE WITH LEARNING DISABILITIES

Generally speaking, there are two main types of factor responsible for learning disabilities: genetic and environmental. The latter are factors that affect mother and/or child, during pregnancy, delivery or after birth. The causes of learning disability are shown, proportionately, in Figure 26.1.

Despite significant advances in molecular biology and genetics, medical scientific knowledge about the causes of learning disabilities is still incomplete and, in as many as one-third of all conditions, no specific cause can be identified.

Due to the progress made in medical science, and to an increased awareness of the influence of environmental factors, there has been a reduction in the number of impaired children being born, but the factors giving rise to learning disability are often difficult to prevent.

Genetic disorders

Some genetic disorders can be detected through screening tests during early pregnancy. Amniocentesis is one such test, carried out during the 18th–20th weeks of pregnancy to detect chromosomal abnormalities such as Down's syndrome. Chorionic villus sampling (CVS) has recently enabled a diagnosis to be made as early as 8 weeks, allowing the option of termination.

The fragile X syndrome is now second only to Down's syndrome as a cause of learning disability.

Despite this, between 2% and 20% of males with learning disabilities have this disorder undiagnosed. Identification of affected males is vital to enable the determination of risk in other family members. Through genetic counselling, there is potential to prevent this form of learning disability.

Genetic counselling plays a large part in reducing and preventing the incidence of learning disability in all identified genetic conditions. With advances in medical science, more genetic conditions will be identified and therefore more will potentially be prevented.

As yet, there is no method for correcting primary gene defects, despite rapid advances in genetic engineering. Substantial technical and ethical issues remain to be overcome. However, some methods of treatment are now available that can reduce or alleviate the consequences of genetic defects (Table 26.2). For instance, in phenylketonuria (PKU) which, if undetected, leads to severe learning disabilities, neonatal screening (Guthrie test) allows a restriction of the phenylalanine intake in affected children, preventing both intellectual and neurological deterioration.

Environmental factors

Much can now be done to limit environmentally caused abnormalities, that is, those occurring because of events during pregnancy, delivery and shortly after birth. Low birthweight is often associated with an increased risk of abnormality. Improved antenatal care, targeted at factors which

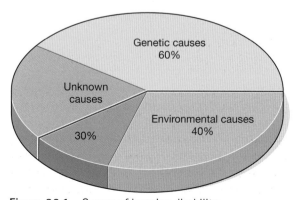

Figure 26.1 Causes of learning disability.

Table 26.2 Reducing the occurrence of genetic defects

Risk factors	Limitation/prevention
Blood relatives, e.g. aunt, grandparent	Genetic counselling
Parent with inherited genetic condition	Screening tests
Women already with a disabled child	Amniocentesis
Women over 35 having first child	CVS Termination

Table 26.3   Environmental factors

Environmental causes	Limitation/prevention
Inadequate education	Health education
Poor maternal diet	Primary health care
Smoking, excess alcohol in pregnancy	Improved living and social conditions
Poor social conditions and low income	Immunisation
Accidents or abuse	Improved obstetric and neonatal care
Maternal or postnatal infection	
Damage during birth	

contribute to lower birthweight, is now common practice. This includes education about maternal diet, alcohol, smoking and poor social conditions. In addition, there is now better monitoring of diabetes and other medical conditions in women contemplating pregnancy.

Maternal infection during pregnancy and early childhood infection increase the risk of a child becoming disabled. Immunisation plays a large part in reducing the occurrence of infections such as rubella, meningitis, whooping cough and measles. The interventions described in Table 26.3 help to reduce the risk of environmentally caused defects.

Other environmental factors which influence the incidence of abnormalities are obstetric and neonatal care. Obstetric complications and birth injuries at time of delivery are thought to account for 10% of all cases of severe learning disabilities.

Other causal factors are accidents, in the home or on the road, and child abuse.

McGrother et al (2001) described 2% of the population (UK) as comprising people with intellectual disabilities, which they attributed to socioeconomic conditions, neonatal care and longevity. The increase in longevity is giving rise to specific services for people with learning disabilities, particularly for people with Down's syndrome, who are at an increased risk of developing dementia (Watchman 2003).

Relevance to occupational therapy practice

In order to inform occupational therapy practice, it is essential to have an understanding of the factors causing learning disability. Symptoms produced by genetic conditions will remain fixed, and it is part of the challenge for the occupational therapist to find ways to modify or compensate for these symptoms (Gilbert 1996).

Environmental factors are perhaps now even more important, as people with learning disability increasingly lead more independent lives, contemplate their own relationships and have children of their own. There is, therefore, an increasing role for occupational therapists to be more involved in health promotion and education surrounding the issues described in Tables 26.2 and 26.3. As with any woman choosing to have a child, women with learning disability have the right to understand what they can do to encourage the development of a healthy baby. There are no definitive numbers available regarding the number of learning disabled people in the UK who are parents, but anecdotal evidence suggests that these numbers are on the increase. Occupational therapy staff must therefore be aware of relevant legislation and child protection issues.

THE OCCUPATIONAL THERAPY PROCESS IN LEARNING DISABILITIES

There is no theoretical framework that cannot be applied to this population. Models of intervention are adequately addressed elsewhere (for example, Chapter 4 and Hagedorn 1997) and each therapist will choose an approach from which to work. This will probably be arrived at and applied by following the occupational therapy process, as shown in Figure 26.2.

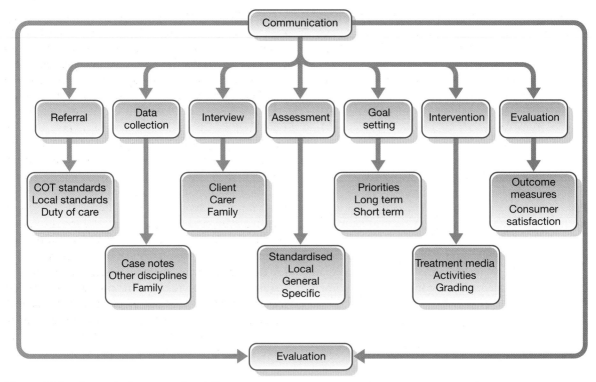

Figure 26.2 Stages in the occupational therapy process.

A case study format has been used to clarify the different stages of the occupational therapy process in a practical way.

REFERRAL

Case study: part 1

Jane was referred to the occupational therapist in the community learning disability team (CLDT), by the consultant psychiatrist in learning disabilities, for assessment. This consultant was liaising with his counterpart in adult psychiatry in accordance with a local interface agreement between the two services.

Jane had been admitted under section 24 of the Mental Health Act (Scotland) (Scottish Office 1984), as a result of a hypomanic episode secondary to polydrug misuse. She was 24 years old, with a 4 year old son, living in the parental home with her mother and grandmother (who was now in the latter stages of Alzheimer's).

This referral was accepted in duty of care terms, in accordance with both national and local practice guidance (College of Occupational Therapists 2003). Referrals can be very specific but, as in this instance, may be vague and general so that the therapist may have to apply several skills in determining how best to progress the referral. Referrals may also reflect the priorities of the person referring, and the therapist will need to apply her interview skills effectively when identifying and incorporating the wishes of her client. In some cases, due to lack of capacity or mental health status, these wishes may be communicated by an advocate, guardian, family member or carer.

Many services are now using person-centred planning (PCP) styles to assist in understanding the individual client and their particular circumstances. The government report *Valuing People* (DoH 2001) defines the five key features of PCP as:

- the person is at the centre
- family members and friends are full partners

- planning reflects the person's capacities and what is important to the person, and specifies the support he requires to make a full contribution to his community
- planning builds a shared commitment to action that will uphold the person's rights
- planning leads to continual listening, learning and action and helps the person get what he wants out of life.

Sanderson et al (1997) discussed the more commonly found PCP styles.

- **PATH**: focuses on what the individual perceives as the ideal future and the actions required to make this more attainable.
- **MAPS**: focuses on what is required to bring about change, with a specific section on the person's history, which can influence both their hopes and fears.
- **Essential lifestyle planning**: focuses on day-to-day supports and is a good way of getting to know the individual.

Occupational therapists may find themselves contributing to these valuable sources of information, as well as referring to them as sources of data.

Data collection

> **Case study: part 2**
>
> Jane had had no contact with either learning disability or mental health services prior to admission. In fact, there was some doubt as to whether or not she had a learning disability.
>
> Jane's mother was a very submissive woman, who had difficulty problem solving and bringing about change. She was, however, the primary caregiver to her own mother, Jane and her grandchild. The grandmother lived in the sitting room of the house, and maintained complete control over the family through repeated demands and verbal abuse.
>
> Jane was described by her mother as a happy, chatty person, 'more of a friend than a daughter', prior to the death of her fiancé in a car crash, when their son was 2 years old. She regularly cooked the family evening meal, enjoyed her job as a waitress and liked going out.

Data collection is closely linked with, and may include, interview. As well as revising her knowledge of any conditions detailed, the therapist will want to evaluate the information gathered and take into account the perspective from which it has been gained. Increasingly, this may include accessing the single shared assessment (Scottish Executive 2000b), which aims for agencies to share information, preventing duplication of work and reducing stress for the individuals and carers. Individuals are central to the single shared assessment process and give consent as to whom this information may be shared with. Carers' views are also sought in completion of the single shared assessment and are taken into consideration in action planning. If the person is unknown to services then the occupational therapist may be required to initiate this process, in which case the initial interview will be especially important. A person's first contact can be crucial to their future engagement with services, as well as to the establishment of therapeutic relationships.

Interview

> **Case study: part 3**
>
> An initial interview was arranged to meet Jane within the ward setting. Information was also gained from her nursing key worker at this time.
>
> Nursing staff reported that Jane had been restless since admission and unable to occupy her time independently. She was demanding of staff attention and showed limited awareness of social boundaries, particularly with regard to the need for privacy of others in the ward.
>
> Jane was able to attend to the interview for 30 minutes before becoming agitated. During this time she was able to recall her education and employment background and stated that she would like to work as a waitress again. She was aware that 'things had gone wrong' since the death of her fiancé; however, she said that she enjoyed shopping for clothes for herself and her son. She appeared unable to retain information from the therapist and, while appearing to cope well with conversation (albeit repetitive), had apparent difficulties in comprehending specific terms.

Although the interview format was used with some success with this client, it may be necessary to interview others as representatives of the client. However, one should be cautious about relying solely on this information, and alternative methods of gaining information directly from the client should always be attempted. Interview need not be restricted to questionnaires or pen and paper exercises. Careful clinical observation and reflection are as essential to successful interviewing as the ability to listen (Remington 1997). For this reason, subsequent interviews were held, in which direct observation was used to determine Jane's current functional level in community living skills such as road safety and money handling.

When interviewing profoundly or multiply handicapped clients, the careful selection of activities taken for the interview can yield useful information. Some musical instruments, a small torch and a ball or beanbag can be used to indicate much about the client's interactional skills, leisure interests, previous experiences and opportunities. The therapist should try to ensure that the activities and equipment are appropriate to the age of the client. It is not necessarily wrong to use play, since adults also play, although often with more structure, more rules and more players than children.

It is worthwhile to prepare an interview schedule, listing what information you want to exchange with the client. Box 26.1 shows an example, which readers may wish to adapt for themselves. Determining what it is that she wants to know brings the therapist closer to deciding how to elicit the information. Cameron & Murphy (2002) explored the use of Talking Mats, a light-technology augmentative framework, with young adults with a learning and communication disability. The participants were able to utilise this tool to indicate their likes and dislikes and to express views about the choices available to them, sometimes to the surprise of their carers. The use of symbols, pictures and photographs in this tool makes it very accessible in eliciting information, and very personal to the person with a learning disability as information is built up about their needs and wishes.

Box 26.1 An example of an initial interview format

Purpose of the interview
One of the main reasons for interviewing someone is to begin building rapport. Where possible, the therapist should explain the purpose of the interview, where the request for occupational therapy intervention came from and the client's rights to agree/disagree with that intervention. An initial interview may last from 5 to 30 minutes and should give direction to further intervention. The next step may be, for example: (a) further development of the therapeutic relationship; (b) functional assessment, or (c) closure of an inappropriate referral.

Physical assessment
The therapist may wish to assess posture, gait, movement through position, tremor, deformity, muscle tone, vision, hearing, gross co-ordination and build. Asking the client if he would like to move to a quiet/seated/tabletop area provides an opportunity for observing many of these points, as well as adding insight concerning the client's orientation/familiarity with his environment.

Mental state
This may include emotional stability, mood, attention span, interests, roles, routines, motivation to participate in activity and the client's own perception of his difficulties. If the client is non-verbal or non-vocal, then photographs, foodstuffs and simple remedial games can indicate much about his previous experiences and his reaction to them. The client's own possessions can aid the information-seeking process.

Communication/interaction
Attention should be given to both non-verbal and verbal skills. Hearing, comprehension, response to touch and response to sound should be considered as factors influencing interactional ability. Insight into behaviours, relationships and interests may be gained through both discussion and observation of responses to environmental distractions. A variety of media, such as photographs, pen and paper, music and the therapist, can be used to elicit responses.

ASSESSMENT

Case study: part 4

From the initial interview and observation period, the therapist began to establish a therapeutic relationship with Jane, and identified the following recommendations.

  - Referral to psychology re Jane's learning disability and sexual vulnerability.
  - Referral to learning disability nursing re monitoring of mental health and bereavement counselling, on discharge from the ward.
  - Referral to speech and language therapy re receptive language and ability to self-advocate. The Model of Human Occupation Screening Tool (MOHOST) was used with the following results.
  - **Motivation for occupation**: Jane's participation in occupations was largely inhibited by her difficulty in understanding her own strengths and weaknesses, an ambivalent choice of occupations she wished to resume and an inconsistency being expressed about what was most important to her. Particularly concerning were her pessimism and feelings of lack of empowerment and control.
  - **Pattern of occupation**: Jane was able to articulate what she felt was expected of her, and attached some value to these expectations. However, she had difficulty in organising herself to meet these expectations without support.
  - **Motor skills**: as shown later by an assessment of motor and process skills (AMPS), Jane had minimal difficulties, with the exception of pacing herself throughout tasks.
  - **Environment**: Jane found her participation in activity restricted by the lack of expectation of her held by her family, her own inability to cope with the demands of previously known social groups and her own self-image.

At this point, it was evident that Jane felt she had little ability to change, that her medication was only 'making things worse', due to her consequent weight gain, and that 'nobody needed her anyway'. The last sentiment was not explained, perhaps due to an inability to do so or perhaps due to the loss of roles she had experienced such as fiancé, worker and mother. This combination of factors can be viewed as a maladaptive cycle, contributing to her low mood and lack of self-esteem (see Fig. 26.3).

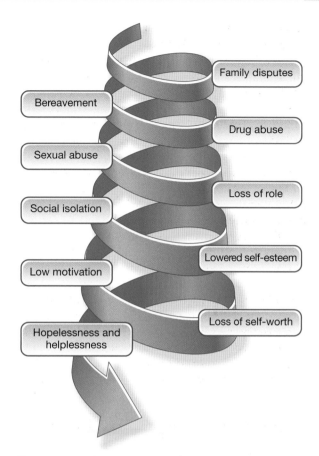

Figure 26.3 Downward spiral.

As already stated, the clinician should also consider who else is assessing the client. It is frustrating for the client to be repeatedly assessed by people from different disciplines, and it may be possible to decrease the overlap in an effective team by sharing results, whether or not a single shared assessment format is being used. An assessment is useless (especially from the client's perspective) unless it leads to interventions that address needs. Principle 1 of the *Principles for Education and Practice for Occupational Therapists Working with Adults with Learning Disabilities* (College of Occupational Therapists 2003) reminds therapists that standardised assessments should be used wherever possible; however, care should be taken to ensure these are appropriate for this population.

GOAL SETTING

Goals do not remain static; instead, they reflect the therapist's evaluation of the assessments and intervention and must be redefined constantly. Goals may be long term, with various short-term objectives being set for their eventual achievement. Even long-term goals should be regularly reviewed to ensure their continuing relevance to the client. Goals should reflect the values of the client and be achievable. The Goal Attainment Scales (GAS) allow the therapist to agree individual goals with the individual and relevant others and to set the criteria against which progress will be measured.

INTERVENTION

Following Jane's discharge under section 33 of the Mental Health Act (Scotland) 1984 (Scottish Home and Health Department 1984) and her grandmother's

---

Case study: part 5

It was recognised that gaining Jane's co-operation and sustaining her motivation to participate in treatment could be difficult. This was due not only to her mental state, and her level of understanding, but also to her past experience when her grandmother had denied access to professionals, deeming them interfering, and her negative experiences of men since her bereavement.

Jane was encouraged to take an active part in goal setting but this was something she found very difficult. This was reflected in her lack of long-term goals, her only objective being to return to the family home. The Interest Checklist identified several areas in which Jane had previously shown both interest and competence, such as decorating, swimming and football, but Jane did not see herself resuming any of these activities.

The occupational therapist decided to focus initially on the preliminary goals detailed in Table 26.4, while completing further assessments at Jane's pace. This would have the effect of increasing her level of independence and her participation in activities within the home. The other purpose of focusing on such skills was that they were highly visible, and would affect not only her self-perception but also her relationships with her mother and son.

---

admission to a nursing home, occupational therapy intervention commenced with a view to Jane:

- developing feelings of self-worth
- regaining the motivation to participate in activity
- adopting an active parenting role
- achieving a healthy lifestyle

(see Table 26.4).

The occupational therapy intervention lasted for 6 months, after which time the further assessments were completed and goals were redefined. Initially, intervention took place within Jane's home and the local community, enabling the therapist and support worker to establish relationships with the remaining residents of the household. It also allowed informal observations of the family dynamics and facilitated assessment of functional performance, participation, interaction and how these impacted on Jane's parenting skills.

Later, the settings used for intervention extended to the wider community, in that contact was re-established with her late fiancé's parents, albeit with support.

All the recommendations and goals were addressed concurrently, with some interventions being episodic, such as psychological testing, and some ongoing, for example, further occupational therapy assessment. However, all were reliant on Jane's agreement and acceptance in order to progress. Therefore, there was a variable degree of success in achieving these goals.

Competence versus independence

'To be competent means to be sufficient or adequate to meet the demands of a situation or task' (White 1971). This definition reflects the person-centred

---

Case study: part 6

1. Referral to psychology
Jane accepted IQ testing, which suggested she was moderately learning disabled. On repetition of this, following a gradual reduction in medication, no statistically significant difference was found.

Jane refused to engage in the assessment of sexual vulnerability, perhaps due to the lack of a female psychologist available to work with her.

2. Referral to learning disability nursing

Again, Jane refused to engage with this, or any other service, offering bereavement counselling.

3. Referral to speech and language therapy

Due to maternity leave this is only being addressed at the time of writing.

4. Promoting a healthy lifestyle

Jane made good progress in attending physical activity sessions, both with and without her son, provided she had support to get to these. She would participate for 30–60 minutes at her own pace; although there was no immediate effect on her mood or expression, both she and her mother reported that these were enjoyed. Despite becoming breathless on exertion, Jane did not wish to stop smoking or explore any smoking cessation options.

Jane's contribution to meal planning was less successful as, whilst she was willing to make suggestions, the majority of shopping and meal preparation activity remained with her mother.

5. Promoting an active parenting role

Jane gradually reduced her dependence on support and succeeded in taking her son to or from nursery and the corner shop on her own 2–3 times per week. She and her son were observed to have a good relationship when jointly involved in activity, but within the house the child initiated most of the interaction.

Jane is currently being supported to clearly express her expectations of the child and to set boundaries where required.

6. Regain the motivation to participate in activity

Jane progressed from not leaving the family home unescorted by either her mother or occupational therapy staff to a few independent outings close to home. She attributed this to being fearful of meeting certain people to whom she felt unable to express her own views and opinions.

Goals were therefore modified to support and encourage Jane to express herself.

Within the house, Jane's mother is encouraged to raise her expectations of Jane with regard to tasks, and to provide positive rather than negative comment on Jane's activity.

7. Developing feelings of self-worth

Jane has been supported to keep an activities diary in order that her achievements to date are recorded and positive reinforcement given. Together with changing her mother's feedback and challenging Jane's negative comparisons of herself to others, some small change is becoming evident.

Supported visits to her late fiancé's parents have been of particular benefit. They had felt excluded from both Jane and their grandchild and were very pleased and positive to have even occasional contact re-established.

approach advocated by occupational therapists, in that excellence is not a prerequisite for an optimal level of independence.

There is a potential misunderstanding that occupational therapists are seeking total independence in all interventions. The aim of occupational therapy intervention does focus on enabling the individual to reach his own optimal level of independence, but the reader must be aware of great differences in the potential levels of independence amongst people with learning disabilities.

Medley (1984) offered the following definitions.

- A competency is 'a single knowledge, skill or professional value'.
- Competence is 'the repertoire of competencies'.

The occupational therapist assists the individual by teaching specific competencies, leading to an overall level of competence which is effective and has relevance to his specific environment. However, this may not reflect an ability to function with complete independence.

Mocellin (1988) advocated that the focus of intervention should be on 'small wins', illustrated in Figure 26.4. A small win is a 'concrete, complete, implemented action of moderate importance' (p5). These small wins, or competencies, are built on by the occupational therapist to enable the person to reach a realistic level of competence in a specific area.

Some people may never realise the optimal level of independence as dictated by professional judgements. However, competence is specified for each person at a level that is realistic and relevant to individual needs and the environments in which they function.

Table 26.4 Occupational therapy goals

Treatment aims	Method/activity	Desired outcome
To encourage Jane to engage with other disciplines and services	Application of the CPA, introducing other supports to her as necessary	Jane accepts support on a regular basis, as appropriate to the needs being addressed
Increase participation in housework	Agreement with Jane and her mother regarding which tasks Jane should do Monitor Jane's motivation to do these	Jane feels a sense of achievement, requires less prompting to initiate tasks and the number of tasks asked of her is increased gradually
Promote a healthier lifestyle	Engage Jane in meal planning, particularly for her son, and similarly support her in attempting leisure activities she/they can do	Jane eats more healthily and takes some exercise to combat the effects of her medication Jane takes a more active parenting role
Promote Jane's participation in activity outwith the home	Support Jane to take her son swimming Support Jane to drop her son off at nursery and collect him again Encourage Jane to go shopping for herself and her son	Jane takes a more active parenting role Jane takes some exercise to combat the effects of her medication Jane initiates one activity herself
Develop self-confidence	Achievement in regaining old skills Positive feedback from occupational therapist, family and other members of the treatment team	Jane is able to dictate the level of support she needs for agreed activities
Encourage Jane to use the functional and organisational skills required to function as a parent	Role modelling through sessions with the occupational therapist, with particular regard to her interaction with her son Support Jane to carry out activities with her son	Jane takes a more active parenting role Jane interacts spontaneously and appropriately with her son Jane learns different strategies for dealing with her son's behaviours, which she finds difficult at present

Treatment media

It would be impossible to outline here all the possible activities that could be utilised within this field. The reader should realise that any activity can be selected and grading the activity enables the therapist to meet individual needs or treatment goals. Analysis, application and grading activities constitute the art of our profession and make us unique among other professions within the health-care environment (see Chapter 6).

While Neistadt (1986) and Llewellyn (1991) referred to 'remedial' and 'adaptive' treatment methods, within this text we refer to 'experiential learning' and 'skills-based learning'. The use of the terms 'remedial' and 'adaptive' could be construed as negative when considering this client group.

They also imply the use of a formal teaching strategy, which may not be the primary method of intervention chosen by the occupational therapist. 'Experiential learning' and 'skills-based learning' are terms more descriptive of the developmental processes through which an occupational therapist can provide stimulation, opportunities and positive experiences for the client group.

These two approaches can be used exclusively or in conjunction with each other, as neither precludes the other from occurring spontaneously. As mentioned earlier, people with learning disabilities may have pockets of particular skills, which are not reflective of their overall performance. For this reason the mix of experiential and skills-based learning is particularly effective within the field of learning disabilities. It should be noted that

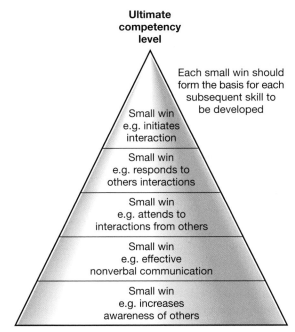

Figure 26.4 Illustration of 'small wins' theory.

experiential learning can produce skills development, although this may not have been the primary goal of intervention. Experiential learning gives people opportunities to develop positive concepts relating to interaction with others and the environment, and this engenders confidence and the motivation to develop further.

EVALUATION

Case study: part 7

Over a 6-month period, small changes have been observed and it is hoped that these gains from occupational participation will lead to further gains. Jane's mood is still of concern, but this may in part be due to external factors, such as a forthcoming court case. Importantly, Jane has begun to express dissatisfaction with her current lifestyle, compared to that previously. Using the Occupational Circumstances Assessment-Interview and Rating Scale (Forsyth et al 2005), it is hoped to help her express this in a more positive way. At this point it may be possible to support Jane in engaging with other services/agencies which can assist her in addressing some of her issues.

No intervention can be shown to be beneficial for the client if it is not evaluated. Evaluation must happen throughout the occupational therapy process in order for it to be effective; for example, evaluation of the referral should enquire whether or not it is appropriate. Many assessments now supply individual learning packages, which include criteria for evaluating progress.

Little is available, however, for evaluating the client's satisfaction with treatment, particularly the client with severe or profound learning disability. A possible solution is to interview the carer, although the therapist should be aware that bias may be present. Another possible solution is to agree with other agencies a checklist of behaviours thought to represent interest and pleasure, and to sample for these behaviours at varying intervals. This can then be used to infer satisfaction or otherwise on the client's part. More able clients can choose not to attend, vocalise their dissatisfaction or be assisted to complete a self-reporting tool.

When designing evaluation tools, the therapist must be careful not to lead the client by verbal or non-verbal cues. Also, the language must be appropriate to the client's communicative abilities and relevant to his sphere of experiences.

SPECIFIC AREAS OF INTERVENTION

A specialist label which this area of work often attracts could be considered a misnomer, as an occupational therapist will utilise all the core skills of the profession and many of the peripheral competencies which are developed during and after training. As discussed earlier in the chapter, the approach used by occupational therapists is primarily person centred. Quality of life is considered at all times and the individual is assisted to function at his optimal level, dependent on a range of factors identified in the assessment process.

The knowledge base in biopsychosocial sciences, environmental adaptation and occupational performance facilitates understanding of the behaviours presented, contraindications for treatment planning and implications of drug side-effects. Skills in assessment provide sound baseline information from which to develop realistic aims and objectives to assist learning and development.

The creative approach of the occupational therapist assists individuals to overcome physical disabilities through learning compensatory methods of functioning. Adaptations and equipment can be provided to assist functional independence.

Occupational therapists are skilled in communication, which will assist clients to develop awareness, interaction and social skills, leading to increased levels of motivation and participation.

The ability to grade activity is the factor which most contributes to the success of the occupational therapist as a clinician. This is particularly true in the field of learning disability where developmental delay, combined with erratic expectations from carers, can result in pockets of skills among major learning deficits. It must be emphasised, however, that the activity chosen, and the setting, are only justifiable if they reflect the needs and wishes of the client. If the occupational therapist is doing more in the session than the client, then either the grading or the activity itself is wrong, and a re-evaluation of the client and the programme should be undertaken.

The occupational therapist must be clear about specific goals and about the teaching necessary for optimal independence and integration with societal activities.

PROFOUND AND MULTIPLE IMPAIRMENT SERVICES

The developmental problems experienced by people with learning disability often combine with auditory and visual impairments to create serious difficulties for those affected. When someone has limited awareness and response to contact, the process of development is slow and laborious. Lack of feedback can demoralise carers who are unsure how to stimulate these people effectively. The occupational therapist can assist in revising the expectations of carers and others to realise the individual's potential for interaction and participation.

When learning is organised into routines or sequentially graded steps that can be accepted and understood by the individual, it becomes clear that the techniques for this group of clients are similar to those used for other groups: that

is, physical intervention and support, practical demonstration, verbal instruction and physical and verbal cueing, reducing as independent sequencing of activity is achieved. In practice, the time-scale for achievement varies from one individual to another. The reader is referred again to Figure 26.4, where the small wins theory is illustrated. The small wins may indeed be very small but, if tasks are graded carefully, progress can be clearly identified, sustaining the therapist and carer and ensuring that the individual's development is consolidated.

This client group has specific needs for:

- a structured environment to facilitate understanding, utilising environmental cues and referencing whenever possible
- consistency of approach to allow trust and self-confidence to develop, since random input will only serve to fuel apprehension and encourage withdrawal from situations
- explanation and assistance in exploration
- time, without which little can be achieved, and
- identification of alternative communication systems that may be necessary to ensure that information is exchanged between the therapist and the client.

Often, the most important piece of equipment is the therapist herself. In establishing rapport and facilitating awareness and understanding of the environment and its opportunities for learning, the therapist may initially need no more than herself, a creative mind and sound observational skills to identify areas where reaction and interaction are positive. Thereafter, equipment can be introduced to allow exploration to develop along more structured lines.

In creating dynamic, structured programmes for individuals with multiple disabilities, it is important to remember that a 24-hour approach is the only way to offer true consistency, and it will therefore be necessary to liaise closely with parents, carers and other professionals when co-ordinating input for these individuals.

One package being used to try and achieve this 24-hour consistency is Active Support (Jones et al 1999, Sanderson et al 2002). This encourages staff to support individuals in participating in activity through: identifying opportunities for activity on a daily basis; ensuring that the correct level of support is given (neither too much nor too little) to support participation; clearly identifying who is responsible for offering this support, and monitoring the participation that results.

SERVICES FOR OLDER PEOPLE WITH A LEARNING DISABILITY

It is important to consider the long-term future of the people who are at present successfully and happily placed in the community. We must be aware that the needs of the person with a learning disability can change considerably as they grow older, and community resources may no longer be appropriate for them. This is already apparent in the case of people with Down's syndrome, who are thought to have a much higher than normal risk of presenile dementia from the age of 40.

Other significant changes can be physical, the onset of mental health problems or even loss of support from family/friends (such as the death of parents), which can reduce the person's ability to remain where they previously lived. The Foundation for People with Learning Disabilities' Growing Older with Learning Disabilities (GOLD) programme emphasises the need for older people with learning disabilities to participate in leisure activities to facilitate and maintain social networks to prevent isolation and maintain a satisfactory quality of life.

Occupational therapy has a significant role to play in anticipating future needs and can play a large part in designing and implementing care facilities and packages that are sustainable over the individual's lifespan.

DUAL DIAGNOSIS

Historically, services have been delivered from either a mental health perspective or a learning disabilities perspective. Over the last 10 years, and particularly since the National Health Service and Community Care Act (1990) was passed, there has been increasing recognition that many people with a learning disability also have one or more diagnosable mental health disorders (Gravestock 1999).

Occupational therapists can contribute to diagnosis as well as to intervention, both through direct client contact and through advice and training for carers and other agencies. Therapists may find themselves working within different service models, such as community-based dual diagnosis teams, inpatient assessment units with outreach function or inpatient mental health acute admission units with designated dual diagnosis beds.

FORENSIC AND CHALLENGING BEHAVIOUR SERVICES

Home at Last? (Scottish Executive 2004a) recommends that health boards and local authorities should ensure that there are local professionals with expertise in working with offenders with a learning disability. This is in recognition of the impact of hospital closures, which traditionally provided an alternative to detention for people displaying a range of antisocial behaviours, from fire raising to severe aggression. Similarly, the hospital closure programme raises concerns for the secure hospitals and the prison service when looking to discharge/release people with a learning disability and offending behaviours, in that there is a shortage of appropriate housing and support packages within the community.

Research has increased into the prevalence of this population. However, the NHS Scotland Learning Disability Needs Assessment Report (Scottish Executive 2004b) concluded that there is a need for a move away from prevalence studies to studies focusing on the development and evaluation of effective interventions and services. Lindsay et al (2004) studied women offenders with a learning disability and suggested that much could be done in addressing psychological issues and mental illness in order to prevent and/or reduce their offending behaviour. This study showed a high incidence of both abuse and mental illness in the women, and the Report of the Inspection of Scottish Borders Council Social Work Services for People affected by Learning Disabilities (Scottish Executive 2004c) suggested that the abuse of people with a learning disability often goes undetected and unaddressed.

This demonstrates the need for health, social work, criminal justice, police and prison services to work closely together to assess and manage the risks of offenders. The multi agency public protection panels (MAPPPs) are seen as providing a model of good practice: offenders who pose a high risk of serious harm, or whose management is difficult or sensitive, are referred to MAPPPs and agencies share information to ensure that accurate assessments of risk are made about potentially dangerous offenders. Plans to manage those risks robustly can then be drawn up and implemented.

Following the legislative principles that demand least restrictive intervention and giving people the right to appeal against excessive security, it is essential that services are configured to provide support to individuals at each tier of the healthcare model set out in *Promoting Health, Supporting Inclusion* (Scottish Executive 2002a). This may include the establishment and/or development of forensic learning disability teams, additional support teams, low secure units and appropriate adult schemes, as well as specialist day and inpatient services.

DAY SERVICES AND WORK PROGRAMMES

Occupational therapists have a valuable role to play in the provision of day services, working to enable people to access community facilities and integrate more effectively. Many clients live alone or with a few hours support each day. Working with staff from social services, voluntary organisations or housing associations, occupational therapists can help to increase clients' self-confidence through broadening their leisure activities, offering opportunities for personal development and helping to create work roles, ultimately reducing their reliance on traditional support centres.

In both the UK and the USA, an increasing demand for employment from people with a learning disability and their carers has arisen from dissatisfaction with traditional adult training centres. Occupational therapists recognise the value of people being engaged to their optimum capacity in purposeful activity which, for most people, includes productive work.

Wilcock (1998) viewed occupation as a central aspect of human experience, with health and survival being strongly related to the innate need to engage in purposeful occupation. From this fundamental professional belief, occupational therapists are ideally placed to provide opportunities that will enable skills development, while encouraging both physical and psychological well-being.

Training or advice to carers may help to alter the perception of their role to one that facilitates individual development and encourages more independence. For individuals requiring increased levels of care and support, the occupational therapist can grade activity, use compensatory techniques to minimise physical limitations and promote interaction and communication to further development. She is also in a strong position to assist those providing activity in adapting their approach to facilitate the involvement of people with a learning disability. This allows individuals to access local activities they have an interest in, at times that are suitable to them, rather than attending a centre that is only open during office hours.

As citizens, people with disabilities have the same rights and responsibilities as all other people to participate in and contribute to the life of the community. The appointment of local area co-ordinators (based on the Australian model of local area co-ordination) has been introduced to much of the country to assist in the fulfilment of this vision, and their role is based on the following principles.

1. People with a learning disability are best placed to determine their own goals and aspirations, supported by their family and, if need be, advocacy.
2. Social networks play a large part in the achievement of a satisfying role in the community.
3. The individual and those important to him need to be central to planning the supports they need. Individuals should be at the centre of decision making about their lives.
4. People can gain more control over their lives if they have access to appropriate and timely information.
5. The inclusion of people with disabilities in a community is of mutual benefit and is supported by the accessibility of amenities, facilities and services.
6. All services and supports can be enhanced by local area co-ordination.

It follows that the occupational therapist needs to work closely with the local area co-ordinator and disability employment advisor in identifying and nurturing opportunities for people with a learning disability in the local community, to progress the social inclusion agenda.

SUMMARY

Occupational therapists will always have a role within the area of learning disabilities. However, in the future they may see their role widen and change as services develop in response to identified need.

The initiation of managed care networks facilitates specialisation to meet these needs (which may not be possible in a small area due to lack of critical mass) and allows the body of evidence for practice to be developed, as well as delivering the appropriate service to any given individual at any given time. This encourages occupational therapists to focus on specific interventions and thus maximise their effectiveness with the different problems encountered by this population.

Similarly, the expansion of particular roles offers opportunities to occupational therapists: in the light of the emphasis on purposeful and meaningful activity in our professional philosophy, who is better placed to take on the role of Active Support implementation or of local area co-ordination? When has there ever been more opportunity, than in this drive for social inclusion, for occupational therapists to influence barrier-free design and manufacture? There is much written about the needs of people with physical disabilities with regard to design of environments, but comparatively little regarding the needs of people with learning disabilities.

Many of our partners are recognising the importance of activity, participation and environment. Also, the individual's voice has never been heard so clearly. As occupational therapists, we have never had more opportunities to lead the way in ensuring that the needs of this population are met.

References

Cameron L, Murphy J 2002 Enabling young people with a learning disability to make choices at a time of transition. British Journal of Learning Disabilities 3(3): 105-112

College of Occupational Therapists 2003 Principles for education and practice for occupational therapists working with adults with learning disabilities. College of Occupational Therapists, London

Cooper S A, Melville C, Morrison J 2004 People with intellectual disabilities. Their health needs differ and need to be recognised and met. BMJ 329(7463): 414

Department of Health 2001 Valuing people: a new strategy for the 21st century. Department of Health, London

Disability Discrimination Act 1995 Stationery Office, London

Fleming A, Mackintosh C 2004 A view from the top. Occupational Therapy News 12(1): 30

Forsyth K, Deshpande S, Keilhofner G et al 2005 Occupational circumstances assessment-interview and rating scale. Version 3.0. UIC Office of Publications Services, Chicago

Gilbert P 1996 The A–Z reference book of syndromes and inherited disorders; 2nd edn. Chapman and Hall, London

Gravestock S 1999 Adults with learning disabilities and mental health needs: conceptual and service issues. Tizard Learning Disability Review 4(2): 6-11

Hagedorn R 2001 Foundations for practice in occupational therapy, 3rd edn. Churchill Livingstone, Edinburgh

Jones E, Perry J, Lowe K et al 1999 Opportunity and the promotion of activity among adults with severe intellectual disability living in community residences: the impact of training staff in active support. Journal of Intellectual Disability Research 43(3): 164-178

Lindsay WR, Smith AHW, Quinn K et al 2004 Women with intellectual disability who have offended: characteristics and outcome. Journal of Intellectual Disability Research 48(6): 580-591

Llewellyn G 1991 Occupational therapy treatment goals for adults with developmental disabilities. Australian Journal of Occupational Therapy 38(1): 233-236

McGrother C, Thorp C, Taub N, et al 2001 Prevalence, disability and need with severe learning disability. Tizard Learning Disability Review 6: 4-13

Medley D 1984 Cited in: Ellis R (ed) 1988 Professional competence and quality assurance in the caring professions. Croom Helm, London, pp43-58

Mocellin G 1988 A perspective on the principles and practice of occupational therapy. British Journal of Occupational Therapy 51(1): 4-7

National Assembly for Wales Learning Disability Advisory Group 2001 Fulfilling the promise: proposals for a framework for services for people with learning disabilities. Stationery Office, London

Neistadt ME 1986 Occupational therapy treatment goals for adults with developmental disabilities. American Journal of Occupational Therapy 40(10): 672-677

Remington R 1997 Verbal communication in people with learning difficulties, an overview. Tizard Learning Disability Review 2(4): 6-14

Sanderson H, Kennedy J, Ritchie P 1997 People, plans and possibilities: exploring person centered planning. SHS, Edinburgh

Sanderson H, Jones E, Brown K 2002 Active support and person centred planning: strange bedfellows or ideal partners. Tizard Learning Disability Review 7(1): 31-38

Scottish Executive 2000a The same as you? A review of services for people with learning disabilities. Stationery Office, Edinburgh

Scottish Executive 2000b Community care: a joint future. Stationery Office, Edinburgh

Scottish Executive 2000c Adults with Incapacity (Scotland) Act. Stationery Office, Edinburgh

Scottish Executive 2001 Patient focus, public involvement. Stationery Office, Edinburgh

Scottish Executive 2002a Promoting health, supporting inclusion. Stationery Office, Edinburgh

Scottish Executive 2002 Community Care and Health (Scotland) Act. Stationery Office, Edinburgh

Scottish Executive 2003 Mental Health (Care and Treatment) (Scotland) Act. Stationery Office, Edinburgh

Scottish Executive 2004a Home at last? The same as you implementation group – report of the sub-group on progress with hospital closure and service reprovision. Stationery Office, Edinburgh

Scottish Executive 2004b Health needs assessment report – summary. People with learning disabilities in Scotland. Stationery Office, Edinburgh

Scottish Executive 2004c Investigation into Scottish Borders Council and NHS Borders services for people with learning disabilities: joint statement from the Mental Welfare Commission and the Social Work Services Inspectorate. Stationery Office, Edinburgh

Scottish Home and Health Department 1984 Mental Health Act (Scotland). Scottish Office, Edinburgh

Watchman K 2003 Critical issues for service planners and providers of care for people with Down's syndrome and dementia. British Journal of Learning Disabilities 31: 81-84

White R 1971 The urge towards competence. American Journal of Occupational Therapy 25(6): 271-274

Wilcock AA 1998 An occupational perspective of health. Slack, New Jersey

World Health Organization 2001 International classification of functioning, disability and health. World Health Organization, Geneva

Further Reading

Booth T 1994 Parenting under pressure: mothers and fathers with learning disabilities. Open University Press, Buckinghamshire

Bright K, Di Giulio R 2001 Inclusive buildings – design and management of accessible environments. Blackwell Science, Oxford

Forsyth K, Lai JS, Kielhofner G 1999 The assessment of communication and interaction skills (ACIS): measurement properties. British Journal of Occupational Therapy 62(2): 69-74

Janicki MP, Dalton AJ (eds) 1998 Dementia, aging, and intellectual disabilities. Hamilton, New York

Magalini S II, Magalini SC 1997 Dictionary of medical syndromes. 4th edn, Lippincott-Raven, Philadelphia

Murphy J 1998 Talking Mats: speech and language research in practice. Speech and Language Therapy and Practice Autumn: 11-14

NHS Scotland 2004 Health needs assessment report. People with learning disabilities in Scotland. NHS, Glasgow

Whitman B, Accardo P 1990 When a parent is mentally retarded. Brookes, Baltimore

Chapter **27**

Community mental health

Jon Fieldhouse

INTRODUCTION

This chapter aims to enthuse and inform therapists and undergraduates who are engaged in, or interested in, community mental health work, which is the largest field of psychosocial occupational therapy (Finlay 2004). It hopes to shed light on some of the main features of the landscape, so practitioners can navigate their way through this very diverse area of practice. It does not presume to offer a *How to...* guide, but hopes to encourage therapists to think for themselves. Above all, it aims to demonstrate how fascinating and rapidly developing this area of practice is; how contested many of its issues still are; and how relevant and potent the core principles of occupational therapy are in relation to these.

The chapter focuses on services for working-age adults with mental health problems. It has five sections. *Working in the Community* explores the shift from institutional to community care, and the implications for occupational therapy; *Working with Service Users* highlights the importance of person-centred working; *Working in a Policy Context* presents some of the structures and policies guiding community care that influence our profession; *Working in Teams* looks at how services are configured and explores issues arising for therapists working in co-ordinated teams; and, finally, *Looking after Yourself* examines some of the resources available for addressing these issues. It ends with conclusions about the continued, or indeed renewed, relevance of occupational therapy to current national agendas and priorities in community mental health.

WORKING DEFINITIONS AND TERMINOLOGY

It may be helpful to give working definitions or background to the following key terms used in this chapter: severe and/or enduring mental health problems, service user, team, and occupation.

Severe and/or enduring mental health problems

The Department of Health (1995) outlined the elements that comprised a definition of severe mental illness: disability, diagnosis, duration, safety issues, and the need for formal or informal care, anticipating that a more precise definition would emerge from using this framework at a local level. However, as Brooker & Repper (2003) note:

> Perhaps nowhere is the potential conflict in the agendas of key stakeholders more manifest than in the question of how to define 'serious mental health problems'. (p312)

If no answer has yet been found, it may be because of a growing consensus that such an absolute right answer does not exist.

This chapter takes serious or severe and/or enduring mental health problems to refer to schizophrenia, bipolar affective disorder (or manic depression), severe depression, severe anxiety, and personality disorders which are of such intensity that they prevent a person from functioning in an adequate and satisfying way as determined on the basis of his culture and background (Sainsbury Centre for Mental Health 1998). Although serious mental health problems can last for several years, 'enduring' means lasting for at least 12 months, which is also how 'long term' is defined under the Disability Discrimination Act (Great Britain Parliament 2005) (www.opsi.gov.uk).

Focusing on mental health problems as lived experience, Finlay & McKay (2004) have suggested three themes that might be familiar to many mental health service users. The first is feeling out of control, in relation to the intrusiveness of overwhelming psychotic symptoms such as voices or visions, in terms of a lack of self-determination as life events or relationships unfold or in terms of extreme emotional states of fear and loss. The second is the struggle beyond the illness, referring to the hardships beyond symptomatology that may characterise daily life and which, were it not for personal strengths and commitment, would otherwise prevent individuals from fulfilling or recovering their life roles, such as parent, worker or friend. The third is the power of the social context, referring to the huge significance of the social world as a factor in both the creation of the mental health problems and the recovery process, particularly in relation to issues such as social inclusion/exclusion, stigma, employment and occupation in general.

Service user

The conflicting agendas of stakeholders are also reflected in the terms used to refer to people who use mental health services. These include survivor, patient, client and service user. Each of these terms has a history and a context.

'Survivor' is a political term used by people who feel they have recovered in spite of the mental health system and often have a negative experience of it (Sainsbury Centre for Mental Health 2003). 'Patient' was the generic term until the 1980s but may imply a passive role and the medicalisation of care, although some people may feel need to adopt a passive patient role at times (Morgan 2004). 'Service user' is widely used in social care, and came out of the push for consumerism in the 1980s which gave people choices and a right to have expectations of services. It has become the most widely used term and is increasingly used in legislation and policy documents. 'Client' is widely used by health professionals but has been criticised for its implicit assumption that people who use services have exercised a choice in doing so (which may not be the case) and also for its reciprocal bolstering of the professional status of practitioners and all the associated power dynamics that go with that (Whalley-Hammell 2006). Most fundamentally, community practitioners are urged to see the people they work with as citizens of their community (Stein & Test 1980). This chapter refers to a person using services as the individual or person or occasionally, where making the distinction helps clarity, as the service user.

Team

The chapter concentrates on occupational therapy delivered through various forms of community mental health team (CMHT), all of which employ occupational therapists. For simplicity's sake, the word 'team' or CMHT will be used throughout this chapter to describe 'any team providing co-ordinated multidisciplinary input in community settings through a team process' (Onyett 2003, p7).

Consequently, the chapter will not focus on occupational therapists working with a unidisciplinary orientation, whose practice may occasionally involve interdisciplinary working or loose networking. The emphasis on co-ordinated care is put in context throughout the chapter.

Occupation

Occupation here means any goal-directed, repeatable activity which carries personal and cultural meaning, and is perceived as doing by the doer (McLaughlin Gray 1997).

WORKING IN THE COMMUNITY

A BRIEF HISTORY OF COMMUNITY CARE

Over the past quarter of a century a huge shift has taken place whereby the vast majority of mental health care is now provided by community-based mental health services, to service users living at home. Rather than being geographically or even conceptually tied to these community-based services, the psychiatric hospital is now generally viewed as one of a range of resources available in care planning.

The community is, and of course should be, a defining characteristic of community-based services and working *with* the community is a central theme in this chapter. The gradual evolution of services, as they have adapted to their 'new' environment, has been characterised by: the development of co-ordinated care planning; the prioritisation of services for people with serious mental health problems; co-ordinated teamworking; and, perhaps most importantly, a widening acknowledgement of the social model of disability and an increasingly sharper focus on social inclusion and access issues. These factors will now be discussed, concluding with some implications for ourselves as occupational therapists.

Co-ordinated care planning

Whereas the old institutions at least provided a kind of seamless range of services by being all under one roof, community care initially presented a bewildering array of fragmented and geographically dispersed services that clients simply were unable to access. Additionally, the needs of clients in relation to this access issue were poorly understood because they had not been encountered before (Stein & Santos 1998).

> Where users lived might be miles away from where they collected their welfare benefit, which again would be a long way from a community mental health centre, which users might need to attend during the day - 'community care' had an inbuilt tendency to become disjointed and fragmentary. The implication of this was that the existence of a service in the community did not necessarily mean that it would be used, particularly by severely disabled clients who often found accessing such diverse and fragmented services more of a challenge than they could manage. It began to be apparent that severely institutionalised service users with long-term and severe disabilities were also substantially disadvantaged in the community. Service users often lived in poverty and severe social isolation and were subject to being stigmatised and rejected by the neighbourhood where they lived.... Also, mental health professionals were not necessarily particularly well equipped to work with severely disabled service users who had previously stayed quiet in mental hospitals year after year. (Ryan 2004, p13–14)

In short, symptom alleviation was being eclipsed by the accessibility of ordinary services as the key indicator of a client's ability to manage in the community.

The Care Programme Approach

The Care Programme Approach (CPA)(DoH 1990) was introduced to prevent vulnerable clients falling out of care in this way and now provides the structure for addressing the full range of an individual's needs. It is integrated with the care management of social care and bestows on the care co-ordinator the authority to operate across professional and agency boundaries to knit together the relevant services. It usually has two distinct levels of care, standard and enhanced, depending on how comprehensive and complex the package of care has to be (DoH 1999b). It is, clearly, more than being a keyworker – which is a looser term normally used to describe someone who acts as the link person for a particular provider agency or resource within the broader care plan – and should not be confused with that role.

Prioritising severity

Throughout the 1990s services were expected to prioritise people with severe and enduring mental health problems because it was recognised that their needs were not being met. In the 1980s practitioners were largely able to choose who they worked with but with the advent of the CPA this had to stop (Ryan & Morgan 2004a). Community mental health services now focus on people with serious mental health problems and on delivering a co-ordinated, individualised package of care to each person.

Co-ordinated teamworking

Teamwork is not, itself, a clinical intervention but it does provide a platform for the effective delivery of care. In community mental health work the focus on severity and the complexity of challenges faced by service users mean that professional skills are pooled and services are generally provided through a process of co-ordinated multidisciplinary teamworking, in which the team becomes the conduit for all multiprofessional (and, for that matter, uniprofessional) interventions. The team, therefore, *is* the resource and effective teamworking between its members is the key to positive outcomes for clients; or, as Onyett (2003) puts it: 'Teams should be used when teamworking is required' (p.2).

In other words, teamworking is not the be-all and end-all of clinical intervention but when required, it must be effective and that requires both clarity of role and commitment to that role.

Onyett (2003) summarises the functions that any community mental health service must fulfil, as follows.

> We do need to be clear about the range of functions that need to be delivered locally. These include early intervention, assertive outreach for people who are difficult to engage, home treatment for people in crisis, services addressing the needs of people with dual diagnosis, culturally appropriate services for black and minority ethnic communities, and services for homeless people and mentally disordered offenders. All these services need to be able to address people's housing, income, occupational and social needs. (p.7)

These functions are usually performed by specific teams and are explored in detail later in *Working in Teams*.

The concept of a family of interconnected but autonomous teams, each with a specific function, is one way in which a traditional service-centred model of care has evolved into a more modern service user-centred model. Instead of the old-style hospital-based services serving a local population of generic mental health service users (that is, people with all types of mental health problem) with separate referral routes to different professional specialisms within that service, there is now a range of specialised community-based teams. Each has its own in-house range of professionals, and each addresses the particular needs of a more specialised service user population who access the relevant team via clear, unique acceptance criteria.

This represents an important evolutionary stage in community mental health practice. The problems of the former model are well documented and included multiple (often duplicated) assessments and care plans, confusion for service users and services, poor communication between the different specialties, and no single evaluation framework. The modern model means teams can be more responsive and hence more adaptive,

developing new kinds of knowledge and skills by focusing their collaborative problem solving on the specific presenting problems associated with particular service user groups.

The social model of disability

If the history of community service provision is the story of a move from fragmented to co-ordinated services, then a similarly overarching theme is an awakening sense of the restorative potential of community participation.

Many people have ongoing symptoms that cannot be removed by traditional treatment and the social inclusion agenda has highlighted that community living cannot be contingent on people ceasing to have problems. There is now far more of a consensus on the need for a broad interpretation of health and what sustains or restores it.

The social model of disability makes a distinction between impairment and disability. It sees disability as being imposed by society on top of any impairment (Oliver 1996). This shifts the emphasis from facilitating change in the disabled individual to changing the community in which they function. Perkins & Repper (2003) describe the importance of facilitating access to ordinary resources and relationships, noting that people with disabilities arising from mental health problems differ from others not in terms of their needs, but in terms of their ability to meet these needs with the ordinary resources available to them. It puts the onus on practitioners to facilitate access to the ordinary means by which people meet their needs, such as work, a home, a reasonable income, a social network and social activities, rather than treating an illness as such. Intervention must focus on a person's life as it is being lived and be compatible with it.

Implications for occupational therapy

From this brief history it is clear that a specifically occupational perspective of health is now highly relevant to the needs of people with serious mental health problems. Confidence in articulating the relevance of this to team goals is likely to be a crucial factor in the evolution of our practice.

The development of skills through an ongoing dynamic relationship with one's environment is fundamental to occupational therapy. We know occupation is contextual and does not happen in a vacuum; neither does occupational therapy. Nothing is context-free. If we apply open dynamic systems thinking to ourselves as practitioners and develop our understanding of how our unique occupational perspective of health and our professional skills can harmonise with our environment (referring to both the community and the teams we work in), it is likely that we will enhance the effectiveness of our practice in innovative ways.

HARNESSING THE RESTORATIVE POTENTIAL OF THE COMMUNITY

This section now concentrates on how an occupational perspective of the community can guide therapists in unlocking its restorative and therapeutic potential, and includes an exploration of how community partnerships can facilitate this. It also explores an occupational perspective of social inclusion and recovery as these are central themes in the College of Occupational Therapists' Mental Health Strategy (COT 2006a).

Occupational science

Occupational science can be influential in community mental health practice because of its emphasis on the role of the environment in the creation and maintenance of mental health problems, through occupational risk factors. These offer practitioners an inclusive language and portrays the essentially occupational nature of society and communities.

Occupational risk factors

There is growing evidence that the incidence and course of major mental health problems like schizophrenia are affected by environmental factors at individual, domestic and societal levels (Warner 2000). Occupational risk factors –occupational deprivation, occupational alienation and occupational imbalance (Wilcock 1998a) – offer a way of understanding the impact of broad-based issues such as poverty or racism on individuals' occupational opportunities and also the vulnerability of particular populations and groups. These factors describe disruptions to the relationship between an individual's occupations and his or her health, and the ongoing unresolved stress that this causes (Townsend & Wilcock 2004, Wilcock 1998a, b).

Significantly for community practitioners, this disruption can arise at any or all of the four interconnected, but distinct, levels at which occupation is organised and has meaning: the individual, the family, society and the population (Molineux & Whiteford 2006). This underlines the importance of macro- and micro-level clinical reasoning and intervention which is now strongly advocated within our professional literature. Krupa et al (2002), for example, describe three roles for therapists in creating occupational opportunities for individuals. These are: one-to-one work with service users and their social networks, brokering within mental health resources and, most importantly, working with the broader community.

Language

Using the terminology of occupational risk factors not only clarifies and legitimises a complex set of ideas and experiences as a coherent topic, but does so in an inclusive way that can be understood by non-occupational therapy colleagues (van Niekerk 2005). The term 'occupational deprivation' may not have the same depth and resonance for a social worker, nurse or psychiatrist as it would for an occupational therapist but it is, in the author's experience, an accessible concept that allows different bodies of knowledge about mental health and deprivation to converge. It fosters the cross-pollination of ideas within a team and can support interprofessional and interagency working, as explored later.

The occupational nature of the community

Wilcock (1993, 1995) has described how early humans, through their occupations, built communities and society over evolutionary time and how occupations are therefore built-in or implicit to social relations, and to communities themselves, as a result. Communities consist of people who do things together. This has implications for how occupational therapists answer the fundamental question, 'How do I ensure I'm using meaningful occupation with service users?'.

Negotiating meaning

The wide range of occupational forms available to community-based therapists includes, essentially, whatever is *out there* in the community. This allows the therapist to go with the service user's interests and frame his occupational choices as therapeutic media, using activity analysis.

The analysis of an occupational form involves considering its performance components and their complexity, understanding how they are sequenced, and acknowledging the social and cultural associations in order to evaluate its therapeutic potential (Duncan 2006). Once analysed in this way, a range of approaches can be applied so that, effectively, any occupation can be harnessed to meet therapeutic ends.

The efficacy of naturally occurring occupations is one of the greatest assets which the community-based therapist has (Yerxa 1994). They often carry particular social and cultural resonances for individuals, which can give the meaningfulness of the occupation, the transferability of skills acquired, and hence the effectiveness of the therapy, a huge head start;

> The knowledge and skill that is gained during the intervention will better carry over to life when it is gained in the natural setting. Therefore our interventions typically take place in the consumer's home, at a local grocery store, or other community settings. (Wollenberg 2001, p108)

These locked-in meanings not only act as a powerful motivator to engage but, once unlocked by the doer, can also become a powerful intrinsic reward to carry on doing, offering much reinforcement of an individual's personal and social identity. Because meaning is therefore both ascribed and derived from the occupation in a uniquely personal way (Kielhofner & Barrett 1998), it cannot be bestowed by the therapist alone. It has to be negotiated and verified jointly.

Using natural settings also helps therapists answer a second underlying question: 'Should the goal of occupational therapy be to help clients acquire the discrete skills and behaviours needed to manage in the community first; or should it be to help clients acquire those skills by living in the community?'.

The former approach is usually characteristic of inpatient or day hospital programmes, where *synthetic* occupations are created with specific therapeutic outcomes in mind, such as addressing deficits in specific performance components. The latter approach is usually the approach adopted by community therapists and is based on naturalistic or real-life occupations in their normal, mainstream settings (van Niekerk 2005) which may also be more acceptable because they are less stigmatising. It brings person centredness and skilled activity analysis to the fore and supports socially inclusive practice.

SOCIAL INCLUSION

Adults with mental health problems are one of the most marginalised, stigmatised and socially excluded groups in society (Office of the Deputy Prime Minister 2004). Social inclusion for mental health service users has long been advocated by the service user movement (Dunn 1999). It is now a government priority (Care Services Improvement Partnership 2006b) and a professional one too (College of Occupational Therapists 2006a).

Burchardt et al (2002) describe social exclusion as non-participation in the key activities of the society in which a person lives. This not only suggests that inclusion is an essentially occupational phenomena, echoing Wilcock (1993, 1995, 1998b), but highlights that solutions to the problems of social exclusion must involve the whole of society. Socially inclusive mental health practice is just one piece of the jigsaw puzzle. Equally important is macro-level work aimed at creating more accepting communities, and much leverage (described later) exists to support therapists in doing this. In this sense social inclusion relates closely to occupational justice (Townsend & Wilcock 2004) because it is about recognising and providing for the occupational needs of individuals and communities as part of a fair and empowering society.

It is particularly important now, while national agendas are focused on social inclusion and mental health, that these ideas should be embraced by occupational therapists and put to work. Our professional theory and skills equip us well for this task, and for taking up the challenge to operate confidently and effectively as *political* animals (Richards 2005). An overview of social networks and social capital may help to illustrate this.

Social networks

MIND (2004) has shown that 84% of people with mental health problems feel socially isolated, compared with 29% of the general population.

Social networks can have a protective effect, acting as buffers to stressors and adverse life events, can promote help-seeking behaviour, validate and develop an individual's self-concept, enhance a person's self-esteem, mood and world view and provide a structure within which skills can be learned, adapted and reinforced (Langford et al 1997, Nolan 1995).

This efficacy depends on the relationships within a network being reciprocal or two-way (Bates et al 2000, Mitchell & Trickett 1980) so the individual perceives himself as a significant network member who can receive and give support. It also depends on the individual's sense of the connections being built and maintained by his *own* efforts.

Social networking through occupation implicitly promotes these features and may well be more engaging and more effective than traditional programme-based social skills training. Furthermore, because specific occupations often support their own communities or social networks, this clarifies an otherwise hazy notion of what the community actually means. Without an occupational basis, it may mean very little. In *An Open Letter to Mental Health Professionals*, Hart (2003) writes:

> Some people talk glibly about moving on – out into the community. Most sufferers from mental distress don't have a community to go out to, especially when we've been marginalized for years, not only by the general public but also by the very services that purport to help us. (p15)

Occupational engagement can therefore transform the notion of community from being a community of mental health professionals, often the sad truth

for many service users (Bates et al 2000), into something more real and self-determined.

Social capital

Social capital is the glue that holds communities together (Cameron et al 2003). It comprises the networks that are woven into the fabric of a society, the personal identity arising from membership and the norms of trust, support and reciprocal help that gradually build up from participating in them (Puttnam, cited in Sainsbury Centre for Mental Health 2000).

Whilst stretching out through a community, social capital actually relies on the personal and idiosyncratic social contacts and activities that make up a person's day-to-day life, however mundane they may seem. Again, it is an occupational phenomenon.

The social inclusion traffic lights

The National Development Team's inclusion traffic lights system (Bates 2005) was devised to clarify thinking about the relative social inclusiveness of the various settings where mental health staff work with service users. Red refers to places used only by mental health service users and providers such as inpatient units or day hospitals; amber refers to service user sessions taking place in venues regularly used by the wider community (such as a day service sports group at a local leisure centre); and green refers to activities where clients are shoulder to shoulder with the general public.

It is perhaps most helpful to view the function of these metaphorical traffic lights as being the same as the real ones, which is to facilitate movement and allow people to make their journeys successfully. Because each colour will have particular qualities regarding issues of safety, supportiveness, opportunity, challenge and integration, it follows that all three colours are necessary in a comprehensive mental health service. For some individuals there will need to be a continuum that allows movement and progress. So, arguably, the most accurate answer to the question, 'What colour is inclusion?' would be that it is brown; that is, all the colours combined.

Occupational therapists as travelling companions

Occupational therapists are well equipped to accompany service users on a recovery journey through the traffic lights because occupation, in being both a means and an end of therapy, can be the consistent vehicle for that journey. Its emphasis can change from having a primarily therapeutic function to ultimately acting as a conduit for social participation, perhaps through adult education, vocational training, volunteering or employment, as the service user makes progress.

Deitchman (1980, cited in Morgan 2004) suggests service users want a travel *companion* because they can share experiences with them, as opposed to a travel *agent* who merely gives directions and makes bookings. In practical terms, this often means doing things alongside service users; that is, sharing an occupational engagement with them. As an informal assessment process, this not only allows therapists to get to know service users and their occupational performance well, and in a way that appears to be more equal from the service user's perspective, but it also allows the therapist to understand some complex psychosocial challenges that can arise for them on the journey.

Understanding stigma

Influential work on social stigma by Goffman (1968) highlighted the complex dilemma facing many mental health service users in the community:

> ... it is not that he must face prejudice against himself, but rather that he must face unwitting acceptance of himself by individuals who are prejudiced against persons of the kind he can be revealed to be. (Goffman 1968, p58)

This description of walking a knife's edge between participation and the possibility of provoking a stigmatising response creates enormous tension for many people. The constant vigilance for potentially disclosing information, or stigma management (Goffman 1968), is not only stressful but can be (quite literally) preoccupying, in that it can prevent occupational engagement.

Whilst the occupational therapy profession is familiar with environmental adaptation, assistive technology and antidiscriminatory legislation in promoting the occupational engagement of people with physical challenges, these complex psychosocial barriers are comparatively less well understood (Rebeiro 2001, van Niekerk 2005).

Affirming environments

Rebeiro (2001) has shown that a key feature of affirming environments, where these barriers are lowered, appears to be the empathic and accepting attitudes of the other people also present. Significantly, it is other people who are felt by an individual to share his stigma who are uniquely qualified to provide this. People appear to value the opportunity to undergo a gradual and reciprocally supportive destigmatising process at their own pace, which in turn promotes experimentation and skill acquisition.

So, in addition to social inclusiveness, therapists need to consider this affirming and restorative dimension of environments in their clinical reasoning and care planning.

COMMUNITY PARTNERSHIPS

As well as a wide range of occupational forms available to harness the community, there are many opportunities to forge community partnerships across the sectors and agencies that host occupational opportunities in the community. This kind of macro-level work, creating access points for service users, can create a range of colleagues with new skills, perspectives and material resources and can be very rewarding. It can, in the author's experience, feel as if a wall is being dismantled from both sides.

There are several reasons why managers may support therapists' time commitment to project work like this. For example, a therapist tackling the occupational deprivation of her clients may find this occupies common ground with a widening participation agenda within the local further education (FE) community. The perceived added value, to the therapist's time, in co-working with partners outside statutory services may be a decisive factor in managers' support. Similarly, there is an economy of scale. If a project builds a bridge with a local college, the bridge can be used by more than one service user. It adds to the resources of the team by creating a move-on pathway that would otherwise require time-consuming casework on an individual-by-individual basis. Collectivising the need is an example of working with a population. Furthermore, such work may open up opportunities for joint bidding for funds from, for example, the government's New Deal for Communities or national bodies such as the Learning and Skills Council (LSC) or charities.

The potential benefits for service users are substantial. The experience of doing a pottery session, for example, as a *student* may be more meaningful and more motivating than doing pottery as part of a day service programme, where the *patient* status is reinforced (Westwood 2003). Also, introducing non-mental health staff into the team's resources can diversify and normalise an individual's support network. Through joint working the relative amounts of therapist/tutor input can be graded to offer both amber and green (traffic light) environments in the college setting so the therapeutic dimensions of the session are retained. The key to service users taking such a step may well be the availability of an amber starting-point or *base camp*, which can be affirming in the ways described and allow people to acclimatise and prepare for the next step. The skill of the therapist may lie in asserting the need for this, if the overall project is to work.

Crucially, there are also incentives for the education service, which is effectively drawing in expert assistance in fulfilling its remit of widening the participation of local citizens as learners. Indeed, the LSC specifically aims to build the capacity of the FE system to support the learning of people with mental health problems (Learning and Skills Council 2006).

Developing the rehabilitative function of the normal, mainstream community is a fundamental social inclusion issue (Care Services Improvement Partnerships 2006a). It extends the navigator or travel companion role and involves the therapist straddling the divide from services to occupations with her clients. Working with the community in this way is likely to assist therapists in developing new skills which may be highly useful to service users, and also highly valued by managers and commissioners of services.

RECOVERY

Recovery is not a therapy, or an intervention, or a type of team (Perkins 2005). It is another aspect of the paradigm shift in mental health away from an overexclusive focus on treatment, to an emphasis on the individual's subjective experience. It does not mean service users should not also be offered the most effective psychiatric treatment that is available, but it does focus on the context in which that happens.

Recovery has been described as the lived experience of people as they accept and overcome the challenge of their disability and experience themselves recovering a new sense of self and of purpose within and beyond the limits of their disability (Deegan 1988).

Historically, people diagnosed with serious mental health problems have been seen as suffering with lifelong disabilities. However, it has been shown that many people are able to recover and lead satisfying lives. Much of the evidence for recovery has come from the personal accounts of service users who have described their journeys from despair to empowerment (Ralph 2004). Mancini (2006) notes the contrast between descriptions of institutional care, characterised by diagnostic labels and a passive patient role, and descriptions of a recovery process, rich in metaphors of growth and transformation, characterised by an active participation in treatment, engagement in occupations and a renewed social life. Indeed, social inclusion has been described as the culmination of a recovery-orientated health service (Sayce 2000).

Deegan (2001) describes how her own renewed identity had to be asserted in the face of unwitting stigmatisation by practitioners (including occupational therapists). She highlights a simple truth about the unproductiveness of this stigmatising process: 'Of course, the great danger of reducing a person to an illness is that there is no one left to do the work of recovery' (Deegan 2001, p9).

Recovery involves committing to a process rather than setting an endpoint as a goal (Deegan 2001).

This point is frequently taken up by service users who perceive that the term 'recovery' is sometimes used by services as a cloak to cover up cuts or to discharge people inappropriately from overstretched and underfunded teams: Some service users have felt threatened by professionals' adoption of recovery because they fear it will mean an additional and unwelcome expectation is placed on them (Roberts & Wolfson 2004). Consequently, recovery needs to be seen in terms of hope and opportunity.

Hope and opportunity

The recovery literature highlights hope and opportunity as the resources that fuel an individual's journey, and describes the important role of other individuals in being holders of hope on the recovering individual's behalf. This role can only exist within a non-hierarchical relationship based on an in-depth knowledge of the person built up over time. Glover (2001) describes the need for a delicate balance within a robust relationship:

> Getting the balance right is the difference between mollycoddling and helping people discover life in a way that they drive their own journey. Knowing when to do for someone... or with someone... and when to kick butt... are the intuitive competencies we must all learn to struggle with and fine tune. (p5)

For practitioners, Perkins (2004) suggests this all-important in-depth knowledge of a service user will include an awareness of his relapse signature, pre-agreed strategies for managing early warning signs, close liaison with crisis and other out-of-hours services when needed, in-reach with the hospital ward if the individual is admitted to hospital, and person-centred goal setting, which is explored in the next section.

Occupational therapy and recovery

There is much common ground between recovery and occupational therapy. Both are concerned with a fundamental, subjective, human experience that is unique for each person; both are responses to the dominant medical paradigm in health care; both cite 19th-century moral treatment as

an influence; both focus on strengths rather than symptoms; both are person centred and promote self-management and autonomy; both stress the importance of choice; both are interested in an individual's story or personal narrative; and both describe themselves in terms of their transformative potential (see Chapters 22 and 23).

Rebeiro (2005) describes particular overlap on issues such as self-esteem, self-efficacy, empowerment, self-determination, quality of life, hope, insight, social support, spirituality, inclusion, belonging, friendships, community and affirming environments. Similarly, she observes that countering stigma is increasingly being acknowledged as a pivotal factor in community integration, meaningful occupation and recovery.

WORKING WITH SERVICE USERS

This section looks at ways of developing and maintaining a person-centred, facilitative approach to one-to-one work in community practice and begins with an outline of some of the issues on which there appears to be a consensus within the service user movement.

THE INFLUENCE OF THE SERVICE USER MOVEMENT

The *NHS Plan* (DoH 2000) advocates service user influence at all levels of the planning and delivery of NHS services, and the notion of a patient-led NHS is widely promoted (DoH 2005).

However, it is still unclear how far this is being implemented within mental health services (Rose 2001). A tension exists between service users' wish to be included in service planning in a real sense, and the worry that it can easily become tokenistic or caught up in the minutiae and cease being a critical eye on the bigger picture. As Alison Faulkner (an independent service user researcher and formerly of the Mental Health Foundation) has observed, when service users are invited to join committees or decision-making bodies:

> ... users will find themselves faced with long documents which they find really boring and all

they will be able to do is comment on paragraphs 11 to 17. They won't be able to say 'Scrap it and start again'. The worry is that all we will be able to do is tinker at the margins. (Laurance 2003, p87)

A striking feature of the service user movement, and which arguably has no parallel in any other aspect of health care, is the strength of its opposition to many existing mental health practices. There is a consensus on what is perceived to be a general devaluing of the service user experience, in terms of both their accounts of living with mental health problems and of using and evaluating mental health services (Laurance 2003).

There is now an increasing obligation on mental health professionals to learn about service users' experiences of them, and to use that information to shape their own practice (Cameron et al 2003). Indeed, if occupational therapists value client-centredness, we will need to listen to the service user movement as well as our individual clients. Significantly, most professional literature on client-centred practice approaches it from only the professionals' point of view (Whalley-Hammell 2006).

WORKING WITH PERSONAL STRENGTHS

Often, the greatest asset to a therapist's work is the service user's own momentum and working with personal strengths gives this full rein. As enablers of occupation, therapists' work should primarily be based on the premise that, for each person or group of people, there will be things they need and want to do in order to grow, flourish, and experience well-being (Wilcock 1998a).

Consequently, any assessment of a service user's *needs* should also include what a service user *wants*. After all, in our personal lives we do not consider ourselves as having friends and partners as a means of *support*, primarily. Nor do we consider what activities will allow us to *structure our weekend*. Though mutual support may be a feature of the important relationships in our life, they do not owe their existence to *needing support*. Similarly, a common short-circuiting of therapists' clinical reasoning is when *needs* are automatically framed in terms of *services*, as Ryan & Morgan (2004b) point out:

For example, a service user who is deemed to be socially isolated may be assessed as having 'problems socialising' and therefore 'needing' a social skills training group. This is a service-led response in that a problem the client is perceived as experiencing is defined as being met by what the service has to offer, whether or not it is actually what the user themselves really wants, and regardless of the actual aspirations the user may have in terms of social contact. (p159)

PERSON-CENTRED GOAL SETTING

As described, recovery requires collaborative and person-centred goal setting. This process has implications for where expertise is perceived to exist or rather, whose expertise is most valued. Biomedical and earlier mental health models prioritised the professional's clinical judgement in prescribing interventions. However, if we accept the primacy of the service user's experience of living with his challenges, this places service users in their rightful position as experts on their own lives. Importantly, this can allow the expertise of the therapist to come to the fore too: 'The empowerment of the consumer empowers the occupational therapist to use his or her clinical reasoning to develop effective interventions' (Wollenberg 2001, p107).

It is a win–win situation that plays to the unique strengths of each partner in the relationship. Also, because goal setting springs naturally from situations where people feel their skills are being used effectively and can be mobilised at will (Forysth & Kielhofner 2006), person-centred goals are likely to breed more goals. It is one way of instilling and holding hope. Significantly, the occupational therapist's expertise is regarded as being the clinical reasoning not the selection of occupational form, echoing the point made earlier about framing and harnessing real-life occupations in the community.

WORKING WITH CULTURAL DIVERSITY

It may be tempting for occupational therapy to assume that, with person-centredness at its core, it would be less prone to slipping into service-centred practices. However, it has been noted that occupational therapy theory may, itself, conceal tacit standards and ideals for what is considered good practice, but which may not be experienced as culturally safe by all our service users: 'Will our existing theories and methods of application, which reflect middle-class Western-centric norms, change to meet these diverse societal needs?' (Iwama 2005, p225).

It is widely acknowledged that services users from black and minority ethnic (BME) communities often carry the double burden of living with a mental health problem and discrimination by the very service providers whose help they need (Rankin 2005). Significantly, during the consultation process for the College of Occupational Therapists mental health strategy, most BME respondents had a negative view of occupational therapy and described being offered irrelevant activities, disconnected from their situation, in both hospital and community settings (College of Occupational Therapists 2006b).

Working with people from distinct and diverse cultural backgrounds, often in their own homes, requires not only awareness of diverse occupational forms but also an openness to different perspectives of what occupation can mean to different people. This may challenge one's assumptions about occupational therapy but it is an opportunity for reflection that must be grasped. It is an important way in which community occupational therapy can develop.

CONFIDENTIALITY

Confidentiality is, obviously, a precondition for trust and a therapeutic relationship and is always *team confidentiality*. In the community, working with a high degree of autonomy can expose a therapist to situations where a service user may presume that an absolute one-to-one confidentiality exists. He may disclose sensitive information which the therapist knows should be shared with the team. This can place an unnecessary burden on the therapeutic relationship, particularly if the service user feels let down when he learns that what was believed to be a secret has been shared. Openness about team confidentiality from the beginning at least gives the service user the choice about what to disclose and provides clear ground rules for the relationship.

POSITIVE RISK MANAGEMENT

The role of mental health services is shaped by the society of which they are part, and it is important to acknowledge the different agendas they therefore serve. In addition to helping people with mental health problems, services also undertake a role in controlling or managing behaviour that is not socially accepted, such as posing a risk to oneself or others through violence or self-neglect (Onyett 2003).

Services have tended to err on the side of caution and instinctively play it safe in terms of what clients are supported to do. Positive risk management acknowledges that some degree of risk, or challenge, is essential to skill acquisition, self-esteem and progress (College of Occupational Therapists 2006a). Positively managing risk does not mean being complacent about risk, but encourages a person-centred approach to evaluating it. Being risk averse can be seen as part of the lack of hopefulness on the part of practitioners and a barrier to recovery (Deegan 2001, Perkins 2004).

Risk management issues may arise in relation to working with service users in mainstream public settings or in the community partnership work described earlier. It is important that therapists clarify these quickly so services do not get stuck in the default position of being risk averse. The notion of public liability may be helpful to consider and trusts will have a risk manager (usually a senior manager at board level) who can advise on risk issues related to particular projects that therapists may want to develop in consultation with their team manager.

THE THERAPEUTIC USE OF SELF

The therapeutic use of self is arguably the most important skill a therapist has. (Duncan 2006, p47)

The therapeutic use of self means knowing oneself and being oneself in a conscious and disciplined way so that personal qualities and attributes can be harnessed in the service of one's professional role (Hagedorn 2000).

Yarwood & Johnstone (2002, cited in Duncan 2006) list the establishment of rapport, respecting the client's wishes, personal honesty and good communication skills as the foundations for the therapeutic use of self and for developing a therapeutic relationship. Similarly, Parker (2006) notes that person-centred therapists are likely to be approachable, welcoming, genuine and spontaneous in their interactions with service users. They are able to instil a sense of security and trust, listen well and offer non-judgemental, non-authoritarian comments. They allow ownership of change to remain with the client and are able to acknowledge their own mistakes openly. (See chapter 13.)

WORKING IN A POLICY CONTEXT

In considering potential new ways of working in mental health the College of Occupational Therapists notes the influence of the *National Service Framework for Mental Health* (NSFMH) (DoH 1999a), the *Social Exclusion Unit Report* (Office of the Deputy Prime Minister 2004), and the *Mental Health Policy Implementation Guides* (MHPIG) (DoH 2001, Ormston 2006).

A summary of each is presented here so that a knowledge of the policy context can help therapists identify allies and champions, levers and buttons in support of their role as political animals when lobbying for occupation. Similarly, an understanding of the overall structure of service commissioning should clarify where and how decisions about services are made.

It is always advisable to get to know the local structure within which one operates as a therapist but as a general overview, primary care trusts control about 80% of the NHS budget and cover all aspects of health care. They are local so they can understand and be responsive to the needs of their local community, whilst strategic health authorities monitor performance and standards. In all areas a local implementation team, bringing together the views of commissioners, providers and users of local mental health services, will be monitoring the implementation of the NSFMH by trying to develop services to match local needs (Cameron et al 2003).

NATIONAL SERVICE FRAMEWORK FOR MENTAL HEALTH (DoH 1999a)

The NSFMH set out a 10-year strategy to tackle issues of public mental health by not only seeking health improvements for service users, but also challenging stigma and discrimination and promoting understanding of mental health issues in the wider population. It lists seven standards spanning five areas: health promotion and stigma; primary care and specialist services; the needs of people with severe and enduring mental health problems; their carers' needs; and suicide reduction.

Its first standard on health promotion specified three levels to this work: strengthening the individual by building personal resilience; strengthening communities by increasing participation; and reducing barriers by increasing access (Sainsbury Centre for Mental Health/mentality 2001).

As a complex intervention (Creek 2003), with biopsycho-sociocultural dimensions, occupational therapy operates at each of these levels and the NSFMH provides ample leverage for occupational therapists to bring an occupational perspective to the fore in their own practice setting.

SOCIAL EXCLUSION UNIT REPORT (OFFICE OF THE DEPUTY PRIME MINISTER 2004)

In order to promote social inclusion, this report set out an action plan to challenge stigma and discrimination, to clarify the role of health and social care in promoting social inclusion, to promote employment, to support families, to promote community participation, to address iniquities in housing and finances and to develop a cross-departmental national programme to maintain the momentum of change (Office of the Deputy Prime Minister 2004).

This agenda covers many occupational therapy issues such as day service modernisation, education, volunteering, community participation and employment (Care Services Improvement Partnership 2006b) and there has been an occupational therapist on the national programme team (seconded from the COT). It sets objectives to guide practice and offers much support for therapists' advocacy of an occupational perspective of social inclusion.

MENTAL HEALTH POLICY AND IMPLEMENTATION GUIDE (DoH 2001)

Mental health is a government priority for service improvement (DoH 2000) and a direct approach to shaping the local delivery of national policy is evident in this guide which provides team specifications, examined below.

WORKING IN TEAMS

The following overview of the teams described in the MHPIG (DoH 2001) sets the scene for the majority of therapists' practice in community settings. Additionally, this section looks at outcome measurement and care co-ordination from an occupational therapist's point of view, and examines some teamworking issues that may arise for therapists also.

TYPES OF TEAMS

There is a range of community teams and services to meet the specific requirements of service users.

Crisis resolution and home treatment teams

These teams provide a 24-hours/7days per week service offering an alternative to inpatient care, as far as possible, for working-age adults who are in an acute mental health crisis. They will also gatekeep by rapidly assessing people and referring them on as necessary. This may happen, for example, if the crisis is related to a primary diagnosis of alcohol or substance misuse or has occurred solely in the context of relationship problems. The aim is to respond to referrals rapidly and work with service users in the least restrictive environment possible – usually the service user's home, alongside their existing support and social networks. Practitioners will be aiming to maximise the service user's self-monitoring and coping strategies, and offering both education and practical assistance. Contacts are frequent (potentially several times per day) but the overall episode of care may be comparatively brief compared to the longer term input from other teams to which the service user may be referred once the crisis is resolved.

Assertive outreach teams

These teams are designed to cater for the small number of working-age adults within any population who have severe mental health problems and complex health and social care needs but who either do not wish to use services or have difficulty doing so. They also operate a 7-day per week service, with flexibility to extend out of hours where necessary.

Assertive outreach service users will often have entrenched difficulties in several areas of life and the input from teams may be intense in terms of both frequency of contact (sometimes daily) and duration (often years). This involves much commitment on the part of practitioners to the quality of their relationship with service users, which needs to be engaging and facilitative, and which requires a conscious focus on the therapeutic use of self.

Practitioners are likely to need a long-term perspective of recovery and social inclusion and may address needs related to accommodation, occupational deprivation and alienation, dual diagnosis, risks related to self-neglect, challenging behaviour or a history of violence or offending.

A generic, problem-solving process is funnelled through a whole-team approach which operates across professional boundaries and requires frankness and openness with colleagues so decisions can be owned by the whole team.

Early Intervention in Psychosis Service

These teams work specifically with people who are in the early stages of developing psychotic symptoms. The range of potential referrers includes Child and Adolescent Mental Health Services and GPs. Often, the onset of psychosis is at a crucial developmental stage in an individual's life (the majority occur between 14 and 35) and timely help has been shown to improve long-term outcomes and recovery. Interventions are aimed at minimising stigma and dislocation of valued social and familial roles and occupations, such as education and employment.

Skilled work is required to address early problems that may be indistinguishable from the normal emotional upheaval of adolescence, and possibly occurring in the midst of difficult family dynamics.

Primary care liaison teams (PCLTs)

As the name suggests, these teams are a support and resource to primary care (GPs) and have the option of referring on to more specialised tertiary services, such as those above, where necessary. They provide the bulk of care to mental health service users in the community. As CMHTs have prioritised severity of need, the role of GPs in treating people with a wide range of mental health problems has increased, and GPs will rely on a prompt referral and assessment relationship with the PCLT. This is via a single point of entry to the team as a whole and not to a specific profession. In some cases a full, needs-led PCLT assessment and advice is the main purpose of the referral, with the assessed person not actually being taken on by the PCLT at all.

PCLTs provide services to people with time-limited problems who can be referred back to their GPs after a few weeks or months and also to a substantial minority with serious mental health problems whose contact with the team may last for years, and whose care will be co-ordinated using the CPA.

PCLTs are expected to address the full spectrum of people's needs including physical and psychiatric care; practical help and advocacy with the whole range of basic living needs such as personal care, budgeting, shopping, income entitlements, and accommodation; help in accessing occupation, work, education and/or training; emotional support; liaison and support for families and carers; and specific psychological therapies if appropriate (DoH 2001).

About 80% of PCLT service users will be on an 'enhanced' level of CPA (DoH 2001). The team will comprise a skill mix that can address all the above interventions and be made up of practitioners whose sole responsibility is to work in that team. This would usually include 1 or 1.5 occupational therapists, 1 or 1.5 clinical psychologists, 2 or 3 social workers and 3 or 4 nurses, all of whom would act as CPA care co-ordinators. Other clinical team members such as medical staff and support workers would not normally undertake enhanced care co-ordination.

Other occupation–based services

The range of services employing occupational therapists is diverse and likely to diversify further. The College of Occupational Therapy's 10-year mental health strategy envisions extending occupational therapy's scope beyond statutory health and social care services (College of Occupational Therapists 2006a). Two aspects of current service provision which routinely employ occupational therapists, but which are not classed as CMHTs, are day services and vocational services. Here the emphasis is usually on providing a particular facility that may be incorporated into care planning, though a care co-ordination role may also be undertaken with people using the service over the long term.

Day services

These can serve the dual functions of acting as a bridge from inpatient units into the community and as a resource that may help an individual avoid a hospital admission. They usually offer an occupation-based programme aiming to help people retain or develop social roles and relationships, and access mainstream social, leisure and vocational opportunities. Much development work is focused on transforming traditional, buildings-based day hospitals into more outward-looking day services which can promote recovery and social inclusion, and develop the rehabilitative function of mainstream occupations (Care Services Improvement Programme 2006a).

Vocational services

Vocational rehabilitation refers to a range of approaches that may help a person overcome practical and psychosocial barriers in accessing, retaining or returning to work. It can take place in and across statutory and voluntary mental health services, mainstream employment services, and open employment. Vocational rehabilitation is prioritised as a social inclusion issue (Office of the Deputy Prime Minister 2004) and, perhaps conflictingly, as part of the reform of incapacity benefits (Department of Work and Pensions 2006, Meacher 2006).

MEASURING OUTCOMES WITHIN TEAMS

The clinical governance and evidence-based practice agendas have a high profile in community mental health because serious mental health problems generate high degrees of disability and distress and draw heavily on the resources of health and social care (Brooker & Repper 2003).

All professions appear to encounter practical difficulties in measuring outcomes (Slade 2006). Godden et al (2006) found that factors influencing occupational therapists' use of outcome measures in mental health settings included perceived time constraints, ease of use, and the culture of managerial and peer support. Concerns about the client-centredness of the measurement tool, the nature of the therapeutic relationship this fostered, and the availability of specific training in outcome measurement were also factors.

Additionally, in the community, because multi-professional teams offer a single co-ordinated package of care to individual clients, the question of which outcomes may be attributable to which intervention may be a difficult one to unpick.

To guide occupational therapists, Finlay (2004) has outlined four approaches to measuring mental health outcomes. These are: comparing progress against clear, specific behavioural objectives; employing a standardised measure; using quality of life measures, which are gaining ground within mental health generally and may also (because of their social and occupational focus) be appropriate for occupational therapists; and, finally, using person-centred, subjective measures, or self-ratings, of an individual's own perception of progress.

Although none of these approaches represents the elusive solution for resolving all outcome measurement dilemmas, any or all can be tried out locally. Significantly, the National Institute for Mental Health in England recognises the widespread difficulties in measuring outcomes and suggests that bottom-up solutions from the local level offer the best way to meet top-down policy

requirements from government (National Institute for Mental Health in England 2005).

OCCUPATIONAL THERAPY AND CARE CO-ORDINATION

From the MHPIG (DoH 2001) it is clear that, as core CMHT members, occupational therapists are expected to take on a care co-ordination role. This has generated much discussion in our professional literature, often producing a rather polarised debate which may be bewildering for new graduates. So, in keeping with the stated aim of providing a navigational aid to inform therapists' own judgement, what follows is an attempt to contextualise care co-ordination within a broad occupational perspective of health. This brings into view several reasons why occupational therapists are entitled to feel confident and positive about taking on this role.

Skills required for care co-ordination

First, the skills needed to make a good care co-ordinator are not owned by any single profession but are, nevertheless, essential to a team's functioning, and are well within occupational therapists' reach. They are said to include: a therapeutic optimism and person-centredness when working with service users, including an ability to form empathic and effective partnerships with users and carers; a preparedness to focus on the minutiae of daily living; a flexible, solution-focused approach; an awareness of the need for positive risk taking; an ability to plan, implement and evaluate interventions; a capacity for holistically assessing needs, and for recognising changing needs; an ability to co-ordinate and review a care plan based on this; an up-to-date knowledge of relevant legislation; and the ability to make use of a team (Onyett 2003, Ryan & Morgan 2004b).

Congruence of roles

However, there is a second and more fundamental reason why a care co-ordination role can feature prominently in therapists' practice, which contains potential benefits to their teams, to their service users, to themselves as practitioners, and to their profession. It is the congruence between occupational therapy skills and the needs of people with serious mental health problems. This is another facet of the evolution of community care, seen as the *prioritisation of practicality* (Morgan & Ryan 2004). A historical perspective may prove to be illuminating here. When community mental health teams were developing in the 1990s a review of existing practice stated:

> The presence of occupational therapists is strongly associated with activities of particular relevance to people with severe and long-term mental health problems, such as training in activities of daily living and assisting clients in achieving satisfying work and leisure...occupational therapists may offer the best model for professional input to CMHT's currently available. (Onyett et al 1995, p38)

Similarly Peck & Norman (1999) cited occupational therapy's focus on the functional consequences of illness and adaptive skill acquisition, its use of strengths to address deficits and its use of occupation as an assessment, intervention and evaluation medium as characterising its highly valued role in community mental health.

This congruence means that therapists do not have to regard decisions about how to combine profession-specific and team roles as an awkward dilemma or a dichotomous choice between polar opposites. Occupation is central to both roles and allows both roles to be mutually informing. Indeed, the most pertinent contemporary question might be 'How can an occupational perspective of health be integrated into the broader work of the CMHT?' (Corrigan 2002, Fowler Davis & Ilott 2002, Harrison 2003).

Integrating an occupational perspective into teamwork enables occupational therapy theory and practice to adapt and develop in harmony with national, evidence-based agendas, and to respond positively to the need for all professions to accommodate to new multidisciplinary environments (Ormston 2006).

The congruence between professional skills, service user needs and team goals is an asset to occupational therapists in a rapidly changing working environment. Allen (2005) suggests that some professions have sought care co-ordination roles because they have been liberating and

offered a greater breadth of responsibility and autonomy whilst also allowing the perspective of the care co-ordinator to express itself. Where this is an occupational perspective, care co-ordination can become a powerful lens bringing diverse interventions into a single, practical focal point – that is, the service user's daily living and his aspirations about it.

Similarity of process

A third point of similarity between care co-ordination and occupational therapy relates to the process of each. Care co-ordination can be very similar to Hagedorn's (1992) notion of the triadic or triangular relationship between the service user, the therapist and the service user's occupations. Hagedorn suggests that, in contrast to other dyadic or two-way relationships between professionals and service users, occupational therapists have a third territory where the therapist can *do* with the service user, and be informed by both her observations and by the service user's reports on that doing. It is the same pattern in care co-ordination, except it is a triad formed between the service user, the therapist and the activities encompassed by the care plan which, as described above, is an essentially occupational domain.

A final reason for promoting a care co-ordination role – which is pragmatic but nonetheless important – is that, as whole-team effectiveness is increasingly prized by purchasers and commissioners of services, the different professions' preparedness to undertake care co-ordination will increasingly inform recruitment decisions (Harrison 2003, Hyde 2002). It does not mean that professions' unique skills are not also prized, but simply that a balanced commitment to both is expected. Indeed, the New Ways of Working (NWW) initiative (www.nimhe.csip.org.uk), which aims to foster an evolutionary process among services, regards effective teamwork as the best way to deliver specialist input where it is needed most.

PERSON-CENTRED CARE PLANNING

To be effective, care planning must engage the service user as an active partner. Care planning usually means assembling a package of care that co-ordinates input from a range of sources. For example, a particular individual's care plan may include the following:

- specific interventions from members of the CMHT
- input from the service user's GP
- a drop-in centre or support group, perhaps run by MIND (www.mind.org.uk) or by Rethink (www.rethink.org)
- a self-help group such as a Hearing Voices Group (www.hearing-voices.org)
- sessions with a vocational rehabilitation service
- some aspect of the service user's ordinary occupations, such as an adult education class or a local walking group
- the role of the support worker at the service user's housing association
- a particular input from the service user's family or carer
- the service user's own contribution and agreement to the plan.

The care plan should be recorded in straightforward language and the service user should be given a copy. At best, it can be written by the service user himself. Efforts to make the care-planning experience as user-friendly and meaningful as possible should include consultation with the service user about the time and place of the meeting; negotiation well in advance regarding who will attend; and the provision of an independent interpreter if necessary. In addition, it may be important to offer to get an independent advocate to support the service user if there are contested issues. Various organisations, such as MIND, run such advocacy schemes.

It is important to bear in mind that care planning is an *approach* to care. It is an ongoing cycle of planning, action, reflection and modification. Focusing all the efforts into a single and unnecessarily over-populated meeting can be damaging to the care-planning process and the therapeutic relationship. It must work for the service user and not become just another procedure of the service system (Ritchie 2000). However, and perhaps not surprisingly, it is often experienced as a daunting ordeal by service users. When done in a tokenistic way, care planning can degenerate into a 'rubber-stamping' process for professionals' input with the client obliged to remain passive and asked only to comment on a *fait accompli*.

The power dynamics of a heavily populated CPA meeting must be appreciated. Care should be taken that only those people directly involved in the care plan are present. It may also help to deconstruct the care-planning process into two or more sub-meetings. For example, the care co-ordinator and service user may need to meet the housing worker to iron out certain issues before the main meeting. This allows time for important preliminary discussions to take place fully whilst still feeding into the central care-planning process. Planning these meetings with the service user beforehand and giving feedback to the central CPA meeting afterwards will ensure this approach is helpful deconstruction rather than unhelpful fragmentation.

TEAM DYNAMICS, ROLES AND BOUNDARIES

Having established that a balance between profession-specific and team roles is needed, a further question might be, 'How can balance be achieved?'. There will undoubtedly be many different ways in which a balance is found. Much will depend on the individual therapists' abilities and preferences (Harries & Gilhooly 2003).

However, since it is likely that a CMHT will have a single therapist, or possibly two (DoH 2001), some reflections on the potential team implications of this balancing act are now offered because it can be a significant factor in therapists' job satisfaction (Parker 2001, Reeves & Summerfield Mann 2004).

As described, an occupational perspective of health encompasses and appreciates both roles. Acknowledging this broader view allows therapists to seize the opportunity to negotiate boundaries whilst committing to both rather than baulk at the choice. This chapter hopes to equip therapists with a greater understanding of the relevance of their knowledge and skills to the service's and team's goals so they can negotiate more confidently and gain clarity. Being flexible does not mean being muddled.

Failing to define one's occupational therapy role means it may be defined by others (Hughes 2001). This can marginalise therapists whose potential contribution to the team's work is then underestimated and/or misunderstood, and whose clinical reasoning is then absent from the main care-planning and decision-making forum of the team.

When occupational therapy clinical reasoning is expressed in team meetings, the team as a whole takes on an increasingly occupational focus. Not only is this beneficial for service users (Hughes 2001, Krupa et al 2002, Onyett et al 1995) but it also creates a benign cycle of job satisfaction and staff retention amongst therapists. In other words, teamwork is likely to have the occupational focus that a skilled practitioner brings to the team *if* that practitioner commits to the team.

Just as clarity is vital, so is the confidence to demonstrate utility. As Finlay (2004) suggests:

> We are being given an ideal opportunity to explore new ways of interprofessional working that aim to provide integrative, needs-led care. It is time to celebrate the way that occupational therapy ideals are being embraced across different health care professions and contexts. It is, also, more than time to end any angst about our role... It is time, finally, to replace defensive practice with defensible practice. (p19–20)

NEW WAYS OF WORKING

In response to the NWW initiative, the College of Occupational Therapists acknowledges that collaborative, flexible, recovery-orientated practice and widened professional roles are likely to be pointers to the future of occupational therapy in mental health, as long as they are consistent with the profession's ideals (College of Occupational Therapists 2006a, Ormston 2006). It lists these ideals or values as: a view of humans as occupational beings; an occupational perspective of health and well-being; a continued focus on the individual's potential, action, strengths and self-determination; and the centrality of client-centredness, positive risk taking, cultural sensitivity and ethical practice (Ormston 2006).

The intention of this chapter has been to illustrate the congruence between these values and the wider agendas and team structures of community mental health practice. Drawing again on the notion of open systems thinking, the form which occupational therapists' input will take in any given team should reflect the function of the team as a whole.

LOOKING AFTER YOURSELF

Having highlighted some of the potential pitfalls and stresses of teamworking, it may be helpful to consider some of the resources available to therapists to minimise these stressors and maximise the enriching experience that community mental health practice can be.

YOUR OWN TEAM

Working as a team, and the culture of support this can create among colleagues, is highly valued by community staff. Not only will a team's weekly round of formal clinical reviews help to support practitioners' clinical skills, but the more immediate need to spontaneously share the personal impact of challenging work is met, and indeed fostered, when teams work well together (Onyett 2003).

SUPERVISION

Individual professional supervision, as well as team management, will provide opportunities to discuss role issues (Craik et al 1999). The MHPIG (DoH 2001) states that, where there is only one member of a discipline in a CMHT, adequate professional support and supervision must be provided, and therapists are encouraged to demand it if it is not offered (College of Occupational Therapists 2006a). This can include the option of incorporating three-way discussions that include one's professional supervisor and one's functional manager together in the same room, perhaps as part of an appraisal process. This will promote congruence between roles, avoid role ambiguity and role conflict (Hughes 2001, Onyett 2003) and also avoid the stress associated with isolated clinical roles (Knapp et al 1992).

It will also be an opportunity to discuss an occupational perspective of health in relation to service users' needs, and to agree how occupational therapy will best fit the team's priorities and one's own skills. An occupational perspective of health may be unfamiliar territory for team managers who are not occupational therapists (Harries & Gilhooly 2003) but, if framed in the terms described in this chapter, connections can be highlighted between therapists' day-to-day practice and the key issues which all CMHTs must now address.

Significantly, many contributors to the debate on generic and specialist working identify the need for interprofessional training, and this may well be a professional development issue to take up in supervision (Harrison 2005a, b, Hughes 2001, Reeves & Summerfield Mann 2004).

SUMMARY

A clear-sighted occupational perspective of health and well-being combined with a person-centred approach is crucial in community mental health work. These characteristics will help to ensure that community occupational therapy practice continues to evolve from an appreciation of human occupation. In the rapidly changing field of community mental health, the occupational therapy interventions that worked in the past cannot be assumed to be applicable in the future.

In exploring the issues presented in this chapter; social inclusion, social capital, recovery and person-centredness, it is striking how, conceptually, they all converge and reinforce one another and how, in practice, they all have an occupational basis.

Translating this into occupational therapy is the challenge. A recurrent theme here has been the need to apply open, dynamic systems thinking to ourselves as community-based therapists, so that working *with* the community maximises our effectiveness *within* the community. This will, arguably, ensure the efficacy and acceptability of our practice to the widest range of service users, and promote it as a valuable asset to commissioners and managers of services.

References

Allen R 2005 Challenges of case management. In: Whiteford G, Wright-St Clair V (eds) Occupation and practice in context. Elsevier, Marrickville, NSW

Bates P 2005 Accidents at the inclusion traffic lights: mistakes and misunderstandings in supporting people to achieve social inclusion. A National Development Team Emerging Themes Paper. Available online at: www.ntd.org.uk

Bates P, Miller C, Taylor P Defining things: defining inclusion. In: Bates P (ed) Working for inclusion: making social inclusion a reality for people with severe mental health problems. Sainsbury Centre for Mental Health, London

Brooker C, Repper J 2003 Serious mental health problems in the community: future directions for policy, research, and practice. In: Brooker C, Repper J (eds) Serious mental health problems in the community: policy practice and research. Baillière Tindall, Edinburgh,

Burchardt T, Le Grand J, Piachaud D 2002 Degrees of exclusion: developing a dynamic, multidimensional measure. In:Hills J, LeGrand J, Piachaud D (eds) Understanding social exclusion, Oxford University Press, New York

Cameron M, Edmans T, Greatley A et al D 2003 Community renewal and mental health. King's Fund, London

Care Services Improvement Partnership 2006a From segregation to inclusion: commissioning guidance on day services for people with mental health problems. Department of Health, London

Care Services Improvement Partnership 2006b National social inclusion programme: 2nd Annual Report. Department of Health, London

College of Occupational Therapists 2006a Recovering ordinary lives: the strategy for occupational therapy services 2007–2017 – a vision for the next ten years. College of Occupational Therapists, London

College of Occupational Therapists 2006b Recovering ordinary lives: the strategy for occupational therapy services 2007–2017 – results from service user and carer focus groups. College of Occupational Therapists, London

Corrigan K 2002 CMHTs: embedding the occupational perspective (letter). British Journal of Occupational Therapy 65(2): 100

Craik C, Austin C, Shell D 1999 A national survey of occupational therapy managers in mental health. British Journal of Occupational Therapy 62(5): 220-228

Creek J 2003 Occupational therapy defined as a complex intervention. College of Occupational Therapists, London

Deegan PE 1988 Recovery: the lived experience of rehabilitation. Psychosocial Rehabilitation Journal 11(4): 11-19

Deegan PE 2001 Recovery as a self-directed process of healing and transformation. Occupational Therapy in Mental Health 17(1): 5-21

Department of Health 1990 The care programme approach for people with a severe mental illness referred to the specialist psychiatric services. HMSO, London

Department of Health 1995 Building bridges: a guide to arrangements for inter-agency working for the care and protection of severely mentally ill people. Department of Health, London

Department of Health 1999a National service framework for mental health. Department of Health, London

Department of Health 1999b Effective care coordination in mental health services: modernising the care programme approach. Department of Health, London

Department of Health 2000 NHS national plan. HMSO, London

Department of Health 2001 The mental health policy implementation guide. Department of Health, London

Department of Health 2005 Creating a patient-led NHS: delivering the NHS Improvement Plan. Department of Health, London

Department of Work and Pensions 2006 A new deal for welfare: empowering people to work. HMSO, London

Duncan EAS 2006 Skills and processes in occupational therapy. In: Duncan EAS (ed) Foundations for practice in occupational therapy, 4th edn. Elsevier, Edinburgh

Dunn S 1999 Creating accepting communities – report of the Mind Inquiry into social exclusion and mental health problems. Mind Publications, London

Finlay L 2004 The practice of psychosocial occupational therapy, 3rd edn. Nelson Thornes, Cheltenham

Finlay L, McKay E 2004 Mental illness: listening to users' experience. In: Finlay L (ed) The practice of psychosocial occupational therapy, 3rd edn. Nelson Thornes, Cheltenham

Forsyth K, Kielhofner G 2006 The model of human occupation: integrating theory into practice and practice into theory. In: Duncan EAS (ed) Foundations for practice in occupational therapy, 4th edn. Elsevier, Edinburgh

Fowler Davis S, Ilott I 2002 Mental health update (letter). British Journal of Occupational Therapy 65(5): 251-252

Glover H 2001 A series of thoughts on personal recovery. Unpublished pamphlet

Godden A, McMahon S, Montgomery S et al 2006 An investigation of the factors that influence the use of outcome measures by occupational therapists practising in mental health. Unpublished BSc (Hons) dissertation, University of the West of England, Bristol

Goffman E 1968 Stigma. Penguin, Harmondsworth

Great Britain. Parliament 2005 Disability Discrimination Act 2005. HMSO, London. Available online at www.opsi.gov.uk/ACTS Accessed 12 November 2007

Hagedorn R 1992 Occupational therapy: foundations for practice. Churchill Livingstone, Edinburgh

Hagedorn R 2000 Tools for practice in occupational therapy: a structured approach to core skills and processes. Churchill Livingstone, Edinburgh

Harries P, Gilhooly K 2003 Generic and specialist occupational therapy casework in community mental health teams. British Journal of Occupational Therapy 66(3): 101-109

Harrison D 2003 The case for generic working in mental health occupational therapy. British Journal of Occupational Therapy 66(3): 110-112

Harrison D 2005a Context of change in community mental health occupational therapy: part one. International Journal of Therapy and Rehabilitation 12(9): 396-400

Harrison D 2005b Context of change in community mental health occupational therapy: part two. International Journal of Therapy and Rehabilitation 12(10): 444-448

Hart L 2003 Recovery? Let's get real: an open letter to mental health professionals. Openmind 124: 15

Hughes J 2001 Occupational therapy in community mental health teams: a continuing dilemma? Role theory offers an explanation. British Journal of Occupational Therapy 64(1): 34-40

Hyde P 2002 Occupational therapists as case managers: the service user's experience. Mentalhealth OT 7(2): 12-15

Iwama MK 2005 The Kawa (river) model: nature, life flow, and the power of culturally relevant occupational therapy. In: Kronenberg F, Algado SA, Pollard N (eds) Occupational therapy without borders – learning from the spirit of survivors. Churchill Livingstone, Edinburgh, pp213-227

Kielhofner G, Barrett L 1998 Meaning and misunderstanding in occupational forms: a study of therapeutic goal setting. American Journal of Occupational Therapy 52(5): 345-353

Knapp M, Cambridge P, Thomason C et al 1992 Care in the community: challenge and demonstration. Gower, Aldershot

Krupa T, Radloff-Gabriel D, Whippey E et al 2002 Reflections on occupational therapy and assertive community treatment. Canadian Journal of Occupational Therapy June: 153-157

Langford CPH, Bowsher J, Maloney JP et al 1997 Social support: a conceptual analysis. Journal of Advanced Nursing 25: 95-100

Laurance J 2003 Pure madness: how fear drives the mental health system. Routledge, London

Learning and Skills Council 2006 Improving services for people with mental health difficulty. Learning and Skills Council, Coventry

Mancini MA 2006 Consumer-providers' theories about recovery from serious psychiatric disabilities. Rosenberg J, Rosenberg S (eds) Community mental health: challenges for the 21st century. Routledge, Taylor and Francis, New York, pp15-24

McLaughlin Gray J 1997 Application of the phenomenological method to the concept of occupation. Journal of Occupational Science: Australia 4(1): 5-17

Meacher M 2006 Mental health problems – is employment the answer? Mental Health Review 11(3): 4-7

MIND 2004 Not alone? Isolation and mental distress. MIND, London

Mitchell RE, Trickett EJ 1980 Task force report: social networks as mediators of support. Community Mental Health Journal 16: 27-44

Molineux M, Whiteford G 2006 Occupational science: genesis, evolution, and future contribution. In: Duncan EAS (ed) Foundations for practice in occupational therapy. Elsevier, Edinburgh

Morgan S 2004 The purpose and principles of a 'strengths' approach. In: Morgan S, Ryan P (eds) Assertive outreach – a strengths approach to policy and practice, Churchill Livingstone, Edinburgh

Morgan S, Ryan P 2004 Assertive outreach – a strengths approach to policy and practice. Churchill Livingstone, Edinburgh

National Institute for Mental Health in England 2005 Outcome measures implementation best practice guidance. National Institute for Mental Health in England, Leeds

Nolan P 1995 Survey of the social networks of people with severe mental health problems. Journal of Psychiatric and Mental Health Nursing 2: 131-142

Office of the Deputy Prime Minister 2004 Mental health and social exclusion – Social Exclusion Unit Report. Office of the Deputy Prime Minister, London

Oliver M 1996 Understanding disability. MacMillan, London

Onyett S 2003 Teamworking in mental health. Palgrave Macmillan, Bristol

Onyett S, Pillinger T, Muijen M 1995 Making community mental health teams work: CMHTs and the people who work in them. Sainsbury Centre for Mental Health, London

Ormston C 2006 New ways of working for occupational therapists in mental health: the underlying value base for occupational therapy practice: a constant in a changing environment. Mental Health Occupational Therapy 11(3): 102-103

Parker D 2006 The client centred frame of reference. In: Duncan EAS (ed) Foundations for practice in occupational therapy, 4th edn. Elsevier, Edinburgh, pp193-215

Parker H 2001 The role of occupational therapists in community mental health teams: generic or specialist? British Journal of Occupational Therapy 64(12): 609-611

Peck E, Norman IJ 1999 Working together in adult community mental health services: an interprofessional dialogue. Journal of Mental Health 8(3): 217-230

Perkins RE 2004 Recovery and rehabilitation. Paper presented at the Avon and Wiltshire Mental Health Partnership Annual Rehabilitation Service Conference, January 23, Vassal Centre, Bristol

Perkins RE 2005 Recovery and social inclusion. Workshop presentation at the Multi-Disciplinary Continuing Professional Development Workshop, February 25, University of Bristol Psychology Department

Perkins RE, Repper J 2003 Principles of working with people who experience serious mental health problems. Brooker C, Repper J (eds) Serious mental health problems in the community: policy, practice and research. Baillière Tindall, Edinburgh

Ralph R 2004 Verbal definitions and visual models of recovery: focus on the recovery model. Ralph R, Corrigan P (eds) Recovery in mental illness: broadening our understanding of well-ness. American Psychological Association, Washington DC

Rankin J 2005 Mental health in the mainstream. Institute of Public Policy Research, London

Rebeiro KL 2001 Enabling occupation: the importance of an affirming environment. Canadian Journal of Occupational Therapy 68: 80-89

Rebeiro KL 2005 Reflections on The recovery paradigm: should occupational therapists be interested? Canadian Journal of Occupational Therapy 2(72): 96-102

Reeves S, Summerfield Mann L 2004 Overcoming problems of generic working for occupational therapists based in community mental health settings. British Journal of Occupational Therapy 67(6): 265-268

Richards S 2005 Keynote speech delivered to South West Region COT Conference at Buckfastleigh, Devon, May 17.

Ritchie P 2000 Modernising services: person-centred planning. In: Bates P (ed) Working for inclusion: making social inclusion a reality for people with severe mental health problems. Sainsbury Centre for Mental Health, London

Roberts G, Wolfson P 2004 The rediscovery of recovery: open to all. Advances in Psychiatric Treatment 10. Available online at: http://apt.rcpsych.org/

Rose D 2001 Users' voices: the perspective of mental health service users on community and hospital care. Sainsbury Centre for Mental Health, London

Ryan P 2004 The origins of and evidence for case management. In: Ryan P, Morgan S (eds) Assertive outreach: a strengths approach to policy and practice. Churchill Livingstone, Edinburgh

Ryan P, Morgan S 2004a Targeting: who is the client? In: Ryan P, Morgan S (eds) Assertive outreach: a strengths approach to policy and practice. Churchill Livingstone, Edinburgh

Ryan P, Morgan S 2004b Care planning and care co-ordination. Ryan P, Morgan S (eds) Assertive outreach: a strengths approach to policy and practice. Churchill Livingstone, Edinburgh

Sainsbury Centre for Mental Health 1998 Keys to engagement. Sainsbury Centre for Mental Health, London

Sainsbury Centre for Mental Health 2000 On your doorstep: community organisations and mental health. Sainsbury Centre for Mental Health, London

Sainsbury Centre for Mental Health 2003 Primary solutions: an independent policy review on the development of primary care mental health services. Sainsbury Centre for Mental Health, London

Sainsbury Centre for Mental Health/mentality 2001 An executive briefing on mental health promotion: implementing Standard One of the national service framework. Sainsbury Centre for Mental Health/mentality

Sayce L 2000 From psychiatric patient to citizen: overcoming discrimination and social exclusion. MacMillan, London

Slade M 2006 Commissioning outcome-focused mental health services. Mental Health Review 11(3): 31-36

Stein LI, Santos AB 1998 Assertive community treatment of persons with severe mental illness. WW Norton, New York

Stein L, Test A 1980 Alternatives to mental hospital treatment: conceptual model, treatment program and clinical evaluation. Archives of General Psychiatry 37: 392-397

Townsend E, Wilcock A 2004 Occupational justice. In: Christiansen CH, Townsend EA (eds) Introduction to occupation: the art and science of living. Prentice-Hall, New Jersey

van Niekerk L 2005 Occupational science and its relevance to occupational therapy in the field of mental health. In: Crouch R, Alers V (eds) Occupational therapy in psychiatry and mental health, 4th edn. Whurr, London

Warner R 2000 The environment of schizophrenia. Innovations in practice, policy and communications. Brunner-Routledge, London

Westwood J 2003 The impact of adult education for mental health service users. British Journal of Occupational Therapy 66(11): 505-510

Whalley-Hammell K 2006 Perspectives on disability and rehabilitation: contesting assumptions, challenging practice. Churchill Livingstone Elsevier, Edinburgh

Wilcock AA 1993 A theory of the human need for occupation. Occupational Science: Australia 1(1): 17-24

Wilcock AA 1995 The occupational brain: a theory of human nature. Journal of Occupational Science: Australia 2(1): 68-73

Wilcock AA 1998a Occupation for health. British Journal of Occupational Therapy 61(8): 340-345

Wilcock AA 1998b An occupational perspective of health. Slack, Thorofare, New Jersey

Wollenberg JL 2001 Recovery and occupational therapy in the community mental health setting. Occupational Therapy in Mental Health 17(3-4): 97-114

Yerxa E 1994 Dreams, dilemmas, and decisions for occupational therapy practice in a new millennium: an American perspective. American Journal of Occupational Therapy 48(7): 587-588

Chapter **28**

Forensic occupational therapy

Edward A. S. Duncan

INTRODUCTION

This chapter provides an introduction to forensic occupational therapy. It commences with a historical overview of forensic care and compares contemporary definitions of mentally disordered offenders. The chapter then continues by exploring whether forensic occupational therapy is a discrete specialism within mental health. Following on from this is an overview of the environments in which forensic occupational therapists work. The chapter then examines the role of security in forensic care and discusses different approaches that can be taken to security by therapists working in this area. The differing forms of security that define forensic services are then described.

Having examined some of the structural elements of forensic care, the chapter continues with a section on occupational therapy assessment and risk assessment within this environment. This is followed by an examination of interventions in this area and the chapter focuses on understanding what one model of practice offers to the conceptualisation of offending behaviour from an occupational perspective. In doing so, a tentative theoretical conceptualisation for occupational therapy interventions to address offending behaviour is provided. The chapter concludes with an exploration of the research priorities for forensic occupational therapy and an examination of the professional issues that arise when working in this area.

HISTORICAL OVERVIEW

This section describes the legislative changes and development of services for mentally disordered offenders. Mentally disordered offenders, as a specific category, have a relatively brief history – approximately 200 years. This period has witnessed remarkable developments in the context of the legal framework, health-care systems and society in general.

MENTALLY DISORDERED OFFENDERS

Prior to the 1800s in England, mentally disordered offenders were legislated for by means of the Vagrancy Acts of 1714 and 1744. These Acts stipulated that such individuals should be housed by family, in bridewells or in poorhouses (McComish & Paterson 1996). During the Middle Ages the life of 'lunatics', as they were then known, was not an easy one whether they offended or not. However, development of moral philosophy, history and economics during the Scottish Enlightenment (1740–1790) had a significant impact on societal attitudes. It is perhaps not surprising, therefore, that the period following the Scottish Enlightenment heralded a series of developments in the care of criminal lunatics, as mentally disordered offenders were then termed. These philosophical advancements coincided with a series of events which brought the criminal lunatic to the forefront of public scrutiny and resulted in significant changes in the society's understanding of the criminal lunatic.

James Hadfield

On 15 May 1800, James Hadfield was arrested after he fired a pistol at King George III whilst the King was attending the theatre in Drury Lane, London. The attempt on the King's life failed when the bullet narrowly missed its mark, as the King was bowing to the audience (Partridge 1953). As the trial progressed, the motivation behind the attack became apparent. Hadfield believed that he was acting on direct instructions from God, who had commanded him to sacrifice his own life in order to save the world. As Hadfield found the thought of suicide too wicked, he plotted to assassinate the King, or at least to commit high treason. This would result, he believed, in a swift execution and the accomplishment of his mission. The task of Hadfield's lawyer (Thomas Erskine) was not easy. Although common law had included a defence on the grounds of insanity as far back as the ancient Greeks, an individual would only be considered insane if they suffered from total deprivation of memory (Skilling 1999). As this was clearly not the case with Hadfield, Erskine argued that an individual suffering from delusions was the true character of insanity. Erskine's speech, described as '... one of the most eloquent and able speeches, probably that was ever delivered at the bar' (Robinson 1998), was obviously convincing. Hadfield was judged as being insane and not responsible for his actions.

This case resulted in a significant shift in legislation. It also placed the court in a dilemma, as the traditional place of disposal for lunatics was Bethlem Hospital, London. Whilst this wasn't considered a safe environment for Hadfield, there were no legislative structures for the detaining of such an individual. Within 1 month of Hadfield's conviction, the Criminal Lunatics Act (1800) was hurriedly passed through Parliament. This enabled individuals acquitted on the grounds of insanity to be held in close custody, 'until His Majesty's pleasure be known'. Although no specific accommodation was provided for such individuals (Faulk 1994), Hadfield was held under this legislation until his death on 23 January 1841, aged 69. The new legal construct of insanity was shortly to be challenged in another high-profile case of a criminal lunatic attacking a well-known member of society.

Daniel McNaughton

Daniel McNaughton, a Glaswegian, was charged with murdering Edward Drummond (private secretary to the then Prime Minister Robert Peel) on 20 January 1843. The offence was committed by shooting Mr Drummond in the back of the head with a pistol. Drummond was fatally wounded and died 5 days later (Partridge 1953). Essentially, the murder was a case of mistaken identity, as McNaughton had intended to kill the Prime Minister. McNaughton was clearly viewed as insane at the time of his trial and had longstanding delusions of personality (McComish & Paterson 1996). After a 2-day trial, McNaughton was found not guilty due to insanity. He was taken to the Bethlem Hospital

from where, in 1864, he was transferred to Broadmoor Hospital of special security which had opened in 1863. McNaughton died there the following year, aged 52, from heart failure (Partridge 1953). The verdict caused a political outcry, not least from Queen Victoria, who had recently been subjected to a pistol attack whilst in her carriage. In order to resolve the matter, the House of Lords invited the judicial system to clarify the stance on criminal insanity. The judges' response became known as the 'McNaughton rules'. These rules state:

> The defendant cannot be held responsible for his or her actions because of the severity of his or her mental illness. By reason of such defect of disease of the mind, it is held that the defendant did not know the nature or quality of his or her own act (i.e. did not realise what he was physically doing at the time). Or, by reason of such defect from disease of the mind, he or she did not know that the act was wrong (i.e. did not know that it was forbidden by law). Or, a person suffering from an insane delusion that prevents true appreciation of the nature and quality of an act has the same degree of responsibility as if the acts were as he or she imagined them. (McComish & Paterson 1996, p154)

The McNaughton Rules are widely quoted and remain an influential test of insanity (Elliot 1996).

FORENSIC CARE

With the birth of the 'lunatic hospitals', the medical establishment took on board the care of mentally disordered offenders (although it would be over 100 years before they were known as such).

DEFINING FORENSIC MENTAL HEALTH AND FORENSIC OCCUPATIONAL THERAPY

Several perspectives of forensic mental health exist.

One perspective focuses on the relationship of law to mental health and views forensic mental health as being concerned with the relationship of law to psychiatric practice and frequently to work with mentally disordered offenders. However, whilst the connection between law and mental health is clear the relationship is not and there can often be competing tensions between both parties. An alternative perspective is provided by Gunn & Taylor (1993) who focus Forensic Mental Health on the prevention, amelioration and treatment of victimisation which has occurred due to person's mental illness.

The above perspectives offer differing views of forensic mental health. These outline various perspectives of its role in health care:

- The application of law to practice
- The relationship of crime and society
- The treatment of mentally disordered offenders
- The victimisation perspective.

DEFINING FORENSIC OCCUPATIONAL THERAPY

Where does forensic occupational therapy fit in these definitions? Any definition of forensic occupational therapy must comfortably relate to a broader occupational therapy definition. However, succinctly defining the profession is challenging, and notoriously difficult (Creek 2003). One definition suggests that 'Occupational therapy enables people to achieve health, well-being and life satisfaction through participation in occupation' (College of Occupational Therapists 2004). However, all definitions of the profession are likely to be partial and the brevity of the College of Occupational Therapists definition is paid for by its lack of breadth of vision. An important aspect omitted from the College of Occupational Therapists (2004) definition is the role of the environment. The World Federation of Occupational Therapists offers a more lengthy definition and consequently also provides a focus on the importance of the environment in occupational therapy. It states that 'Occupational therapists believe that participation can be supported or restricted by physical, social, attitudinal and legislative environments ... Therefore occupational therapy practice may be directed to changing aspects of the environment to enhance participation' (World Federation of Occupational Therapists 2002).

Forensic occupational therapy can be seen not only as a form of intervention for people who offend with mental health problems but also as a method of addressing offending behaviour. The distinct physical and social environments of forensic hospitals and prisons also highlight differences in forensic occupational therapists' roles.

Couldrick (2003), in a core text for forensic occupational therapy, defined the specialism as follows: 'Helping people to engage in occupation that gives their lives meaning and value and connects them to the society and culture in which they live not only promotes health but may mitigate alienation and antisocial behaviour' (p13). This definition, like that of the College of Occupational Therapists, is brief and consequently suffers from similar drawbacks.

In a keynote lecture to the 2004 National Forensic Occupational Therapy Conference, Duncan (2004) offered a definition that attempted to address the challenges of occupational therapists working in secure environments:

> Forensic occupational therapy engages people and facilitates their participation in meaningful life activities whilst assisting in the development of their increased personal capacity and pro-social values, identity and skills.

> Forensic occupational therapists use engagement in occupation as their therapeutic medium. They also analyse and adapt the physical and social environment to maximise individuals' and groups' meaningful life participation. Where adaptation is impossible (e.g. for reasons of safety and security), occupational therapists actively report the impact of the environment on each individual within their care.

WHERE DO FORENSIC OCCUPATIONAL THERAPISTS WORK?

Forensic occupational therapists work in a variety of environments. The nature of their work and the patient population means that the majority of therapists work in varying degrees of secure accommodation. These include special hospitals, regional secure units, low secure units and prisons.

A growing number of forensic occupational therapists are now also being employed in community forensic teams, a challenging area ideally suited for forensic occupational therapists who are central professionals in assisting patients to adjust to community life and both obtain and maintain a meaningful and offence-free lifestyle. Recently, new government policy has seen the development of four new units (two in prisons and two in special hospitals) in England for people with dangerous and severe personality disorders. These units do not exist in Scotland, where separate service developments for such individuals are under consideration.

SPECIAL HOSPITALS OR HIGH-SECURITY HOSPITALS

The first special hospital within the UK (Broadmoor, just north of London) was founded in 1863, following the Criminal Lunatic Asylums Act (1860) and in the wake of both Hadfield and McNaughton. Broadmoor was followed by Rampton, Nottinghamshire (1912), and Moss End, now known as Ashworth Hospital (1914), near Liverpool (Walsh & Ayres 2003). Whilst Scotland had been considering the development of an equivalent institution for some time, it was not until 1948 that the State Institution for Defectives (for people with learning difficulties) was opened. In 1957 the State Mental Hospital (for people with mental illnesses) was opened, and the two bodies later became known as The State Hospital, Carstairs.

Patients are resident in hospitals of special/ high security due to their immediate potential dangerousness. Consequently security needs to be as significant as that required to house the most dangerous category A prisoner. Patients are detained in special hospitals (now referred to as hospitals of high security) against their will, through the use of either mental health or criminal justice legislation. Some patients are admitted for assessment and discharged after a relatively brief period, whilst at the other end of the spectrum there are some patients who have been resident in special hospitals for more than 30 years, some of whom, due to their ongoing dangerousness, are unlikely to ever be transferred or released.

Patients are admitted to a high-security hospital from three sources: other secure and general mental health hospitals, from prison or direct from court. Patients are likely to be transferred from other secure units or general hospitals due to a real or perceived increase in the risk of violent behaviour. Such a transfer will often follow a violent or aggressive incident in a unit of lesser security, although it may also result from a patient breaching the conditions of his stay in less secure units, for example bringing in or using banned substances or absconding.

Since 1989 in England and Wales and 1995 in Scotland and Northern Ireland, the high-security hospitals have come completely within the remit of the NHS/Scottish NHS. There is now a focus of care within all these environments and an aim to rehabilitate all patients to a level where they can be deemed to be not of an immediate risk of violence or danger. To enable this to occur, special hospitals are generously staffed with a variety of professional groups: nurses, occupational therapists, psychiatrists, clinical and forensic psychologists and social workers.

Forensic occupational therapists working in secure units have a dual task: the rehabilitation of individuals so that they no longer require to be detained in conditions of high security and the development of a meaningful quality of life for individuals resident in such conditions. The latter issue is of particular importance as patients' length of stay within secure environments is certainly longer than the average length of admission to a general mental health environment; a few individuals may never be considered safe to be transferred from a high-security hospital and thus the environment becomes their 'home' and the development of a meaningful pattern of activities becomes ever more important.

REGIONAL SECURE UNITS

Despite an initial suggestion for the development of regional secure units (RSUs) in England in 1961, it was not until 1974 that their concept was reintroduced and developed in the Butler Report (Home Office and Department of Health and Social Security 1975). This report suggested that each regional health authority should provide secure care. Regional secure units are specifically designed to accommodate individuals who are potentially dangerous and difficult, but do not require the conditions of high security.

Neither the Butler Report (Home Office and Department of Health and Social Security 1975), which recommended provision of medium (or regional) secure units in England and Wales, nor the Reed Report (Department of Health 1994), which recommended an increase in medium secure provision, were adopted within Scotland. Consequently, until very recently, there have been no staged levels of secure psychiatric provision within Scotland. In 1999, a policy statement and framework of services for mentally disordered offenders in Scotland was published (Scottish Office 1999) which stated that patients should be cared for '... under conditions of no greater security than is justified by the degree of danger they present to themselves or to others' (p3). In 2000, the Orchard Clinic in Edinburgh, Scotland's first medium secure unit, was opened. There remains, however, a substantial shortfall of medium secure provision. Future models of secure forensic services have been developed (Scottish Office 1999) and legislation has enshrined the rights of patients to be detained at the lowest appropriate level of security (Scottish Office 1999). Plans for the development of a series of medium secure units in Scotland are now in place.

The length of stay in existing RSUs is notably shorter than the average length of stay of a patient in a high-security hospital. Ideally, it is envisioned that a patient would remain in a RSU for no longer than 18–24 months; however, such ideals are often not achieved and the reality has been suggested to be closer to 5 years (Rogowski 2002).

Patients can be admitted to RSUs from a similar range of environments to high-security hospitals and transfers of patients, in both directions, between RSUs and high-security hospitals are regular occurrences. RSUs are staffed with similar professionals to those found in special hospitals. Similarly, intervention programmes also occur to assist in patients' rehabilitation. A novelty of this process in RSUs is, however, the increased use of community facilities by patients, with both escorted leave from the unit and, through time and following detailed risk assessments, increasing levels of unescorted leave and access to community educational and vocational services.

Low secure units are often used for individuals who require longer term residential care in secure settings, but do not pose an immediate or grave risk to themselves or to others. Individuals in low secure units may have frequent escorted and at times unescorted leave from the unit to participate in community activities.

COMMUNITY FORENSIC SERVICES

A growing number of forensic occupational therapists are working in community forensic teams. Occupational therapy community forensic service provision can take various forms (Joe 2003):

- as a member of a community forensic mental health team
- as a dedicated member of a specific community resource, for example offender hostels
- as a split post between inpatients and community services.

The central distinction between therapists who work in community mental health teams and those who work in forensic community mental health teams and other forms of community forensic occupational therapy is the degree of legislation under which their services are provided (Joe 2003). The remit for forensic occupational therapists working in the community includes public safety, social inclusion and therapeutic intervention (Joe 2003). Whilst the perceived risk of patients living in the community is lower than individuals resident in secure units, the consequences of patients relapsing can have greater implications for public safety.

PRISONS

There are two types of facilities within prisons: those for prisoners who have yet to be convicted, called remand prisoners, and those who have been convicted. Prisons are segregated according to gender as well as by age, with adult prisons being for people older than 21 whilst young offender prisons are for 17–21 year olds (Rogowski 2002). Prisoners are placed in prisons according to their security requirements. There are four separate levels of prisons with differing levels of security. Category A prisons have the highest level of security and are intended for the most dangerous individuals. At the other end of the spectrum, category D prisons are open prisons and are often populated by prisoners who are coming to the end of a life sentence and may be undergoing a vocational or educational opportunity in the community.

The prevalence of psychiatric disorders within the prison population is high, with a lifetime prevalence of 71% amongst remand prisoners, with difficulties of anxiety, depression, psychosis and alcohol and substance misuse frequently found (Birmingham et al 1996). Prison healthcare services have only significantly developed since 1990. Whilst health services within prisons have significantly progressed in the intervening years (Hills 2003), the sheer volume of the problems faced by the prisoner population means that many prisoners with mental health problems may not come to the attention of prison health services. Some individuals who do come to the attention of prison health services can be deemed to be too ill to remain within the prison environment and so are transferred to RSUs or high-security hospitals according to risk. When the mental health of such individuals improves they may be returned to the prison environment. Alternatively, the clinical team for a patient may deem that a return to prison would be counterproductive to their mental health and consequently arrange for them to be transferred to the forensic system and remain in hospital. There are some prisoners, however, who remain in prison despite their mental health problems. For such individuals, occupational therapists working in prisons should aim to offer services equal to those that would be found in the community (Hills 2003).

Imprisonment can have a profound effect on an individual's occupational functioning. Prisoners may be locked up for several hours a day and have significant restrictions placed on them in terms of personal and self-care activities such as slopping out (going to the toilet in a cell occupied by another prisoner), having restricted access to their razor and more productive occupations.

A prisoner's routine is not dictated by him but by the institution and this too can affect the prisoners' volition and sense of capacity, leading to difficulty in goal setting and achievement (Hills 2003).

In 1998, it was known that 18 prisons had occupational therapists working in them (College of Occupational Therapists 1998). This figure has undoubtedly increased in the intervening period, although more recent statistics are unavailable. Within the prison environment, occupational therapists endeavour to develop programmes for prisoners that address their current occupational needs within their impoverished environment and to prepare them for their future release into the community. Frequently occupational therapists in prisons are part of a local forensic service. This arrangement has two distinct advantages. First, it enables therapists easily to transfer prisoners' intervention packages if they are moved to the local forensic service and second, it maintains therapists' professional links with other occupational therapists, in what might otherwise be a professionally remote experience.

DANGEROUS AND SEVERE PERSONALITY DISORDER HIGH SECURE SERVICES (DSPD)

The purpose of the DSPD services is to provide a new service for people who present a high risk of committing a serious violent or sexual assault due to their severe personality disorder (Dangerous and Severe Personality Disorder (DSPD) High Secure Services 2004). Four DSPD units have been opened (two in high secure hospitals and two in prisons). The key outcomes of such units are better protection for the public, the provision of new services to improve mental health and reduce risk and to increase knowledge regarding what works in the treatment of such individuals. Underpinning all of these outcomes is the overriding importance of public protection. Occupational therapists are being included within the development of these services; however, it is too early to state precisely what their role in DSPD units will be. Undoubtedly, it will develop the role of occupational therapists in working with individuals with personality disorders. Perhaps occupational therapists in such units will be able to develop the evidence for occupational therapy and personality disorders which to date has no proven efficacy (Couldrick 2003).

SECURITY – THERAPEUTIC FRIEND OR FOE?

Undoubtedly, one of the key characteristics of working in forensic environments is the presence and importance of security. It is a defining feature in differentiating between levels of security, yet paradoxically these differences are not well defined (Crichton 2005). Security features in forensic environments are often striking, for example the high perimeter fence or wall, and this can give rise to a range of feelings for therapists who enter such an environment for the first time. There are a range of levels of security and various ways in which the issue of security can be considered by an occupational therapist.

THE RELATIONSHIP BETWEEN THERAPY AND SECURITY

How can you be client centred in a secure environment? Does security place excessive restrictions on practice? Can you carry out security checks on patients, such as searching them, and maintain your therapeutic role? These questions, and others, are often faced by forensic occupational therapists, whether as a natural reflexive component of their practice or by students or other therapists. Essentially, these questions relate to a therapist's conceptualisation of the relationship between the various forms of security and her therapeutic role as an occupational therapist. The relationship between security and therapy is certainly not immediately natural but the challenges this presents depend greatly on the perspective that is taken of the relationship, Fundamentally three models outline the ways in which security and therapy relate to each other: the oppositional model, the inclusive model and the environmental model.

The oppositional model (Fig. 28.1)

The oppositional model of security and therapy views both components in competition and suggests that the presence of security inhibits

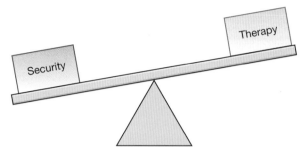

Figure 28.1 An oppositional model of security.

therapy and that being therapeutic lessens the security of a situation. Therapists who hold an oppositional model are likely to find working in forensic care challenging. The challenge of the limited therapeutic media available for therapy is often highlighted by therapists who hold an oppositional model of security and therapy. Control and restraint policies may be viewed as in conflict with the development of a therapeutic relationship. In this model, client-centred practice is often viewed as impossible. Practising forensic occupational therapy from this perspective can be very challenging, as Walsh & Ayres (2003) illustrated, stating 'Working within a high secure setting often presents a dilemma for occupational therapists trying to balance a therapeutic approach with the demands for security' (p95).

An inclusive model (Fig. 28.2)

The inclusive model of security and therapy places security firmly within the sphere of therapy. This model emphasises the requirement for safe practice in order to be therapeutic and recognises the necessity of security. This more optimistic model supports therapists to practise within secure conditions. Taking such a perspective, occupational therapists may be happier to engage in control and restraint practices and feel less challenged by working in such an environment. Supporting an inclusive model, Neeson & Kelly (2002) stated 'Security is an intrinsic part of the treatment of mentally disordered offenders, not only to protect

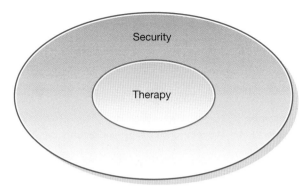

Figure 28.2   An inclusive model of security.

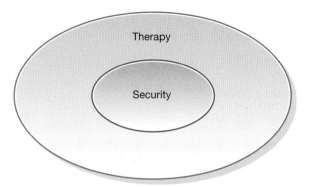

Figure 28.3   An environmental model of security.

the individual, but also to protect staff, other patients and the public' (p127).

However, this model is not without its limitations. An inclusive model of security and therapy places the focus of a patient's behaviour on the individual and the illness, in what is essentially a biomedically supported perspective. In doing so, this model ignores the impact of the secure environment on patients' functioning and behaviour.

An environmental model (Fig. 28.3)

An environmental model of security and therapy is presented here as a proposed resolution to the challenges of both the oppositional and the inclusive models previously outlined. The environmental model places security within context of therapy and in doing so emphasises the requirement for safe practice and does not reject the importance of security. But in doing so the model also highlights the importance of the environment within practice, providing a more holistic perspective of illness/behaviour, and is in greater keeping with the profession's philosophy which works with patients in the context of their physical and social environment. Within forensic occupational therapy, therapists are required to engage in security procedures, but should also recognise the effects that these have on individuals and groups. It is in recognition of the environmental model of security and therapy that Duncan (2004) presented his definition of forensic occupational therapy outlined above.

THE LEVELS AND FORMS OF SECURITY

Levels of security are linked to the categories of the units whereas the forms of security are found in all forensic environments.

Levels of security have been well reviewed in England and Wales and specific standards of security have been set for high-security hospitals (Tilt 2005). No such standards have yet been set for the State Hospital in Scotland.

Broadly, three categories of secure hospitals/units exist: high, medium and low. Defining and distinguishing between these categories is challenging as no succinct definitions exist within the literature. Often such units can be distinguished by comparing them to higher or lower secure units and observing the differing levels of security. One attempt at defining levels of security has been made by Collins & Davies (2003) and is outlined in Table 28.1.

Fundamentally three distinct forms of security are found in forensic environments (Crichton 2005) (Fig. 28.4):

- physical
- procedural
- relational

Physical security

Physical security in secure environments varies according to the level of security. Generally, such security is composed of external or perimeter security, such as a fence or wall, and entry security, which may range from a locked door to 'airport-style' security where each person passes through

Table 28.1 A brief definition of levels of security (Collins & Davies 2003)

High security	The level of security necessary only for those patients who pose a grave and immediate danger to others at large. Security arrangements should be capable of preventing even the most determined absconder. High secure services should only be provided in secure hospitals with a full range of therapeutic and recreational facilities within the perimeter fence, acknowledging the severe limitations on the use of outside services and facilities.
Medium security	The level of security necessary for patients who represent a serious but less immediate danger to others. Patients will often have been dealt with in the Crown courts and present a serious risk to others combined with the potential to abscond. Security should therefore be sufficient to deter all but the most determined. A good range of therapeutic and recreational facilities should be available within the perimeter fence to meet the needs of patients who are not ready for off-site parole, but with the emphasis on graduated use of ordinary community facilities in rehabilitation whenever possible.
Low security	The level of security deemed necessary for patients who present a less serious physical danger to others, often dealt with in magistrates/sheriff courts and identified by court assessment/diversion schemes. Security measures are intended to impede rather than completely prevent absconsions, with greater reliance on staffing arrangements and less reliance on physical security measures.

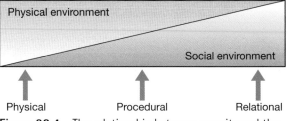

Figure 28.4 The relationship between security and the environment.

essential to ensure that patients do not feel as if they are living in a goldfish bowl, whilst maximising safe design. The entrance to a secure forensic establishment is an obviously vulnerable site and various checks take place ranging from assuring visitors' identities to full airport-style security. Internally secure hospitals may also use a range of physical facilities including CCTV, airlock-style entrances/exits to wards and other areas, locked doors and innovative furniture designed to minimise risk of violence and escape.

From an occupational perspective the architectural barriers to successful occupational adaptation are perhaps the most striking feature of a secure hospital. These barriers frequently increase patients' experiences of occupational deprivation which has been described as 'a state of preclusion from engagement in occupations of necessity and/or meaning due to factors that stand outside the immediate control of the individual' (Whiteford 2000, p200).

Procedural security

Procedural security is a term used to describe the various control processes that are regular features of life in secure environments and have been developed to minimise risk of harm to all individuals within the environment. Essentially there are three areas that comprise procedural security: control of communications, control of items and control of people (Crichton 2005).

Control of communications

Unlike in general hospitals, forensic environments often place greater control on patients' confidentiality of access to other people. Phone calls may be monitored by a member of staff, outgoing and

a metal detector and all baggage is scanned for prohibited items and substances. Internal physical security may comprise locked doors, secure window fittings and personal attack alarms. Central to good internal security is the safe design of wards and off-ward activity areas, so that patients can easily be observed. Sensitive architecture is incoming mail may, with a few exceptions, such as contact with an MP or lawyer, be read and use of the internet/email is often restricted or prohibited. The extent of such communication prohibitions depends on the level of security. With the advent of the European Human Rights Act clinical teams should clearly document why such rights are being refused and review such decisions on a regular basis.

Control of items

The control of items is an issue that directly affects anyone who enters a secure forensic environment. Frequently, such units have a list of prohibited items that are not allowed to enter the site, regardless of whether a person is a patient, member of staff or visitor. If visiting a forensic unit, it is worth enquiring as to what is/is not allowed before you visit. In order to maintain the control of items, staff, patients and visitors may be searched according to the unit policies and procedures. Screening tests for drugs and alcohol may also form part of a secure unit's control of items, with the frequency of screening often dictated by a patient's perceived risk. Similarly patients' access to pornography is often restricted by clinical teams.

It is impossible to create a functioning environment without the inclusion of various items, which have the potential to be misused. Perhaps nowhere is this more obvious than in the occupational therapy department or other activity centres. Cutlery, sharp knives, tins and jars, paint brushes and craft tools are frequently located in forensic occupational therapy departments. Their use in this context should be dependent upon individual risk assessment but it is of paramount importance that such items should be accounted for at regular intervals. Depending on the level of security, such items may be counted, often by two people, once per day or before and after each session with a patient and before they leave the environment. Such processes can often appear cumbersome and are disruptive to the normal form of activities but they constitute a vital element of procedural security. Limits are often set on the number of personal items patients may hold at any time both on their person and in their rooms.

The control of items undoubtedly limits the occupational opportunities of patients within secure environments. Occupational therapists have an important role to maximise the occupational opportunities for patients within the limitations of safety and security. At times this will mean that patients cannot have access to items that would, if used properly and not for illicit purposes, assist their occupational competence. At other times this may mean that occupational therapists challenge the perceived norms of an institution regarding possession of specific items due to the needs of the patient and therapists' perceived risk to themselves and others.

Control of people

Movement within secure environments is controlled in a variety of manners. Hospital visitors may require special permission to attend and visits to patients may be observed by a member of staff. In particular, child visiting may be restricted for some patients and hospitals now have an overriding responsibility to the welfare of any visiting child. Patients' movements may be further controlled within the forensic environment with specific permissions required to move between units or access the grounds for unescorted walks. Similarly staff movement may also be controlled and monitored through the use of CCTV, ID cards, radios and keys.

Outings from secure units are a regular occurrence and can occur for reasons of patient health care, such as hospital appointments, for court appearances, for compassionate reasons such as visiting a sick relative or as part of a patient's rehabilitation programme. All outings require careful planning with consideration being given to the aims of the outing, the environment that is being visited and the appropriate level of staffing.

Relational security

Relational security describes the effect and importance of developing a therapeutic relationship with this patient group. Aspects that can be viewed as relational security include developing positive therapeutic relationships, the management of violence and aggression, patients' responses to therapeutic interventions and security intelligence.

Building a therapeutic relationship

Therapeutic relationships are built on partnership, trust and co-operation (Murphy et al 1998). Undoubtedly such issues are more challenging in secure forensic environments. Neeson & Kelly (2002) describe these challenges, stating:

> ... Staff must be very aware of the 'us and them' syndrome, in the knowledge that the balance of power does lie with the multidisciplinary team. Patients often feel they cannot trust staff or they view staff as the people who hold the keys that keep them 'locked away'. (p127)

Fortunately, the nature of the forensic occupational therapist's role in such environments is such that they carry out fewer overt and humiliating security procedures, such as locking patients in their rooms at night or observing urine being given for analysis for illicit drug use, than their nursing colleagues. Consequently the forensic occupational therapist's security role is less evident, though certainly not non-existent. Perhaps because of this and the collaborative nature of occupational therapy, it would appear that occupational therapists in the forensic environment are often amongst the professionals with the most positive therapeutic relationships with this patient group. Undoubtedly this supports the relational security element of practice and coupled with the active engagement of patients in activity, decreasing their occupational deprivation, explains why violent incidents appear to occur less frequently when patients are engaged in occupational therapy than in other tasks (Garman 2000).

The management of violence and aggression

Due to the volatile and potentially aggressive client group, it is necessary to be equipped to deal with physically violent episodes. Prevention is certainly better than cure in this context and therapists working in secure settings should ensure they receive training in de-escalation techniques. Self-awareness and an understanding of the impact of both verbal and non-verbal interactions are also useful in this context (Neeson & Kelly 2002). Breakaway techniques are usually a core part of induction for therapists and students working in secure environments. Control and restraint techniques, where individuals learn safe methods of physically restraining patients, are also often taught. Control and restraint should be viewed as a method of last resort (Neeson & Kelly 2002). However, when used appropriately, it can be the most effective way to provide a safe environment for the patient and other people.

Patients' responses to therapeutic interventions

As patients progress through their therapeutic interventions, medical, psychological and occupational, they can become less prone to violence. With careful review from the multidisciplinary clinical team, it is often possible to grade patients' access to environments of potentially great risk such as woodwork or outings out of the hospital.

Security intelligence

Security intelligence forms a further component of the necessary background information for a patient in the forensic environment. Such information is often gathered by specific security personnel within the hospital, but is made available to clinicians working in direct contact with a patient. Security intelligence includes information about previous criminal convictions, past drug abuse, incidents that have occurred whilst within the hospital and any specific relationships the patient has with other patients or individuals outside the hospital that may pose a specific risk.

USE OF ASSESSMENT IN FORENSIC OCCUPATIONAL THERAPY

As in all areas of occupational therapy, assessment forms an important early stage of the therapeutic process and is ongoing throughout therapy. This section of the chapter outlines the forms of assessment commonly used within secure care, examines the process of conducting assessments in secure conditions and explores the assessment and management of risk.

FORMS OF ASSESSMENT

As in other areas, forensic occupational therapy uses well-recognised methods: structured observation, performance checks, self-rating scales, structured, semi-structured and unstructured interviews and standardised assessments (Barton 2003).

In 2002, as part of the national research priority setting survey, the frequency and type of assessments used in forensic occupational therapy were examined (Duncan et al 2003a). Sixty-six percent of forensic occupational therapists who responded to the survey (n=44) stated that they used standardised assessments as outcome measures in practice. Respondents were requested to list the top five measures they used. Two issues arose from this question. The overwhelming majority of assessments listed were occupational therapy-specific measures, reinforcing the occupation-focused nature for forensic occupational therapy practices, and the majority of these assessments (74%) were based on the Model of Human Occupation (MOHO) (Kielhofner 2002). Further to the MOHO assessments listed, respondents also reported using assessments linked to other conceptual models of practice and, to a lesser extent, a range of general mental health assessments (Duncan et al 2003a). The popularity of MOHO theory and the use of its associated assessment in practice is also emphasised by other authors in the field (Barton 2003, Lloyd 1987, Urquhart 2003).

Whilst several forensic occupational therapy units do appear to be using standardised assessments, their use is not without challenges. Barriers to using assessments in practice include (Duncan et al 2003a):

- time constraints (n=27)
- the complex client need and complexity of the cases (n=8)
- the lack of measures that are sufficiently sensitive or appropriate (n=8)
- lack of availability of measures (n=7)
- clients' lack of tolerance to standardised assessments (n=5)
- lack of training (n=4)
- lack of evidence regarding validity and reliability in forensic care (n=2)
- lack of managerial support (n=1).

Due to the small numbers of respondents, little can be definitively stated from these findings. Since this research, occupational therapy measures and their reliability and validity within the forensic context have improved (Parkinson et al 2006, Forsyth et al 2005).

CONDUCTING ASSESSMENTS WITHIN SECURE CARE

Barton (2003) outlines several factors that are important to consider when implementing assessments within a secure environment.

Information gathering

Whilst some therapists prefer to meet patients first, before reading their notes, Barton (2003) importantly acknowledged that this may not be the most appropriate method within secure environments. It is important to read patients' notes prior to meeting them as this enables the therapist to be aware of identifying particular risk factors, potentially sensitive areas of questioning, such as asking about family history when the patient has killed a close family member, and to gather any additional relevant information that could shape the assessment process.

Communication

Patients in secure settings often have access to several professionals, all of whom are carrying out assessments. Communication with other members of the team can avoid a patient being repeatedly asked similar questions by a range of professionals, an experience that can be frustrating for the patient and may limit their co-operation in the assessment process.

Preparation

Ensure that everything needed is brought to the assessment session. It is often not possible to leave a patient unsupervised in order to collect forgotten items.

Assessment environment

The choice of room in which an assessment is conducted, even if it is as straightforward as a brief interview, is very important. The room should be appropriate to the nature of the task and be centrally located so that other staff can attend should you require any assistance. Select a room that is spacious enough to allow for personal space and in order not to create an intense atmosphere. Avoid environments in which you are likely to be unnecessarily interrupted.

Risk management

In the assessment context, risk management refers to the safe conduct of the assessment session. In practice, the principles described in this section are as relevant to any session as they are to assessment sessions in particular.

- Prior to any session, therapists should seek a handover or update on the patient's behaviour from a relevant member of staff to ensure that an assessment session would be appropriate/safe; what appears safe and sensible one day may not be so by the next day.
- All staff should be aware of patient's current risk assessment and management plans.
- Staff should always ensure they have a personal attack alarm in their possession or know where the attack alarm buttons are located in the room.
- When preparing a room for a session, therapists should always place themselves closest to the door. This enables them to make a swift exit if necessary and reduces the potential for a hostage situation.
- Always inform staff in the environment of the session where you are and who you are with.
- Throughout the session, continue to monitor the patient for any changes in behaviour or presentation.

Engaging the patient in the assessment process

It is important that the patient understands why he is being assessed, what the information will be used for and who it will be communicated to. Sometimes, patients can be very hesitant to share information as they believe that such information may then be used against them and result in longer periods in secure care. At times, this may result in patients withholding information that would be of use in their intervention programme. Therefore, it is important that each patient understands the purpose and relevance of the assessment process to his life. Whilst great care should always be

given to ensuring confidentiality, safety concerns may override individual patient rights. Therapists should also ensure that each patient understands that any information he shares, which may have an impact on the safety of the patient or others, will be reported to other members of the clinical team. Some of the patients' anxieties surrounding this can be limited by informing the patient that the therapist will always inform the patient if she is going to do this.

Sharing information

Assessment processes can raise issues that a patient has not previously considered or that are emotionally sensitive. But it can be some time before the patient reacts to these issues. It is important therefore that the therapist feeds back information regarding the session to the members of staff who will continue to spend time with the patient after the session has ended. This may often be the patient's ward-based nursing staff. Such feedback need not necessarily be detailed; however, any changes in a patient's behaviour or presentation should always be noted and discussed.

RISK ASSESSMENT

Risk assessment is the assessment of an individual's dangerousness. The term can be used to relate to the potential for both immediate violence and longer term violence. Dangerousness, however, is a difficult concept to define, with some people viewing the tendency as unpredictable and untreatable (Scottish Office 1999) and others disagreeing (Tidmarsh 1982).

The requirement to accurately assess risk has resulted in an abundance of risk assessment measures. Hollin (2002) provides an overview of a range of such assessments. Some risk assessments are actuarially based, some are based on clinical assessment and yet others use a mixed method approach. Actuarial assessment is the use of past events to predict future behaviour mathematically. It originates from the insurance industry, which tries to predict future risks of car accidents or burglary on the frequency of known risk factors. Whilst the superiority of actuarial processes compared to clinical judgement has been comprehensively

Table 28.2 Potential outcomes of risk assessment

	Actual 'yes'	Actual 'no'
Predict 'yes'	True positive (hit)	False positive (miss)
Predict 'no'	False negative (miss)	True negative (hit)

- The precipitating factors for previous violence, for example psychosis, alcohol or drugs.
- Any new potential precipitants such as upcoming court appearances or rejected appeals.
- Level of engagement in services in general.
- Is there any potential for use of weapons in the session? Can such risks be managed?
- Are the patient's risk factors well known? Examples could include use of weapons, physical or sexual violence, previous history or risk of hostage taking, drug or alcohol misuse, fire raising, previous history or current risk of absconding.
- Does the therapist feel safe at the prospect of conducting the session?

This list is not comprehensive and various factors will need to be considered on an individual basis. The importance of risk assessment is such that it should not be conducted in isolation and the therapist who is working with the patient should always share her assessment with other members of the multidisciplinary or occupational therapy team. Some settings will insist that this occurs. Such sharing of information, whilst important, can create a different challenge – agreeing the outcome.

proven (Grove & Meehl 1996), the controversy of such procedures in clinical practice remains.

Essentially, when assessing a patient's risk, four potential outcomes are possible (Table 28.2). The desired outcome from any risk assessment, according to the table, is the correct prediction of risk. False negative means that a person was not deemed to be of risk and went on to be violent; the media are swift to publicise such events. False positive refers to occasions when a person is deemed to be of risk, and perhaps has their detention continued on this basis, but would in fact not be of danger. Human rights, moral issues and unnecessary public spending are all important issues in such cases. Whilst the frequency of false positives remains unknown, the human tragedy of such events which statistically must occur is enormous; sadly this issue does not command similar degrees of public attention.

Assessment of immediate risk

Whilst occupational therapists often form part of the multidisciplinary team that completes an assessment of future risk for patients, it is perhaps the assessment of immediate risk that is a more pressing issue for therapists. Occupational therapists are often involved in engaging patients in activities of increased risk such as cooking with sharp knives, using tools in the garden or woodwork or taking patients on rehabilitation outings. Accurate risk assessment in such activities is of vital importance and can only be partly informed by standardised risk assessments. There are several important risk factors that require careful consideration prior to patients engaging in occupational therapy in secure environments.

- Knowledge of previous personal, psychiatric and criminal history.
- Current factors surrounding the patient's mental state.

Variables in risk assessment

Determining a patient's readiness for transfer to another unit or for engaging in a therapy session is not always clear cut. Undoubtedly, there are cases at both ends of the spectrum where the risk of an individual is clear to all. Not all cases, however, are so apparent and different judgements can be made by various members of the multidisciplinary or clinical team. This can occur for two reasons. First, the individuals may be using differing variables in their risk assessment or placing differing weights on the same variable. Second, individuals may have differing thresholds for acceptable risk. A variety of factors can affect the level at which an individual's threshold for acceptable risk is placed such as personal perspectives, previous experiences, position and responsibilities within the organisation or recent adverse events.

When faced with disagreements in judgements about a patient, it is useful to consider whether this is due to differing risk assessments or differing personal risk thresholds. Differences in risk assessment can be resolved by agreeing the risk factors and appropriate weighting. Differences in personal risk thresholds are more challenging to resolve as they reflect strongly held personal perspectives and are less flexible to change. Regardless, it can be helpful when discussing such decisional conflicts to realise that the disagreement in judgement is not necessarily about the risk of the patient himself, but of the differing perspectives and thresholds of the professionals involved.

INTERVENTIONS IN FORENSIC OCCUPATIONAL THERAPY

As the majority of mentally disordered offenders have major mental illness, the form and range of occupational therapy interventions are the same as interventions with similar populations in general mental health settings. Engaging with patients and developing their motivation to engage in activities is an important first stage of occupational therapy intervention and one where the therapeutic use of media appears to assist (Chacksfield 2003). Group work is a popular mode of intervention in secure settings. Duncan et al (2003a) reported on the type of group work carried out in secure units; 86% of respondents (n=87) stated that they had developed protocol-driven group manuals to guide their interventions and 16% (n=16) stated they used published intervention manuals. Several of these appeared to have been developed using a cognitive behavioural approach. Popular group interventions within secure services include effective communications/social skills groups, life skills groups such as domestic skills or budgeting, drug and alcohol addiction groups and anxiety management (Duncan et al 2003a).

A THEORETICAL CONCEPTUALISATION OF OFFENDING BEHAVIOUR REHABILITATION

One area of intervention which differs at least in its conceptualisation from general mental health occupational therapy is offending behaviour rehabilitation and its associated interventions. Offending behaviour is a pervasive issue within forensic services, which has been targeted within national agendas (Scottish Office 1999). Occupational therapy is rarely discussed in the literature as a potential solution to this social issue. It could be argued, however, that, through engagement in occupation, occupational therapy has a unique role to play in lowering recidivism rates amongst offenders.

The Model of Human Occupation (MOHO) is a popular conceptual model of practice within forensic occupational therapy (Duncan et al 2003a). Forensic mental health involves clinicians working with individuals with a broad range of occupational deficits, which may result from mental illness, developmental disorders or offending behaviour. Whilst the first two categories have previously been addressed within the MOHO, offending behaviour, to date, has not.

A conceptual model of practice such as MOHO assists clinicians to develop intervention strategies that are evidence based, theory driven and client focused. To date, however, occupation-focused models have not addressed offending behaviour and have focused instead on specific client groups with diagnosed illnesses: schizophrenia, depression, stroke and intellectual and developmental disorders. However, within forensic occupational therapy, it is not uncommon to work with individuals whose psychosis is controlled through medication or, perhaps in the case of personality disorder, do not have an Axis I diagnosis. Such individuals often remain functionally impaired due to their offending behaviour life patterns and consequent functioning.

A tentative theoretical conceptualisation of offending behaviour using MOHO is, by its nature, general and the specific nuances of individuals cannot be adequately represented within the confines of this chapter. It is important, however, to develop this conceptualisation as, in doing so, a theoretical understanding of such a challenging population can begin to be developed and in time be tested for rigour. Understanding patients in this way, it is postulated, assists in understanding how best to work with and assist offenders to develop more functional pro-social occupational choices and identities (Duncan et al 2003b).

Individuals unfamiliar with the MOHO are recommended to carry out further reading (e.g. Forsyth & Kielhofner 2005) in order to understand the model in greater depth. Essentially, the MOHO conceptualises a person as a dynamic system which explains how human occupation is motivated, patterned and performed (Kielhofner 2002). The model comprises three dynamic systems, all occurring within the context of a person's social and physical environment. These systems are volition, habituation and performance capacity (Kielhofner 2002).

VOLITION

This component of the MOHO is composed of three separate but interlinked components: personal causation, values and interests.

Personal causation

Personal causation relates to individuals' view of their own personal capacity and how effective they are. It relates to the choices people make in activities and occupations and how these are experienced and interpreted. In examining personal causation in individuals who present with offending behaviour histories, it can be seen that such people may:

- have difficulty identifying many things to be proud of
- be unable to set realistic goals based on their own abilities
- often state that the future will be different and present unrealistic plans in response to the challenges which face them.

Values

Values are the things that a person places importance upon and they affect the choices, experience, interpretation and experience of the things a person does. In looking specifically at the values of people with offending behaviour, it can be observed that these often centre around:

- their family
- patterns of occupation centred on drugs and drink
- criminal lifestyle choices
- focusing on values held by peers who often pursue similar criminal lifestyles.

In summary, the values held by such individuals frequently do not support pro-social occupational choices and identities.

Interests

Interests relate to the things that people like to do and how such activities or occupations affect choices of participation, experience, interpretation and future anticipation. Interests are highly individualised but central interests can be observed. These relate to individuals' interests before admission to forensic environments and whilst resident in such situations. Drink and drugs are often cited as central interests by people with offending behaviour and frequently play a central role in consequent offending.

- People with offending behaviour are recognised as individuals who seek immediate gratification and often display a reluctance to engage in an activity which does not have an immediately clear benefit.
- The activities on offer within forensic residential settings are often limited, due to environmental restrictions and risk assessment. This results in patients frequently being offered a limited range of activities and demands a high degree of creativity and collaboration between the therapist and patient.
- Despite all the limitations described above, clients will often talk about a desire to undertake adaptive choices on discharge; however, they often have little adaptive history on which they can build and are really attempting to create a pro-social occupational identity and lifestyle.

HABITUATION

Habituation refers to the routine and familiar patterns of occupation carried out by individuals and is governed by people's roles and habits (Forsyth & Kielhofner 2005).

Roles

Roles relate to both the past and present and life roles affect what a person routinely does or plans to do on discharge. Frequently, offenders:

- display limited life roles
- focus on family roles
- have often not held down stable employment or developed a role as a worker
- have difficulty in identifying future pro-social and realistic life roles on discharge.

The issue of occupational identity – who a person is – is central here. Individuals with offending behaviours who wish to change often appear to struggle to develop or consider how to develop a pro-social future identity for themselves. This is unsurprising as it often requires a change of identity and underlines the importance of occupational therapy in such interventions.

Habits

Habits relate to the patterns of occupation and routines a person engages in such as going to work or regular leisure activities. Individuals with offending behaviour histories are frequently observed to have lacked a meaningful structure to their routine prior to admission. Any existing routines may have centred around drink, drugs and gaining money for their supply. Frequently such routines are maladaptive and have been unhelpful in assisting individuals to develop the pro-social identity they say that they desire.

PERFORMANCE CAPACITY

Individuals' performance capacity enables patients to actually do things in life. Individuals with offending behaviour histories may show some of the following strengths and weaknesses.

- Motor skills are not usually problematic.
- Poor problem solving is a recognised deficit within offending behaviour and can be observed to have an impact on the choices and patterns of occupations.
- Communication and interactions amongst such a population can frequently be confrontational and unsupportive of their longer term life desires. Frequently, interactions can be hostile and based on individuals' poor perception of themselves, how others view them and how they view others.

THE ENVIRONMENT

Within the MOHO the environment is considered to include both social and physical components. The past and present environments have a strong effect on patients' participation in pro-social lifestyle choices.

Social environment

In the past, individuals may have socialised within a criminal peer group. Such behaviour can often continue in forensic settings where people with offending behaviour will often group together, thus reinforcing some of their choices, routines and expectations for the future. Dysfunctional family relationships are common and unlikely to be supportive of change. This, however, is challenging as individuals place great importance on family relationships and they often form the core of occupational roles and identities. Finally, within forensic settings, patients often have restricted access to significant others in their life and this can be a source of stress and difficulty in maintaining positive close relationships that could support future pro-social life choices and the creation of a positive occupational identity.

Physical environment

The impoverished residential setting of a forensic unit can make it difficult to develop and achieve positive occupational choices. Individuals have often come from a limited income/itinerant criminal lifestyle and have experienced exclusion from work/school.

WHY IS THIS THEORETICAL CONCEPTUALISATION OF OFFENDING BEHAVIOUR NECESSARY?

- It develops an occupation-focused way of conceptualising patients' offending behaviour histories. This reinforces occupational therapy's unique contribution to the health of the forensic population.

- It provides a starting point to developing and validating standardised assessments for the forensic setting. This has already started with the development of a specific forensic version of OCAIRS (Forsyth et al 2005), and a significant proportion of the data for the validation of the MOHOST (Parkinson et al 2006) was collected within a high-security forensic service in Scotland.
- It provides a language with which to talk about our perspectives in multidisciplinary contexts and highlights to others our role in the rehabilitation of people with offending behaviours.
- It provides a theoretical framework to support the clinical reasoning of occupational therapists' working in this challenging setting.

RESEARCH IN FORENSIC OCCUPATIONAL THERAPY

The evidence base for forensic occupational therapy, like so much of occupational therapy and mental health, is sparse. Whilst much of the evidence required in forensic mental health can be gathered from general mental health publications, there are some issues that would benefit from research specifically in forensic environments.

RESEARCH PRIORITIES

A survey of research priorities in forensic occupational therapy was conducted by Duncan et al (2003a). The survey drew on key themes that had arisen at two previous national forensic occupational therapy conferences to identify potential research priorities in the identified list.

- The development of reliable and appropriate outcome measures.
- The development of effective group work programmes.
- The development of effective risk assessment tools.

Since this research was carried out, the potential for occupational therapists to work specifically with people who have personality disorders has developed in line with government policy and the creation of units in England for people with dangerous and severe personality disorders. Greater priority might now be given to developing a consensus statement for the role of occupational therapy with this group.

Contemporaneously with the above research study, another list of research priorities for forensic mental health was developed by the National Forum for Forensic Head Occupational Therapists (College of Occupational Therapists 2002). This list bears close resemblance to the previous survey but also included the development of outcome studies, the impact of security policies on practice, the impact of the environment on therapy, vocational rehabilitation and staff recruitment and retention.

COLLEGE OF OCCUPATIONAL THERAPISTS RESEARCH AND DEVELOPMENT PLAN

In recognition of the importance of developing research in this area, the College of Occupational Therapists, together with the National Forum for Forensic Head Occupational Therapists, published a research and development strategic vision and action plan (College of Occupational Therapists 2002). The forensic research and development strategic vision and action plan recognised that there were both opportunities and challenges in developing research in this area.

Research opportunities include the established network of forensic occupational therapists already in existence (see Useful Websites), the proactive nature of professionals within this specialism, existing managerial supports, the recognition by funding bodies that forensic occupational therapy required development and finally that there were existing groups of occupational therapists within forensic environments already developing research expertise. However, challenges were also noted. These included the lack of research leadership, the small patient numbers which would make larger scale studies more challenging, significant competition for limited research funds and the lack of development of clinicians as research consumers, let alone research collaborators or leaders.

PROFESSIONAL ISSUES

Working in forensic occupational therapy can bring therapists face to face with individuals with whom the client-centred values of unconditional positive regard, empathy and congruence are challenged. Perhaps working with sexual offenders is the obvious example of such a challenge but similar situations could occur with a range of patients. There are several reasons for this.

- Society and the media are repulsed by violent acts and are swift to condemn such events.
- Offenders may communicate in both a verbally and non-verbally challenging manner. Frequently, self-protection strategies may be consciously or unconsciously employed, such as ignoring difficult patients. These defensive strategies are unhelpful as it is more useful to evaluate difficult patients' communication strategies than the subjective responses of the therapist. Such communication difficulties may be indicative of clinical or personal deficits in the patient: 'When framed in this manner, the difficult communication style of the individual can be reformulated and understood as an indication of his difficulties and occupational performance deficits' (Duncan 2003, p204).
- Personal reasons can also make working with such patients challenging. Offenders' victims may be similar to friends or relations of the therapist or the offences may resemble events or relationships in the therapist's life.

Whatever the challenges faced by forensic occupational therapists, it is crucial that appropriate use is made of clinical supervision and such issues are openly acknowledged, explored and where possible resolved.

CONCLUSION

Duncan (2003) acknowledged the difficulties that exist when working with offenders, and particularly sexual offenders, but also referred to Martin Luther King for inspiration as he stated:

> When we look beneath the surface, beneath the impulsive evil deed, we see within our enemy-neighbour a measure of goodness and know that the viciousness and evilness of his acts are not quite representative of all that he is. We see him in a new light.

References

Barton C 2003 Assessment. In: Couldrick L, Alred D (eds) Forensic occupational therapy. Whurr, London, pp30-44

Birmingham L, Mason D, Grubin D 1996 Prevalence of mental disorder in remand prisoners: consecutive case study. BMJ 313(7071): 1521-1524

Chacksfield J 2003 Forensic addictive behaviours. In:. Couldrick L, Alred D (eds) Forensic occupational therapy. Whurr London, pp182-194

College of Occupational Therapists 1998 Occupational therapy in prisons. Report of the study day held at the College of Occupational Therapists, 2 December. College of Occupational Therapists, London

College of Occupational Therapists 2002 Research and development strategic visions and action plan for forensic occupational therapy. College of Occupational Therapists London

College of Occupational Therapists 2004 Definitions and core skills for occupational therapy. College of Occupational Therapists, London

Collins M, Davies S 2003. Security needs assessment profile. Rampton Hospital

Couldrick L 2003 So what is forensic occupational therapy. In: Couldrick L, Alred D (eds) Forensic occupational therapy. Whurr London, pp11-21

Creek J 2003 Occupational therapy defined as a complex intervention. College of Occupational Therapists, London

Crichton J 2003 (Chair) 2005 Definition of security levels in psychiatric inpatient facilities in Scotland. Forensic Mental Health Services Managed Care Network. The State Hospital, Carstairs

Dangerous and Severe Personality Disorder (DSPD) High Secure Services 2004 Planning and delivery guide. Home Office, London

Department of Health 1994 Report of the Working Group on High Security and Related Psychiatric Provision (the Read Report) Department of Health, London

Duncan EAS 2003 Occupational therapy and the sexual offender. Couldrick L, Alred D (eds) Forensic occupational therapy. Whurr, London, pp207-221

Duncan EAS 2004 Defining forensic occupational therapy. Keynote address at the 6th Annual National Forensic Occupational Therapy Conference, Leeds

Duncan EAS, Munro K, Nicol M 2003a Research priorities in forensic occupational therapy. British Journal of Occupational Therapy 66(2): 55-64

Duncan EAS, Walker K, Forsyth K, et al 2003b Understanding offending behaviour through an occupational therapy conceptual model of practice. Paper presented at the College of Occupational Therapists Annual Conference, Harrogate

Elliot C 1996 Rules of insanity: moral responsibility and the mentally ill. State University of New York, Albany

Faulk M 1994 Basic forensic psychiatry, 2nd edn. Blackwell Science, Oxford

Forsyth K, Deshpande S, Kielhofner G et al 2005 The Occupational Circumstances Assessment Interview and Rating Scale (OCAIRS) Version 4.0. The Model of Human Occupation Clearing House, Chicago

Forsyth K, Kielhofner G 2005 The model of human occupation: embracing the complexity of occupation by integrating theory into practice and practice into theory. In: Duncan EAS (ed) Foundations for practice, 4th edn. Churchill Livingstone, Edinburgh

Garman G 2000 Reported incidents at the Oxford Clinic: a 13 month study of incidents. Unpublished paper

Grove WM, Meehl PE 1996 Comparative efficiency of informal (subjective, impressionistic) and formal (mechanical, algorithmic) prediction procedures: the clincial/statistical controversy. Psychology, Public Policy and Law 2: 1-31

Gunn J, Taylor PJ 1993 Forensic psychiatry: clinical legal and ethical issues. Butterworth Heinemann,Oxford

Hills R 2003 The occupational therapist working in prison. In: Couldrick L, Alred D (eds) Forensic occupational therapy. Whurr, London, pp98-106

Hollin C 2002 Risk-needs assessment and allocation to offender programmes. In: McGuire J (ed) Offender rehabilitation and treatment: effective programmes and policies to reduce re-offending. John Wiley and Sons, Chichest p 309-332.

Home Office and Department of Health and Social Security 1975 Report of the Committee on Mentally Abnormal Offenders (Butler Report). HMSO, London

Ilott I, White E 2001 College of Occupational Therapists research and development strategic vision and action plan. British Journal of Occupational Therapy 64(6): 270-277

Joe C 2003 The development of community forensic occupational therapy. In: Couldrick L, Alred D (eds) Forensic occupational therapy. Whurr, London, pp107-116

Kielhofner G 2002 Introduction to the model of human occupation. In: Kielhofner G (ed). Model of human occupation: theory and application. Lippincott, Williams and Wilkins, Philadelphia, pp1-9

Lloyd C 1987 The role of occupational therapy in the treatment of the forensic psychiatric patient. Australian Occupational Therapy Journal 34: 20-25

McComish AG, Paterson B 1996 The development of forensic services in Scotland 1800–1960. Psychiatric Care 3(4): 153-158

Murphy E, Dingwall R, Greatbatch D et al 1998 Qualitative research methods in health technology assessment: a review of the literature. Health Technology Assessment 2(16):

Neeson A, Kelly R 2002 Security issues for occupational therapists working in a medium secure setting. In: Couldrick L, Alred D (eds) Forensic occupational therapy. Whurr, London, pp126-138

Parkinson S. Forsyth K, Kielhofner G 2006 The Model of Human Occupational Screening Tool (MOHOST) Version 4.0. The Model of Human Occupation Clearing House, Chicago

Partridge R 1953 Broadmoor – a history of criminal lunacy and its problems. Chatto and Windus, London

Robinson DN 1998 Wild beasts and idle humours. Harvard University Press, Cambridge, Massachusetts

Rogowski A 2002 Forensic psychiatry. In: Creek J (ed) Occupational therapy and mental health. Churchill Livingstone, London, pp491-510

Scottish Office 1999 Health, social work and related services for mentally disordered offenders in Scotland. The Scottish Office, Edinburgh

Skilling G 1999 The State Hospital at Carstairs, 1948–1999. The insanity plea and the development of forensic services in Scotland. Unpublished manuscript, The state Hospital, Carstairs

Tidmarsh D 1982 Implications from research studies In: Hamilton JR, Freeman H (eds) Dangerousness: psychiatric assessment and management. Gaskell, Oxford, pp12-20

Tilt R (Chair) 2005 Report of the review of security at the high security hospitals. Department of Health, London

Urquhart G 2003 Setting up a forensic occupational therapy service. In: Couldrick L, Alred D (eds) Forensic occupational therapy. Whurr, London, pp117-125

Walsh M, Ayres J 2003 Occupational therapy in a high-security hospital – the Broadmoor perspective. In: Couldrick L, Alred D (eds) Forensic occupational therapy. Whurr, London, pp87-97

Whiteford G 2000 Occupational deprivation: global challenge in the new millennium. British Journal of Occupational Therapy 63(5): 200-204

World Federation of Occupational Therapists 2002 Definitions of occupational therapy. World Federation of Occupational Therapists, Forrestfield, Western Australia

Useful Websites

Forensic e-discussion group

An email-based discussion group for anyone interested in forensic occupational therapy. Established in January 2003, it has over 500 members (predominantly forensic occupational therapists) who regularly use the group for a range of clinical, research and educational purposes. Group membership is open and can be joined by sending a blank email to: forensic_occupational_therapy-subscribe@yahoogroups.co.uk

National Forensic Occupational Therapy Conference

Established in 1998, this annual conference is the major forum for occupational therapy clinicians, researchers, managers, students, support workers and educators with an interest in forensic occupational therapy. This conference is organised by the College of Occupational Therapists specialist section mental health. It is jointly supported by the National Forum for Forensic Head Occupational Therapists. Details regarding forthcoming conferences are posted as emails and attachments in the above discussion group and are available from: www.cot.org.uk/specialist/aotmh/intro.php

Chapter 29

Substance misuse

Jenny Lancaster, John Chacksfield

INTRODUCTION

Occupational therapists in all fields of practice are likely to meet clients who have problems with substance misuse. This chapter is intended as a starting point for occupational therapists interested in the specialism of substance misuse as well as those who work in other areas of mental health and encounter substance use alongside psychiatric disorder. It discusses the nature and extent of substance misuse in the UK. An occupational perspective is offered on why people take drugs and the types of problems that the individual drug user may experience. The treatment process is outlined and the role of the occupational therapist highlighted. Treatment approaches are described as well as specific occupational therapy intervention strategies available for problem drug and alcohol users.

DEFINITIONS OF SUBSTANCE MISUSE

Substance use and misuse are widespread within our society and culture. Ninety percent of the adult UK population drink alcohol and about 10% of the population drink above recommended daily guidelines (Strategy Unit 2004). It is estimated that 30–50% of people with severe mental health problems misuse substances (Cabinet Office 2004). The prevalence of illegal drug misuse is harder to assess but it is estimated that 1% of the UK population use heroin or cocaine (NTA 2002).

The term 'substance use' generally means the consumption of alcohol or psychoactive drugs that have the potential to be addictive. Substance misuse has been defined as drug and/or alcohol taking that causes harm to the individual, his significant other or the wider community (NTA 2002). Substance dependence is a specific diagnostic term describing what is commonly termed addiction. Although there are myriad substances that are used and abused due to their psychoactive properties, this chapter will primarily focus on those which cause the most harm: heroin, cocaine and alcohol.

HISTORY OF SUBSTANCE MISUSE

The use of addictive substances has been intertwined with human occupation for a considerable proportion of mankind's history. Some examples are descibed below.

Alcohol

According to Nunn (1996), archaeological evidence exists for the use of alcohol in ancient Egypt from as early as 6000 BC. In Britain in the 17th century, due to the lack of drinking water, beer and gin were commonly drunk by the whole population throughout the day, starting at breakfast (Allen 2001, Tyler 1995). One-third of England's farmland was devoted to growing barley for beer and one in seven buildings was a tavern. In the second half of the century, 2000 coffee houses sprang up in London. This had a sobering effect on the population. Instead of getting drunk in taverns, coffee houses provided a safe place to read, play games and for political debate. Indeed, the first ballot box was used in the Turk's Head Coffee House in London. This change from the use of one depressant substance (alcohol) to a stimulant (caffeine in coffee) has been associated with increased literacy, political change and improved standards of living (Allen 2001).

However, with the changes in the occupational lives of workers during the Industrial Revolution, alcohol use dramatically increased in response to days toiling in factories and mines and increasing urbanisation (Tyler 1995). From 1951 to 2001 per capita alcohol use increased by 121% (Strategy Unit 2003). Currently 40% of alcohol use is binge drinking, i.e. drinking over twice the recommended guidelines in a single day. Binge drinking has been associated with a range of socially and physically harmful situations.

Opiates

It is believed that the opium poppy has been used for the last 6000 years (Tyler 1995). Opiates have been widely available in a variety of forms: opium, laudanum, morphine, heroin and methadone. Typically new forms of opiates were developed to 'cure' dependence on the previous form of opiate. Morphine was developed to treat opium addiction, heroin was introduced as a safe, non-addictive miracle drug to cure morphine addiction (Gossop 2000). Currently heroin addiction is typically treated by prescribing methdaone.

In the 17th century laudanum, a tincture of alcohol and opium, was used to treat a variety of ailments, incuding period pains and colic in babies. Controls were not introduced until 1868 due to concerns regarding the numbers of infant deaths through opium overdose (Drugscope 2007). This control led to a clearer distinction between medical and recreational use (Tyler 1995). Opiate use outside the medical context became seen as deviant. Even so, non-medical use of opiates was not an offence until the 1920s following the intervention of the Rolleston Committee (Tyler 1995) but doctors were still able to prescibe opiates to those who had become dependent.

In the 1960s, due to the creation of an illegal market in heroin created by a number of over-prescibing private GPs, the 1967 Misuse of Drugs Act led to the creation of the first drug dependency clinics in the NHS. However, in the 1970s and 1980s a massive increase in illegal availability of heroin and high unemployment rates led to a 'working class epidemic' (Tyler 1995). This, combined with a rapid increase in drug-related crime, has led to opiate dependence being viewed as an issue of social deviancy which needs to be controlled. Opiate use has been associated with unemployment and poverty over recent years. It can be viewed as a means of escape from an occupationally deprived life.

Cocaine

Cocaine comes from the coca leaf which has been used as an aid to work among Peruvians Indians for thousands of years (Gossop 2000). Currently, impoverished Peruvian miners chew coca leaves as a substitute for food to help them cope with work (Tyler 1995). Cocaine was first extracted from the leaves in 1855 and became a popular medicine and tonic and in fact, Coca Cola contained cocaine until 1904. It differs from opiates and alcohol in that, although powerfully psychologically addictive, it is not possible to become physically dependent on cocaine. Cocaine became popular in the UK in the 1970s. It was common among the affluent classes and developed a somewhat glamorous image. However, in the mid-1980s a more powerful, cheaper form of cocaine known as crack was developed. Unlike cocaine, crack use is associated with deprivation, crime and co-existing heroin use (Home Office 2002a). Crack use typically follows a binge pattern

where once people start using, they become completely consumed with using more and engage in activities to obtain more crack. Users frequently stay awake for over 24 hours, becoming increasingly more paranoid and aggressive. The binge is followed by a 'crash' in which users experience extreme exhaustion and emotional lability. This pattern of binging and crashing completely disrupts users' daily lives and routines.

CULTURAL CONTEXT

Culture mediates views of drugs in terms of how dangerous they are, how legal they should be and how good or bad they are. For example, the Christian, moralist, Temperance movement in 19th-century Britain set out to reduce alcohol consumption (Berridge 2005). At the end of the 19th century, cocaine was highly popular and recommended by doctors such as Sigmund Freud and Sir Clifford Albutt. At the same time, Albutt (cited in Gossop 2000) held a different view of another drug, popular today, as illustrated in a quote from his medical textbook: 'The sufferer is tremulous and loses his self-command, he is subject to fits of agitation and depression. He loses colour and has a haggard appearance. As with other such agents, a renewed dose of the poison gives temporary relief, but at the cost of future misery'. The drug described was coffee.

Many cultures use and have used drugs in social ritual or religious ceremony, to enhance skill in war and for pleasure. In some, the cultivation of drug crops, though often illegal, is a major industry that offers considerable employment opportunities and contributes to the national economy (Henman 1985). Drug profits have been known to drive political movements, such as the suggested use of heroin trafficking by the People's Republic of China to fund Communist Party activities (Musto 1993).

Alcohol has long been considered to be the dominant drug of European culture, whereas in the Americas plant-based drugs unknown in Europe, such as nicotine and cocaine, were widely used for centuries before alcohol was popularised with the coming of immigrants from Europe (Gossop 2000).

Substance misuse from the 18th to the early 20th century was primarily seen as a sin. The drunk and the 'opium sot' were seen as morally degraded. The turn of the 20th century saw this attitude change towards a much more disease-oriented concept that offered a cure. In the 1960s came the idea of dependence as a concept that acknowledged psychological reliance on a drug and, in the 1970s, this was developed into the modern dependence syndrome. More recently, social models of substance misuse have been developed that take into account wider cultural, economic and psychological factors.

SUBSTANCE MISUSE

Currently, in the UK, substances misused are generally categorised as either legal or illegal, are subject to restrictions according to age or cultural acceptability, and are either natural plant extracts or manufactured.

Substance misuse can lead to social, psychological, physical or legal problems related to intoxication or regular excessive consumption and/or dependence (NTA 2002). Most of the results of problem use of substances or dependence on them can be observed in the patterns of human occupation exhibited by the user and their impact on the user's quality of life. Some of these effects are described later in the chapter. It is important to remember that the myriad problems that substance misusers experience do not occur in isolation. Frequently people develop substance misuse problems in an attempt to deal with problems in their lives, e.g. the breakdown of a relationship. It has been proposed that it is important to consider the interrelation of three factors in relation to substance misuse (Ghodse 2002, Gossop, 2000):

- the drug
- the individual
- the environment.

Examining the relationship between the individual and the environment in relation to human occupation is a core component of occupational therapy practice. When working with substance-using clients, occupational therapists consider how the substance use or abstinence from a previously habitually used substance affects occupation, e.g. the woman whose drinking increases due to changes in work environment or the ex-heroin user who, having given up a large network of drug-using friends, feels he doesn't have the confidence to engage in new leisure activities alone.

Substance misuse has been described as a chronically relapsing condition (NTA 2002). Research indicates extremely high relapse rates following an episode of substance misuse treatment, between 75% and 90%, and that relapse is most likely within a short period following initial treatment (Hunt et al 1971, Milkman et al 1984, Stephens and Cottrell 1972). However, the largest multi-site trial in the UK has proved the long-term effectiveness of drug treatment (Gossop et al 2003).

The costs of illegal drug misuse for communities are high. The National Treatment Outcome Research Study (Gossop et al 2003) calculated that for every £1 spent on drug treatment, £3 was saved in costs to the criminal justice system and victims of crime. Consequently illegal drug misuse has been high on the government's political agenda since 1998 with the publication of the national strategy *Tackling Drugs to Build a Better Britain* (HMSO 1998) and the Updated Drugs Strategy in 2002b (Home Office). Numerous policies and initiatives have followed. The website www.drugs.gov.uk/is a useful resource for finding out about current initiatives and the national policy.

NATIONAL POLICIES

In 2001 the government created the National Treatment Agency (NTA) for Substance Misuse. The NTA is a special health authority for England designed to improve effectiveness of treatment for drug misuse (NTA 2002). It has published *Models of Care*, a national service framework to guide the development of treatment services (NTA 2006). This document summarises the evidence base of all aspects of drug treatment. The NTA aims to double the number of people in effective, well-managed treatment from 100,000 in 1998 to 200,000 in 2008 and to increase the proportion of people who successfully complete or, if appropriate, continue treatment. It also stresses the importance of community integration, enabling service users to consolidate treatment gains through access to training and employment (NTA, 2006). In Scotland the Effective Interventions Unit was set up in June 2000 to identify and disseminate effective practice to support the implementation of the drug misuse strategy *Tackling Drugs in Scotland: Action in Partnership* (Scottish Office 1999). Wales has its own 8-year drugs strategy, *Tackling Substance Misuse in Wales: A Partnership Approach*, which was launched in 2000 (National Assembly for Wales 2000).

There has been less activity at a policy level in relation to alcohol. The first national alcohol strategy, the Alcohol Harm Reduction Strategy for England, was published in 2004 (Cabinet Office 2004). There are more people dependent on alcohol than illegal drugs – 2.9 million compared to 250,000 (Alcohol Concern 2007, NTA 2002) – and alcohol-related harm costs the country an estimated £20 billion per year (Strategy Unit 2004). The alcohol market is worth £30 billion per year and provides 1 million jobs (Strategy Unit 2003). However, the relationship between alcohol use and harm is not straightforward as it is related to occupational form. For example, the UK has a culture of binge drinking – going out specifically to get drunk, associated with harm – whereas other European countries drink similar weekly amounts but the alcohol is consumed in more moderate amounts as part of the daily evening meal.

Research into addictive substances and their management has evolved over the last 200 years from being a fragmented and underdeveloped area of science to becoming a frontier subject with its own identity (Edwards 2002). Some of the developments which have led to addiction being taken seriously as a manageable issue, as opposed to a 'sin', have included the landmark research into the relationship between smoking and lung cancer, and the importance given to research in treating the massive heroin problem in the USA among GIs during the Vietnam war.

Where alcohol and drugs are used by people with mental health diagnoses, they can severely exacerbate symptoms and disrupt treatment. They are associated with disrupted lifestyles, suicide (Duke et al 1994) and violent behaviour (Swanson et al 1990). The issue of 'dual diagnoses', i.e. substance misuse by people with a mental health problem, has been highlighted as important within UK government policy (DoH 2002).

WHAT ARE DRUGS AND OTHER SUBSTANCES?

Drugs and other substances are usually grouped according to psychotropic action or legality.

Drug action

The action of drugs on the human brain determines whether they are considered an opiate, a stimulant, a depressant, a hallucinogen or a minor tranquilliser. Some drugs, such as cannabis, nicotine and volatile inhalants, do not conform to any of these classifications.

It should be noted that drug action and effect can be influenced by: the route of administration, e.g. smoking, drinking or injecting; personality characteristics of the user; cultural expectations; and the immediate setting and expectations. Taking a drug together with another drug, or taking drugs when mentally ill, can also influence drug action and effect.

Alcohol and drugs act on specific centres of the brain. For example, opiates (e.g. heroin) act on the opiate receptor in areas of the brain such as the limbic system, specifically the nucleus accumbens and the ventral tegmentum (Stellar & Rice 1987). Changing the state of these receptors by using drugs results in pleasurable experiences.

Many drugs are thought to act on the dopamine system. Dopamine is a chemical messenger which plays an important role in the brain's reward centre. It is released when we do pleasurable things, from eating good food to having sex. Drugs such as cocaine and heroin cause a massive surge of dopamine to be released, and this extra dopamine leads to the sensation of pleasure. Over time, repeated drug use can lead to dopamine receptor sites in the brain being reduced or shut down. Therefore, the drug user finds less effect from using a drug, which leads to an increase in the amount used. The other significant effect is that the drug user is likely to experience a decreased ability to feel pleasure or satisfaction in activities of daily life. This can lead to further drug use or thrill-seeking activities. It is important for occupational

Table 29.1 Drugs and substances according to psychoactive quality and legality

	Drug name	Method of consumption	Legal class/status
Stimulants	Nicotine	Smoking in cigarette, cigar, pipe	Legal if aged 16+
	Cocaine	Heated and inhaled or smoked	Illegal: Class A
	Crack cocaine	Smoked or injected	Illegal: Class A
	Amphetamines	Tablets or injected	Illegal: Class A
Depressants	Alcohol	Oral ingestion via carrier substance	Legal if aged 18+
	Benzodiazepines	Tablet form, oral or injection	Legal if prescribed
Opiates	Heroin	Injected or smoked by heating and inhalation ('chasing the dragon')	Illegal: Class A
Hallucinogenics	Lysergic acid diethylamide (LSD or 'acid') Psilocybin ('magic mushrooms') MDMA ('ecstasy')	Manufactured as 'tabs', small squares of paper which are placed on the tongue Infusion (tea) or smoked after drying Tablet form	Illegal: Class A Illegal: Class A if prepared for use, e.g. by drying Illegal: Class A
Other	Cannabis	Smoked, inhaled	Illegal: Class C

therapists to be aware of this in their clinical work as clients who have recently stopped using and have reduced dopamine levels may struggle to feel satisfaction from the occupations selected in occupational therapy.

Alcohol has a variety of complex actions but is generally a nervous system depressant. The reason alcohol appears to produce euphoria is that it depresses frontal cortex functioning, resulting in loss of inhibition.

Legality

Alcohol is legal for use by people over the age of 18. The legality of other drugs is determined in the UK by the Misuse of Drugs Act (HMSO 1979). This classifies drugs as Class A, Class B or Class C. Each class carries particular penalties for use and supply of the drug.

Table 29.1 illustrates some of the most common substances in terms of legal classification and psychoactivity.

Measurement

Alcohol is measured in units of 10 mg. One unit of alcohol can be found in a single measure of spirits, a glass of wine or a half pint of ordinary-strength beer.

Drugs are also measured in terms of amount purchased or mode of delivery. Heroin, cocaine and cannabis (resin or leaf forms) are generally measured by weight, although for non-cannabis drugs in powder form, the purity of what is purchased is variable according to what the powder has been mixed (or cut) with. LSD and Ecstasy are sold in units or 'tabs'.

WHY DO PEOPLE USE SUBSTANCES?

People are known to use substances for many and varied reasons (Edwards 1987, Gossop 2000). Alcohol, for example, is widely used as a social lubricant, to reduce tension, to intoxicate as a way of coping with negative feelings or as a sedative.

Drugs such as cannabis are used to remove the symptoms of glaucoma, to relax, bring pleasure, alter consciousness or as part of initiation into a social group. Heroin use is described as offering a warm, dreamy 'cocoon' and, for many users, it serves as an antidote to emotional pain and the stress of a life lacking in meaning (Tyler 1995).

Reasons for substance use: an occupational perspective

Substance use is often closely tied to human occupational behaviour. It could be said that the most common reasons for the use of substances lie in their ability to either enhance or disrupt human occupation. Some of the reasons for substance use can be categorised under the headings listed below. These reasons can be applied to almost all substances, including alcohol, nicotine, caffeine and tranquillisers as well as illegal drugs. It is important to note that each individual drug user will have his own very specific reasons and the following list is unlikely to be exhaustive.

Enabling occupation

- By reducing tension
- By removing inhibition
- By stimulating mental alertness
- By imitating others' drug use

Avoiding occupation

- Through intoxication
- Through stimulus seeking via drug use
- Through escape into drug culture
- Through denial of responsibility by drug use

As a coping mechanism

- To cope with anxiety
- To relieve or avoid facing pain
- To mask distress
- To increase confidence and peer acceptance
- As self-medication for mental health problems

To alter perception

- In order to develop wider understanding of life
- For desired spiritual attainment
- As part of religious ritual
- To assist creativity

- Because drug-induced perception is considered more pleasant than normality

To develop meaning in life

- Through the ritual of drug-taking behaviour
- Through the routine of drug obtaining or dealing activities
- Through the excitement of avoiding legal services
- Through interacting and sharing a culture with associates in a drug-using network

To enhance occupation

- By celebrating positive events
- By enhancing good feelings
- By removing negative emotional states

To cope with occupational imbalance

- To cope with boredom – 'kill time' (occupational deprivation)
- To cope with the pressure of too many demands on one's time

Applying some of these ideas, using the Human Open System (Kielhofner 2002), a possible model of their interaction can be constructed (Fig. 29.1).

WHEN DOES DRUG USE GO WRONG?

In general, it is likely that most people can regulate their use of alcohol, caffeine and other drugs without this use leading to damage to themselves, others or their occupational behaviour patterns. However, the use of alcohol and other drugs can and does lead to a considerable range of physical, psychological and social problems.

User surveys reported by the Department of Health (1996) suggest that drug use cannot be tackled in isolation. It is often associated with factors such as unemployment, family break-up and crime. Failure to address the wider life context issues can slow down or reverse progress in treatment of the drug problem itself.

Research has shown that substance users have higher rates of psychiatric disorder than the general population (DoH 2002). Either the disorder may be induced by drug use or drugs can be used to self-medicate the symptoms. Other studies show that drugs and crime are interlinked (Forshaw & Strang 1993). A major American study

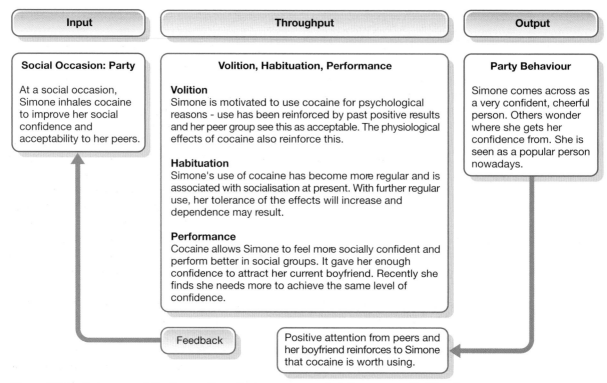

Figure 29.1   Drug use and the Human Open System: an example (all names are fictitious).

revealed that violent behaviour is approximately three times more likely in people who both use drugs and have a mental disorder than those who do not suffer either (Swanson et al 1990).

Problems and dependence

Two issues represented in the academic literature on substances are problems and dependence. These are illustrated in Figure 29.2. The quadrants in Figure 29.2 do not represent distinct categories but each axis lies on a continuum (Drummond 1992).

- Sector A: those who experience problems related to non-dependent use (e.g. often young people)
- Sector B: a group who experience both dependence and problems (typical in the clinical setting)
- Sector C: a group in the population who take a substance but experience neither significant dependence nor problems
- Sector D: those who are significantly dependent but do not experience problems

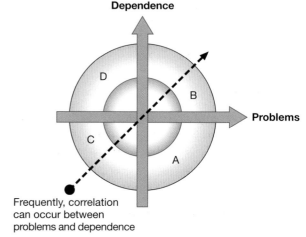

Figure 29.2   Diagram to show how problems and dependence coexist (after Edwards et al 1977).

Research by Drummond (1990) suggested that people who are more dependent on alcohol experience more problems, but that certain problems are more closely related to dependence than others. Also, dependence can lead to abnormal drinking patterns. Where alcohol problems may be subject to sociodemographic effects, dependence is more likely to exist independently of most sociodemographic variables. Dependence and problems can be seen as coexisting and interrelated but not as separate entities (Drummond 1992, Gossop 1994a).

Problems

Alcohol or drug problems can be said to occur when their use severely disrupts a person's normal lifestyle balance or physical state.

- Consumption of more than 50 units of alcohol per week for men and over 35 units weekly for women is likely to cause problems (Gossop 1994a).
- Patterns of drug use can be problematic, such as binge use of a particular drug, or drug use as the only way to cope with difficulties.
- Physical problems can range from malnutrition to heart problems and lung, liver and gastric disease. Between 50% and 80% of injecting drug users are infected with the hepatitis C virus (British Liver Trust 2007).
- Psychological problems include anxiety, depression, memory loss, neurological damage, chronic psychotic symptoms and dementia. National figures show that drug and alcohol users die younger than non-users.

Dependence

Dependence on substances is diagnosed using the dependence syndrome (Edwards et al 1981). This consists of a list of seven problems, three of which at least have to be present in a greater or lesser degree to indicate dependence.

1. Subjective awareness of compulsion to use a drug or drugs.
2. A desire to stop using the drug in the face of continued use.
3. A stereotyped drug-taking habit; that is, a narrowing of the repertoire of drug-taking behaviour.
4. Experience of withdrawal symptoms (evidence of neuroadaptation/tolerance).
5. Use in order to relieve withdrawal symptoms.
6. Primacy of drug use over other activities in life (salience).
7. Rapid reinstatement of dependence after a period of abstinence.

The dependence syndrome is the most widely used method of diagnosing substance dependence and is used within the major diagnostic classification systems, such as ICD10 and DSMIV. It consists of both physical and psychological aspects and aims to emphasise the importance of psychological dependence on a substance as well as physical symptomatology. Edwards (Edwards & Gross 1976, Edwards 1987), who developed the dependence syndrome concept, emphasised the need to take a clinical picture in its social and environmental context and to tailor the picture to the individual.

Dependence on alcohol is generally identified either through interview or by using questionnaires such as the Severity of Alcohol Dependence Questionnaire (SADQ) (Stockwell et al 1979). The SADQ is the instrument recommended by the World Health Organization (Anderson 1990).

Other concepts of dependence include the addictive personality concept, which suggests that addiction is a form of personality disorder, or that people dependent on a drug are predisposed towards this because of their personality characteristics. The validity of this view has been largely dismissed on the research evidence (Gossop 1994a). Another approach to understanding drug dependence is the conditioning approach, first developed by Wickler (1948) which suggests that drug-related behaviours occur because they become paired with the reinforcing effect of the feelings a drug produces. Other conditioning models exist, as do social models and the basic biomedical approach.

TREATMENT OF SUBSTANCE MISUSE

A MODEL OF CHANGE

Before considering drug and alcohol treatment in context, it is useful to present a transtheoretical model of change that can be used with clients with any addictive behaviour (or any client working towards behaviour change). The stages of change model is a useful tool for guiding the selection of treatment goals and interventions (Fig. 29.3). Therapeutic intervention can be targeted to help clients progress through the stages of change.

Prochaska & DiClemente (1982, 1986; Prochaska et al 1992) first developed this model with cigarette smokers, who they found reported movement through different stages of change as they attempted to give up. These same stages have since been observed in all other addictive disorders (Gossop 1994b). It reflects the reality that it is normal for an individual to go through all the stages several times before achieving lasting behaviour change. Most of us can relate to attempting behaviour changes ourselves, for example, dieting, starting regular exercise or stopping smoking, where we have not succeeded in maintaining the change at the first attempt. In fact, Prochaska & DiClemente's initial research was with smokers who went round the cycle between three and seven times before finally giving up for good.

Addiction can be viewed as a chronic, relapsing condition in which relapses are viewed as normal events that can be learned from rather than seen as failure. Although represented as a cycle, it is now conceptualised as a spiral acknowledging that each time the person goes through the stages, they are learning from the experience of previous attempts to change.

Stages of change

The central concept of this model is that behaviour change takes place through the following discrete stages.

- **Precontemplation**. These are people who do not recognise that they have a problem, therefore they are outside the 'model of change'. 'Precontemplators' rarely present for treatment. However, when they do, it is in order to assuage the concerns of others.
- **Contemplation**. In this stage, the person recognises that his behaviour is problematic and considers doing something about it. This change is characterised by ambivalence. Motivational enhancement therapy or motivational interviewing is a useful, evidence-based approach to use during this stage.
- **Preparation** The person prepares to change.
- **Action**. Making the change, implementing the plan.
- **Maintenance**. Sustain the change, integrating the change into the individual's lifestyle.

Due to the nature of this model, it follows that a person may slip back a stage or exit the cycle into precontemplation at any time.

By using this model the therapist can establish which stage the client is at and use this to select the most appropriate treatment. For example, a client in the maintenance phase may benefit from learning stress management and developing satisfying occupations in day-to-day life which are important in preventing relapse into drug or alcohol use. This would boost self-confidence and reduce the risk of relapse. However, these strategies would probably be wasted on someone in the precontemplation phase. The use of this framework to guide occupational therapy service delivery is described by Buijsse et al (1999).

The model of change is an effective means to assess readiness for treatment. Research indicates that effective treatment matching based on an

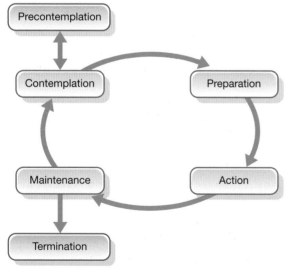

Figure 29.3   A model of change (adapted by Jenny Lancaster from Prochaska & DiClemente 1982, 1986).

assessment of treatment readiness is a significant predictor of engagement and retention (Project MATCH 1993, Simpson et al 1997). If the client has an alcohol problem a standardised assessment, the Readiness for Change questionnaire (Heather et al 1991), can be completed. For drug users the stage of change can be ascertained through self-reported drug use, urine analysis and client consultation.

In addition to assisting in treatment matching, this model is helpful for both client and therapist in setting realistic and achievable goals; that is, to move to the next stage in the cycle rather than try to stop the behaviour immediately. Also, it is a more optimistic approach in that relapse is viewed as a normal part of the process of achieving long-term behaviour change rather than as failure. Occupational therapy input is ideally placed when the client has reached the maintenance phase. However, the reality is rarely that straightforward. The occupational therapist needs to be able to assess what stage the client is in and respond accordingly.

SUBSTANCE MISUSE TREATMENT IN CONTEXT

Drug and alcohol treatment services are operated by the NHS, Social Services and prisons, private clinics and the voluntary sector. Treatment settings include hospital and community locations, and treatment can commence in either.

Triggers to treatment entry

Entry into treatment is usually triggered by a crisis. For example, a family seeks help from their general practitioner as they can no longer tolerate their daughter's growing drug habit; a young person is caught breaking into houses to fund a growing crack cocaine habit; a patient is admitted to hospital because his liver is failing as a consequence of his drinking; a City of London businesswoman is taken to a private clinic by her partner out of concern for the amount of whisky she drinks at work; a vulnerable, homeless person with schizophrenia has been sexually assaulted when incapacitated on tranquillisers; or a sex worker seeks help

during her latest attendance at a needle exchange in a Manchester treatment facility.

Referral

People with alcohol problems are frequently referred for treatment by their GP, self-refer or are referred after an alcohol-related physical problem is identified, e.g. in A&E. Those with drug problems tend to self-refer or are referred as a result of initiatives within the criminal justice systems, i.e. arrest referral schemes whereby people arrested for a drug-related crime are offered an assessment or a 'community sentence' as an alternative to prison. Some referrals will come from employers or employee assistance programmes.

MULTIDISCIPLINARY ASSESSMENTS

Assessments are initially adisciplinary. The person at the first point of contact may be a nurse, a doctor or a duty drug worker of any profession. The assessment needs to be tailored, needs led and an ongoing progress (NTA 2002). The goal of the assessment is to discover the primary issues surrounding the client's substance use, his motivation to change his habit and how long and how severe the habit is. During this time the client will be monitored for withdrawal symptoms. He may also be breathalysed or have urine and/or blood tests to monitor the alcohol or drug content and assess liver functioning. A risk assessment will also form a part of the procedure.

During the assessment period, a number of assessment techniques may be used, including:

- screening assessments
- structured questionnaires
- interviews
- observation
- self-assessment
- physiological assessments (for example, blood analysis, ECG).

Screening assessments

A number of screening assessments can be used. The widely used CAGE questionnaire (Box 29.1; Mayfield et al 1974) or the S-MAST (Pokorny et al

---

Box 29.1 The CAGE questionnaire

1. Have you ever felt you ought to CUT DOWN on your drinking?
2. Have people ANNOYED you by criticising your drinking?
3. Have you ever felt bad or GUILTY about your drinking?
4. Have you ever had a drink first thing in the morning to steady your nerves or get rid of a hangover? (EYE-OPENER)

Two or more affirmative replies are said to identify the problem drinker. Research has supported this assertion.

1972) provide fast, rough guides to the extent of drinking problems. For drug use there is the Severity of Dependence Scale (Gossop et al 1995), which is designed to be generic for a range of drugs. It is essential to monitor withdrawal (Edwards 1987) and assessments are often used to assist this, such as the Short Opiate Withdrawal Scale (Gossop 1990).

Interview techniques

Interviews add to the assessment. These can follow a standard mental health interview approach but should also include questions about the client's substance use such as:

- number of different drugs used
- amount used
- a typical day of use
- history of use, including first drug use occasion and changes in use over time.

Structured assessments

Multidisciplinary, structured questionnaires aim to investigate the severity of dependence, the range and complexity of problems associated with substance use and motivation to engage in treatment or change substance use behaviour. Other issues may include measurement of specific symptoms, such as anxiety, and rehabilitation potential, using occupational therapy assessments.

OCCUPATIONAL THERAPY ASSESSMENT

Occupational therapy investigates three domains (American Occupational Therapy Association 1994).

Performance areas

Categories of human daily activity, such as activities of daily living, leisure, self-maintenance and work/productivity. Substance use affects each of these areas in different ways.

Occupational therapists are concerned that substance misuse and dependence disrupt the balance of work, self-care and leisure (Busuttil 1989, Lindsay 1983, Chacksfield 1994, Morgan 1994, Nicol 1989, Rotert 1990). Quantitative research by occupational therapists such as Mann & Talty (1990), Scaffa (1991), Stoffel et al (1992) and Chacksfield & Lindsay (1999) has highlighted poor use of leisure by alcohol-dependent clients as a key problem area.

Performance components

Fundamental human abilities are required for successful engagement in performance areas including sensorimotor, cognitive, psychosocial and psychological components. Drug action can create both short- and long-term effects on performance components.

Occupational therapy research has suggested that low motivation and low self-esteem are significant in substance misusers (Stoffell et al 1992, Viik et al 1990).

Performance contexts

Environmental factors and situations that influence the client's engagement in performance areas. These are significant in substance-using clients due to the way environmental cues can impact and trigger substance use, called 'environmental press' by Kielhofner (2002).

This idea has been supported by a growing body of research into cue exposure (Drummond et al 1995). Cue exposure concerns environmental cues or stimuli that trigger addictive behaviour in individuals. A client returning to the same lifestyle on discharge is likely to relapse to substance use and will need work on coping strategies to counteract environmental effects.

Occupational therapy assessment tools

Occupational therapists will wish to supplement the standard initial interview with open questioning to obtain information about how substance use is impacting on the client's occupational performance areas, components and contexts.

The Occupational Circumstances Assessment Interview and Rating Scale (OCAIRS) (Forsyth et al 2005) is a semi-structured interview often used by occupational therapists with this client group. Other appropriate tools include:

- Occupational Self-Assessment (OSA)
- Rosenberg Self-Esteem Inventory
- Self-Efficacy Scale
- Volitional Questionnaire
- Coping Responses Inventory (CRI)
- Interest Checklist
- Role Checklist
- Assessment of Motor and Process Skills (AMPS)
- Internal/External Locus of Control Scale
- Occupational Performance History Interview.

Use of these instruments will be limited by the time available.

INTERVENTIONS

Substance dependence is typically a chronically relapsing condition. Therefore interventions often do not follow a linear path. Using the model of change to assess treatment readiness and motivation (described above) combined with an accurate picture of the person's current substance use is important in selecting the most appropiate intervention.

ENGAGEMENT

Many people with substance misuse problems struggle to engage with treatment services. Feelings of ambivalence, anxieties about change, fluctuating levels of motivation and a chaotic lifestyle are part of an addiction or dependence. Enhancing engagement and retention is key in achieving positive outcomes of treatment (NTA 2004). The importance of establishing rapport, empathy and motivational enhancement techniques from the initial assessment onwards must not be underestimated (NTA 2004).

PRINCIPLES OF INTERVENTION

Intervention is a complex process in the field of substance misuse due to the complex needs presented by clients; therefore, a multidisciplinary, multimodal, multiagency approach works best (DoH 1996, Edwards 1987). Some principles of intervention include:

- tailoring treatment to the individual client
- fostering a relationship between the client and the treatment institution
- setting achievable goals for intervention
- involving the family or carers
- emphasising empowerment of the client in overcoming substance problems or dependence.

Treatment strategies

Strategies tend to aim towards the following goals:

1. detoxification
2. rebalancing external and internal problems not directly related to substance use
3. reducing external and internal problems that are related to drug use
4. reducing harmful or hazardous behaviour associated with the use of drugs (for example, sharing dirty needles)
5. developing the internal resources (self-esteem, motivation, knowledge) to address the drug problem or dependence
6. establishing a safe, controlled pattern of drug use that is not harmful or dependent
7. establishing abstinence from the problem drug (or drugs)

8. establishing abstinence from all drugs
9. establishing an independent lifestyle.

These goals are not mutually exclusive and can be carried out in combination. For instance, many physical problems, such as muscle atrophy or memory loss, may continue to require treatment during many of the other stages.

Occupational therapists contribute to the intervention programme by enhancing occupational performance via activity-based and other related interventions.

TREATMENT OPTIONS

Alcohol misuse

Detoxification or detox followed by abstinence is recommended for people who are physically dependent on alcohol. Detox involves the prescription of decreasing doses of librium to manage withdrawal symptoms. Those who are at risk of withdrawal fits will be offered inpatient detox, others may be offered a community detox.

Those with less severe alcohol problems and binge drinkers may opt for 'controlled drinking'. This means keeping alcohol consumption within safe levels by adhering to a set of personal rules, e.g. not drinking alone, not having more than two drinks a day, not drinking on consecutive days.

After becoming abstinent or successfully controlling alcohol, people are typically offered a range of psychosocial interventions, in particular relapse prevention which will be discussed later.

Drug misuse

A hierarchy of goals has been developed for drug treatment (DoH 1996, NTA 2002). These are:

- reduction of health, social and other problems directly related to drug misuse
- reduction of harmful or risky behaviours associated with the misuse of drugs (e.g. sharing injecting equipment)

- reduction of health, social or other problems not directly attributable to drug misuse
- attainment of controlled, non-dependent, or non-problematic, drug use
- abstinence from main problem drugs
- abstinence from all drugs.

This hierarchy of drug treatment goals endorses the principle of harm minimisation, which refers to the reduction of the various forms of drug-related harm (including social, medical, legal and financial problems) until the drug misuser is ready and able to come off drugs (DoH et al 1999). Harm reduction interventions include safer injecting advice and needle exchange schemes.

Substitute prescribing

Many opiate-dependent users require prescription of a substitute drug, methadone. This aims to stop the user experiencing unpleasant withdrawal symptoms but does not provide a 'high'. The rationale behind substitute prescribing is that the drug user no longer has to inject street heroin, with its associated health risks, or be involved in illegal activities in order to fund a habit. Long-term prescription of methadone, or methadone maintenance, aims to allow users to stabilise their drug use and therefore their lives and, combined with psychological and social support, enables users to make positive lifestyle changes. It is often considered after a user has tried to detoxify and failed, and requires close monitoring due to the risk of overdose or harm related to illicit drug or alcohol use.

Physical and mental health treatment

Many clients also have physical, social, legal and psychological problems which need to be addressed as part of a comprehensive treatment plan.

APPROACHES TO INTERVENTION

There are numerous models of substance misuse treatment and it is beyond the scope of this chapter to cover all of them. However, those approaches that occupational therapists are most likely to come across and those of most relevance to occupational therapists are described below.

The Twelve Steps

Alcoholics Anonymous (AA) and its associate Narcotics Anonymous (NA) is a self-help movement that offers an extensive international support network for substance users and their families. Meetings of these organisations occur at various times during the day and are supplemented with Step Meetings, for those serious about abstinence, and individual support from a sponsor. The sponsor is a person who has been successful in his abstinence for a significant length of time and who has worked his way through the Twelve Steps (Box 29.2). As it is so comprehensive, this approach is widely advocated and some research evidence exists to show it works for about 26% of members (Bebbington 1976).

Criticism has been made of the requirement that those who attend have to adhere to the idea that dependence is a disease and that people attending have to constantly remind themselves that they are alcoholic, even when they have been abstinent for many years. Additionally, criticism is directed at the idea that a higher power is responsible for an AA or NA member's abstinence, suggesting that this removes the responsibility for sobriety from the individual.

Relapse prevention

Based on the model of change, relapse prevention (RP) (Marlatt & Gordon 2005) has become one of the most widely used intervention approaches in the field of addiction. Marlatt (Marlatt & Gordon 2005) suggested that RP is a self-management programme that is designed to enhance the maintenance phase of the model of change.

Relapse prevention can be defined as 'a wide range of strategies to prevent relapse in the field of addictive behaviours' with an emphasis on 'self management and the techniques and strategies aimed at enhancing maintenance of habit change'. It is a self-control programme that combines behavioural skills training, cognitive interventions and lifestyle change procedures' (Wanigaratne et al 1990, p1). There is a growing body of evidence supporting the effectiveness of RP interventions (Carroll 1996, Irvin et al 1999).

The RP approach uses cognitive behavioural strategies to help clients who are trying to stop or reduce drug or alcohol use to learn how to anticipate and cope with situations and problems that might lead to a relapse (Wanigaratne et al 1990). The model focuses on the notions of high-risk situations and coping strategies available to the individual.

Box 29.2 The Twelve Steps of Alcoholics Anonymous

1. We admitted we were powerless over alcohol – that our lives had become unmanageable.
2. Came to believe that a Power greater than ourselves could restore us to sanity.
3. Made a decision to turn over our will and our lives to the care of God as we understood Him.
4. Made a searching and fearless moral inventory of ourselves.
5. Admitted to God, to ourselves, and to another human being the exact nature of our wrongs.
6. We were entirely ready to have God remove all these defects of character.
7. Humbly asked Him to remove our shortcomings.
8. Made a list of all the persons we had harmed, and became willing to make amends to them all.
9. Made direct amends to such people wherever possible, except when to do so would injure them or others.
10. Continued to take a personal inventory, and when we were wrong promptly admitted it.
11. Sought through prayer and meditation to improve our conscious contact with God as we understood Him, praying only for knowledge of His will for us and the power to carry it out.
12. Having had a spiritual awakening as a result of these steps, we tried to carry this message to alcoholics, and to practise these principles in all our affairs.

Research has shown that people who are aware of potential relapse situations and use specific strategies can effectively reduce their risk of relapse (Kirby et al 1995, Litman 1980). Boredom and negative mood states are most likely to precipitate a relapse. Second comes social pressure and being offered, or talking about, drugs. Other risk factors beyond these include alcohol use, interpersonal conflict and environmental cues.

Environmental cues or triggers to relapse are important factors in prognosis, therefore these are given high significance in relapse prevention. Initial stages of relapse prevention focus on enabling the client to develop good awareness of internal and external triggers to craving. Methods used include diary keeping, where clients regularly chart substance use and the antecedent and consequent feelings, activity and location of use. Clients are encouraged to identify possible relapse triggers unique to themselves and work on these with the therapist. The therapist, either in a group setting or individually, can help the client to analyse these situations. The client will also be taught how to analyse situations for himself. Structured problem-solving techniques are used as well as role-play or rehearsal of relapse situations.

Specific cognitive techniques (Marlett & Gordon 2005, Wanigaratne et al 1990) used to assist the client in preventing relapse include:

- **seemingly irrelevant decisions (SIDs)**: this works on how to identify and prevent covert planning that may lead to relapse, such as *happening* to go into the local pub to buy cigarettes and eventually obtaining alcohol
- **urge surfing**: this is a technique for coping with craving. When craving is experienced, the client must allow the feeling to *wash over* and beyond him. Coping strategies, such as relaxation methods, distraction, biofeedback or other approaches, may assist this technique.

In addition to specific coping techniques RP stresses the importance of 'global lifestyle change'. It aims enable clients to:

- arrive at a balanced lifestyle
- learn effective time management (to fill up the vacuum left by giving up the substance use)

- discover and take up positive activities
- identify and change unhealthy habit patterns.

Therefore it can be seen that relapse prevention is an approach that fits well with occupational therapy, in particular because it focuses on lifestyle and real situations that cause relapse. Here, occupational performance areas, components and contexts are critical to treatment success. Developing psychological performance components, such as self-esteem and volition, for example, can help an individual cope with environmental triggers to relapse, also called environmental press (Kielhofner & Forsyth 1997).

OCCUPATIONAL THERAPY AND SUBSTANCE MISUSE

The earliest papers describing occupational therapy with alcoholics highlight areas for concern that are close to those identified by modern occupational therapists after research and the experience of time. For example, a Canadian occupational therapist, Hossack, writing in 1952, highlighted reduction in former interests and activities as well as social connections, difficulty concentrating, tension and family problems. She suggested that the alcoholic 'must look to a more fully rounded life with a balance of activity'. Doniger, in 1953, suggested unpredictability, elusiveness, relationships, leisure and motivation as areas for concern.

The issues raised by these two pioneers of occupational therapy in the field of addiction remain key throughout much of the subsequent occupational therapy literature.

Occupational therapy can have a significant impact in preparing a client for change and in changing from substance misuse to a more controlled or abstinent life. Substance dependence has an inherent occupational nature as illustrated by these diagnostic criteria for substance dependence:

> A great deal of time is spent in activities necessary to obtain the substance, use the substance or recover from its effects.

> Important social, occupational or recreational activities are given up or reduced because of substance abuse. (American Psychiatric Association 1994, p181)

For many clients with substance misuse problems, prior to treatment their lives have completely centred around their drug/alcohol use. After becoming abstinent or engaged in treatment, clients may experience a vacuum in their day-to-day lives which leaves them de-skilled, vulnerable and bored. Occupational therapy can help clients to develop skills and coping strategies, as well as a more satisfying, balanced lifestyle.

Some of the general issues occupational therapy can address are divided under the three occupational performance area headings of work, self-care and leisure. Intervention is usually via individual work and group work. It can involve both task-oriented and person-centred activities aimed at developing performance components in a range of contexts, for example learning to cope with anxietys without alcohol or saying 'no' if offered drugs. Group contexts and community locations can provide the chance for try-outs of performance components. Individual work can focus on enhancing very specific components through counselling and/or role-play.

LEISURE

Leisure is one of the key problem areas for substance misuse clients. This is principally because leisure activities and contexts are where alcohol and drugs are most commonly used. Negative mood states, such as boredom, and social pressure are the two most common factors in relapse. Many people who have become dependent on substances will know few or no other leisure activities apart from those that involve substance use.

The importance of leisure as an effective component of relapse prevention has been highlighted in a wide range of research literature (Bennett et al 1998, Burling et al 1992, Cheung et al 2003, Hodgson & Lloyd 2002, Mcauliffe 1990), including occupational therapy literature (Hodgson & Lloyd 2001). Leisure activities are particularly useful in reducing the frequency of negative thoughts and alcohol craving (Bennett et al 1998) as well as building self-confidence (Cheung et al 2003), therefore reducing the risk of relapse.

The use of physical activities in particular for a variety of therapeutic goals is described in research literature (Burling et al 1992, Donaghy & Mutrie 1999) and provides a small but promising evidence base. Ussher et al (2000) describe the development of a physical activity programme as part of an occupational therapy programme within a community alcohol service.

The goals of occupational therapy will focus on learning how to use leisure time and how to counteract negative mood states. During treatment, new or forgotten leisure activities can be tried out. Sport and fitness-related activities will raise self-esteem and confidence and counteract negative affect. Discovering or rediscovering leisure can help develop motivation to change and move clients round the process of change, in conjunction with other therapies.

Group work can be used to explore leisure-seeking and leisure replacement techniques and self-motivation. As part of a relapse prevention programme, rehearsal and role-play around leisure-based relapse situations can be useful. This can be linked to cue exposure therapy programmes, in which role-play is carried out in the environment where substances may have been used or obtained.

Leisure intervention may form an important part of family therapy, where family-oriented leisure has been involved with or affected by substance use. In the authors' clinical experience, activities that help a substance user to engage in adaptive interactions with family members are often highly successful. This is especially so where the client enjoys and can remember the activity and where it stimulates both client and relative. Examples include practising magic tricks (as described in the case vignette in Box 29.3), cooking group meals, learning day trip locations, swimming, playing racket sports, bowling and visiting theatres, cinema or art galleries. Activities that individuals can take up as a hobby and talk about with the family are effective. The impact of substance misuse on family is often highly significant.

Box 29.3 Case vignette (based on a case in a London alcohol unit)

Brian was a 32-year-old alcoholic man who had a history of verbal and sometimes physical violence towards his two young children. He valued his role as a father but felt he did not know what to talk to his children about.

Occupational therapy involved attendance at six weekly group sessions on magic tricks. After the third week his children visited him and he showed them one of the coin tricks he had learned. They were delighted and spent an hour talking to him about it and trying to learn what he could do.

He took magic up as a hobby and obtained the admiration of family and friends for his abilities. He remained sober for over a year.

WORK/PRODUCTIVITY

Work and productivity in substance misuse cover two distinct areas of discussion:

- drug use during everyday, legal employment
- drug use or dealing following similar patterns to paid work and providing similar rewards and meaning to life
- helping service users gain employment.

Work–based substance use

Where substances are used during a job, this can be very subtle and often either linked to peer pressure or for coping with work pressure. Substance use can be considered a part of work when the entertainment of business clients is part of the working day. Substances are often hidden at work and used covertly. Initial experiences of high achievement reinforce this pattern of substance use but errors of judgement usually ensue and crises occur. Jobs are often affected negatively or lost altogether once substance misuse patterns become established.

Other non-paid work, such as housekeeping and voluntary work, will exhibit similar features to the above.

Occupational therapy goals focus on helping a client cope with work without using the drug.

In addition, intervention aims to develop resistance to relapse triggers in work settings. Work may involve liaison with an employer to develop graded re-entry into work and to identify coping strategies and support strategies for both employer and employee. People who, owing to their substance use, have lost work or have been unable to hold down a job may need to start with low-pressure, voluntary work until they have developed the confidence, tolerance and skills to enter full-time employment.

Substance–based productivity

Where maintaining a drug habit becomes work, an individual's effort can be directed to obtaining a regular supply of the substance, selling the substance or engaging in regular criminal activity in order to fund the drug habit.

These three types of behaviour can follow patterns and display characteristics that are very similar to legal employment. A certain amount of a product will have to be obtained during the day. Where dealing is involved, this product will have to be sold to obtain money to either buy more or maintain a regular supply of drugs. In order to achieve this, and avoid arrest by the authorities or violence from peers, a considerable repertoire of specialised dealing, trading and bargaining habits can be developed. Alcoholics often describe a daily routine of waking, drinking, obtaining money, going to purchase alcohol and drinking it. When withdrawal occurs, more alcohol is purchased. This pattern can be as regular as the routines in a 9-to-5 office job.

Occupational therapy can focus on identifying habit-maintaining skills and transferring these to non-drug related activities, such as voluntary work, training or employment. Clients can be encouraged to enrol in training to develop business skills or apprenticeship-type work where a gradual skill transfer can occur. This type of intervention should ideally occur in conjunction with appropriate support. Alcoholics Anonymous and Narcotics Anonymous offer opportunities for members to engage in voluntary work to help run the organisation. This can work well, as support from peers with experience of abstinence is available.

Vocational Rehabilitation.

There is an increasing focus in treatment services on helping service users gain employment. This is part of a wider policy initiative aimed at reducing the number of people receiving benefits but also acknowledging the positive link between employment and recovery from substance dependence (NTA, 2006, McIntosh & McKeganey, 2000, Scottish Executive, 2000). Occupational therapists have a key role in enabling services work towards meaningful employment.

SELF-MAINTENANCE

Self-maintenance activities tend to decrease the more substances are used. The compulsion to use a drug eventually supersedes any awareness of nutrition, health, cleanliness, safety or responsibility for finances and daily life becomes chaotic.

Drug users, once abstinent or stabilised in treatment, often feel particularly de-skilled to cope with day-to-day household activities such as budgeting or basic time management.

EVALUATION OF OUTCOMES

Outcome measurement is possible through a wide range of occupational therapy-specific and other questionnaires or assessment tools. Some of these are described in the assessment section (above). Most of those described are used as before and after measures of blocks of intervention. Others can be used on a sessional basis, such as the General Health Questionnaire (Goldberg 1986).

In addition all drug services in England are implementing the Treatment Outcomes Profile or TOP. This is a outcome measure that has developed by the NTA that measures:

- Drug and alcohol use
- Physical and psychological health
- Social functioning
- Offending and criminal involvement.

SUMMARY

This chapter has focused on the range of issues presented by people who misuse substances and the intervention strategies open to them.

It is clear that there is considerable scope for occupational therapists to contribute to substance misuse treatment. Substance misuse occurs at the very centre of human occupation, in work, leisure and self-care, and it gradually takes over as the most central driver of occupational behaviour, changing and damaging performance components as it progresses.

Occupational therapy methods work well with the key clinical approaches already developed in the field of addiction. Furthermore, occupational therapists can learn and enhance practice through their work with the subtle and complex issues that clients in this field present.

Further research is recommended in this area, as is further education, especially as substance use exists within all areas of mental health practice and is more likely to increase than decrease in everyday practice.

References

Alcohol Concern 2007 Available online at: www. alcoholconcern.org.uk/servlets/doc/282

Allen SL 2001 The devils's cup – coffee's driving force in history. Ballantine Books, New York

American Occupational Therapy Association 1994 Uniform terminology for occupational therapy, 3rd edn. American Journal of Occupational Therapy 48(11): 1047-1054

American Psychiatric Association 1994 Diagnostic and statistical manual of mental disorders, 4th edn (DSMIV). American Psychiatric Association, Washington

Anderson P 1990 Management of drinking problems. WHO Regional Publications, European Series, No. 32. World Health Organization, Geneva

Bebbington PE 1976 The efficacy of Alcoholics Anonymous: the elusiveness of hard data. British Journal of Psychiatry 128: 572-580

Bennett LW, Cardone S, Jarczyk J 1998 Effects of a therapeutic camping program on addiction recovery: the Algonquin Relapse Prevention Program. Journal of Substance Abuse Treatment 15(5): 469-474

Berridge V 2005 Temperance: its history and impact on current and future alcohol policy. Joseph Rowntree Foundation, York

British Liver Trust 2007 Available online at: www. britishlivertrust.org.uk/content/diseases/hepatitis_c.asp

Buijsse N, Caan W, Davis SF 1999 Occupational therapy in the treatment of addictive behaviours. British Journal of Therapy Rehabilitation 6(6): 300-307

Busuttil J 1989 Setting up an occupational therapy programme for drug addicts. British Journal of Occupational Therapy 52(12): 476-479

Burling TA, Seidner AL, Robbins-Sisco D et al 1992 Batter up! Relapse prevention for homeless veteran substance abusers via softball team participation. Journal of Substance Abuse 4(4): 407-413

Cabinet Office 2004 Harm eduction strategy for England. Cabinet Office, London

Carroll M 1996 Relapse prevention as a psychosocial treatment: a review of controlled clinical trials. Experimental and Clinical Psychopharmacology 4(1): 46-54

Chacksfield JD 1994 Occupational therapy: the whole in one treatment for alcohol dependent clients. Paper presented at the World Federation of Occupational Therapists, 11th International Congress. Congress Summaries 3: 995-997

Chacksfield JD, Lindsay SJE 1999 The reduction of leisure in alcohol addiction. Paper presented at College of Occupational Therapists Conference.

Cheung C, Lee T, Lee C 2003 Factors in successful relapse prevention among Hong Kong drug addicts. Journal of Offender Rehabilitation, Special Issue: Treating substance abusers in correctional contexts: New understandings, new modalities 37(2–4): 179-199

Department of Health 1996 The task force to review services for drug misusers: report of an independent review of drug treatment services in England. Department of Health, London

Department of Health 2002 Mental health policy implementation guide: dual diagnosis good practice guide. Department of Health, London

Department of Health, Scottish Office Department of Health, Welsh Office, Department of Health and Social Security in Northern Ireland 1999 Drug misuse and dependence: guidelines on clinical management. Stationery Office, London

Donaghy ME, Mutrie N 1999 Is exercise beneficial in the treatment and rehabilitation of the problem drinker? A critical review. Physical Therapy Reviews 4: 153-166

Doniger J 1953 An activity program with alcoholics. American Journal of Occupational Therapy 7(3): 110-112, 135

Drugscope 2007 Available online at: www.drugscope. org.uk/druginfo/drugsearch/ds_results.asp?file=\ wip\11\1\1\heroin_opiates.html

Drummond DC 1990 The relationship between alcohol dependence and alcohol-related problems in a clinical population. British Journal of Addiction 85: 357-366

Drummond DC 1992 Problems and dependence: chalk and cheese or bread and butter? In: Lader M, Edwards G, Drummond C (eds) The nature of alcohol and drug related problems. Oxford University Press, Oxford, pp61-82

Drummond DC, Tiffany ST, Glautier S et al 1995 Addictive behavior: cue exposure, theory and practice. Wiley, New York

Duke PJ, Pantelis C, Barnes TRE 1994 South Westminster schizophrenia survey. British Journal of Psychiatry 164: 630-636

Edwards G 1987 The treatment of drinking problems. Blackwell Scientific, Oxford

Edwards G (ed) 2002 Addiction: evolution of a specialist field. Blackwell Science, Oxford

Edwards G, Gross MM 1976 Alcohol dependence: provisional description of a clinical syndrome. BMJ 1: 1058-1061

Edwards G, Arif A, Hodgson R 1981 Nomenclature and classification of drug-and alcohol-related problems: a WHO memorandum. Bulletin of the World Health Organization 59: 225-242

Forshaw DM, Strang J 1993 Drug, aggression and violence. In: Taylor PJ (ed) Violence in society. Royal College of Physicians, London.

Forsyth K, Deshpande S, Kielhofner G et al 2005 The Occupational Circumstances Assessment Interview and Rating Scale (OCAIRS) Version 4.0. University of Illinois at Chicago

Ghodse H 2002 Drugs and addictive behaviour – a guide to treatment. Cambridge University Press, Cambridge

Goldberg D 1986 Use of the general health questionnaire in clinical work. BMJ 293(6556): 1188-1189

Gossop M 1990 The development of the short opiate withdrawal scale (SOWS). Addictive Behaviours 15: 487-490

Gossop M 1994a Drug and alcohol problems: investigation. In: Lindsay SJE, Powell GE (eds) The handbook of clinical adult psychology, 2nd edn. Routledge. London

Gossop M 1994 Drug and alcohol problems: treatment. In: Lindsay SJE, Powell GE (eds) The handbook of clinical adult psychology, 2nd edn. Routledge, London

Gossop M 2000 Living with drugs, 5th edn. Ashgate, Aldershot

Gossop M, Darke S, Griffith P et al 1995 The Severity of Dependence Scale (SDS): psychometric properties of the SDS in English and Australian samples of heroin, cocaine and amphetamine users. Addiction 90(5): 607-614

Gossop M, Marsden J, Stewart D et al 2003 The National Treatment Outcome Research Study (NTORS): 4-5 year follow-up results. Addiction 98(3): 291-303

Heather N, Gold R, Rollnick S 1991 Readiness to change questionnaire: user's manual. Technical Report 15. National Drug and Alcohol Research Centre, University of New South Wales, Kensington, Australia

Henman A 1985 Cocaine futures. In: Henman A, Lewis R, Malyon T (eds) Big deal: the politics of the illicit drugs business. Pluto Press, London

HMSO 1979 Misuse of Drugs Act. HMSO, London

HMSO 1998 Tackling drugs to build a better Britain. HMSO, London

Hodgson S, Lloyd C 2001 The leisure participation of clients with a dual diagnosis. British Journal of Occupational Therapy 64(10): 487-452

Hodgson S, Lloyd C 2002 Leisure as a relapse prevention strategy. British Journal of Therapy and Rehabilitation 9(3): 88-91

Home Office 2002a Tackling crack – a national plan. Stationery Office, London

Home Office 2002b Updated drugs strategy 2002. Tackling drugs. Stationery Office, London

Hossack JR 1952 Clinical trial of occupational therapy in the treatment of alcohol addiction. American Journal of Occupational Therapy 6(6): 265-282

Hunt WA, Barnett LW, Branch LG 1971 Relapse rates in addiction programs. Journal of Clinical Psychology 27(4): 455-456

Irvin JE, Bowers CA, Dunn ME et al 1999 Efficency of relapse prevention: a meta-analytic review. Journal of Consulting and Clinical Psychology 67(4): 563-570

Kielhofner G 2002 A model of human occupation: theory and application, 3rd edn. Williams and Wilkins, Baltimore

Kirby KC, Lamb RJ, Iguchi MY et al 1995 Situations occasioning cocaine use and cocaine abstinence strategies. Addiction 90(9): 1241-1252

Lindsay WP 1983 The role of the occupational therapist in the treatment of alcoholism. American Journal of Occupational Therapy 37(1): 36-40

Litman G 1980 Relapse in alcoholism. In: Edwards G, Grant M (eds) Alcoholism treatment in transition. Croom Helm, London

Mann WC, Talty P 1990 Leisure activity profile: measuring use of leisure time by persons with alcoholism. Occupational Therapy and Mental Health 10(4): 31-41

Marlatt GA, Gordon JR 2005 Relapse prevention: maintenance strategies in the treatment of addictive behaviors, 2nd edn. Guilford Press, New York

Marsden J, Farrell M, Bradbury C et al 2007 The Treatment Outcomes Profile (Top): A Structured interview for the evaluation of substance misuse treatment. National Treatment Agency for Substance Misuse, Londan

Mayfield D, McLeod G, Hall P et al 1974 The CAGE questionnaire: validation of a new alcoholism screening instrument. American Journal of Psychiatry 131: 1121-1123

Mcauliffe WE 1990 A randomised controlled trial of recovery training and self-help for opioid addicts in New England and Hong Kong. Journal of Psychoactive Drugs 22(2): 197-209

McIntosh J, McKeganey 2000 The recovery from dependent drug use: addicts' strategies for reducing the risk of relapse. Drugs: eduction, prevention and policy. Vol 7 No 2, pp 179-192

Milkman H, Weiner SE, Sunderwirth S 1984 Addiction relapse. Advances in Alcohol and Substance Abuse 3(12): 119-134

Morgan CA 1994 Illicit drug use: primary prevention. British Journal of Occupational Therapy 57(1): 2-4

Musto DF 1993 The rise and fall of epidemics: learning from history. Edwards G, Strang J, Jaffe J (eds) Drugs, alcohol and tobacco: making the science and policy connections. Oxford Medical Publications, Oxford

National Assembly for Wales 2000 Tackling substance
misuse in Wales: a partnership approach. National
Assembly for Wales, Cardiff

Nicol M 1989 Substance misuse – who cares? British Journal
of Occupational Therapy 52(1): 18-20

Nunn JF 1996 Ancient Egyptian medicine. British Museum
Press, London

NTA 2002 Models of care for the treatment of drug misusers
– promoting quality, efficiency and effectiveness in
drug misuse treatment services in England. Part 2: Full
reference report. Department of Health, London

NTA 2004 Research into practice no. 5 – engaging and
retaining clients in drug treatment. Department of
Health, London

NTA (2006) Models of care for treatment of adult drug
misusers: Update 2006. NTA, London

Pokorny AD, Miller BA, Kaplan HB et al 1972 The brief
MAST: a shortened version of the Michigan Alcoholism
Screening Test. American Journal of Psychiatry 129: 342-
345

Prochaska JO, DiClemente CC 1982 Transtheoretical
therapy: towards a more integrative model of change.
Psychotherapy Theory, Research and Practice 19:
276-278

Prochaska JO, DiClemente CC 1986 Towards a
comprehensive model of change. In: Miller RJ, Heather
N (eds) Treating addictive behaviours: processes of
change. Plenum, London

Prochaska JO, DiClemente CC, Norcross JC 1992 In search of
how people change: applications to addictive behaviors.
American Psychologist 47(9): 1102-1114

Project MATCH Research Group 1993 Project MATCH:
rationale and methods for a multisite clinical trial
matching patients to alcoholism treatment. Alcoholism:
Clinical and Experimental Research 17: 1130-1145

Rotert D 1990 Occupational therapy and alcoholism. Journal
of Occupational Medicine 4(2): 327-337

Royal College of Psychiatrists 1987 Drug scenes: a report
on drugs and drug dependence by the Royal College of
Psychiatrists. Gaskell, London

Scaffa ME 1991 Alcoholism: an occupational behaviour
perspective. Occupational Therapy in Mental Health
11(2/3): 99-111

Scottish Executive 2001 Moving On: Education, training
and employment for recovering drug users. Effective
Interventions Unit, Edinburgh

Scottish Office 1999 Tackling drugs in Scotland: action in
partnership. Scottish Office, Edinburgh

Simpson DD, Joe GW, Brown BS 1997 Treatment retention
and follow-up outcomes in the Drug Abuse Treatment
Outcome Study (DATOS). Psychology of Addictive
Behaviour 11: 239-260

Stellar JR, Rice MB 1987 Pharmacological basis of
intracranial self-stimulation reward. In: Royal College
of Psychiatrists (eds) Drug scenes: a report on drugs and
drug dependence by the Royal College of Psychiatrists.
Gaskell, London

Stephens R, Cottrell E 1972 A follow-up study of 200
narcotic addicts committed for treatment under the
narcotic addict rehabilitation act (NARA). British Journal
of Addiction 67(1): 45-53

Stockwell T, Hodgson R, Edwards G et al 1979 The
development of a questionnaire to measure severity of
alcohol dependence. British Journal of Addiction 74: 79-
87

Stoffel VC, Cusatis M, Seitz L et al 1992 Self-esteem and
leisure patterns of persons in a residential chemical
dependency treatment program. Occupational Therapy
in Health Care 8(2/3): 69-85

Strategy Unit 2003 Alcohol Harm Reduction Project: interim
analytical report. Cabinet Office, London

Strategy Unit 2004 Alcohol harm reduction strategy for
England. Cabinet Office, London

Swanson JW, Holzer CE, Ganju VK et al 1990 Violence and
psychiatric disorder in the community: evidence from
the epidemiological catchment area surveys. Hospital
and Community Psychiatry 41(7): 761-770

Tyler S 1995 Street drugs. Hodder and Stoughton, London

Ussher M, McCusker M, Morrow V et al 2000 A physical
activity intervention in a community alcohol service.
British Journal of Occupational Therapy 63: 219-231

Viik MK, Watts JH, Madigan MJ et al 1990 Preliminary
validation of the assessment of occupational functioning
with an alcoholic population. Occupational Therapy in
Mental Health 10(2): 19-33

Wanigaratne S, Pullin J, Wallace W et al 1990 Relapse
prevention for addictive behaviours – a manual for
therapists. Blackwell, London

Wickler A 1948 Recent progress in research on the
neurophysiologic basis of morphine addiction. American
Journal of Psychiatry 105: 329-338

Useful Contacts

**College of Occupational Therapists, Specialist Section
– Mental Health** Website: www.cot.org.uk/

Drugscope Tel: 0207 928 1211 Website: www.drugscope.org.
uk Provides information on drugs and drug misuse.

Alcohol Concern Tel: 0207 928 7377 Website: www.
alcoholconcern.org.uk Alcohol Concern is a national
alcohol misuse agency.

Drinkline 0800 917 8282

Alcoholics Anonymous (AA) Tel: 0207 352 3001 Website:
www.alcoholics-anonymous.org.uk

Alcohol Harm Reduction Strategy Website: www.strategy.
gov.uk/workareas/alcohol_misuse

National Treatment Agency Website: www.nta.nhs.uk/

Narcotics Anonymous (NA) Tel: 0207 730 0009 Helpline:
0207 251 4007 Website: www.ukna.org/

National Drugs Helpline 0800 776600 Website: www.
talktofrank.com

Chapter 30

Working with people on the margins

Nick Pollard, Frank Kronenberg

INTRODUCTION

Occupational therapists profess to work with all people who can benefit from their expertise, without discrimination against anybody on the basis of culture, religious beliefs, lifestyle or other characteristics (Creek 2003). However, in practice, the majority of occupational therapists work with people who are referred by physicians or with those people who can pay for our services. In other words, there seems to be a discrepancy between who we say we are (our rhetoric of change) and what we do (our practice of change) in the world. Should occupational therapists deal simply with the problems at hand, or is our role also to question the conditions that produce disability and deprivation?

When occupational therapists are asked to devise activities to meet problems such as limited attention span, lack of social opportunity, institutionalisation or its threat, restricted opportunities for expression or disempowerment, they are confronting restriction of occupations and experiences of marginalisation. These experiences have been called occupational apartheid (Kronenberg & Pollard 2005a), occupational injustice (Townsend & Wilcock 2004) and occupational deprivation (Whiteford 2000, Wilcock 1998).

TERMINOLOGY OF MARGINALISATION

Occupational apartheid is the segregation of groups of people through restriction or denial of access to dignified and meaningful participation in the occupations of daily life on the basis of race, colour, disability, national origin, age, gender, sexual preference, religion, political beliefs, status in society or other characteristics (Kronenberg & Pollard 2005a). The product of political forces, its systematic and pervasive social, cultural and economic consequences jeopardise the health and well-being of individuals, communities and whole societies. The term is intended to confront the production of stigma and marginalisation, for example, surrounding the experience of mental illness (MIND 2004).

Occupational injustice arises from the natural tendency of people to answer their needs through occupation. In the pursuit of their own interests, people begin actions which result in injustice for others by depriving them of occupational resources or means; for example, the colonisation and cultivation of land by one group of people may interrupt traditional access to naturally occurring food sources for other groups living in the same area.

Occupational deprivation occurs where people are unable to take part in meaningful occupations; that is, to do things which answer their needs and interests, due to factors that are outside their control. For example, someone who is confined in a prison may experience occupational deprivation if the regime does not allow access to activities and exercise.

When occupational apartheid, injustice and deprivation occur, there is usually a lack of awareness and knowledge about the needs of the people who experience these problems. Occupational therapists negotiate with people about how they wish to reaffirm their cultural identity, represent their realities to others and develop their own

structures and systems, and when they do so the line between personal and political development is crossed (Fransen 2005, Galheigo 2005, Kronenberg & Pollard 2005b, 2006). Occupational therapists engage with marginalised people to make connections with the community at large, and have the potential to benefit the wider society as well as helping the individual. By providing concrete examples of good practice, occupational therapists can demonstrate to policy makers that people need occupation. By proving the value of their input to the communities with which they are working, occupational therapists pave the way for participation in further developments (Letts 2003).

A WIDER ROLE FOR OCCUPATIONAL THERAPY

In many countries, the agenda of how and for whom occupational therapy is to build its future has been both facilitated and, increasingly, limited by established systems, structures and practices. However, this conservatism is being challenged by new ideas and innovative practices that are described in recent books from South Africa (Watson & Swartz 2004), Australia/New Zealand (Whiteford & Wright St Clair 2005) and Europe (Kronenberg et al 2005a). These publications advocate a re-examining of occupational therapy to recognise a broader, global and social responsibility and acknowledge a need for the profession to address inequality and poverty. Enabled by developing theories, which address occupational injustice and deprivation, occupational therapy practitioners, educators, researchers, students and the people they work with are coming to understand and face up to the political nature and potential of the profession (Kronenberg & Pollard 2005a, 2006).

Tackling the problems arising from the social, political, economic and environmental contexts in which occupational therapists work requires an approach that builds the future with people rather than for them (Kronenberg & Pollard 2005a, b).

Because occupational therapy deals with how people function in their environment and community, it strives to take a more comprehensive, holistic approach. Rather than emphasising biomedical intervention, it focuses on underlying social and community concerns, at least in theory. In practice, however, the occupational therapy profession too often falls short of its more holistic, egalitarian goals. And, as with the other health professions, the poorest and neediest often fall between the cracks (Werner 2005).

A key to widespread improvement in health is strong political commitment to equity in meeting all people's basic needs (Kronenberg & Pollard 2006, World Federation of Occupational Therapists 2006, World Health Organization 1978, 2001). Occupational therapists are developing a critical awareness and understanding about this reality (Kronenberg & Pollard 2006, Letts 2003), but recognition of inequalities in access to occupation is in its infancy. Research and literature on the political nature of occupational therapy are very limited; until recently occupational therapy seems to have been perceived as an apolitical profession by its practitioners (Kronenberg 2003, Kronenberg & Pollard 2005a, 2006).

Sinclair (2005, pxiv) argued that:

> Occupational therapists must develop their roles as agents of social change, taking the profession to a new level that makes a difference to entire communities as well as to the individuals we treat and encourage. To enable them to become effective agents of change, the way in which occupational therapists are educated must come under sweeping review. The future trend in professional education must include a strong component on enablement, advocacy and social reform.

Sinclair is one of an increasing number of occupational therapists who are arguing for activities to be developed in surroundings other than health and social care settings (Creek 2003, Fransen 2005, Galheigo 2005, Rebeiro et al 2001, Ryan & Pollard 2002). In some situations, practitioners are obliged to go into the community to find and engage with their clients (Duncan & Swartz 2004, Kronenberg 2005, Letts 2003, Pollard et al 2005, Thibeault 2002). For example, many mental health services have developed teams that are proactive in maintaining links with those people who, because of their mental health problems, require regular contact and follow-up when they do not attend sessions or miss appointments (Burns & Firn 2002, Stein & Santos 1998).

This chapter will describe the process of marginalisation and how this applies to people with mental health problems, those living in poverty and asylum seekers. It will then examine the broadly political aspect of occupation, introducing the political reasoning tool. The implications of this discussion for the work of occupational therapists and those they work with will be explored through a series of real case examples. These have been developed and worked through for this chapter in co-operation with participants in the cases. Particular emphasis is given to ways in which occupational therapists can work co-operatively and participatively with communities, especially in negotiating practice with local populations according to their needs. Community-based rehabilitation is offered as a means of realising these objectives and attending to global responsibilities. Finally, there is a review of the implications of this approach for practitioners, offering a new vision of a profession without borders.

MARGINALISATION

Care in the community is not a new concept, although an effective community care policy has proved difficult to achieve (Parry Jones 1981, Warner 1994). Care in the community offers the appearance of being fiscally popular, particularly in the era of closing hospitals and selling off the land for redevelopment but, in the UK, its implementation may even be in retreat (MIND 2004). As far back as the mid-19th century, the experimental lodging of small concentrations of people with mental health problems amongst the wider populace was thought to be detrimental to local residents' property values, while lunacy commissioners thought the seemingly cost-effective practice of placing mentally ill people as lodgers in Highland crofts would be difficult to monitor and, consequently, prone to abuse (Parry Jones 1981).

Thus, economic factors are closely linked to quality of care. Warner (1994) explored the relationship between the performance of economies, the growth of industrialisation and levels of unemployment in relation to care provision for mental health. Generally he found that mental health deteriorates with decreasing prosperity because less money is spent on care in a declining economy. The growth of industrial society during the 19th century exposed many more people to poverty as the boom and bust economic swings of industrial capitalism reduced the value of wages or made large numbers unemployed.

Poverty is well established as a factor that increases the risk of premature death from numerous causes, including poor diet, poor housing and increased exposure to a risk of violence. People living in impoverished environments are more likely to experience a range of socially disruptive life events, including more exposure to crime and accident, which are causes and the consequences of stress, depression and addictive behaviours. Poverty and disability are inextricably linked and, for large sections of the world's population, disaster, war, trauma and chronic deprivation have an enduring and intergenerational detrimental effect upon mental health.

In the global community, extremes of poverty can be found in every society. The effects of policy or corporate decisions in one part of the world can quickly determine living conditions and impose occupational injustices thousands of miles away. For example, company decisions to relocate can have significant effects on those communities which depend on a local industry. Often, problems that affect individuals cannot be separated from those prevailing in surrounding social, economic, political and spiritual conditions, in which participation in a normal range of occupations is denied.

Those marginalised groups who may be experiencing occupational apartheid within a community include people with mental health problems, those with learning disabilities, people living in poverty and asylum seekers. All these groups may be afraid of drawing attention to themselves from other members of the community who will exploit or oppress them because of their difference or vulnerability. For example, many people in receipt of disability benefits for mental illness will potentially have more cash in their possession than other people receiving jobseekers' allowances. In areas of chronic poverty, where alternative economies have developed around criminal activities, people with mental health problems or learning difficulties are sometimes targeted as a source of cash, or as people who will be less likely to complain if their homes are used as places for drug dealing.

MENTAL ILLNESS

A key problem in the development of suitable approaches to working with people with severe and enduring mental ill health lies in the tendency for mental illnesses to be reduced to diseases with medical solutions, an approach that belies the complexity of the interrelationship between illness and social factors, such as poverty and urban living. The problems experienced by people with schizophrenia, for example, are more to do with the symptoms and the way they affect an individual's functioning than with the illness itself (Thomas 1997).

People with schizophrenia may find that they cannot make effective occupational choices and cannot access services or do not know how to because, for example, social skills and educational attainments at key points of their development have been compromised by the onset of psychosis. They are likely to experience reduced functioning and tend to find themselves living in poor housing because they are unable to retain jobs or maintain the social attributes which will preserve their starting position in society. Thomas (1997) suggested that the relatively high numbers of people with schizophrenia in urban areas may be due to a downward social drift. People with more wealth and earning power have moved to the suburbs and the poorer social groups have moved into the town centres.

Poor physical and social environments can have an adverse effect on mental health (MIND 2004, Warner 1994) and additional stresses arise from living in poor housing or in situations which are lacking in amenities. The social environment can be affected by a concentration of people with social difficulties arising from poverty, high levels of drug dependency and related crime. However, although there is documentation of higher rates of alcohol and drug abuse amongst some groups of people with schizophrenia, many abuse alcohol and drugs less than the norm because they are less sociable and, hence, less subject to social pressure (Burns & Firn 2002).

It is difficult to draw clear conclusions about the occupational behaviours of people with long-term, severe mental illness because of a lack of social information concerning the lives of these people as a group (Christiansen et al 1999). The absence of, or potentially confusing information about, the needs of people with such illnesses reinforces the need to respond to people as individuals.

POVERTY

An individual needs money to be a person in this world: 'If you don't have money you don't exist' (Mohammed Yunus, quoted by Robertson 2001). Access to many occupations is dependent on income and there is a pattern of social exclusion which stems from the high degree of financial insecurity amongst people with mental health problems (Bradshaw et al 2004). Of all disabled groups, those with mental health problems are the least likely to be in employment: in the UK, only 21% are employed compared to a national employment rate of 74.7% amongst people of working age (National Statistics 2004). Twelve percent of these people are concerned about the security of their housing. Despite these problems, fewer adults with mental illness access services such as banking. Many of them will be considered a financial risk by insurance companies and so cannot obtain loans, life insurance or other means of achieving financial security.

Lack of money is just as important a factor in social exclusion, and a contributor to occupational apartheid and deprivation, in a wealthy society as it is in a poor one, and potentially more so. In a wealthy society, there are many more institutions and services which cost money and without which individuals cannot do other things. For example, not having a bank account makes it difficult either to save or access money safely. A bank account is one source of identity, required in order to receive benefits or wages. However, without a permanent address an individual cannot open a bank account and is therefore denied access to many of the things needed to survive as a citizen. A permanent address has to be rented or bought, requiring access to sufficient money or social security benefits. Having a place to live brings a whole range of taxations and charges for services, which must be maintained,

and ignoring a few reminder letters may lead to eviction. Some people are quite socially skilled and yet unable to deal with the paperwork involved in personal finance issues.

The globalisation of poverty and limitations of occupational opportunity go hand in hand with the effects of public service cutbacks to produce social, political and economic marginalisation (Boyce & Lysack 1997).

ASYLUM SEEKERS

In the rapidly developing social contexts of Britain's communities, new groups of people are finding it difficult to engage with the society around them. For example, due to war, disaster and oppression elsewhere in the world, numbers of people are arriving who, unlike more established groups of migrants, do not have bridgehead communities to offer them support in finding work and accommodation (Katz 1958).

The situations from which they have come have often lacked facilities or services, due to poverty or through the destruction brought about by conflict. These asylum seekers may well have experienced multiple traumatic events, both prior to leaving their original homes and in making their way to their host countries. On arrival, as their entry is being approved and processed, they may experience occupational deprivation as they are between communities and held in a compound or other temporary housing (OOFRAS 2006).

Often, asylum seekers are unable to continue with many of the roles they held previously. Adolescents become bored and depressed and women are unable to perform the activities through which they hitherto maintained relationships within their families, because the institutional environment prevents this (Wilson 2004). Once they have been placed in housing in host communities, asylum seekers may find themselves culturally and socially isolated and experience the disenfranchisement that occurs when people are struggling to acquire the language skills and cultural competencies to access their rights in the host society (Centre for Economic Policy Research 2001, OOFRAS 2006). They may encounter hostility promoted by the media, including the popular misconception that housing is not being as swiftly allocated to local people (Sriskandarajah 2004). These circumstances can quickly degenerate into situations of occupational apartheid, in which occupational opportunities are restricted or denied by the fact of living in social isolation.

Furthermore, these circumstances compound any traumas which remain unaddressed (Searle 1997). For example, children who shortly beforehand may have experienced torture or witnessed murder and rape have to fit into a school life and a new culture alongside children who cannot imagine such events. People have to adjust to a society where domestic security measures are against antisocial neighbours who have marked you out as a vulnerable target, rather than against a wider conflict in which your neighbours share the hardships.

ACTIVITIES WITHOUT SOCIAL OR ECONOMIC VALUE

The experience of restriction or denial of access to chosen activities is often felt by people to deprive their life of aspects of its meaning. For example, if a person has no time for leisure or social activities, she may feel that she is working merely to exist and some of the meaningfulness of life is lost to her. In *The Informed Heart* (1970), Bruno Bettelheim explained how the systematic enforcement of petty rituals for almost every action was combined with intensification of labour in the Nazi concentration camps at Dachau and Buchenwald. This made life unbearable to the point that many inmates lost the will to live.

The term *occupational absurdity* is used to describe situations in which people are expected to produce articles that are clearly not needed, simply for the purpose of having something to do (Kronenberg & Pollard 2005a). Bettelheim (1970) gave several examples of nonsensical labour, such as downing shovels to fill a barrow with sand by hand, performed simply at the whim of prison guards, for the purpose of deliberate humiliation. This might include people knitting squares in an old asylum occupational therapy department, while in the same room other people unpick them. It might mean overproducing goods, which have to be dumped on the market, or increasing productivity to an extent that overworks people so that the quality of what they produce is poor. Overwork

can lead to taking time out due to illness and, hence, to an inability to enjoy leisure time.

A POLITICAL ROLE FOR OCCUPATIONAL THERAPY

Aristotle (1962) thought that human beings are naturally political animals. Cardona (2001) described politics as 'the people's capacity and power to construct their own destiny'. Politics can, therefore, be seen as an occupation and all occupations can be seen to have a political aspect. Each of the above examples of marginalised groups shows a conflict and co-operation situation (Kronenberg & Pollard 2005a). According to the Dutch political scientist van der Eijk (2001), this dialectic tension between conflict and co-operation 'is the motor of all political engagement'.

Van der Eijk (2001) claimed that it is impossible to pose and maintain a single definition of politics because the word belongs in the category of controversial terms, as does the term *occupation*, the core construct of occupational therapy. According to van der Eijk, descriptions of the concept of *politics* can be classified into two main types:

- the broad aspect approach, which views politics (with a small p) as an aspect of human occupation and human relationships that can be found everywhere
- the domain approach, which views Politics (with a large P) as a particular, defined sphere of human relationships, indicated by such terms as the state, government, public administration or a political party.

Recognising the political in our personal lives is not always easy, but civilised society depends on its members taking an active political interest (Aristotle 1962). The Brazilian educationalist Paulo Freire (1972) maintained that a prerequisite of democracy is a critical literacy, a level of awareness he called *conscientisation*, which is essential to the communication of ideas and action that underpins effective co-operation.

Occupational therapy students can be taught to appreciate the motives of policy, power and governance that inform medical and social approaches to health and disability, and to adjust their practice orientations accordingly (Hocking & Ness 2002, Kronenberg 2004 unpublished lecture). Political literacy provides the health professional with a frame of reference for understanding and responding to the organisational processes affecting authority, status and organised forms of society (Kronenberg 2004, unpublished lecture).

Politics is concerned with:

- conflicts between groups of people
- the development of conflict
- the development of co-operative strategies to influence the outcome of conflict in one or other group's desired direction, and
- the resolution of conflict (van der Eijk 2001).

Conflict and co-operation are characteristics of the political interactions that occur everywhere, in all sorts of situations and relationships. These terms do not mean that conflict is bad or that co-operation is good, but rather refer to the aims and actions of individuals and groups.

Conflict occurs when individuals or groups work against each other to realise their own goals and interests, when these are mutually incompatible. Conflict is inevitable and often cannot be fully resolved. Co-operation can be viewed as the reverse of conflict, and it can also be viewed as inevitable. Reaching solutions for society as a whole requires co-operation.

Bettelheim (1970) explored several situations where, by setting different groups of prisoners and even individuals against each other, the Nazi concentration camp regime was able to prevent sufficient co-operation occurring to threaten their power. By the promotion of conflict between groups, individual prisoners were so concerned by the continual threat to their own existence that they battled for survival against fellow inmates and were prevented from working together against their oppressors.

The next section describes a tool that can be used for analysing the political nature of any conflict and co-operation situation.

A POLITICAL REASONING TOOL (KRONENBERG & POLLARD 2006)

This political reasoning tool has been designed to help the therapist to understand the political nature of occupation (Kronenberg & Pollard 2005a). This was originally termed the 'political activities of daily living (pADL) framework' but has been renamed because practitioner feedback suggested that the title was confusing. The six questions in the tool are interrelated and interdependent, meaning that the answer to one question will have implications for the other questions.

- What are the characteristics of the conflict and co-operation situation?
- Who are the actors? (who are the people and organisations or groups?)
- How do actors conduct themselves? What are their aims, motives, interests, perceptions and attitudes?
- What are their means?
- What does the political landscape look like?
- What is the broader context for conflict and co-operation?

What are the characteristics of the conflict and co-operation situation?

Bettelheim's (1970) account of his experiences in concentration camps is particularly concerned with aspects of human behaviour he witnessed, the means by which people organised their survival and the principles which appeared to govern these situations.

Bettelheim described the context for conflict and co-operation as one in which the Gestapo and the SS, the German forces who ran the camps, systematically employed every means to break the human spirit of the prisoners. The concentration camps were initially for the internment of people from races the Nazis wanted to eliminate, such as Jews, Slavs and Poles, religious minorities such as Jehovah's Witnesses, homosexuals, people with mental illnesses, political opponents and a range of people who had been caught up in the repression, as well as criminals. All these people, prison guards and prisoners, were the actors, whose motives were taken up with either breaking the human will or surviving.

Those prisoners who succumbed to the pressures of hard labour and terrible conditions died, having lost the will or even the ability to live. Some people survived while they believed that there was hope of getting out of prison or the regime changing, but when that hope was lost they died. Those who survived did so by maintaining themselves through the means of preserving some aspect of their occupational being, maintaining an activity – which in Bettelheim's case was making a study of the behaviour of his fellow prisoners. One of the stories he tells is of a group of Jewish bricklayers who recognised that their skills were in short supply and so co-operated to work together as a skilled team at the camp. They took a professional pride in their work but continued to hate the inhumanities of the regime which imprisoned them and with which they were in conflict. However, their survival depended on their co-operation with the actors to whom they were opposed and who appeared to have control of the political landscape. As a consequence, most of the bricklayers survived through the war to be liberated, when most of the other Jewish prisoners had been killed.

Case example 1: People Relying On People

People Relying On People (PROP) is a group of people with early onset of dementia who have been involved in developing a service to meet their own needs, beginning with meetings in local pubs in Doncaster. These younger people with dementia, and their carers, found that they needed an informal and inclusive environment which would be a place to meet and a resource centre as well as providing a base. After successful lobbying of the local authority and health trust, a house in the grounds of a hospital was leased to the group.

The group conducts most of its meetings informally, on the pattern of a social gathering or house party, at a pace which allows everyone in the group to participate at their own level. The domestic environment is suited to the requirements of people who want to carry out activities such as baking or gardening, which they are not able do at home due to carers' fears they may be at risk.

Members of PROP, both service users and carers, felt that they had lost confidence, social skills and even the art of conversation through their experiences of dementia and dementia services. Involving them in decision making about the local young people with dementia service enabled the group to move from being a social support network into advocates for themselves, using their disability as

a lever to open doors by illustrating their problems. One of the group gives a powerful presentation to potential funders, in which he pulls items such as a calculator, diary, toy car and mobile phone out of an executive briefcase, showing the functions that people with dementia have lost. Members of PROP confront the issue of alienating and disabling professional jargon by demanding explanations which they can understand (Chaston et al 2004, Jubb et al 2003).

Members of the group have also developed a robust sense of humour. Just as in a prisoner of war film, an escape committee revises the answers for mini-mental state examinations to avoid the stress and anxiety of the regular tests that may mean an individual being moved into care. Members are reminded to maintain functioning by such maxims as 'use it or lose it'. Funders have been told, when querying an application, 'we can't remember applying for it last year, we've got dementia' (Jubb 2004, personal communication).

Situations of conflict, based in exclusion, can be met through co-operation with actors who are often part of the apparatus that has been partly responsible for that exclusion and marginalisation, such as health-care institutions. For example, the People Relying On People, in case example 1, co-operated to form an 'escape committee', which enables the group to reduce their anxiety about the mini-mental state examination test. This co-operation arises from the conflict between the interests of a care regime providing institutional care and the individuals' fear of losing their independence and personal identity. Although staff working with the PROP group represent the care system, they recognise the value of the escape committee in promoting and maintaining independence through encouraging members to feel confident in their abilities.

Who are the actors?

The political reasoning tool is concerned not so much with actors as with the co-operation or conflicts that develop between them. The question could be reworded as 'Who is the ally, partner or opponent of whom?'. This recognises that actors may co-operate in some areas and come into conflict in others. Allies or partners do not agree about everything but will be on the same side in some conflicts, to their mutual benefit.

Relationships between actors can become a source of power and influence through co-operation in conflict situations (Kronenberg & Pollard 2005a). In case example 2, a group of people with learning difficulties and the volunteers and support workers working with them developed a writing activity into a powerful means for expressing individual needs through group action. The co-operation they have built up with each other in order to produce a publication and to arrange launch events to publicise it has given the group a positive local profile against a context of poor funding. Rather than enter into conflict with the local authority, the group has used its co-operative abilities to work with the local council and generate good news stories about itself and its achievements. The group and those working with it have enabled the project to continue because the positive profile it has gained has been a means for power and influence.

Case example 2: Voices Talk and Hands Write

A community publishing organisation, the Federation of Worker Writers and Community Publishers (FWWCP), began working with a group of people with learning difficulties in a day centre in Grimsby, with input from an adult learning educator and an occupational therapist (Pollard et al 2004). Many of the group were socially isolated and found it difficult to do the things that they would really like to do.

Over a 3-month period of weekly meetings, the group began writing creatively, supported by a number of support workers and volunteers from community publishing groups, including two from a local writers' workshop. The group, which became Voices Talk and Hands Write (VTHW), produced a community publication of their work (Voices Talk and Hands Write 2004) that was given a civic launch at the town hall. They also gave public performances of their work and, when input from the FWWCP ended, continued to meet with the local volunteers and support workers. During this time they made their own decisions about their progress, such as choosing the name of the group,

planning a social occasion to round off the sessions and celebrate achievements and meeting as a group with the council press officer. They continued to write, putting together another anthology of their work, and developed a logo for the group, which was printed on a T-shirt for performances. The group has recruited new members and published a second anthology of group poetry.

Volunteers and support workers have gained from participation in this activity in various ways (White 2004). This was the first time that the FWWCP had set about creating a new community publishing group. None of the support workers had prior experience of community publishing, and some had not tried creative writing before. Some of the volunteers, many of whom were themselves disabled, travelled over a hundred miles to participate in the group. Those who came from the local writers' workshop had never before worked with people with learning disabilities, but one of them has since begun developing workshops with mental health service users and has learned how to obtain funding.

Actors may be people within the institutions or other agencies that have a relationship to a project, for example, because they allocate funding or enable access to resources. The actors in this case example include all the people involved: service users, the occupational therapist, the adult educator, support workers, volunteers and additional others, such as the press officer and the audiences for performances.

How do actors conduct themselves?

In any conflict and co-operation situation, there will be a complex range of aims, motives and interests, for each actor and between actors, together producing both conflict and co-operation. *Aims* refers to what the actors are consciously striving for, *motives* refers to actors' less conscious or less publicly expressed desires and *interests* refers to what actors strive for consciously in a way that is clear to others (Kronenberg & Pollard 2005a). It is necessary to recognise the aims, interests and motives of the actors in any situation in order to get an idea of what they are trying to achieve.

Actors may seek to develop several different aims, motives and interests within a single situation, thus increasing the likelihood of conflict. For example, an institution may have the aim of providing care but, in doing so, simultaneously serves the motive of contributing to social order by preventing people being exposed to risk through behaviours associated with their illness. In order to fulfil this motive, it may use methods that are experienced as restrictive by the people who use the service, denying them the opportunities they want for social participation or meaningful activity.

Case example 3 illustrates some of the different aims, motives and interests that interacted to create a successful dance project.

Case example 3: A dance project

A group of dance therapists and psychologists have been working in Italy with a number of people with psychosis and autism since the mid-1990s. A few years ago, the group began to work with dancers towards developing public performances. The therapeutic group began to develop its technical abilities and, with some funding from private sources and the commune of Florence, created a stage production, 'Il filo del tempo' (The cord of time). This dance performance, based on the group interpretation of the four seasons, was eventually staged at the Teatro di Riffredi in Florence and in Tuscany.

The participants discovered a range of abilities, for example, working together, paying attention to the music, performing, adapting and changing their choreography to suit different theatre stages. These experiences added up to 'being the protagonists of their lives' (Pouliopoulou 2004, personal communication). They acquired a professional attitude to their work as dancers or as actors, in that they were actors or dancers, not patients acting or dancing.

There were also significant outcomes for the dancers and clinical staff involved in the project. The dance therapist had to develop a demonstrative approach which enabled people with a more concrete perception of the world to understand and follow the dance and to learn to express themselves through it. The dancers and stage technicians learned to work to realise creative possibilities with people with psychosis and autism. These processes were facilitated by a voluntary framework that focused on the creative expression, enjoyment and presentation of dance. This enabled spontaneity, the emergence and expression of humour and the growth of friendship among all the participants.

Each of the groups involved in this project had their own aims, motives and interests, such as the search for fun. One motive for the dancers and clinical staff was to see what was possible for the people with whom they were working, through exploring opportunities for them to express their creativity. Actors had to learn new ways of being either practitioners or patients, and boundaries began to disappear as human interaction took over from the traditional and professional borders between the two. People, irrespective of which side of the border they started from, realised new possibilities in themselves and were enabled to exercise these through this interaction.

What are their means?

This key question is concerned with phenomena that deal with influence, power and related notions. *Influence* is the capacity of actors to determine or change the availability to other actors of a range of behaviours or choices. *Power* is often viewed as the capacity of actors to determine or change the behaviours or choices of others.

The capacity indicated by the term *power* is based on:

- the means of power, including force and coercion. *Means* refers to everything that actors can use to realise their political aims in conflict and co-operation situations (van der Eijk 2001)
- the resources of power, such as connections, money, information or means of communication.

Asking the question 'What are their means?' gives insight into the actors' means of power and the power that these means yield. Means refers to anything which may be turned to the actors' advantage, including other actors, as well as resources and opportunities. Case example 4 illustrates a variety of means that were employed in the development of a theatre project.

Case example 4: A theatre group

An occupational therapist working in a closed and isolated psychiatric hospital in a mountainous part of Greece began a theatre group with some of her 350 patients. The group was formed with the aim of using stage productions as a bridge between the institution and the outside world. Initially, this was difficult as there were inadequate facilities and many of the patients were institutionalised and apathetic. There were other, pressing demands on the therapist's time, some staff were apprehensive that the group would worsen patients' conditions and administrators were concerned about the expense involved. Developing the group took much work, both with individuals and in groups, because the patients lacked social and community living skills and their past experiences led them to fear rejection.

Despite these problems, the group met twice a week, outside the hospital in the local town centre, with support from the city council. Between 1999 and 2004, three plays were developed for performance to school children and communities in several cities, including a visit to Crete. After the success of their first play, the patients themselves requested more opportunities to rehearse in the community, and the therapist was able to present evidence of the need for more occupational therapists at the hospital.

In 2003, in a climate of deinstitutionalisation, the occupational therapists approached Voulgaris, a well-known film director in Greece, to see if there was a possibility of the actors participating in films. Voulgaris and one of the hospital doctors agreed a proposal for patients to become involved in films for therapeutic purposes. Subsequently, one actor from the group appeared in 'Brides', a film by Voulgaris, and another in 'A Dog's Dream', a film by Frantzis (Pouliopoulou 2004, video presentation).

The group had to learn initially to trust each other and to work together. They developed ways of working to produce a performance despite the lack of theatre space and equipment. They learned to resolve disagreements about which parts to play or which play to act, and to adapt their performances around problems such as poor concentration through the use of intervals and music. The two members who became film actors were paid at the going rate, and they had to be able to integrate and respond to the professional demands of working with other actors and film crew. As a result, some of them began to take more initiative in their own lives, for example,

travelling independently. One of the actors describes his experience in case example 7.

Some staff felt that these changes might be harmful, for example that those who had been in films would have unrealistic ideas about their status as stars and that their psychiatric condition would be affected. However, through making a video about their activities, the actors showed that this was clearly not so. They had, in fact, become more enthusiastic about participating in the theatre group.

Prestige is a valuable ally and, clearly, having a film director involved provided a source of power. Through the mediation of the film director, the evidence of the film and subsequent participation in evaluation of the theatre group by the patient/actors themselves, those who were initially dubious about the benefits of the theatre and film project eventually accepted its success.

However, it is important to note that even earlier in the project, important work was done to build up a source of power through a relationship with the city council.

What does the political landscape look like?

Conflict and co-operation take place within political systems. How they arise and develop is partly dependent on the organisation of the system, which includes, among other things, institutions and rules. Political institutions are more or less established forms for the organisation of behaviour. They include:

- concrete institutions, such as the House of Commons, the United Nations, the College of Occupational Therapists and the World Federation of Occupational Therapists, and
- procedural institutions, such as regular and free democratic elections, annual general meetings and World Federation of Occupational Therapists' Council meetings.

Besides institutions, the political landscape also includes *rules*, which are codes for what is and is not allowed or appropriate in the conduct of conflict and co-operation. Rules should not here be confused with legal principles but instead refer to the methods for conducting political activity.

In the arena of politics, rules are often vague and there is no external referee, yet rules present an important source of conflict and co-operation. Knowledge of these rules, and awareness of how they are continuously subject to changes and reinterpretations, enables participants to better understand and deal with situations of conflict and co-operation (Kronenberg & Pollard 2005a).

Case example 5 illustrates some of the methods that are used in the production of a local newsletter, a complicated and demanding process.

Case example 5: Southwark MIND's newsletter (by Lynne Clayton)

This local rag for mental health service users is now in its seventh year, during which time it has come out without fail every month, with a current print run of 800. Incredible stuff, especially when you think it's not funded and is produced and distributed entirely by volunteer service users from Southwark MIND.

Actually, I remember the early days, when Robert Dellar was Southwark MIND's first development worker. The newsletter was one of the first things he started, as he wisely realised that we could reach loads more people in the Borough that way. Anyway, the editorial subgroup would meet in our tiny office to decide on what would go into it each month. Pete Shaughnessy was very much involved – one of my favourites was his 'Lily Largactil' series – hilarious! Rob would cut and paste most of it by hand – when I politely pointed out that he could use the computer for all that nowadays, he laughed and said he liked the 'amateurish, zany' feel to it! We still cut and paste some of it – bet you can tell! (It reminded me of my earlier involvement with another, what we used to call 'underground', rag, 'The Peckham Jemmy', produced by the Peckham squatters in the '70s. That thrived on air, too, though it didn't last as long.)

The editorial subgroup are all unpaid volunteers from Southwark MIND. We meet twice a month, once to decide on the content of that month's edition and once to distribute it. The subgroup has strong links with the Writing Club, which supports users who want to write but don't feel confident enough, or who want to improve their writing skills, etc.

The 'Contents' meeting is usually very lively, as we have a lot to juggle, and sometimes it's hard to choose from all the contributions that we get. So we've got a sort of priority list, though this is flexible. We're also aware that many of our readers feel isolated and so we try to make it a mixed bag, not just up-to-date information and reports but also creative stuff, mostly poems and artwork (with the proviso that it can only be reproduced in black and white). Sometimes we get upset when we read a submission and we might decide not to put it in as we don't want to make anyone feel sad! (We do have obituaries, though, to honour our dead.) If we think something's offensive, we throw it out, usually, unless we think it'll offend the right people! What we don't do is to interfere with someone's work. If we like it, we put it in as written, except for spellings (even this is hard, sometimes) and the odd, hopefully helpful, full stop. Sometimes we put things in that sound nice, even though we're not quite sure what it means – perhaps our readers will get it!

When we've finally made all these choices, a couple of us work hard to get it print-ready ('Oh, well, at least you can read it') and it goes off to our wonderful Catford Printers who miraculously send us back 800 copies within a few days. Then we all get together again, with lots of tea, coffee and biscuits, and mail them all out. How do we manage to do all this? With love and pride.

Lynne Clayton's description reveals the balancing acts which are required in order to meet the demands of the political landscape against which the group publishes. The landscape provides no funding for a community publication of a considerable size but, through good relations with a writing club who provide source material, as well as the resources which come from the unpaid volunteers, the newsletter can be sustained.

Another important feature of the political landscape is the readers, without whom the occupational benefits of participating in the newsletter would have no value. It is this landscape of readers that the volunteers have continually in view as they work on the publication. They have had to evolve an editorial strategy which does not interfere too much with contributors' material, judges what will offend and what can be allowed to offend and is balanced with information and illustration according to a range of interests. The final aspect of the political landscape is the volunteers themselves – the mailing out of the newsletter is presented as an enjoyable collective occasion which celebrates the product of their co-operation. It is a political landscape which, perhaps because it produces an atmosphere of difficulties which have to regularly be overcome and worked with, enables the volunteers to co-operate 'with love and pride'.

What is the broader context for conflict and co-operation?

This question is intended to elicit what else is going on at the time in the world around the situation. Politics is not a spare-time or academic activity and, if the personal is the political, we have to pay attention to the broader context question in order to see how what we do fits in.

Case example 6: Survivors' poetry group

A member of a survivors' poetry group (that is, people who have survived the mental health-care system) invited an occupational therapist to bring some of his service users with severe and enduring mental health problems to Scotland, on holiday, where members of the group would act as guides. Funding from the Learning Skills Council enabled this proposal to be developed into a weekend course on Scots literature in Dumfries, home of Robbie Burns. The weekend was followed by a residential course at Northern College, a residential adult education college in South Yorkshire, for both the service users and the survivors' poetry group (Pollard & Steele 2002). A further course in Dumfries was organised around Scots history.

These three events produced numerous outcomes. All the service users had individual learning objectives to achieve during the courses, some of which were as broad as learning about Scots literature while others were about developing social and communication skills (Ryan & Pollard 2002). A key aspect of these activities was the opportunities they gave for service users, some of whom led quite isolated lives, to make friends with people who were not professional staff. The spontaneity of poetry group members added a natural richness to the experience for everyone. This was facilitated by 'keeping strongly to the here and now ... [for example] like children, we sat on the shingle shore of St Mary's Loch and bounced the stones from wave to wave' (Peter and Frances Grant 2004, personal communication).

At Northern College, the service users wrote and performed their own poems and made a video, activities which none of them had done before (Pollard & Steele 2002). The staff involved had not worked with mental health service survivors as volunteers, and the success of the first visit to Scotland encouraged other staff members to participate in a second. The series of events also led to local providers offering other opportunities for service users to identify barriers to education with them and to find out about access to learning (Pollard 2003). Some of the survivors' poetry group, who themselves had not facilitated such a course before, have since given presentations on the work they did (Davidson & Pollard 2003), including seminars with occupational therapy students at the University of Vic, in Spain (Davidson 2004).

While it may have been of therapeutic value to a patient group to have a holiday in Scotland, the availability of external funding enabled the original exchange between the service users and the survivors' poetry group to take place and allowed the project to be developed into a richer learning experience.

The poetry group have gained local media publicity for the project and are regularly featured in the local press. This has led to the group being perceived as part of the community, or broader context. As the leader of the group, Davidson, says: 'The editor told me that a good local paper should make sure that everyone in the community appears in it at least once a year, and I hold him to make sure that we do'.

An awareness of the political landscape makes it possible to use experiences in other ways, such as lobbying funders to persuade them to finance further activities. For example, all local publicity states who sponsored the activity and made it possible.

WORKING WITH MARGINALISED POPULATIONS

From the six case examples given in the last section, it is possible to identify some of the features of the people who are able to work successfully on the margins of health and social care.

The first feature is that staff and service users are prepared to work outside the borders of established institutions, using social participation as both a means and a goal (World Health Organization 2001). By stretching the borders of the occupational therapist's or other health professional's work settings in this way, a bridge can be made to the outside world (Pouliopoulou 2004, personal communication). This approach to practice is essentially health promoting at both individual and social levels.

The second feature is that professionals are prepared to learn from their patients, clients or service users and can thus develop through their work. Under conditions of collaboration and mutual education, adverse circumstances such as poverty, the constrictions of institutional frameworks, occupational apartheid, injustice and deprivation become reframed as opportunities for community development, and disability becomes a vehicle for personal development.

Third, in all the projects described, new links had to be made in order for the activities to develop. These links depended on the receptivity of the people who were approached to support them but, in all of these examples, there were conflicts which arose from presenting institutional frameworks with opportunities that they had not previously had to accommodate. For example, it was a challenge for clinical staff to work with people from outside agencies, without clinical qualifications, and to find ways of making the different approaches work together. Conflicts sometimes arose from problems of accommodation, when the unsuitability of rooms and spaces became a barrier to the activity being carried out. Service changes prevented one of the initiatives being developed further because staff were no longer available to support the project. Traditional approaches to the explication of professional therapeutic rationales to clients were too complex for clients to comprehend.

Finally, a key feature is that means were established to work with survivors, service users or clients as colleagues in a collaborative way. This is not simply a matter of finding professionals who are prepared, or able, to work in a co-operative way, but also of having people who are prepared to work with them. It can be easy to suppose that

where programmes do not develop the cause is a lack of motivation, a judgement which is usually made by the professional part of a failed partnership. However, working with other people outside the usual professional group requires positive risk taking and efforts to ensure sustainability. It involves evidencing a degree of commitment.

Community-based activities are precarious. They often lack funding and every resource has to be begged, borrowed or persuaded, such as a meeting space in the local community centre. At first, a lot of people are enthusiastic but this wanes, and it is easy to think that the activity no longer has value. Sometimes, persistence is needed through these slack periods. The first author ran a creative writing group for several years. Every summer, numbers dwindled from 15 regular attenders to two or three. However, the continuation of the group depended on its regularity. People would drop in again after 3 months expecting it still to be there, and each winter it would grow in membership. It continues today, with the same fluctuation, but answering a local need and local patterns for a creative and expressive outlet. Taking a long-term view, and understanding the needs of the members, the group has sustained numerous individuals over a 25-year history of regular meetings.

COMMUNITY–BASED REHABILITATION

Similar questions of sustainability are central to community-based rehabilitation (CBR), an approach which occupational therapists are using to address problems in impoverished communities (Fransen 2005, Kronenberg et al 2005b). Originally developed around the needs of populations in the developing world, alongside primary health care, its applicability in the developed world is being increasingly recognised. Community-based rehabilitation requires occupational therapists to negotiate solutions with communities rather than with individuals or groups within them.

Many of the people who inhabit rural and urban communities lack places in which they can meet, receive education, form networks or build themselves into the kind of groups who can co-operate and negotiate for a stake in the community

(Commission for Rural Communities 2006). Often, facilities are unavailable because they have been destroyed, vandalised or simply closed down for economic reasons. Community-based rehabilitation is an approach which harnesses people's capacity to work out their own strategies for accessing and developing the resources of their communities. Thus, it has the potential for giving individuals occupational opportunities for discovering their own self-worth and appreciating the contributions and needs of others.

NEW APPROACHES

This section offers a summary of approaches that have been found to be effective when working with people in marginal positions. Reference is made to the case examples in the previous section to illustrate how these approaches have been used in real situations.

Helping people to meet their own needs

Where is the border between personal development and the political development which is often necessary to enable the continuity that is needed for the types of projects described here? Often, this continuity can only be provided by the people who are being served by the project, therefore they have to be enabled to address their own needs. Letts (2003) argued for occupational therapists to work with the people they serve to develop their own grassroots organisations and the skills to run them, to enable them to meet their own community needs, such as transportation, and to address issues such as isolation.

Building bridges into the community

The case examples given so far share common characteristics, including the apparent limitations imposed both by cognitive disabilities and by individual and social perceptions of how to respond to them. A feature of each example is an emergence into the community by way of a bridge that enables activity to take place. Groups of service users are able to assert their membership of the society which has excluded them through cultural actions.

The theatre group PROP, Voices Talk and Hands Write, the dance group and the meetings between survivor poets and mental health service clients are all examples where, like the first author's creative writing group, people have developed activities around their own needs. The PROP group and survivor poets were already established as features of their local community but, even where these activities were initially facilitated by professional health workers or educators, service users, patients and survivors have developed further initiatives of their own. In so doing they have put their own stamp on the project and demonstrated their ownership of the activity through their performance or through taking a hand in some aspect of the organisation.

It is possible for everyone involved to determine learning outcomes from their experiences of conflict and co-operation, whether it is a new experience of education or working with mental health service users as colleagues for the first time.

Opening new opportunities

The activities of the various groups have produced changes in the organisations with which they are connected, including new flexibilities and new opportunities. Several of the activities mark a true emergence of the participants into the community as people with highly visible products of their abilities, such as taking part in a film, giving presentations based on their activities to professional and student audiences and producing community publications and performances. The impact of one of the projects described in this chapter on one of the participants is described in case example 7.

If context can be affected by action, then actors can use their means to effect change. As Chomsky said, 'out of activities and organisation come opportunities for interaction among people' (Chomsky, in Cogswell 1996, p142). A spiral of development can be brought about by demonstrating the achievement of clear outcomes, through products such as film, performance or publication (including the use of mass media and professional publications).

Sometimes, circumstances cannot be altered by action, because the resources available are not enough to affect the context or because the context

Case example 7: 'Brides' (by Vassilis)

Although I wanted very much to participate, when I was told that I had a part in 'Brides' I didn't understand where we were going or know what I would find. I was afraid of Athens. I pictured it as a beast with a big figure and teeth that eats people, because I grew up in a village in Kilkis. When we got into the bus with the other extras and actors I wondered what they would all do when we got to the film set at Piraeus harbour. The first thing that I wanted to do was to meet the director. Before leaving my hometown I asked everybody who he was, I didn't know about him. I wanted to see how he lives, how he makes films.

At first I smiled and said 'Good morning'. I met his family. We talked in the simple way people in small towns speak. Mrs Ioanna, the wife of Mr Voulgaris and scriptwriter of the film, asked me what I enjoy doing. I said that I love birds. For a long time nobody had paid attention to what I was saying – she gave me a bird mobile. The filming started, I tried to do my best. I became attached to the other actors – both old and young. I forgot everything, all of my problems and my illness and I felt that if anything happened the other actors would stand by me. The weather was hot and that was quite tiring. Water was offered to everyone. We drank a toast to Mr Voulgaris and Mrs Ioanna. These two are so close to one another – I realised that he wouldn't do anything just by himself. I wish I could do something in my life that will endure too. I made new friends, I talked with men and women and learned something different from everyone.

There were fewer people in my second scene. I remember the dancing at the wedding party and the table full of food. Mr Voulgaris encouraged us. My bride and partner helped me a lot, we danced together. The actors told me 'Take courage, don't feel embarrassed, let yourself feel free' and I told myself, 'Vassilis, you are not ill, prove it'. I gave myself to the camera and to the role.

Miranda discreetly and carefully explained to me what I should do. She gave me courage. Gradually she left me by myself and I liked that. I felt that I could work independently. We caught each other's eyes a few times. I knew that she was there and proud for me.

When I got back home, at first I felt very calm. I started to talk to other people about my experiences. I was proud of myself. I am grateful to Mr Voulgaris and Mrs Ioanna for inviting me to take part in the film. I'd like to be in a film with them again. I also hope that other people will have the opportunity, because it is good for their health. It revitalised me.

Following the film premiere in Thessaloniki

I enjoyed seeing Thessaloniki where I went to meet Mr Voulgaris and the actors. I saw my photograph with the grooms in the film brochure. Once the film people arrived we had photos taken. I watched the press conference and I liked what they said. I enjoyed the film, it was very good, very emotional, although I don't know much about films. Mr Voulgaris introduced me to people from the arts, I met a lot of people. I had a very good time. It didn't matter how much I appeared on the screen, when I saw the other actors – my friends – acting, it was as if they were me. When I saw our names at the end I cheered, but I would like to see the film again. I felt proud that I was lucky enough to be among those people. I will tell my friends and relatives to go and see it. I will send them the brochures with my photograph with the grooms.

is fixed. It is important to recognise when change is not going to happen and, if possible, to transfer resources to other projects.

Challenging stereotyping and stigma

The issue of property values in relation to exclusion is a similar argument to the reasons given for opposing the settlement of asylum seekers in a community, the fear that accommodating people with differences will pose a threat to the economic and social stability of a society (Rattansi 2004). However, *difference* can be an asset to the wider community, it can produce opportunities to realise things which have not been realised before – challenging public perceptions of mental illness or learning difficulty.

In each of the examples given above, people were enabled to find new means of expression, of creating meanings for themselves through occupation and of challenging the limitations under which they previously lived. Through public self-representation in theatre, performance, print, film and talks, they generated evidence of their abilities and raised awareness of their situations. These actions can be seen

as part of a political process of empowerment that is fundamental to active citizenship
(Tansey 2000).

Crossing professional boundaries

Clinical distance, important to therapeutic objectivity and impartiality, is questioned when the
practitioner develops a collaboration with the
people being worked with. The power relationship between client and practitioner is changed
through the needs arising from and met by the
activity process. Practical considerations that arise
from working together can result in changes
in relationships and, through the dynamics of
working with people in non-clinical settings,
participants can become friends, as in case examples 2, 3 and 6.

Carrying out the activities described in the
case examples challenged professional roles. For
example, in case example 3, staff did not initially
realise that working with patients in dance situations would require their own active participation.
This participation was also an essential part of the
development of the writing activity with VTHW,
in case example 6 (Pollard et al 2005). In case
example 4, the lack of transportation required that
staff crossed professional boundaries in drawing upon their friends to provide transport for
participants.

THE ROLE OF PROFESSIONAL ORGANISATIONS

The scope of individual action is already large and
could be made larger (Goldstein 1996). Occupational
therapists are developing the apparatus to enable
them to achieve this; the Council of the World
Federation of Occupational Therapists (WFOT) has
approved position papers on community-based
rehabilitation (World Federation of Occupational
Therapists 2004) and on human rights (World
Federation of Occupational Therapists 2006). This
shows that the WFOT is starting to raise its voice,
taking an official stance on issues of global relevance. Such overt action exceeds what many
view as traditional professional interests but it is
fundamental to the needs of the people with whom
occupational therapists work.

SUMMARY

It is a mark of civilisation to wish to join in the
political life of the community (Aristotle 1962).
If occupational therapists are to confront the
stigma, exclusion and prejudice which support
the occupational injustice and occupational apartheid experienced by people affected by mental
ill health, then we must enable these people to
exercise their rights. As demonstrated in the case
examples, it is possible to have learning difficulties, dementia or mental health problems and still
be a responsible political actor, enjoying full rights
as a citizen.

Full citizenship means more than the limited participation and narrow view of politics offered by the nation-state, and ordinary
citizens can do more than vote every 5 years
(Letts 2003, Tansey 2000, Ward 1985). There is
great satisfaction to be had, and much to be
achieved, not only through discussing political issues in the abstract but also by helping to
build a better world through active membership of voluntary organisations that attempt to
influence events (Chomsky 2002), from Green
Peace to Amnesty International. Occupational
therapists can participate more fully through
becoming involved in the work of national and
international professional organisations, such as
the Council of Occupational Therapists in the
European Community (COTEC), the European
Network of Occupational Therapy in Higher
Education (ENOTHE) and the World Federation
of Occupational Therapists.

Important political decisions can be made at
work, within educational and leisure organisations, by local and regional authorities, through
voluntary interest groups and by international
co-operation.

Throughout the development of our profession, the political implications which arise from
a concern with occupation have often been
neglected as we have accepted a medical understanding of therapy which has little to do with
the world outside the hospital or health centre.
But occupational therapists can be key to revealing an understanding of local actions in terms
of global responsibilities and to addressing local

problems in a participative and democratic way with the people they aim to serve (World Federation of Occupational Therapists 2004). This will require a broader and fuller focus for the occupational therapy profession and its practitioners, working across or even outside traditional settings, without borders (Kronenberg & Pollard 2006).

ACKNOWLEDGEMENTS

Miranda Pouliopoulou, Dimitra Pouliopoulou, Brunelle, Vassilis Voulgaris, Maria (translations), Eric Davidson, Peter and Frances Grant, Dennis Jubb, Denise Chaston, Caroline Kendrew, Michelle and the PROP Group, Lynne Clayton, Jim White, Voices Talk and Hands Write.

References

Aristotle 1962 The politics. Penguin, Harmondsworth

Bettelheim B 1970 The informed heart. Paladin, London

Boyce W, Lysack C 1997 Understanding community in Canadian CBR: critical lessons from abroad. Canadian Journal of Rehabilitation 10(4): 261-271

Bradshaw J, Kemp P, Baldwin S et al 2004 The drivers of social exclusion. Social Exclusion Unit, London, Office of the Deputy Prime Minister. Available online at: http://216.239.59.104/search?q=cache:oRhGUzrwkvEJ:www.socialexclusionunit.gov.uk/impactstrends/pdfimptre/driversreport.pdf+&hl=en

Burns T, Firn M 2002 Assertive outreach in mental health: a handbook for practitioners. Oxford University Press, Oxford

Cardona C E 2001 Que es y para que sirve la politica? Educación para la Paz. Documento interno, Edicion 1. Oficina Pastoral Social Arzobispado de Guatemala, Guatemala

Centre for Economic Policy Research 2001 Labour demand, education, and the dynamics of social exclusion. Available online at: www.pjb.co.uk/npl/bp38.doc

Chaston D, Pollard N, Jubb D 2004 Young onset dementia: a case for real empowerment. Journal of Dementia Care 12(6): 24-26

Chomsky N 2002 Understanding power: the indispensable Chomsky. The New Press, New York

Christiansen A, Dornink R, Ehlers S L et al 1999 Social environment and longevity in schizophrenia. Psychosomatic Medicine 61: 141-145

Cogswell D 1996 Chomsky for beginners. Writers and Readers, London

Commission for Rural Communities 2006 Rural disadvantage: reviewing the evidence. Commission for Rural Communities, London

Creek J 2003 Occupational therapy defined as a complex intervention. College of Occupational Therapists, London

Davidson E 2004 Adopt-a-FED-group-be-a-friend-get-internationale. Federation 28: 12-14

Davidson E, Pollard N 2003 Mental health and social inclusion. RED Journal Summer: 20

Duncan M, Swartz L 2004 Transformation through occupation: towards a prototype. In: Watson R, Swartz L (eds) Transformation through occupation. Whurr, London, pp301–319

Fransen H Challenges for occupational therapy in community based rehabilitation. In: Kronenberg F, Simo Algado S, Pollard N (eds), Occupational therapy without borders: learning from the spirit of survivors. Elsevier/Churchill Livingstone, Oxford, pp166–182

Freire P 1972 The pedagogy of the oppressed. Penguin, Harmondsworth

Galheigo S M 2005 Occupational therapy and the social field: clarifying concepts and ideas. In: Kronenberg F, Simo Algado S, Pollard N (eds) Occupational therapy without borders: learning from the spirit of survivors. Elsevier/Churchill Livingstone, Oxford, pp87–98

Goldstein J 1996 International relations in everyday life. In: Zemke R, Clark F (eds) Occupational science: the evolving discipline. FA Davis, Philadelphia

Hocking C, Ness N E 2002 Revised minimum standards for the education of occupational therapists. World Federation of Occupational Therapists, Perth

Jubb D, Pollard N, Chaston D 2003 Developing services for younger people with dementia. Nursing Times 99(22): 34-35

Katz F E 1958 Occupational contact networks. Social Forces 37(1): 52-55

Kronenberg F 2003 In search of the political nature of occupational therapy. Unpublished MSc pilot study, Linköping University, Sweden

Kronenberg F 2005 Occupational therapy with street children. In: Kronenberg F, Simo Algado S, Pollard N (eds) Occupational therapy without borders: learning from the spirit of survivors. Elsevier/Churchill Edinburgh pp261–276

Kronenberg F, Pollard N 2005a Overcoming occupational apartheid: a preliminary exploration of the political nature of occupational therapy. In: Kronenberg F, Simo Algado S, Pollard N (eds) Occupational therapy without borders: learning from the spirit of survivors. Elsevier/Churchill Edinburgh, pp58–86

Kronenberg F, Pollard N 2005b Introduction: a beginning. In: Kronenberg F, Simo Algado S, Pollard N (eds) Occupational therapy without borders: learning from the spirit of survivors. Elsevier/Churchill Edinburgh, pp1–13

Kronenberg F, Pollard N 2006 The political dimensions of occupation and the roles of occupational therapy. American Journal of Occupational Therapy 60(6): 617-625

Kronenberg F, Simo Algado S, Pollard N (eds) 2005a Occupational therapy without borders: learning from the spirit of survivors. Elsevier/Churchill Livingstone, Oxford

Kronenberg F, Fransen H, Pollard N 2005b The WFOT position paper on community-based rehabilitation: a call upon the profession to engage with people affected by occupational apartheid. WFOT Bulletin 51: 5-13

Letts L 2003 Enabling citizen participation of older adults through social and political environments. In: Letts L, Rigby P, Stewart D (eds) Using environments to enable occupational performance. Slack, New Jersey

Lorenzo T, Duncan M, Buchanan H et al 2006 Practice and service learning in occupational therapy, enhancing potential in context. Wiley, Chichester

MIND 2004 Not alone? Isolation and mental distress: executive summary. Available online at: www.mind.org.uk/About+Mind/Mind+week/isolationsummary.htm

National Statistics 2004 Labour market statistics 15 December 2004. Available online at: www.statistics.gov.uk/pdfdir/lmsuk1204.pdf

OOFRAS 2006 The IdiOT's guide to working with refugees. OOFRAS, Brisbane

Parry-Jones W L 1988 The model of the Geel lunatic colony and its influence on the nineteenth century asylum system in Britain. In: Scull A (ed) Madhouses, mad-doctors, and madmen: the social history of psychiatry in the Victorian era. University of Pennsylvania Press, Philadelphia, 201–217

Pollard N 2003 Making adult learning fun. Occupational Therapy News 11(3): 30

Pollard N, Steele A 2002 From Doncaster to Dumfries. Occupational Therapy News 10(11): 31

Pollard N, Smart P, Diggles T, Voices Talk and Hands Write 2004 Occupational benefits of community publication. Poster presentation at the Seventh European Congress of Occupational Therapy, Athens

Pollard N, Smart P, Voices Talk and Hands Write 2005 Voices Talk and Hands Write. Kronenberg F, Simo Algado S, Pollard N. (eds) Occupational therapy without borders: learning from the spirit of survivors. Elsevier/Churchill Livingstone, Oxford, pp287–301

Rattansi A 2004 New Labour, new assimilationism. Open Democracy. Available online at: http://64.233.183.104/search?q=cache:q5LIB35p7swJ:www.opendemocracy.com/debates/

Rebeiro K L, Day D G, Semeniuk B et al 2001 Northern Initiative for Social Action: an occupation-based mental health program. American Journal of Occupational Therapy 55: 493-500

Robertson C 2001 Grameen Bank: servicing the poor world-wide. Available online at: http://marriottschool.byu.edu/emp/wpw/2001-3-21%20Grameen%20Bank%20-%20Microenterprise%20Conf.pdf

Ryan H, Pollard N 2002 Poetry on the agenda for Scottish weekend. Adults Learning 13(5): 10-11

Searle C 1997 Living community, living school. Tufnell Press, London

Sinclair K 2005 Foreword. In: Kronenberg F, Simo Algado S, Pollard N (eds) Occupational therapy without borders, Elsevier/Churchill Livingstone, Oxford, ppxiii-xv

Sriskandarajah D 2004 Stock taking – the real impacts of migrants on housing. Institute for Public Policy Research. Available online at: www.ippr.org.uk/articles/index.asp?id=428

Stein L I, Santos A B 1998 Assertive community treatment of persons with severe mental illness. Norton, New York

Tansey S D 2000 Politics: the basics. Routledge, London

Thibeault R. 2002 Muriel Driver memorial lecture. In praise of dissidence: Anne Lang-Etienne (1932–1991). Canadian Journal of Occupational Therapy 69(4): 197-204

Thomas P 1997 The dialectics of schizophrenia. Free Association Books, London

Townsend E, Wilcock A 2004 Occupational justice and client-centred practice: a dialogue-in-progress. Canadian Journal of Occupational Therapy 71: 75-87

van der Eijk C 2001 De kern van de politiek. Het Spinhuis, Amsterdam

Voices Talk and Hands Write 2004 Voices Talk and Hands Write. Federation of Worker Writers and Community Publishers, Stoke on Trent

Ward S 1985 Organising things. Pluto, London

Warner R 1994 Schizophrenia: psychiatry and political economy. Routledge, London

Watson R, Swartz L (eds) 2004 Transformation through occupation. Whurr, London

Werner D 2005 Foreword. In: Kronenberg F, Simo Algado S, Pollard N (eds) Occupational therapy without borders: learning from the spirit of survivors. Elsevier/Churchill Livingstone, Oxford, ppxi-xii

White J 2004 Grimsby writing pilot project. Federation 27: 40

Whiteford G 2000 Occupational deprivation: global challenge in the new millennium. British Journal of Occupational Therapy 63(5): 200-204

Whiteford G, Wright St Clair V 2005 Occupation and practice in context. Elsevier, Marrackville

Wilcock A 1998 An occupational perspective of health. Slack Thorofare, New Jersey

Wilson C 2004 Occupational opportunities for asylum seekers. OOFAS Newsletter, March

World Federation of Occupational Therapists 2004 World Federation of Occupational Therapists position paper on CBR. World Federation of Occupational Therapists, Perth, Australia

World Federation of Occupational Therapists 2006 World Federation of Occupational Therapists position paper on human rights. World Federation of Occupational Therapists, Perth, Australia

World Health Organization 1978 Declaration of Alma Ata. Available online at: www.who.int/hpr/NPH/docs/declaration_almaata.pdf

World Health Organization 2001 International classification of functioning, disability and health. World Health Organization, Geneva

Useful Websites

Film 'Brides: www.nyfes.gr
Occupational Opportunitiesfor Refugees and Asylum Seekers www.oofras.com

Glossary

Ability: measure of the level of competence with which a skill is performed.

Activity: 'a structured series of actions or tasks that contribute to occupations' (ENOTHE 2006).

Activity adaptation: adjusting or modifying an activity to suit the client's needs, skills, values and interests.

Activity analysis: 'a process of dissecting an activity into its component parts and task sequence in order to identify its inherent properties and the skills required for its performance, thus allowing the therapist to evaluate its therapeutic potential' (Creek 2003, p49).

Activity grading: adapting an activity so that it becomes progressively more demanding as the client's skills improve, or less demanding as the client's function deteriorates.

Activity sequencing: 'finding or designing a sequence of different but related activities that will incrementally increase the demands made on the individual as her/his performance improves or decrease them as her/his performance deteriorates' (Creek 2003, p38).

Activity synthesis: combining activity components into new activities to achieve therapeutic goals.

Approach: 'the methods by which theories are put into practice and treatment is administered' (Creek 2003).

Assessment: 'the process of collecting accurate and relevant information about the client in order to set baselines and to monitor and measure the outcomes of therapy or intervention' (Creek 2003).

Autonomy: 'the capacity to think, decide, and act on the basis of such thought and decision freely and independently and without ... let or hindrance' (Gillon 1985/1986, p60).

Client: 'a person who engages the professional services of another [who] has the right to demand information and is free to voice an opinion' (Sumsion 1999, p28). The client could be a group of people, such as the family, carers or a community agency.

Client–centred approach: embraces the possibility that the client's beliefs and attitudes may be different from those of the therapist.

Client–centred practice: a collaborative process in which the therapist, client and other interested parties negotiate and share choice and control.

Clinical audit: a cyclical process of systematic review of care against written standards or guidelines in order to improve the quality of services to patients.

Clinical effectiveness: using interventions that are known to work, whether for a particular patient or for a population, in the real-life situation so as to achieve the greatest possible health gain within available resources.

Clinical governance: 'a framework through which ... organisations are accountable for continuously improving the quality of their services and safeguarding high standards of care by creating an environment in which excellence in clinical care will flourish' (DoH 1998).

Clinical reasoning: 'the mental strategies and high level cognitive patterns and processes that underlie the process of naming, framing and solving problems and that enable the therapist to reach decisions about the best course of action' (Creek 2003, p51).

Community development: a population approach that involves the therapist working in partnership with the community to bring about internal and external change (Watson 2004).
'Community consultation, deliberation and action to promote individual, family and community-wide responsibility for self sustaining development, health and wellbeing' (Wilcock 1998, p238).

Competence: 'skilled and adequately successful completion of a piece of performance, task or activity' (Hagedorn 2000, p308).

Context: 'a set of circumstances or conditions' (Creek 2003, p51).

Continuing professional development: 'a range of learning activities through which health professionals maintain and develop throughout their career to ensure that they retain their capacity to practise safely, effectively and legally within their evolving scope of practice' (Health Professions Council 2006, p1).

Creative therapies: a range of interventions that aim to tap into the client's own creative potential.

Creativity: a natural process resulting in the production of novelty in form, appearance or relationship.

Cultural competence: 'an awareness of, sensitivity to, and knowledge of the meaning of culture, including a willingness to learn about cultural issues, including one's own bias' (Dillard et al 1992, p722).

Culture: 'the patterns of values, beliefs, symbols, perceptions and learnt behaviours shared by members of a group and passed on from one generation to another' (Hasselkus 2002, p42).

Discrimination: 'attitude, policy, or practice that knowingly excludes a person or group of persons from full participation and benefits' (Wells & Black 2000, p279).

Dysfunction: 'a temporary or chronic inability to meet performance demands adaptively and competently and to engage in the repertoire of roles, relationships and occupations expected or required in daily life' (Creek 2003, p52).

Enablement: the process of helping the client to identify what is important to him, set his own goals and work towards them, thus taking more control of his life.

Engagement: 'a sense of involvement, choice, positive meaning and commitment while performing an occupation or activity' (ENOTHE 2006).

Environment: 'the human and non-human surroundings of the individual, including objects, people, events, cultural influences, social norms and expectations' (Creek 2003, p52).

Environmental adaptation: assessing, analysing and modifying physical and social environments to increase function and social participation.

Ethical reasoning: a process of thinking about the moral dimension of a situation in order to reach the best decision.

Ethnicity: a cultural concept that is shared by a group which has a common religious belief, genealogy, language, culture or traditions. This term is used to refer to a group of individuals with shared racial origins, cultural norms and language that are ethnically rooted but not governed by nationality.

Evidence–based practice: the process of seeking, appraising and implementing the most recent research findings to ensure that patients receive interventions that have been demonstrated to be effective.

Extrinsic motivation: 'the drive to avoid harm and meet needs' (Creek 2007, p129).

Flow: an experience of harmony that occurs when an individual is immersed and totally absorbed in an activity (Emerson 1998).

Frame of reference: 'a collection of ideas or theories that provide a coherent conceptual foundation for practice' (Creek 2003, p53).

Function: 'the underlying physical and psychological components that support occupational performance' (ENOTHE 2006). The 'ability to perform competently the roles and occupations required in the course of daily life' (Creek 2003, p53).

Functional assessment/ functional analysis: part of the assessment process that looks at how the individual manages the normal range of daily life activities; a wide-spectrum assessment that allows the therapist and client to identify the client's strengths, problems, sociocultural environment and personal view of life.

Goal: 'a concise statement of a desired outcome or specific result to be attained at particular stage in an intervention' (Creek 2003, p54).

Habit: 'a performance pattern in daily life, acquired by frequent repetition, that does not require attention and allows efficient function' (ENOTHE 2006).

Health: 'a dynamic, functional state which enables the individual to perform her/his daily occupations to a satisfying and effective level and to respond positively to change by adapting activities to meet changing needs' (Creek 2003, p54).

Health promotion: 'improving quality of life and potential for health rather than the amelioration of symptoms and deficits' (World Health Organization 2002, p8).

Humanistic approach: involves the therapist attempting to understand how clients feel, and viewing their problems and the intervention used from their perspectives.

Independence: 'the position of not being dependent on authority; not relying on others for one's opinions or behaviours; being able to do things for oneself; having choice, control and participation in society' (Creek 2003, p54).

Institutional racism: 'a collective failure of an organisation to provide an appropriate and professional service to people because of their colour, culture or ethnic origins' (Macpherson 1999, p4262-i).

Interest: the expectation of pleasure in an activity, which is aroused by a combination of experience and some degree of novelty.

Intrinsic motivation: 'the drive to act for the enjoyment of exercising one's capacities, for learning and for taking pleasure in activity' (Creek 2007, p130).

Lifestyle: the configuration of an individual's activities that links with both personal needs and the expectations of society.

Meaning: the significance or importance that an activity has for an individual or a social group.

Mental health: 'the emotional and spiritual resilience which enables us to survive pain, disappointment and sadness' (Health Education Authority 1997).

Model: a simplified description or representation of something.

Model for practice: 'a simplified representation of the structure and content of a phenomenon or system that describes or explains certain data or relationships and integrates elements of theory and practice' (Creek 2003).

Motivation: 'a drive that directs a person's actions towards meeting needs' (ENOTHE 2006).

Occupation: 'a group of activities that has personal and sociocultural meaning, is named within a culture and supports participation in society. Occupations can be categorised as self-care, productivity and/or leisure' (ENOTHE 2006).

Occupational alienation: engagement in activity which is not in accordance with the occupational nature of the species or the individual.

Occupational apartheid: 'the segregation of groups of people through the restriction or denial of access to dignified and meaningful participation in occupations of daily life on the basis of race, colour, disability, national origin, age, gender, sexual preference, religion, political beliefs, status in society, or other characteristics' (Kronenberg & Pollard 2005, p67).

Occupational behaviour: the entire developmental continuum of play and work that evolves throughout the life cycle (Reilly 1969).

Occupational choice: the process of choosing a job or career.

Occupational deprivation: external circumstances prevent the individual from using his capacities to the full, leading to imbalance and failure to develop or maintain normal functioning.

Occupational disruption: 'a transient or temporary condition of being restricted from participation in necessary or meaningful occupations, such as that caused by illness, temporary relocation, or temporary unemployment' (Christiansen & Townsend 2004, p278).

Occupational form: the established format of rules, procedures, equipment and environment for performing an occupation.

Occupational genesis: 'the evolving adaptive process in which humans engage in purposeful activities that are meaningful to their lives as their world and their experiences change' (Breines 1995).

Occupational imbalance: a lack of balance between work, rest and play causing a loss of harmony between internal bodily systems and between the person and the environment.

Occupational injustice: the many ways in which participation in occupations can be 'barred, confined, restricted, segregated, prohibited, undeveloped, disrupted, alienated, marginalized, exploited, excluded or otherwise restricted' (Townsend & Wilcock 2004, p77).

Occupational justice: 'justice related to opportunities and resources required for occupational participation sufficient to satisfy personal needs and full citizenship' (Christiansen & Townsend 2004, p278).

Occupational performance: 'the task-oriented, completion or doing aspect of occupations, often, but not exclusively, involving observable movement' (Christiansen & Townsend 2004, p278).

Occupational science: an academic discipline that studies people as occupational beings (Yerxa 2000).

Occupational therapy ethics: 'the analytical activity in which the concepts, assumptions, beliefs, attitudes, emotions, reasons and arguments underlying medicomoral decision making are examined critically' (Gillon 1985/1986, p2).

Occupational therapy process: recognisable sequence of steps or actions taken by the therapist towards achieving desired outcomes.

Outcome: the intended or expected results of intervention.

Outcome goal: 'an agreed, clearly defined, expected or desired result of intervention' (Creek 2003, p56).

Outcome measurement: 'evaluation of the nature and degree of change brought about by intervention, or the extent to which a goal has been reached or an outcome has been achieved' (Creek 2003, p56).

Paradigm: 'the profession's world view that encompasses philosophies, theories, frames of reference and models for practice' (Creek & Feaver 1993).

Participation: 'involvement in a life situation through activity within a social context' (ENOTHE 2006, World Health Organization 2001).

Performance enablers: intrinsic factors that enable or support occupational performance (Christiansen & Baum 1997).

Play: the medium through which the child is able to learn and rehearse a wide range of skills that will enable him to respond appropriately and adaptively in different situations; 'a transaction between the individual and the environment that is intrinsically motivated, internally controlled and free from many of the constraints of objective reality' (Bundy 1991 p59).

Problem formulation: 'the process of identifying and recording the difficulties an individual is having which may require action' (Creek 2003, p57).

Problem solving: a process involving a set of cognitive strategies that are used to identify occupational performance problems, resolve difficulties and decide on an appropriate course of action.

Professional philosophy: system of shared beliefs and values held by members of a profession.

Purpose: 'the reason for which something is done or made, or for which it exists' (Creek 2003, p58).

Recovery: the lived experience of people as they accept and overcome the challenge of their disability and experience themselves recovering a new sense of self and of purpose within and beyond the limits of their disability (Deegan 1988).

Reflection: subjective awareness and appreciation of activity and its impact on the individual and the environment; a way of making sense of those situations, commonly encountered in practice, that are characterised by complexity, uncertainty and uniqueness.

Role: social constructs that carry behavioural expectations and contribute to a person's self-image and sense of identity.

Routine: 'an established and predictable sequence of tasks' (ENOTHE 2006).

Skill: 'a specific ability or integrated set of abilities (e.g. motor, sensory, cognitive or perceptual) which evolve with practice' (Creek 2003, p59).

Social capital: the networks that are woven into the fabric of a society; the personal identity arising from membership, and the norms of trust, support and reciprocal help that gradually build up from participating in them (Puttnam, cited in Sainsbury Centre for Mental Health 2000).

Social exclusion: non-participation in the key activities of the society in which a person lives (Burchardt et al 2002).

Task: 'a series of structured steps (actions and/or thoughts) intended to accomplish the performance of an activity' (ENOTHE 2006).

Task analysis: discovering the sequence of steps or tasks that make up an activity.

Temporal adaptation: the normal use of time in a purposeful daily routine of activities.

Theory: a conceptual system or framework that is used to organise knowledge and to understand or shape reality.

Therapeutic use of self: the process of the therapist evaluating the effect of her characteristics, values and practice in interactions with others, and the extent to which this brings development and insight for the client (Freshwater 2002). Knowing oneself and being oneself in a conscious and disciplined way so that personal qualities and attributes can be harnessed in the service of one's professional role (Hagedorn 2000).

Thinking skills: 'the mental actions used by the therapist in framing problems and working out the best solutions' (Creek 2007, p4).

Values: the individual's 'personally held judgement of what is valuable and important in life' (Creek 2003, p60).

Volition: 'the skill of being able to perceive and work towards a goal through choosing and performing activities that will achieve desired results' (Creek 2007, p132).

Well-being: a subjective experience consisting of 'feelings of pleasure, or various feelings of happiness, health and comfort, which can differ from person to person' (Schmid 2005, p7).

Wellness: a process of caring for oneself, including care for the body, the emotions, personal identity and the spiritual self.

Work: any productive activity, whether paid or unpaid, that contributes to the maintenance or advancement of society as well as to the individual's own survival or development.

References

Breines EB 1995 Occupational therapy activities from clay to computers: theory and practice. FA Davis, Philadelphia

Bundy A 1991 Play theory and sensory integration. In: Fisher AG, Murray EA, Bundy AC (eds) Sensory integration theory and practice. FA Davis, Philadelphia, pp46-67

Burchardt T, Le Grand J, Piachaud D 2002 Degrees of exclusion: developing a dynamic, multidimensional measure. In: Hills J, LeGrand J, Piachaud D (eds) Understanding social exclusion. Oxford University Press, New York

Christiansen C, Baum C 1997 Person–environment occupational performance: a conceptual model for practice. In: Christiansen C, Baum C (eds) Occupational therapy: enabling function and well-being. Slack, Thorofare, New Jersey, pp47-70

Christiansen CH, Townsend EA 2004 Glossary. In: Christiansen CH, Townsend EA (eds) Introduction to occupation: the art and science of living. Prentice-Hall, Upper Saddle River, New Jersey

Creek J 2003 Occupational therapy defined as a complex intervention. College of Occupational Therapists, London

Creek J 2007 Engaging the reluctant client. In: Creek J, Lawson-Porter A (eds) Contemporary issues in occupational therapy: reasoning and reflection. Wiley, Chichester

Creek J, Feaver S 1993 Models for practice in occupational therapy, part 1: defining terms. British Journal of Occupational Therapy 56(1): 4-6

Deegan PE 1988 Recovery: the lived experience of rehabilitation. Psychosocial Rehabilitation Journal 11(4): 11-19

Department of Health 1998 A first class service: quality in the new NHS. HMSO, London.

Dillard PA, Andonian L, Flores O et al 1992 Culturally competent occupational therapy in a diversely populated mental health setting. American Journal of Occupational Therapy 46(8): 721-726

Emerson H 1998 Flow and occupation: a review of the literature. Canadian Journal of Occupational Therapy 65(1): 37-44

ENOTHE 2006 www.enothe.hva.nl

Freshwater D 2002 The therapeutic use of the nursing self. In: Freshwater D (ed) Therapeutic nursing. Sage, London

Gillon R 1985/1986 Philosophical medical ethics. Wiley, Chichester

Hagedorn R 2000 Tools for practice in occupational therapy: a structured approach to core skills and processes. Churchill Livingstone, Edinburgh

Hasselkus BR 2002 The meaning of everyday occupation. Slack, Thorofare, New Jersey

Health Education Authority 1997 Mental health promotion: a quality framework. Health Education Authority, London.

Health Professions Council 2006 Your guide to our standards for continuing professional development. Health Professions Council, London

Kronenberg F, Pollard N 2005 Overcoming occupational apartheid: a preliminary exploration of the political nature of occupational therapy. In: Kronenberg, F, Algado SS, Pollard N (eds) Occupational therapy without borders: learning from the spirit of survivors. Elsevier Churchill Livingstone, Oxford, pp58-86

Macpherson W 1999 The Macpherson Report. HMSO Command Paper No. 4262. HMSO, London

Reilly M 1969 The educational process. American Journal of Occupational Therapy 23(4): 299-307

Sainsbury Centre for Mental Health 2000 On your doorstep: community organisations and mental health. Sainsbury Centre for Mental Health, London.

Schmid T 2005 Promoting health through creativity: an introduction. In: Schmid T (ed) Promoting health through creativity for professionals in health, arts and education. Whurr, London

Sumsion T 1999 Implementation issues. In: Sumsion T (ed) Client-centred practice in occupational therapy. Churchill Livingstone, Edinburgh

Townsend E, Wilcock AA 2004 Occupational justice and client-centred practice: a dialogue in progress. Canadian Journal of Occupational Therapy 71(2): 75-87

Watson R 2004 A population approach to transformation. In: Watson R, Swartz L (eds) Transformation through occupation. Whurr, London

Wells SA, Black RM 2000 Cultural competency for health professionals. American Occupational Therapy Association, New York

Wilcock A 1998 An occupational perspective of health. Slack, Thorofare, New Jersey

World Health Organization 2001 International classification of functioning, disability and health. World Health Organization, Geneva

World Health Organization 2002 Prevention and promotion in mental health. World Health Organization, Geneva

Yerxa EJ 2000 Confessions of an occupational therapist who became a detective. British Journal of Occupational Therapy 63(5): 192-199

Index